OPERATIVE MANUAL FOR ENDOSCOPIC ABDOMINAL SURGERY

OPERATIVE PELVISCOPY
OPERATIVE LAPAROSCOPY

Operative Manual
for
Endoscopic Abdominal Surgery

Operative Pelviscopy
Operative Laparoscopy

by
o. Prof. Dr. med. Dr. med. vet. h. c. K. SEMM

Director of the Women's Hospital at the Christian Albrechts
University and Michaelis School for Midwives in Kiel, Germany

Introduction by

Prof. Dr. RAOUL PALMER, Paris, France

Translated and Edited by

ERNST R. FRIEDRICH, M.D., F.A.C.O.G.
Professor of Obstetrics and Gynecology
Head, Section of Gynecology
Washington University School of Medicine
St. Louis, Missouri

This volume continues the series of monographs consisting of

Atlas of Gynecologic Laparoscopy and Hysteroscopy (1977) and
Slide Atlas of Pelviscopy, Hysteroscopy and Fetoscopy (1979)

With 387 figures, 7 tables, 2 charts,
an atlas with 384 four-color prints, 2 radiographs, 1 black and white print,
and 379 line drawings.

YEAR BOOK MEDICAL PUBLISHERS, INC.
CHICAGO • LONDON • BOCA RATON

A Year Book Medical Publishers
imprint of Mosby-Year Book, Inc.

Mosby-Year Book, Inc.
11830 Westline Industrial Drive
St. Louis, MO 63146

3 4 5 6 7 8 9 0 CK 91 90

This book is an authorized translation from the German edition published and copyright © 1984 by F. K. Schattauer Verlag GmbH,
Stuttgart, Germany. Title of the German edition: *Operationslehre
für endoskopische Abdominal-Chirurgie: Operative Pelviskopie-
Operative Laparoskopie*

In this book, key words that are also registered trademarks are not
expressly indicated as such. It must not be assumed from the use of
these words that they have not been registered.

Library of Congress Cataloging-in-Publication Data

Semm, K. (Kurt), 1927-
  Operative manual for endoscopic abdominal surgery.

  Translation of: Operationslehre für endoskopische
Abdominal-Chirurgie.
  Includes bibliographies and index.
  1. Gynecology, Operative.   2. Endoscope and
endoscopy.   I. Title.   [DNLM: 1. Abdomen—surgery.
2. Endoscopy.   3. Pelvis—surgery.   WI   900 S472o]
RG104.S4513   1986   618.1'45   86-7804
ISBN 0-8151-7713-5

Sponsoring Editor: James D. Ryan, Jr.
Manager, Copyediting Services: Frances M. Perveiler
Production Project Manager: Max Perez
Proofroom Supervisor: Shirley E. Taylor

Editor's Foreword

Those who have previously been treated to Kurt Semm's unsurpassed color presentations on subjects of gynecologic endoscopy, be it format-filling color slides, exhibits with enlarged color prints of minute anatomical and surgical details, or superb teaching films and videotapes, will know that his latest work, *Operative Manual for Endoscopic Abdominal Surgery: Operative Pelviscopy-Operative Laparoscopy,* will undoubtedly become the gold standard for the next decade or so. This book continues the series of monographs consisting of *Atlas of Gynecologic Laparoscopy and Hysteroscopy,* 1977,* and *Slide Atlas of Pelviscopy, Hysteroscopy and Fetoscopy,* 1979. Whereas the first atlas focused mainly on diagnostic applications of pelviscopy/laparoscopy, the present operative manual and atlas expands on the foundation of the previous one and concentrates mainly on safe, modern techniques of pelvic/intra-abdominal endoscopic operative techniques.

Kurt Semm reminds me of an organist. Not an ordinary organist who plays the instrument only on Sundays and holidays, but one who loves the instrument and lives for the instrument every day of every year. One who plays the instrument extremely well, using all its registers. One who plays his own composition as well as the tunes of others—with his own variations, of course. One who constantly improves his techniques and those of others. Not only the techniques—even the instrument. One who dreams up, designs, distributes, and promotes new instruments whenever the old ones have outlived their usefulness or can no longer satisfy his needs or those of his audience.

Kurt Semm is a designer, engineer, experimental biologist, meticulous surgeon, dynamic teacher, and enthusiastic salesman or even crusader. Crusading for:

Safety: He replaced the high-risk methods of unipolar and bipolar endoscopic coagulation with low-voltage endocoagulation and, more recently, with endosuture, endoligature, and endoloop techniques.

Convenience: He designed, developed, and introduced more convenient instruments and technical equipment for operative pelviscopy, e.g., endocoagulators; grasping, claw, biopsy, and spoon forceps; needleholders; dual-purpose irrigation/suction cannulas; the OP-PNEU Electronic Insufflator, Aquapurator, Pelvi-trainer, etc. Without such instruments, operative pelviscopy/laparoscopy could be a frustrating and risky surgical exercise.

Terminology: Have you tried a computer literature search of "laparoscopy"? It is listed as "peritoneoscopy." Most references listed pertain first to internal medicine. "Operative" is not in the computer's vocabulary. References on "pelviscopy" can be retrieved as such and list the publications of Kurt Semm and his co-workers. This is the only word by which "gynecologic pelvic laparoscopy" can be readily distinguished from all the others.

Recognition: There is no doubt in any gynecologic endoscopist's mind that our diagnostic and especially operative pelviscopic/laparoscopic procedures are of a different order of magnitude than the primarily diagnostic laparoscopy done in internal medicine. All our pelvic endoscopic procedures begin with a laparoscopic evaluation of the mid and upper peritoneal cavity, followed by specifically gynecologic procedures which formerly had required a laparotomy. Health care agencies, insurance companies, and some among our own ranks have not yet fully recognized that pelviscopic operations have the advantage that the patient recovers much more rapidly after an endoscopic operation, although some procedures may take longer than the same operation performed through a lapa-

*German edition, 1976.

rotomy incision. We need our own identity by which we and our specific work can be easily recognized. Therefore, Kurt Semm proposed *Pelviscopy*.

In this era of diagnosis-related groups (DRGs), we have learned to accept eight to ten different categories of office visits, etc. We also need more specific terminology to identify more accurately our specific operative procedures. Therefore, I have decided not to use the more common and broader term ''laparoscopy,'' as translators of Semm's previous works have done, but have retained Semm's more specific term *pelviscopy* in this English language text. This word has been well defined in German medical dictionaries; it will be in our best interest to adopt it in our language, too. It allows us to indicate when we have performed two separate procedures in separate DRG fields: diagnostic and/or operative laparoscopy in the mid and upper abdomen versus diagnostic and/or operative pelviscopy in the classic realm of the pelvic surgeon, respectively.

When Kurt Semm honored me with his request to translate his manual and atlas into English I accepted under the condition that I could mitigate a few of his opinions which in the United States are perceived as unrealistically dogmatic. With his permission, I have, where I considered it appropriate, made editorial comments, which have always been identified as such. I hope that they will be appreciated by the English language reader practicing in the United States, Canada, and other countries.

The chapter on anesthesia has been expanded to include practical instructions for the effective use of local anesthesia and ''volonelgesia.''

Several instruments and devices that have been developed or improved since publication of the German text have been included in this English edition. A completely new chapter has been added about the Pelvi-Trainer, which allows the surgeon to practice new endoscopic techniques on placentas and surgical specimens before applying these new skills in the operating room.

The descriptions of the superb color photographs have been reorganized into a systematic pattern with which North American clinicians are more familiar: history, findings, operative procedure, precautions, comments, and references to other color plates or chapters. The extensive bibliography retains the original language for the reference titles.

I wish to thank James Ryan, Max Perez, and Frances M. Perveiler and the staff of Year Book Medical Publishers for their cooperation in revising text and illustrations and their commitment to make this manual and atlas available to the English speaking audience. I also wish to thank my secretary, Delia Whitehead, for her professional transcription and word processing of the translated text and my nurses: Lora Bell, R.N., Elaine Charlton, R.N., Judy Gamblin, R.N., and Susan Jones, R.N., for their help in proofreading and indexing. Last but not least, I want to express my gratitude to my family: my wife, Marianne, lecturer in German at Webster University, as well as my bilingual children, Andrea and Michael, both students at Washington University, for their substantial participation in the translation, word processing, editing, correction of the manuscript, preparation of illustrations with the English text, proofreading, and indexing.

ERNST R. FRIEDRICH

Preface

A wishful dream of mankind to take a look into the darkness of the body's cavity to diagnose disease has been fulfilled for all areas of endoscopy of body cavities, thanks to the technical development of the instruments necessary. From panintestinoscopy through bronchoscopy, cystoscopy, laparoscopy, hysteroscopy, tubaloscopy, ventriculoscopy, to arthroscopy, all expandable body cavities or spaces have been made accessible to man. Clinically, the endoscopic techniques available today are not competitive but complementary diagnostic modalities to radiologic and ultrasonic imaging. Endoscopy in the abdominal cavity is an invasive diagnostic method. Therefore, during the last decade, it has lost some of its importance compared to the noninvasive imaging of abdominal organs by ultrasound. This is particularly true when findings suspected by palpation, such as a cystic or solid structure, must be confirmed. Today, in such cases a sonogram should be considered first, and possibly only secondarily would endoscopy be indicated.

As this operative manual shows, endoscopic methods for hemostasis in the abdominal cavity were developed in Kiel during the last decade. They will make many indications for a classic laparotomy unnecessary. The operative procedure is more appropriately done endoscopically. This applies, to name only a few indications, to adhesiolysis in the entire abdominal cavity, salpingo-oophorectomy, conservative and nonconservative operations for tubal pregnancy, a variety of operations on the tubal ampulla for the correction of sterility, up to appendectomy.

Hence, a procedure originally developed for diagnostic purposes has reached a new level of importance with its application in the surgical field: after a visual diagnosis has been made, corrective surgery can be performed in the same operation. Thanks to the endoscopic miniaturization of the procedure, not only the hospitalization time but also the patient's perception of the physical impact of the disease process, i.e., the inability to work, is reduced to only a few days.

Therefore, it is a great pleasure that only a few years after publication of my *Atlas of Gynecologic Laparoscopy and Hysteroscopy* I can present an operative manual for endoscopic abdominal surgery. Whereas the first atlas with its subsequent volume of color slides dealt primarily with gynecologic intra-abdominal diagnosis, this present work, which assumes familiarity with the content of the diagnostic volume, is limited only to the new operative procedures.

Individual operative steps which are sometimes difficult to describe in words were again translated by the extraordinary pictorial talents of our graphic artist, Mrs. M. Rabe, from color slides into a symbolic language which everyone can understand. These line drawings, in conjunction with a numerical index, permit easy identification of anatomical landmarks. Thanks to the untiring efforts of our photographer, Mrs. G. Schliemann, in collecting and cataloging my archives of endoscopic illustrations (approximately 30,000 photographs), and in collaboration with the gracious generosity of the F. K. Schattauer publishing house, we succeeded in producing an operative color atlas of unique character.

KURT SEMM
KIEL, GERMANY

Introduction

It is undoubtedly the *bottom line of the current status of pelviscopic surgery* that Dr. Semm presents in his new operative manual of endoscopic abdominal surgery. In succession, he discusses in depth possible indications, instruments, different operative techniques, and postoperative care.

Of a total of 254 pages of text (with 387 illustrations), about 70 are dedicated to a most thorough and detailed description of instruments and their utilization. In endoscopic surgery, Semm considers it even more important than in open abdominal surgery always to have the best-suited instruments at hand (and to keep one or two duplicate instruments available for emergencies).

The instruments consist of two sets:
- One set for diagnostic pelviscopy, with two 30° endoscopes of 6.5 mm diameter and 35 forceps and different other accessories;
- One set for operative pelviscopy, with a straight endoscope of 11 mm diameter with special dilators to replace the 7-mm trocar by an 11-mm trocar, and seven instruments for endoscopic surgery, including, in particular, needleholders of 3 and 5 mm diameter for intra-abdominal sutures and ligatures;
- Not included in this list are equipment and monitors, most notably the one for continuous gas insufflation, the CO_2-PNEU Electronic insufflator, the endocoagulator for hemostasis, the Aquapurator for simultaneous irrigation and suction, etc.
- And not to be forgotten are the instruments for vaginal manipulation and the equipment for photographic and cinematographic documentation.

Most of these instruments have been developed to perfection by Dr. Semm himself, who is a true genius in this field due to his knowledge in physics and mechanical engineering, which most of us are lacking. His imagination and vitality in this area seem to be inexhaustible.

The latest novelty in this field is his perfection of a well-developed technique for intra-abdominal sutures and ligatures with the aid of two special needleholders of 3 and 5 mm diameter so that even microsurgical needles can be handled.

These instruments have allowed Dr. Semm to perform not only fimbriolysis but also salpingostomies and conservative operations for extrauterine pregnancies and ovarian cysts. I personally do not care very much for myomectomy by morcellation; its usefulness is not yet evident to me.

The text is followed by a color atlas with 387 photographs, each accompanied by stylized line drawings and explanations.

The *risks of pelviscopic surgery,* both diagnostic as well as operative, are discussed in depth, including possible ways to avoid or correct them. Above all, one will remember the repeated warnings against unipolar high-frequency coagulation because of the potential risk of indirect intestinal burns. This coagulation technique can be replaced either by ligatures with *endoloops* or by endocoagulation.

The patients are duly informed that pelviscopy may be followed immediately by a laparotomy if their conditions can only be managed after the abdomen has been opened. They are also advised that three, four, or five *mini-incisions* may be necessary for the introduction of accessory instruments at the most appropriate sites.

Operative pelviscopy may only be performed by a surgeon with sufficient training in open abdominal surgery and, if possible, also in microsurgery. He should already have had experience in several hundred diagnostic laparoscopies. Any gynecologic surgeon interested in more than the diagnostic application of the laparoscope or the easy application of the Yoon ring has an obligation to read Dr. Semm's book attentively.

Kurt Semm should be congratulated on this outstanding achievement.

PROF. Dr. RAOUL PALMER
PARIS

Contents

EDITOR'S FOREWORD **BY ERNST R. FRIEDRICH** . . . .   *v*

PREFACE **BY KURT SEMM** . . . .   *vii*

INTRODUCTION **BY RAOUL PALMER** . . . .   *ix*

1. **Introduction** **1**

2. **Historical Review: From Diagnostic Laparoscopy to Operative Pelviscopy** **5**

3. **Informing Patients About Endoscopic Abdominal Surgery** **16**

4. **Timing of Endoscopic Abdominal Surgery** **18**

   4.1. Timing of Endoscopic Abdominal Surgery: Typical Gynecologic Elective
   Procedures   18

   4.2. Timing of Endoscopic Abdominal Surgery: Pelviscopic Tubal Surgery
   for Correction of Sterility   18

   4.3. Timing of Endoscopic Abdominal Surgery: Gynecologic Procedures
   to Treat Pelvic Endometriosis   19

   4.4. Timing of Endoscopic Abdominal Surgery: General Abdominal Surgical
   Procedures   19

5. **Patient Preparation for Endoscopic Abdominal Surgery** **20**

   5.1. Psychological Preparation of the Patient for Endoscopic Abdominal Surgery   21

   5.2. Physical Preparation   22

6. **Medical Requirements for Endoscopic Abdominal Surgery** **24**

7. **The Operating Team for Endoscopic Abdominal Surgery** **27**

8. **Indications for Endoscopic Abdominal Surgery** **28**

   8.1. Catalog of Indications for Endoscopic Abdominal Surgery Based on Diagnostic
   Pelviscopy   28

      8.1.1.   Indications for Endoscopic Operative Procedures on the Uterine Corpus . .   29

8.1.2.   Indications for Endoscopic Operative Procedures on the Adnexa   29

8.1.2.1.   Endoscopic Operation on the Oviduct.   29

8.1.2.2.   Endoscopic Operations on the Ovaries   30

8.1.2.3.   Endoscopic Operations on the Mesovarium/Mesosalpinx   30

8.1.2.4.   Endoscopic Operations on Other Structures in the Pelvis   30

8.1.3   Indications for Endoscopic Surgery for Correction of Sterility   31

8.1.4.   Indications for Endoscopic Abdominal Surgery in the Adolescent
and Infant   31

8.2. Endoscopic Abdominal Operative Possibilities Applicable to General Surgery   32

8.2.1.   Catalog of Indications for Endoscopic Abdominal Surgery.   33

8.3. Emergency Pelviscopy in Gynecology and General Surgery   33

9. Contraindications to Endoscopic Abdominal Surgery **35**

9.1. Absolute Contraindications to Endoscopic Abdominal Surgery   35

9.2. Relative Contraindications to Endoscopic Abdominal Surgery   35

10. Anesthesia for Endoscopic Abdominal Surgery.   **37**

10.1. Anesthesia for Endoscopic Abdominal Surgery That May Be Administered
by the Surgeon   37

10.1.1.   Local Anesthesia.   38

10.1.2.   "Volonelgesia"   38

10.2. Anesthesia for Endoscopic Abdominal Surgery That Requires an Anesthesiologist . .   40

10.2.1.   Regional Anesthesia.   40

10.2.2.   General Anesthesia   40

11. Patient Position for Endoscopic Abdominal Surgery. **42**

11.1. Patient Position for Endoscopic Abdominal Surgery for Gynecologic Indications . . .   42

11.2. Patient Position for General Surgical Indications.   42

12. Instruments and Equipment for Endoscopic Abdominal Surgery **46**

12.1. Endoscopic Light Source.   46

12.1.1.   External Light for Diagnostic and Operative Procedures   46

12.1.2.   Transmission of the Endoscopic Light   47

12.1.3.   External Light for Photographic Documentation.   50

12.1.4.   Endoscopic Light Source for Cinematographic and Videotape Recording . .   51

12.2. Endoscopic Optical Systems   53

12.2.1.   Endoscopes for Intra-abdominal Diagnosis.   53

12.2.2.   Endoscopes for Intra-abdominal Surgery.   54

12.2.3.   Support of the Endoscope for Bimanual Operation   55

12.2.4. Low-Power Loupe Magnification of the Endoscopic Image (Endoscopic
Microsurgery)   57

12.2.5. Endoscope for Intra-abdominal Documentation by Photography,
Cinematography, and Videotape Recording   57

12.2.6. Preparation of the Endoscope for the Intra-abdominal Procedure   58

12.2.7. Sterilization and Maintenance of the Endoscope.   59

12.3. Insufflation Equipment to Establish a Pneumoperitoneum   61

12.3.1. Expansion Media to Establish the Pneumoperitoneum (Selection
of Gas)   64

12.3.1.1. Transabdominal Insufflation of the Pneumoperitoneum
by Blind Puncture and Veress Needle.   66

12.3.1.2. Transvaginal Insufflation of the Pneumoperitoneum
Through the Posterior Vaginal Fornix (Insufflation of the
Cul-de-Sac of Douglas)   69

12.3.1.3. Insufflation of the Pneumoperitoneum by
"Open Laparoscopy"   70

12.3.2. Electronic and Mechanical Control of the Pneumoperitoneum for Intra-
abdominal Diagnosis.   72

12.3.3. Electronic and Mechanical Control of the Pneumoperitoneum for Endoscopic
Abdominal Surgery   75

12.4. Technical Equipment for Intra-abdominal Irrigation   76

12.4.1. Equipment for Endoscopic Abdominal or Pelvic Irrigation   76

12.4.2. Equipment for Tubal or Transuterine Irrigation   77

12.4.3. Equipment for Ovum Aspiration for In Vitro Fertilization   79

12.5. Technical Equipment for Thermal Hemostasis   80

12.5.1. Comments Regarding the Difference Between Hemostasis
by High-Frequency Current in General Surgery and in Endoscopic
Abdominal Surgery   81

12.5.2. Historical Survey of the Utilization of Destructive Heat
for Blood Coagulation.   81

12.5.3. Biophysical Reasons Not to Use High-Frequency Currents in the Closed
Abdominal Cavity   82

12.5.4. Biologic Changes in the Area of the Adnexa After Utilization of
High-Frequency Coagulation: Follow-up of 1,003 Sterilized Patients   88

12.5.5. Compelling Medical Reasons Not to Use High-Frequency Current
in the Closed Abdomen (in Pelviscopy/Laparoscopy).   90

12.5.6. Equipment for Controlled Endocoagulation   92

12.5.6.1. Instruments for Endocoagulation   92

12.5.6.2. Histologic Changes After Heat-Induced Hemostasis   93

12.6. Instruments and Methods for Conventional Hemostasis by Ligature and Suture   95

    12.6.1. Hemostasis by Loop Ligature   95

    12.6.2. Hemostasis by Endoligature and External Tying of Knots   96

    12.6.3. Hemostasis by Endosuture With External or Internal Tying of Knots   98

    12.6.4. Hemostasis by Clips (Absorbable)   102

12.7. Instruments for Vaginal Mobilization of the Uterus   103

12.8. Endoscopic Instruments for Abdominal Surgery   106

    12.8.1. Sleeves for Endoscopes and Operative Instruments   106

    12.8.2. Instruments for Grasping and Holding   107

    12.8.3. Instruments for Aspiration   108

    12.8.4. Instruments for Cutting   111

    12.8.5. Instruments for Morcellation   111

    12.8.6. Instruments for Ligation   113

    12.8.7. Instruments for Suturing   113

    12.8.8. Instruments for Dilatation   114

    12.8.9. Instruments for Coagulation   117

    12.8.10. Instruments for Follicle Puncture   117

    12.8.11. Instruments for Extraction of the Appendix   118

    12.8.12. Instruments for Clamping of Large Vessels (Emergency Instrument Set)   120

    12.8.13. Instruments for Closure of Skin Incisions for Trocar Insertion   120

13. Establishing an Operating Room for Endoscopy **124**

13.1. Preparation of Instruments for Diagnostic Pelviscopy Laparoscopy   124

13.2. Preparation of Instruments for Endoscopic Abdominal Surgery   126

13.3. Seating and Support Possibilities for the Endoscopic Surgeon During the Procedure   128

14. Course of Endoscopic Abdominal Surgery **130**

14.1. Diagnostic Phase   130

    14.1.1. Preparation of the External Genitalia   130

    14.1.2. Preparation of the Abdominal Wall and Umbilicus   131

    14.1.3. Limiting the Risk of Perforation   132

        14.1.3.1. Safety Tests With the Blind Puncture Method   132

            14.1.3.1.1. Needle Test   133

            14.1.3.1.2. Aorta Palpation Test   133

            14.1.3.1.3. Snap Test   133

            14.1.3.1.4. Hissing Phenomenon   134

14.1.3.1.5.   Aspiration Test 134

14.1.3.1.6.   Manometer Test 135

14.1.3.1.7.   Volume Test 135

14.1.3.2.   Insufflation of the Pneumoperitoneum 138

14.1.3.3.   Probing/Sounding Test: Safety Test Before Introduction
of the Trocar for the Endoscope 139

14.1.3.3.1.   Probing/Sounding Test 139

14.1.3.4.   Blind Introduction of the Trocar for the Endoscope 141

14.1.3.5.   Introduction of the Endoscope and First Scan for Orientation . . 144

14.1.4.   Second Diagnostic Scan 147

14.1.5.   Second and Third Punctures to Establish a Diagnosis as an Indication
for the Operative Phase 150

14.1.6.   Transition to the Operative Phase: Exchange of Endoscopes 151

14.2. The Operative Phase 151

14.2.1.   Catalog of Abdominal Procedures Feasible With an Endoscope 151

14.2.2.   Typical Gynecologic Endoscopic Procedures 152

14.2.2.1.   Omental Adhesiolysis in the Upper, Mid, and Lower
Abdomen and Omental Resection 152

14.2.2.2.   Adhesiolysis Without Prior Hemostasis
(Bloody Adhesiolysis) 152

14.2.2.3.   Adhesiolysis After Prophylactic Hemostasis
(Bloodless Adhesiolysis) 154

14.2.2.4.   Omental Resection 156

14.2.2.5.   Pelviscopic Adhesiolysis in Preparation for a Laparotomy
Either During the Same Operation or at Another Time 156

14.2.3.   Endoscopic Operative Management of Superficial Pelvic Endometriosis . . 157

14.2.3.1.   Excision of Endometriotic Implants 158

14.2.3.2.   Coagulation of Endometriotic Implants 161

14.2.4.   Pelviscopic Sterility Operations 163

14.2.4.1.   Endoscopic Salpingo-ovariolysis 163

14.2.4.2.   Endoscopic Fimbrioplasty 163

14.2.4.3.   Endoscopic Salpingostomy 164

14.2.4.3.1.   Distal Salpingostomy 164

14.2.4.3.2.   Isthmic Salpingostomy 168

14.2.4.4.   Endoscopic Tubal Surgery in the Presence of Endometriosis . . 169

14.2.4.5.   Pelviscopic Tubal Surgery in Preparation for Subsequent
Microsurgical Measures to Reestablish Fertility
by Laparotomy 169

14.2.5.   Pelviscopic Ovarian Biopsy 169

14.2.6.   Pelviscopic Puncture and Excision of Ovarian Cysts 171

    14.2.6.1.   Puncture of Ovarian Cysts 171

    14.2.6.2.   Excision of Ovarian Cyst and Ovarian Suture 172

    14.2.6.3.   Removal of Ovarian Cysts by Oophorectomy
                or Salpingo-oophorectomy 175

14.2.7.   Pelviscopic Oophorectomy 175

14.2.8.   Pelviscopic Salpingo-oophorectomy 180

    14.2.8.1.   Transection of the Infundibulopelvic Ligament 180

    14.2.8.2.   Salpingo-oophorectomy 181

14.2.9.   Salpingectomy for Hydrosalpinx 183

14.2.10. Pelviscopic Operations on the Uterus 184

    14.2.10.1. Pelviscopic Enucleation of Myomas 184

    14.2.10.2. Pelviscopic Removal of a ''Lost IUD'' . . . . 188·

    14.2.10.3. Suture of the Uterus After Perforation With a Curette 189

14.2.11. Pelviscopic Operations for Tubal Pregnancy 189

    14.2.11.1. Conservative Management of Tubal Pregnancy 190

        14.2.11.1.1. Ectopic Pregnancy in the Distal Tubal Ampulla . 191

        14.2.11.1.2. Ectopic Pregnancy in the
                      Mid-Segment of the Tube 191

    14.2.11.2. Salpingectomy for Tubal Pregnancy 193

    14.2.11.3. Operation for an Abdominal Pregnancy 195

14.2.12. Excision of Hydatid Cysts of Morgagni 195

14.2.13. Pelviscopic Excision of Parovarian Cysts 197

14.2.14. Aspiration of Oocytes for In Vitro Fertilization 198

14.2.15. Pelviscopic Tubal Sterilization 199

    14.2.15.1. Tubal Sterilization by Destructive Heat 200

        14.2.15.1.1. Tubal Sterilization by Unipolar High-Frequency
                      Coagulation 201

        14.2.15.1.2. Tubal Sterilization by Bipolar High-Frequency
                      Coagulation 202

        14.2.15.1.3. Interval Tubal Sterilization by Coagulation
                      (on the Nonpuerperal Uterus) 203

        14.2.15.1.4. Tubal Sterilization by Coagulation During
                      the Postpartum or Postabortal Phase 205

    14.2.15.2. Tubal Sterilization by Ligation 206

        14.2.15.2.1. Tubal Sterilization by Clip Application 207

14.2.15.2.2. Tubal Sterilization by Silicone Ring
Application 209

14.2.16. Comments and Conclusions Regarding Endoscopic
Tubal Sterilization 210

14.2.16.1. Comments and Conclusions Regarding Endoscopic
Tubal Sterilization by Pelviscopy 211

14.2.16.2. Comments and Conclusions Regarding Endoscopic
Tubal Sterilization by Hysteroscopy 211

14.2.16.3. Counseling of Patients Before Operative
Sterilization 211

14.3. Pelviscopic Monitoring of an Operation to Construct a Neovagina 212

15. General Endoscopic Abdominal Surgery **214**

15.1. Omental Adhesiolysis and Resection 214

15.2. Intestinal Adhesiolysis and Intestinal Suture 215

15.3. Endoscopic Appendectomy 216

15.3.1.   Indications, Requirements, and Selection of Patients for Endoscopic
Appendectomy 217

15.3.2.   Technique of Orthograde Appendectomy 217

15.3.3.   Technique of Retrograde Appendectomy 221

15.4. Instruments for Endoscopic Appendectomy 222

15.5. Biopsy of Peritoneal Metastases 224

15.6. Liver Biopsy 224

15.7. Lysis of Perihepatic Adhesions 224

16. Transition From Endoscopy to Laparotomy in the Same Operation **225**

16.1. Transition From Endoscopy to Laparotomy in the Same Operation:
As a Planned Procedure 225

16.2. Transition From Endoscopy to Laparotomy in the Same Operation:
As an Option Previously Considered 225

16.3. Transition From Endoscopy to Laparotomy in the Same Operation:
As ''Emergency Laparotomy'' 226

17. Postoperative Care After Endoscopic Abdominal Surgery **228**

17.1. Postoperative Care After Diagnostic Laparoscopy 228

17.2. Postoperative Care After Endoscopic Operations for General
Gynecologic Indications 229

17.3. Postoperative Care After an Endoscopic Operation for the Indication: ''Sterility'' . . 231

17.3.1.   General Postoperative Care 231

17.3.2.   Postoperative Care According to the ''Three-Phase Therapy''
for Endometriosis and Sterility 235

17.4. Postoperative Care After General Surgical Endoscopic Abdominal Operations 237

    17.4.1.   General Postoperative Care 237

    17.4.2.   Postoperative Care After Endoscopic Appendectomy or Intestinal Suture . . 238

18. Recovery and Restoration to Working Capacity After Endoscopic Abdominal Surgery. **239**

19. Repeated Endoscopic Abdominal Procedures **241**

20. Documentation of Endoscopic Abdominal Surgery. **242**

20.1. Written Documentation of the Endoscopic Operation (= Operative Report). 242

20.2. Photographic, Cinematographic, and Videotape Documentation of the Endoscopic Abdominal Surgery. 242

21. Assessment of the Operative Risk in Endoscopic Abdominal Surgery. **249**

22. Pelvi-Trainer **251**

22.1 Description of the Pelvi-Trainer 251

22.2 Pelvi-Trainer Practice: Three Steps 251

22.3 Recommended Training Program 253

23. Color Atlas **255**

    12.3.1.   Insufflation Media to Produce the Pneumoperitoneum (Choice of Gas) 256

    12.3.1.2.   Transvaginal Insufflation of the Pneumoperitoneum Through the Posterior Vaginal Fornix (Insufflation of the Cul-de-Sac of Douglas). 256

    12.5.6.2.   Histologic Changes After Heat-Induced Hemostasis 258

    12.6.1.   Hemostasis by Loop Ligature 258

    12.8.1.   Trocar Sleeves for Endoscopes and Operative Instruments 260

    12.8.8.   Instruments for Dilatation 260

    14.1.5.   Second and Third Punctures to Establish a Diagnosis as an Indication for the Operative Phase 262

    14.2.2.2.   Adhesiolysis Without Prophylactic Hemostasis (Bloody Adhesiolysis). 262

    14.2.2.3.   Adhesiolysis After Prophylactic Hemostasis (Bloodless Adhesiolysis) 266

    14.2.2.5.   Pelviscopic Adhesiolysis in Preparation for a Laparotomy Either During the Same Operation or at Another Time 270

    14.2.3.1.   Excision of Endometriotic Implants 276

    14.2.3.2.   Coagulation of Endometriotic Implants 280

    14.2.4.1.   Endoscopic Salpingo-ovariolysis 288

14.2.4.2.   Endoscopic Fimbrioplasty   292

14.2.4.3.   Endoscopic Salpingostomy.   296

14.2.4.3.1.   Distal Salpingostomy.   296

14.2.4.3.2.   Isthmic Salpingostomy   306

14.2.4.4.   Endoscopic Tubal Surgery in the Presence of Endometriosis   308

14.2.5.   Pelviscopic Ovarian Biopsy   308

14.2.6.1.   Puncture of Ovarian Cysts   310

14.2.6.2.   Excision of Ovarian Cysts and Ovarian Suture   314

14.2.6.3.   Removal of Ovarian Cysts by Oophorectomy or Salpingo-oophorectomy . . .   326

14.2.7.   Pelviscopic Oophorectomy.   334

14.2.8.1.   Transection of the Infundibulopelvic Ligament.   342

14.2.8.2.   Salpingo-oophorectomy   344

14.2.9.   Salpingectomy for Hydrosalpinx   354

14.2.10.   Pelviscopic Operation on the Uterus   366

14.2.10.1.   Pelviscopic Enucleation of Myomas.   368

14.2.10.2.   Pelviscopic Removal of a ''Lost IUD''.   380

14.2.10.3.   Suture of the Uterus After Perforation With a Curette.   384

14.2.11.1.2. Ectopic Pregnancy in the Mid-Segment of the Tube   386

14.2.11.2.   Salpingectomy for Tubal Pregnancy   394

14.2.12.   Excision of Hydatid Cysts of Morgagni   398

14.2.13.   Pelviscopic Excision of Parovarian Cysts.   400

14.2.14.   Aspiration of Oocytes for In Vitro Fertilization   402

14.2.15.1.1. Tubal Sterilization by Unipolar High-Frequency Coagulation   406

14.2.15.1.2. Tubal Sterilization by Bipolar High-Frequency Coagulation   408

14.2.15.1.3. Interval Tubal Sterilization by Coagulation
              (on the Nonpuerperal Uterus)   408

14.2.15.2.   Tubal Sterilization by Ligation 412

14.2.15.2.1. Tubal Sterilization by Clip Application 414

14.2.15.2.2. Tubal Sterilization by Silicone Ring Application 416

14.3   Pelviscopic Monitoring of an Operation to Construct a Neovagina 418

15.2.   Intestinal Adhesiolysis and Intestinal Suture 420

15.3.   Endoscopic Appendectomy 434

15.5.   Biopsy of Peritoneal Metastases 444

15.6.   Liver Biopsy 444

15.7.   Lysis of Perihepatic Adhesions 446

24.   Literature References 450

24.1.   Literature Cited in Text 450

24.2.   General Survey of the Literature 455

24.2.1.   Books and Monographs 455

24.2.2.   Journals 459

I.   History 459

II.   Instruments for Pelviscopy 459

III.   Pelviscopy/Statistics/Methods 460

IV.   Diagnostic Pelviscopy 462

V.   Sterility 465

VI.   Pelviscopy and Carcinoma (Tumor Diagnosis) 467

VII.   Hysterosalpingography and Pelviscopy 468

VIII.   Pelviscopy and Tuberculosis 468

IX.   Anesthesia and CO_2-Gas Metabolism 468

X.   Pneumoperitoneum (Without Complications) 470

XI.   Operative Pelviscopy 470

XII.   Operative Pelviscopy—Complications 473

XIII.   Sterilization by Pelviscopy 476

XIV.   Complications With Sterilization by Pelviscopy 481

XV.   Pelviscopy in Children 482

XVI.   Pelviscopy—Appendectomy 482

XVII.   Hystero-fetoscopy 483

XVIII.   Photo Documentation and Training 484

KEY TO THE ENDOSCOPIC COLOR PRINTS 485

INDEX 487

1 _____ Introduction

Every intra-abdominal operative procedure requires an artificial access for the instruments which must, of necessity, in most cases penetrate the abdominal wall. The trauma of establishing such access through the abdominal wall often vastly exceeds that of the actual operative correction of the diseased organ. For example, consider the opening of the abdominal cavity through a longitudinal incision or, preferably, a Pfannenstiel* low transverse incision: the physical stress to the patient from the size and extent of the incision is much greater than that from the microsurgical manipulation of the tube during a fimbrioplasty. Efforts to minimize the trauma to the abdominal wall in general surgery are most evident in an appendectomy: in this case, the patient experiences much more discomfort related to the trauma to the abdominal wall than related to the actual site of the operation, the cecal wound.

We are indebted since 1946 to the gynecologic surgeon Palmer for introducing laparoscopy, which was practiced mainly by internists, into the gynecologic field as "celioscopy." It is understandable that he was stimulated to apply this technique both to the visual diagnosis of pathologic conditions on internal female reproductive organs, and, at the same time, to the endoscopic correction of such conditions. Only his inability to effectively control a possible hemorrhage restricted his activity to procedures with minimal acceptable risks, i.e., blunt lysis of adhesions, biopsy of ovarian tissue, and similar procedures.

Since 1958, the gynecologic laparoscopist H. Frangenheim has practiced and publicized gynecologic laparoscopy in German-speaking countries of central Europe. In 1959, M.R. Cohen became an enthusiastic proponent of this technique in North America. Despite their most meritorious efforts, operative laparoscopic procedures on pelvic organs achieved only limited acceptance, for the following reasons:

1. The initial puncture, i.e., the blind insertion of a needle through the abdominal wall to establish a pneumoperitoneum, constituted an uncontrollable risk to the patient before electronic monitors for gas flow and pressure became available.

2. The insertion of a finger-thick trocar for the endoscope through the abdominal wall into the abdominal cavity, where pressures could not be monitored, was considered a greater risk than an exploratory laparotomy.

3. Since an incandescent light bulb was mounted on the tip of the endoscope, any contact with bowel threatened to cause burns. Such intestinal contacts can hardly be avoided during an exploration of the pelvis (unlike a laparoscopic exploration of the upper abdomen).

4. Mounting the light source at the tip of the endoscope made it necessary to deflect the optical axis to an angle of vision of 90°. This resulted in problems of orientation during operative procedures, particularly in the presence of massive peritoneal adhesions.

5. Since the volume and pressure of the pneumoperitoneum could not be controlled and endotracheal inhalation anesthesia had not been developed at that time, anesthesia presented problems.

6. The insufflation of atmospheric air to establish a pneumoperitoneum and the possibility that the blood vessels could be opened during op-

*H.-J. Pfannenstiel, Chairman in Kiel, 1907–1909.

1

erative procedures always posed an imponderable risk of embolism.

7. Hemostatic methods were practically unknown. Even small but persistent bleeding from omental vessels required a laparotomy for control.

8. A laparotomy resulting from a laparoscopic operation resulted in malpractice suits against the surgeon.

Although Kalk (1929 ff.) had introduced and perfected laparoscopy as a valuable diagnostic method in internal medicine, the above reasons explain why no further progress could be made in gynecology. Today, the clinical value of laparoscopy in the field of internal medicine is much in dispute. Much progress has been made in the development of biochemical tests to evaluate the liver metabolism, to examine the liver and gallbladder by noninvasive sonographic techniques, and to visualize the liver by radioisotope imaging techniques (liver scintigraphy) or, recently, by nuclear molecular response/nuclear magnetic resonance (NMR) imaging. Today, laparoscopy of the liver is much less important and is limited essentially to biopsies of the liver parenchyma under endoscopic vision and to the demonstration of metastatic tumors in the liver.

The inadequacies of the method, enumerated under reasons 1–8 above, have essentially been eliminated by technical improvements in equipment, instrumentation, and methodology (introduction of cold light sources, monitoring of the pneumoperitoneum by a CO_2-PNEU device and similar equipment, and endoscopic procedures for hemostasis). It is logical that active gynecologic surgeons were primarily responsible for progress in the technical development of "laparoscopy." This is also evident from numerous efforts to find a more specific name for the endoscopic inspection of abdominal and pelvic organs, i.e., to replace the etymologically inaccurate term "laparoscopy" (denoting inspection of the flank or abdomen) by terms such as abdominoscopy, celioscopy, abdominal-pelvic endoscopy, gynecologic laparoscopy, gynecologic pelviscopy, koiloscopy, organoscopy, pelvic laparoscopy, pelveoscopy, pelviscopy, peritoneoscopy, splanchnoscopy, and ventroscopy.

The gynecologic surgeon was familiar with the utilization of destructive heat to produce hemostasis by means of a high-frequency current. In 1934, high-frequency coagulation was utilized by Werner in Ahlen, Germany, for tubal sterilization through a laparotomy and in 1936 by Bösch in Switzerland for laparoscopic tubal sterilization. This explains why gynecologists—unaware of the

TABLE 1.

Introduction of Laparoscopic/Pelviscopic Operations in the Federal Republic of Germany and Reduction of Mortality

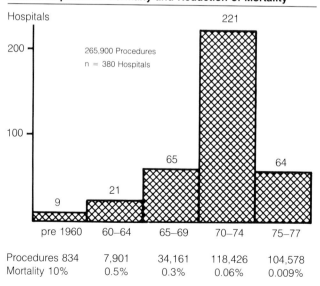

	pre 1960	60–64	65–69	70–74	75–77
Procedures	834	7,901	34,161	118,426	104,578
Mortality	10%	0.5%	0.3%	0.06%	0.009%

On March 8, 1978

unpredictable risk of high-frequency currents (see chapter 12.5. ff.)—utilized this modality without hesitation for intra-abdominal hemostasis.

Although high-frequency coagulation seemed to be well suited for tubal sterilization, this method did not reach significant proportions in France and Germany until the beginning of the 1970s. In those countries, pelviscopy was almost exclusively reserved for preoperative diagnosis in the management of sterility. Operative procedures with a pelviscope were categorically rejected until that time.

The importance of this method or the clinical need for endoscopic diagnosis in gynecology can be seen in Table 1. It indicates the rapid increase in the number of gynecologists utilizing endoscopic methods in Germany once reasons 1 through 6, enumerated above, were no longer considered valid contraindications, approximately since the 1960s.

This method had been developed in Europe primarily for diagnostic purposes; however, after M. Cohen introduced Semm's CO_2-PNEU device and the cold light technique for pelviscopy in the United States at the beginning of the 1970s, it was utilized over 95% of the time for tubal sterilization. Within only a few years, several million laparoscopic tubal sterilization operations had been performed and enormous practical experience had been accumulated with unipolar high-frequency current (see collective statistics by Phillips, 1979).

Numerous incidents during sterilization with high-frequency current (for causes see chapter 12.5.1–12.5.5.) stimulated Semm to study both the causes of thermal blood coagulation and risks from high-frequency currents. Based on physical facts, it was concluded that high-frequency current: (1) when utilized in intra-abdominal endoscopic methods poses a risk that cannot be completely controlled by the surgeon, and (2) therefore is not generally suitable or safe for hemostasis in the closed abdominal cavity.

Out of this need for safer methods, the following program of development was initiated.

On the one hand, we experimented how hemostasis by suture and ligature (well-established methods in general surgery for hundreds of years) could be accomplished through a trocar of 5 mm diameter; on the other hand, we tried to apply to endoscopic abdominal surgery the well-known technique of heat coagulation without utilizing high-frequency currents. In an effort to perform tubal sterilization without utilizing high-frequency current, in 1971 in Kiel we succeeded in replacing

the coagulation of proteins by high-frequency current with a much better method. We also learned from microsurgical techniques which, in the meantime, had been introduced into gynecology. After appropriate methods, instruments, and suture and ligature techniques had been developed for use in general surgery they were adapted to pelviscopic surgery and used on a routine basis and without risk to the patient.

Statistical data on operative pelviscopic procedures performed at the University Women's Hospital in Kiel are compiled in Table 2 (see also Fig 361). They show that the number of these procedures increased in parallel with the development of new techniques, such as techniques for achieving intra-abdominal hemostasis. The development of new techniques for operative gynecology is also spreading into general abdominal surgery (omental and intestinal adhesiolysis, appendectomy, etc.).

These new possibilities in gynecologic endoscopic surgery have brought about a fresh attitude regarding the indications for pelviscopy. Pelviscopy performed for purely diagnostic purposes no longer has the same significance it had in the past because morphological changes in the female reproductive organs can, in general, be investigated by ultrasound. After a tentative diagnosis has been made by ultrasound and the patient has been prepared for a possible laparotomy, the diagnosis is confirmed pelviscopically. If indicated and technically possible, her condition could then be corrected endoscopically under the same anesthesia.

Preparing the patient for a possible laparot-

TABLE 2.

Number and Types of Pelviscopies Performed at the Women's Hospital, Kiel University, 1971–1981 ($n = 8,060$)

YEAR	DIAGNOSTIC	DIAGNOSTIC-OPERATIVE	SURGICAL-THERAPEUTIC
1971	192	30	181
1972	173	23	171
1973	195	19	253
1974	247	26	443
1975	236	30	481
1976	168	66	366
1977	241	78	625
1978	315	78	549
1979	362	107	577
1980	262	118	588
1981	249	91	520
Σ	2,641	666	4,764

TYPE OF PELVISCOPY (spanning header over the three data columns)

omy, including obtaining the necessary informed consent, gives the gynecologic endoscopic surgeon the option to proceed immediately from an endoscopic operation to a laparotomy. With this new attitude in operative gynecology, approximately 40%–45% of all gynecologic operations that only a few years ago required a laparotomy may now be completed by pelviscopy.

The endoscopic operation (salpingo-oophorectomy, conservative or radical treatment of a tubal pregnancy, etc.) is characterized by an extremely short hospitalization time. Another essential benefit is that it constitutes only a minor physical stress to the patient, who is free of symptoms when she leaves the hospital, i.e., fully recuperated. It eliminates the long period of inability to work that is usually necessitated by a laparotomy incision.

The present operative manual concentrates primarily on the description and discussion of the operative phases of endoscopy. The atlas (chapter 23) further expands on the knowledge of techniques and problems of pelviscopy, presented in depth in Semm's color *Atlas of Gynecologic Laparoscopy and Hysteroscopy,* previously published in German (1976) and English (1977).

The technique of diagnostic pelviscopy is only briefly reviewed in a series of illustrations, most of which have been transferred from the first *Atlas.*

Finally, it should be emphasized that endoscopic abdominal surgery requires a solid knowledge of general surgery or gynecologic surgery. This knowledge and experience can only be acquired in an open abdomen. Efficient endoscopic abdominal surgery—or, for that matter, any type of surgery, such as Wertheim's operation—requires that a special set of instruments be available. It should consist of many different types of instruments as well as backup duplicates. If even one essential instrument is unavailable and an emergency, such as hemorrhage—although probably not occurring more than two or three times per thousand pelviscopies—does arise, then a laparotomy may become necessary. This endoscopic operative manual should be augmented by a color slide atlas to represent an appendix and an expansion of the previous color slide atlas, *Pelviscopy, Hysteroscopy and Fetoscopy* (1980 ff.). Arranged in the same order of subjects as the present manual, the color slides are most instructive and well suited for teaching purposes. In addition, the following films can be requested from the author:

"Operative-Therapeutic Pelviscopy"
"Conservative Operation for Tubal Pregnancy"
"Oophorectomy or Salpingo-oophorectomy"
"Endoscopic/Microsurgical Procedures on the Tubal Ampulla"

These films show, better than text, pictures, and slides, the time sequence of operative procedures.

At the conclusion of this chapter and as an introduction to operative pelviscopy, the former "laparoscopist" is presented with a motto:

The endoscopic abdominal surgeon will strive to perform all endoscopic procedures in accordance with the rules and techniques established for laparotomy.

In other words, laparoscopic emergency measures practiced in the past, such as achieving hemostasis in the omentum by coagulation, should be abandoned and replaced. Any hemorrhage should be prevented or managed by ligature or suture.

2

Historical Review: From Diagnostic Laparoscopy to Operative Pelviscopy

The gynecologist who was trained in operative procedures specific for his specialty viewed diagnostic laparoscopy from its earliest beginning as a possible opportunity to utilize this transabdominal procedure for surgical intervention, too. As early as 1936, P.F. Bösch developed into a laparoscopic technique a method of sterilizing women by tubal coagulation with high-frequency current, originally described by R. Werner in 1934. Independently of the previous authors, S.H. Power and A.C. Barnes (1941) of Ann Arbor, Michigan, developed a sterilization method by fulguration of the tubes with the peritoneoscope. H. Frangenheim (1964) introduced this technique into the German-speaking countries of Europe.

Biopsy of the ovaries for the histologic evaluation of their function, practiced by R. Palmer since 1946, and primarily blind adhesiolysis in the area of the internal genital organs comprised the limits of operative procedures that could be performed endoscopically. Although quite limited, these endoscopic operative procedures already surpass all other surgical interventions in any field of endoscopy. In this case, too, one was restricted to only small biopsy specimens for fear of hemorrhage. The only exception was operative cystoscopy in urology. Even in the early stages of development, urologic surgeons removed urinary concrements. An advantage of operative cystoscopy is that it is performed not in a gaseous environment but in a liquid environment, water. This provides an ideal cooling effect, even though extensive hemostasis by destructive heat, or high-frequency current, might be required.

As indicated in Table 2, the number of gynecologic surgeons performing endoscopic procedures in Germany in the early 1970s was very small and in most parts of the world this method was practically unknown. To emphasize the pioneering work of individual investigators, those authors most eminent in the development and dissemination of gynecologic laparoscopy/pelviscopy are named in chronological order in Table 3.

In Europe, this endoscopic method had been developed exclusively for diagnostic purposes. The breakthrough for operative pelviscopy, however, occurred only with the reversal of purpose, when this diagnostic method was adopted in the United States and adapted almost exclusively for the purpose of tubal sterilizaton. In the United States "culdoscopy," developed by A. Decker in 1946, was the predominant method because it did not appear to be as involved and as hazardous as gynecologic laparoscopy. Moreover, it permitted access to the pelvis through the posterior vaginal fornix, a more familiar route to the gynecologist.

As was the case in Europe until 1965, laparoscopy was also rejected by most American colleagues in gynecology because of its unpredictable risk with insufflation. A new era began when M.R.

TABLE 3.
**Chronological Development of Gynecologic Laparoscopy/Pelviscopy (○)
and Culdo-/Douglasscopy (×)**

1927	Korbsch	○	1956	Magendie	○
1929	Kalk	○		Kelly	×
1934	Ruddock	○		Mohri	×
	Werner	○			
1936	Boesch	○	1957	Derjabina	○
1937	Hope	○	1958	Frangenheim	○×
1941	Power and Barnes	○			
1942	Donaldson	○	1959	Cohen	○×
1945	Bismuth	○×	1960	Benaim	○
1946	Decker	×		Daley et al.	×
	Palmer	○×		Gonzalez-Lobo	×
1947	Elert	○		Jamain	○
	Klaften	×		Lenzi et al.	○
	Wildhirt	×		Thoyer-Rozat	○
1948	Endicott	○			
	Te Linde et al.	×	1961	Cittadini	○
	Wenner	○		Golubev	○×
1949	Antonowitsch	×		Neumann	○×
1950	Ravina	×	1962	Albano	○
	Teton	×		Siede et al.	×
1951	Abarbanel	×	1963	Clyman	×
	Doyle	×	1964	Mintz	○
	Thomsen	×		Lübke	○
1952	Botella-Llusia	×		Pye	○×
1953	Hopkins	○×		Schwalm	○
1954	Buxton	×		Semm	○
	Clauss	×		Steptoe	○
	Walch	×	1965	Hayden	○
1955	Gorga	○	1966	Eisenburg	○
	Menken	×	1968	Marchesi et al.	○
1956	Guggisberg	○	1974	Hasson	○

Cohen demonstrated in his 1970 atlas, *Laparoscopy, Culdoscopy and Gynecography*, that gynecologic laparoscopy had matured to a useful modality with the introduction of the cold light and the monitor for the pneumoperitoneum, the CO_2-PNEU device (according to Semm, 1964). This atlas was published at a time when concerns about population dynamics and political pressures were mounting, and gynecology was challenged to develop a sterilization method that would be well tolerated and safe. This initiated an explosive dissemination of laparoscopy in the United States. As early as 1972 the American Association of Gynecologic Laparoscopists (AAGL) was founded, under the chairmanship of J. Phillips. Within a few years, 4,000 members had joined and statistical data on several million laparoscopic sterilization procedures had been published.

However, the record acceptance for purely operative purposes—tubal sterilization—of a method that in Europe was utilized almost exclusively for diagnostic purposes also led to a multitude of unpredictable *complications*.

Gynecologic endoscopists who were responsible for the development of the method in Germany and France had worked only with a small high-frequency coagulation apparatus with a maximum power of 100 W. In America, the Bovie high-frequency apparatus was almost exclusively used for coagulation. It had a maximum power of 350 W and, even at its lowest level of adjustment, delivered 100 W of energy. Because coagulation times of 10–20 seconds were recommended by German surgeons (who did not specify the power intensity), and because users on both sides of the Atlantic were unfamiliar with the technical data of the high-frequency generators they used, unexplained burns of skin, bowel, ureter, and even of the gynecologic

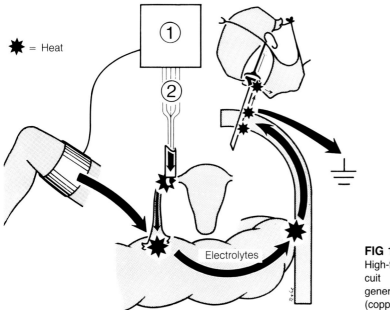

✳ = Heat

FIG 1.
High-frequency coagulation circuit *1*, high-frequency current generator; *2*, first-order conductor (copper wire).

endoscopist occurred in the United States. (A general scheme of the high-frequency coagulation apparatus is diagrammed in Fig 1.)

The danger of unipolar high-frequency current is based primarily on the fact that it flows through the human body in an uncontrollable pattern due to conduction systems with various electrolytic contents (Fig 2). Therefore, in 1970 I tried to introduce the application of bipolar high-frequency currents, which had been previously well established in neurosurgery. The bipolar "tubal set" which I described in 1963 was used for hemostasis during operative procedures on fallopian tubes. It had been used successfully in a technique described by Walz (1959), who performed reconstructive operations on the tube under magnification with a colposcope, i.e., microsurgically. With the bipolar forceps of the "tubal set," described by Fikentscher and Semm, we successfully performed tubal sterilizations in Kiel in 1971.

In consideration of reports from the United States at the beginning of the 1970s about serious complications with tubal sterilizations (sometimes terminating with the death of the patient), and for

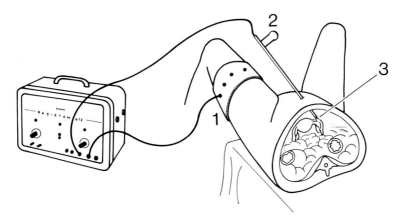

FIG 2.
Unipolar high-frequency current conduction. *1*, negative return electrode; *2*, unipolar instrument; *3*, contact point between instrument and patient's tissue (e.g., fallopian tube).

reasons of liability, no German companies were willing to produce high-frequency equipment for sterilization purposes, not even after the uncontrollable risk had been all but eliminated by utilization of bipolar high-frequency currents. Tubal sterilizations with high-frequency currents were performed by gynecologists with commercially available atraumatic grasping and biopsy forceps (described by Semm). Although the previous decision, based on legal considerations, was revised in 1974–1975 by both German and American industry, it became the prime stimulus for me to search for other ways in which the classic method of coagulating proteins by heat could be utilized as a low-risk technique for achieving hemostasis in abdominal endoscopy.

The first occasion for efforts in this direction was H.-J. Lindemann's proposal, in 1971, of a new technique for transuterine tubal sterilization by hysteroscopy. This technique was based both on the pioneering work of Kocks (1878, blind method, i.e., without hysteroscope) and on studies of transuterine sterilization, initiated by Mikulicz-Radecki and A. Freund in 1927. With transuterine intratubal application of the unipolar high-frequency probe (Fig 3), the level of heat conduction in the surrounding tissues cannot be controlled because the conductivity of these tissues is not known.

Therefore, in a few cases the coagulation effect was not strictly limited to the tubal ostium but was also transmitted to adjacent bowel. To prevent this uncontrollable side effect, I modified the thermoprobe I had developed in 1965 for the treatment of cervicitis. With this new instrument, the electrical current was no longer in contact with the human body (Fig 4).

Here it may be helpful to summarize the historical development of hysteroscopy, which may

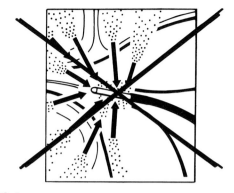

FIG 3.
Transuterine intratubal placement of unipolar high-frequency probe. Heat conduction in surrounding tissues cannot be controlled.

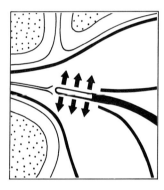

FIG 4.
Modified thermoprobe technique (Semm). The electrical current is no longer in contact with tissue.

TABLE 4.
Eminent Authors in the Investigation of Hysteroscopic Techniques

1864	Aubinais	1956	Mohri
1868	Pantaleoni	1957	Englund and Ingelmann-Sundberg
1879	Nitze	1960	Benaim
1895	Bumm	1962	Silander
1908	David	1966	Schmidt-Matthiesen
1925	Rubin	1968	Marleschki
1926	Seymour	1969	Menken
1927	Mikulicz-Radecki and Freund	1969	Semm
1928	Gauss	1970	Edström
1934	Schroeder	1971	Lindemann
1949	Norment	1974	Rimkus
1951	Izawa		

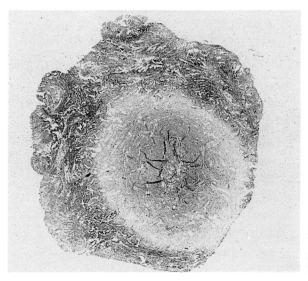

FIG 5.
Tissue cylinder heated by thermoprobe (hysteroscopy). The size of the tissue cylinder is controlled and reproducible.

be considered one of the oldest gynecologic-endoscopic methods (Table 4).

With the newly developed thermoprobe, thermal energy is monitored as it dissipates into surrounding tissues by convection. The size of the tissue cylinder heated in this manner is reproducible at any time (Fig 5).

In the years of experimental development, from 1971 to 1975, it became apparent that this mode of transuterine tubal occlusion by destructive heat was not successful. If there are no postoperative inflammatory reactions in the heated area of the tubal ostium, the heat-induced thermal necrosis, as expected, will heal without obstructing the tubal lumen, and will often result in a larger tubal ostium than before. This was documented for the first time in 1974 by Rimkus and Semm, who reported a postoperative pregnancy rate of more than 20%. These results, confirmed by other investigations, led to the conclusion that, at present, transuterine sterilization is of no clinical importance. The same applies to tissue adhesives and plug methods.

The development by Semm of thermoprobes which are heated with direct current and can be applied by the transuterine route led to the development of heated tubal forceps in 1971 (Fig 6).

The electrical current has no contact with the human body. The tubal tissue is biologically destroyed by thermal conduction and radiation at 100° C.

This tubal grasping forceps was soon replaced by the crocodile forceps (see Fig 327). This instru-

ment, combined with a modern electronic monitor, is now the fundamental device for achieving hemostasis by destructive heat during endoscopic abdominal surgery (endocoagulator with crocodile forceps and point coagulator, see chapters 12.5.6. ff. and 12.8.9.).

The experimental and scientific investigation of thermal coagulation (i.e., achieving hemostasis by protein coagulation) revealed, however, that adequate and risk-free intra-abdominal hemostasis cannot always be achieved with this instrument.

In search of a substitute for endoscopic hemostasis, we found (Semm, 1977) a ligature loop and slipknot technique for tonsillectomy in children, which was described by Roeder at the end of the last century. It requires that the bleeding vessel be pulled through the open loop and then that the loop be closed. However, during an actual operative procedure, not all bleeding vessels can be pulled through a loop, but some must occasionally be ligated before the organ is resected. Therefore, we also developed two more endoscopic techniques: endoligation with external tying of a slip-

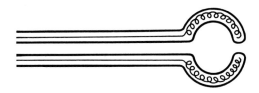

FIG 6.
Heated tubal forceps, developed by Semm in 1971.

knot, and endosuture with external or internal tying of the knot (see chapters 12.6.2. and 12.6.3.).

With these techniques, all classic methods of achieving hemostasis were also available for operative endoscopic abdominal surgery. With the development of the electronic insufflator and monitor for the pneumoperitoneum (see chapter 12.3.3.) and of ideal grasping and cutting instruments that could be introduced through the trocar sleeves of 5 and 11 mm diameter, a compatible set of instruments and equipment has become available for the endoscopic surgeon for the first time. It makes possible the gynecologic and general surgical procedures depicted in Figures 7 through 21.

Typical gynecologic procedures (Figs 7–18)

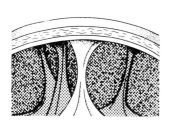 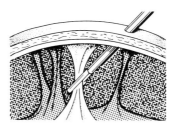 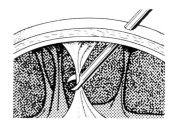

FIG 7.
General intra-abdominal adhesiolysis, including omental resection.

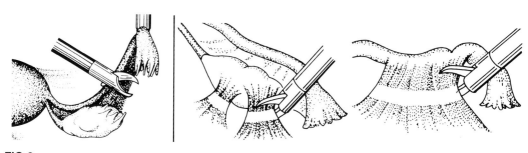

FIG 8.
Ovariolysis and salpingolysis in operations to correct sterility.

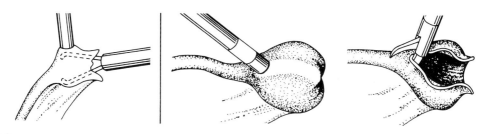

FIG 9.
Fimbrioplasty with blunt dilatation of the distal ampulla or salpingostomy.

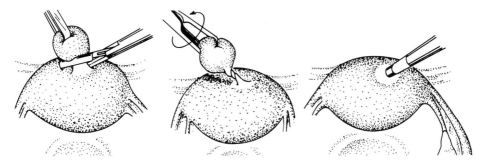

FIG 10.
Excision of pedunculated or subserous myomata (if necessary, with uterine suture) (see Fig 315 and Plates 225 through 232).

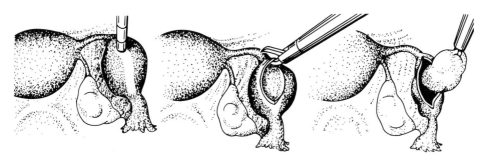

FIG 11.
Conservative (i.e., tube-preserving) operation for tubal pregnancies.

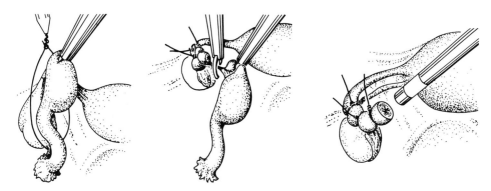

FIG 12.
Salpingectomy, e.g., as a radical operation in the management of tubal pregnancy or hydrosalpinx.

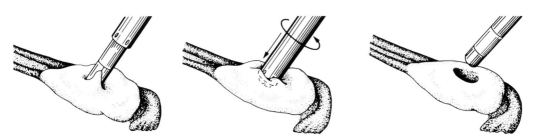

FIG 13.
Ovarian biopsy.

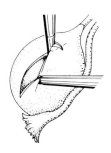 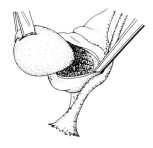 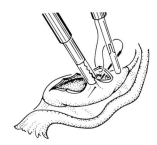

FIG 14.
Excision of ovarian cyst with closure of ovarian wound by endosuture.

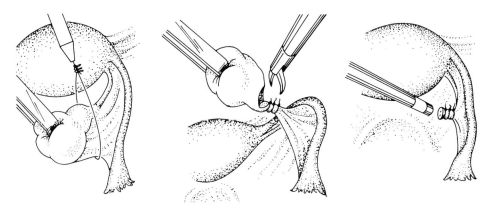

FIG 15.
Oophorectomy (triple-loop technique).

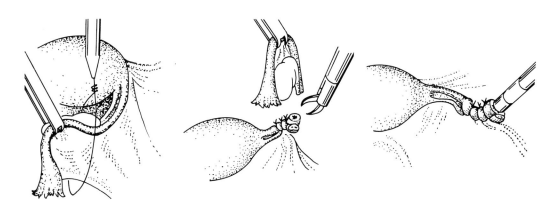

FIG 16.
Salpingo-oophorectomy (triple-loop technique).

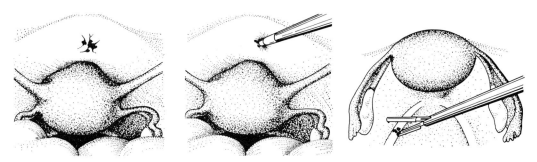

FIG 17.
Coagulation of endometriotic implants.

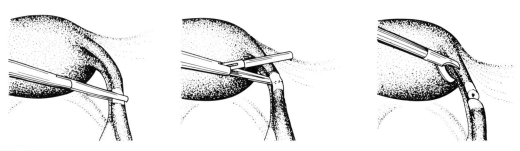

FIG 18.
Tubal sterilization with sharp transection.

General surgical endoscopic intra-abdominal operations (Figs 19–21)

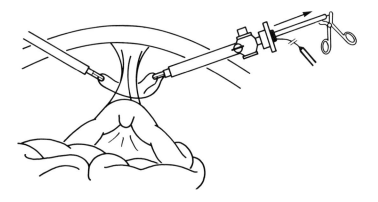

FIG 19.
Adhesiolysis, including omental resection.

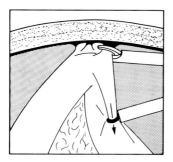

FIG 20.
Postoperative intestinal adhesiolysis (with intestinal suture).

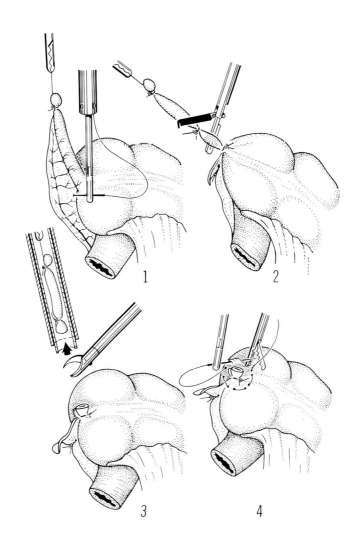

FIG 21.
Appendectomy.

The gynecologic operations illustrated above correspond to 30%–70% (depending on the type and clinical function of the institution) of the formerly classic indications for a laparotomy. If the options for endoscopic surgery are fully utilized, the frequency of laparotomies and the hospitalization times will be reduced. Very important—particularly for third-party payers—is the reduction of hospitalization time by 50%–75%.

In the past four decades, the foundation was laid for a new operative technique in the abdominal cavity. The procedures presented in this operative manual are just the beginning of this new surgical era and will stimulate the development of numerous variations. This is in contrast to the state of instrument technology: as far as optical improvements are concerned, the mechanical and physical limits have been reached. This may also apply to the electronic insufflator and monitor for the pneumoperitoneum. In the field of surgical instruments, considerable improvements can certainly be expected.

3 _____ Informing Patients About Endoscopic Abdominal Surgery

This chapter is placed near the beginning of the text because the changes that have occurred in the use of laparoscopy or pelviscopy are most evident in the information patients are given preoperatively. In the past, laparoscopy in internal medicine was considered a practically risk-free method for the inspection of the upper abdomen, occasionally extended to small biopsy procedures that were necessary for diagnostic purposes, too. If such a laparoscopic procedure terminated in a laparotomy, something went wrong.

This fact has also been established in legal decisions. Every patient and every lawyer will suspect medical malpractice if a laparotomy is performed subsequent to a laparoscopy. In the same context, information in the sense of "laparoscopy, possibly laparotomy" may appear to have a negative connotation. It is therefore advisable not to mention laparoscopy in regard to endoscopic abdominal surgery at all, but to refer only to operative pelviscopy. This term has already been defined in Pschyrembel's Clinical Dictionary (German, 1983) as an operative procedure, whereas laparoscopy has been defined only as "diagnostic procedure." Therefore, a malpractice suit can no longer be based on a declaration that the defendant had not been informed about and had not consented to the possibility of a laparotomy.

Today, operative pelviscopy primarily is undertaken to verify a pathologic condition that has already been diagnosed by bimanual palpation and confirmed by ultrasound; then it can be determined whether the condition can be managed by pelviscopy (i.e., endoscopically), or if instead a laparotomy will be necessary. An explanation and advice in this sense must be fully understood by the patient.

The patient will be informed according to the following train of thought: Your ovarian cyst (ectopic pregnancy, adhesiolysis after a previous laparotomy, etc.) used to require an open laparotomy or repeat laparotomy, respectively. However, new technical developments permit us to carry out many operative interventions through an endoscope. Whether or not this will be possible can only be recognized and decided during the endoscopic procedure.

If the patient has been informed and sufficiently prepared for a laparotomy, she will wake up from the operation content if she has no abdominal incision. On the other hand, she has no reason to complain—as was frequently the case after a classic laparoscopy or pelviscopy—if, indeed, she does have an incision. After informing the patient properly, the endoscopic surgeon has the option to take full advantage of his endoscopic operative skills without the constant fear of a laparotomy. This drastic change in informing the patient of and preparing her for an operative pelviscopy resulted in a 40% reduction of all classic indications for laparotomy and its replacement by endoscopic operations at the University Women's Hospital in Kiel. The indication for sterilization is not even included in this calculation. For other indications, such as peripheral ampullary tubal damage, the classic laparotomy can be replaced in 90% of cases.

The patient must be fully informed of the planned procedure: "initially pelviscopy and possibly subsequent laparotomy." For this, she must give written consent. Information that tends more toward a laparotomy is advisable and certainly an advantage. Even if the patient has not had a laparotomy, she will show a higher appreciation of her surgeon's efforts postoperatively.

[I am in full agreement with Semm that a surgeon should emphasize laparotomy whenever a more extensive endoscopic operation is anticipated, or if the surgeon has had only limited experience in endoscopic surgery. However, if a patient is scheduled for a tubal sterilization and, by history and examination, appears to have a "normal" abdomen and pelvis, her preoperative fears will be substantially relieved if she is informed that the likelihood of a laparotomy being necessary is extremely low (<1/1,000). The preoperative discussion with the patient should also include mention of a multitude of other risks, including allergic reactions to drugs, infections, blood transfusions, anesthesia; injuries to bladder, bowel, blood vessels, or nerves; pregnancy at the time of or following sterilization; the possibility that surgery may have to be terminated before completion of the planned procedure; incomplete success of the operation, and the possibility of recurrence of the same or other conditions postoperatively.

I personally consider it more harmful than beneficial to "scare" every patient with the possibility of death unless the patient inquires about that subject.

If the endoscopic procedure is scheduled under local anesthesia (see chapter 10.1.1.) or "volonelgesia" (see chapter 10.1.2.), there must also be a clear agreement on the level of discomfort that will be acceptable to the patient, and under what circumstances the procedure should be abandoned or general anesthesia should be initiated. If both the gynecologic surgeon and the anesthesiologist participate in the administration of local and systemic anesthetic agents, respectively, it must be ascertained that their individual agreements with the patient do not contradict each other.—*Ed.*]

4 _____ Timing of Endoscopic Abdominal Surgery

According to classic surgical protocol, there is a certain interrelation between the indication (see chapter 8) and the scheduling of the surgical intervention. It is determined partly by the type of the surgical procedure and partly by the availability of certain personnel and equipment within the limits of the routine daily schedule. The transition from a procedure originally scheduled as a laparotomy to an endoscopic operative procedure does affect the schedule.

4.1. TIMING OF ENDOSCOPIC ABDOMINAL SURGERY: TYPICAL GYNECOLOGIC ELECTIVE PROCEDURES

The patient will be informed (see chapter 3) and prepared (see chapter 5) as if she were scheduled for a laparotomy. Scheduling of the operative intervention will follow the guidelines of the classical surgical protocol. A variation may be called for if an inflammatory process is suspected (adnexitis, pyosalpinx, etc.).

In such a case, one is inclined—more so today than in the past—to consider early pelviscopic intervention. When a laparotomy was done in the past, the surgeon was frequently committed to total excision of the ovary or the tubes. Today, intervention is limited to aspiration of pus from the pyosalpinges with simultaneous vigorous irrigation of the pelvis, and the intra-abdominal and intratu-

bal instillation of antibiotics. With these measures, the course of the illness can be shortened considerably—as could be shown in many cases—and the loss of an organ can be prevented. The antibiotic sensitivity test on cultures taken at the same time prevents such cases in which, for example, a *Candida* salpingitis is treated for weeks, or even months, with nonspecific antibiotic regimens that lack antifungal agents.

Prior to operative pelviscopy, and if time permits, surgery should be postponed until the patient's bowels have been thoroughly purged. Distended bowels interfere with inspection of the pelvic cavity, and therefore also interfere with endoscopic operative measures. This applies in particular to operations in the area of the sigmoid colon and the rectal ampulla (see chapter 5.2.).

4.2. TIMING OF ENDOSCOPIC ABDOMINAL SURGERY: PELVISCOPIC TUBAL SURGERY FOR CORRECTION OF STERILITY

The ascending chromosalpingoscopy (see chapters 12.4.2. and 14.2.4.2. ff.) is absolutely necessary for the demonstration of tubal patency. Since the possibility of dissemination of endometrial particles (Sampson's dissemination or implantation theory, 1921) is still under discussion, this procedure should be performed only at the beginning of the proliferation phase. Furthermore, it is recommended that this procedure be performed immediately after the menstrual period has ended, so that another approximately 5 days are available for prolonged hydropertubation (see chapter 17.3.), if indicated.

If a follow-up pelviscopy is indicated after a previous laparotomy for sterility, scheduling depends on the specific intention. After surgical correction of pathologic conditions on the ampullae, the series of hydropertubations is begun on the first postoperative day. After end-to-end operations or tubal reimplantations, hydropertubation should be postponed for 3–4 days to await the complete closure of the surgical wounds in the tubes.

4.3. TIMING OF ENDOSCOPIC ABDOMINAL SURGERY: GYNECOLOGIC PROCEDURES TO TREAT PELVIC ENDOMETRIOSIS

Mild cases of superficial endometriosis of the internal genitalia (Acosta, 1973; AFS, 1985; or EEC, grades I and II) are best recognized endoscopically at the end of menstrual cycles. The less experienced surgeon should schedule the pelviscopic procedure during that phase. However, if a diagnostic evaluation of the patient's sterility is desired, the procedure should be postponed until immediately after the menstrual period to prevent the possibility of dissemination of endometrial particles. At that time, however, the blood contained in the endometriotic implants has been discharged (see Plates 61 and 62) so that they show only a discrete discoloration in comparison to the surrounding healthy peritoneum. Therefore, they are easily overlooked at this time. Only careful inspection of the peritoneal surfaces in the pelvis with a low-power loupe attached to the eyepiece of the endoscope (see chapter 12.2.4.) will reveal the diagnosis! If superficial endometriosis of the internal genitalia is present, one usually finds approximately 5–20 ml of serosanguinous exudate in the cul-de-sac of Douglas (see Plates 52, 59, and 76), which should be an indication for an intensive search for endometriotic implants. In doubtful cases, the diagnosis will be made by a positive thermocolor test (see chapter 14.2.3.2. and Plates 61, 62, 64, and 387). [As an alternative, the peritoneal surfaces could be examined with the endoscope at a very close range of only 1–2 cm, at which the inherent magnifying power of the endoscope is 2–4 X.—*Ed.*]

4.4. TIMING OF ENDOSCOPIC ABDOMINAL SURGERY: GENERAL ABDOMINAL SURGICAL PROCEDURES

In these cases, the time to operate is determined by the same established criteria that apply to laparotomy. However, since a preliminary diagnostic endoscopic exploration constitutes only a minor physical stress to the patient, it is usually carried out sooner than an exploratory laparotomy would have been in cases of, for example, suspected abdominal adhesions or tubal pregnancy, appendicitis, partial intestinal obstruction, and the like. The justification is even stronger, because the diagnostic exploration can be followed immediately by the operative phase of pelviscopy. In the majority of cases (e.g., adhesiolysis), the endoscopic intervention will also have a therapeutic effect without the risk of recurrence.

5 _____ Patient Preparation for Endoscopic Abdominal Surgery

The preparation of patients for endoscopic abdominal surgery differs considerably from previous measures taken before a diagnostic laparoscopy. In addition to the preoperative technical preparation of the patient for the endoscopic operative intervention (which will be discussed further below), it is important to emphasize the psychological and physical aspects of this operative phase

The psychological guidance and education of a patient before endoscopic abdominal surgery and before laparotomy are fundamentally different. The endoscopic procedure always begins as a diagnostic measure to determine if (1) the suspected or established diagnosis is correct and (2) the necessary surgical intervention can be accomplished endoscopically, or (3) a laparotomy will still be required.

Regardless of the indication for the scheduled endoscopic procedure, the surgeon must always consider these three aspects in his psychological guidance of the patient. The patient will be informed that:

- The first phase is only a diagnostic exploration of low risk, and will not be a long, involved operative procedure.
- The surgeon's decision will be based on the findings of the diagnostic exploration and will determine whether further endoscopic operative mea-

sures or a laparotomy will be required; what the final decision will be cannot be predicted precisely.

The patient must be psychologically prepared that her illness, if confirmed, would, according to good surgical practice, require that her abdominal cavity be opened, but that newly developed techniques have provided the option—with this or that probability—to spare her the physically more stressful abdominal incision.

Regarding consent, the surgeon definitely must prepare the patient for a laparotomy. This will allow the surgeon:

- In case of a medical necessity, to proceed, under the same anesthesia, to further operative measures or immediately to a laparotomy.
- In case of failure of the endoscopic operation, to complete the planned procedure by laparotomy, without being blamed by the patient for an unexpected laparotomy.

The patient's preparation should also include all measures necessary for a purely diagnostic laparoscopic procedure.

In summary, it should be emphasized that it is psychologically wrong and detrimental to the excellent reputation of the method to give the patient the impression that there is nothing to an endoscopic operative procedure, that it is "a piece of cake." The patient will have a greater and more objective appreciation of the personal benefits to be derived from these new, combined diagnostic and operative methods once the possibilities and limits of this endoscopic procedure have been fully explained.

Another important aspect in the psychology of correct guidance of the patient is that the patient will retain a favorable memory of the endoscopic intervention. If the patient should again require such diagnostic operative surgical procedure during her lifetime it should be repeated without instigating horrible memories.

5.1. PSYCHOLOGICAL PREPARATION OF THE PATIENT FOR ENDOSCOPIC ABDOMINAL SURGERY

By comparing the advantages and disadvantages of the planned operative intervention by laparotomy or by pelviscopy, the patient will be psychologically prepared for the procedure to be initiated with the endoscopic phase. This phase primarily corroborates or confirms the diagnosis. It is followed by the operative phase, under the same anesthesia, with the intention of completing the entire operation through the endoscope—that is, to spare the patient a laparotomy, which conventionally would have been necessary.

In the psychological preparation of the patient, one must consider the following three main thoughts:

1. The diagnostic phase is the essential one in which it is decided whether a surgical procedure (which appears to be indicated on the basis of the patient's history, physical findings, etc.) is necessary at all. If a surgical procedure is necessary, the surgeon decides whether it can be performed endoscopically or will have to be carried out by laparotomy immediately after the diagnostic endoscopic procedure.

2. The operative measures performed through the endoscope that immediately follow the diagnostic phase are merely an attempt to complete the procedure without a laparotomy (i.e., a large incision in the abdomen).

3. Any additional complications occurring during the endoscopic operation (e.g., intestinal or ureteral injuries) are not mishaps specifically related to the endoscopic operative technique. Such injuries are the same known risks inherent in any general surgical procedure entailing a laparotomy and may occur even with most skillful and meticulous operative techniques.

It is of fundamental importance that these three aspects are covered in the psychological preparation of the patient by her physician. The patient will be informed about the benign nature and low risk of the procedure and of the personal benefits she may expect. However, she must be psychologically prepared to accept fully that the procedure may possibly end with a classic laparotomy.

Therefore, the endoscopic surgeon is well advised to obtain the patient's preoperative consent so that:

1. In case of a medical necessity the surgeon is permitted to perform, under the same anesthesia, the required operation by either pelviscopy or by laparotomy, or

2. If the patient prefers, such a procedure is postponed until a later date.

It has become easier to obtain the patient's consent under the present circumstances than in the past, when the indication for the procedure was strictly a diagnostic one, and no operative intervention was planned.

In this context, it should be repeated that surgeons who have performed laparoscopy in years past will have to undergo some "brainwashing" (cleansing of their minds): the original laparoscopy was exclusively a diagnostic method. It has now been replaced, to a large extent, by the nonaggressive diagnostic techniques of ultrasound. On the other hand, endoscopic abdominal surgery is replacing operations which actually require a laparotomy; this should be replaced by a modern, less aggressive procedure—operative endoscopy.

The patient should also be psychologically prepared for the need for endotracheal anesthesia, which will permit an immediate transition from the endoscopic diagnostic phase to the operative phase. [However, in the editor's experience, in certain selected cases (pelvic-lower abdominal pain of unknown etiology, patient's fear of general anesthesia, etc.), it may be desirable to perform the diagnostic phase under local anesthesia (see chapter 10.1.1.) or "volonelgesia" (see chapter 10.1.2.), and then proceed to general anesthesia if more extensive operative measures are indicated. With this approach, the psychological preparation of the patient before surgery and support during surgery, by both a committed surgeon and a cooperative staff, are absolutely essential.—*Ed.*]

The patient must also be informed that endoscopic operative procedures require that one incision be made for the introduction of the endoscope in the umbilical area, and possibly another three to four perforations for the most favorable placement of additional operative instruments. The exact location of the 5- to 10-mm-long skin incisions cannot be predicted. Unexpected or extensive intra-abdominal adhesions may occasionally make it necessary to select atypical places for the second to fourth punctures, if these are the only sites free of adhesions.

As a rule, the patient should be psychologically prepared that the hospitalization time cannot be exactly defined in advance. Although there is no large abdominal incision to cause much postoperative discomfort, the healing process in the peritoneal cavity will, nevertheless, not be accelerated! The patient should be advised preoperatively that she may feel only little discomfort as early as the first or second postoperative day after an endoscopic operation (e.g., for ectopic pregnancy, salpingo-oophorectomy, appendectomy, etc.); however, because of internal wound healing, she should not leave the hospital immediately.

[In contradiction to the recommended, most cautious approach, the editor and other experienced endoscopic surgeons in the United States have consented to the request by many patients to be discharged from the hospital only several hours after, or on the morning after, quite extensive endoscopic operations. Only on extremely rare occasions were patients readmitted for further observation because of prolonged or more severe postoperative pain.—*Ed.*]

It is psychologically wrong and detrimental to the excellent reputation of the method to give the patient the impression that there is nothing to the endoscopic operative procedure; that it is "just a piece of cake."

It bears reemphasis that the great advantage of endoscopic abdominal surgery is not only a reduction in the hospitalization time. The benefit for the patient lies in the fact that she is usually free of complaints when she leaves the hospital and is able to return to work.

Proper psychological guidance of the patient is extremely important: she should retain good memories of the endoscopic abdominal procedure even after extensive intra-abdominal operations. This applies, for instance, to the aspiration of follicles, when it is expected that a single procedure rarely will accomplish the desired goal, or to the "three-phase therapy" of endometriosis (see chapters 14.2.3. and 17.3.2.), in which repeat pelviscopy is scheduled after several months of therapy.

5.2. PHYSICAL PREPARATION

After the patient has been informed about and has consented to a laparotomy (see chapter 3), her preoperative preparation for endoscopic abdominal surgery is the same as for a laparotomy. The procedure is begun with the full realization that the usual and customary approach would be a laparotomy. If possible, however, the patient should be spared the physical stress of a laparotomy, although, for technical reasons, the indication for one may arise at any time.

If the indication for the procedure is the correction of abdominal adhesions after a previous laparotomy, a 3- to 4-day liquid diet (occasionally an astronaut diet) is recommended. Intestinal loops adherent to the anterior abdominal wall can be dissected more easily and microsurgically [i.e., under low-power loupe magnification (see chapter 12.2.4.)] if they are empty, that is, not distended by gas. Complete purging of the intestinal tract is an important requirement for the success of every pelviscopic procedure.

Distended loops of bowel not only obstruct the view, but also restrict the movement of instruments. This applies in particular to a distended sigmoid colon and a full rectal ampulla. Both will limit the view into the small pelvis and take up so much space that any operative procedure on the left adnexa is difficult. If necessary, a rectal tube may be placed during the pelviscopic procedure to aspirate gas from the lower intestinal tract.

To prevent such manipulations for the evacuation of bowels during the operation, we recommend to the patient that she restrict her diet to fluids only on the day prior to hospitalization. In addition, on the morning of the operation, an enema is given to promote another evacuation of stools and gas from the sigmoid colon and rectal ampulla before the operation begins.

Before a gynecologic operation, and particularly before pelviscopy for the operative correction of sterility, any vaginal infection should be treated in order to prevent an ascending infection that may be caused by chromosalpingoscopy. A wet-mount preparation of vaginal secretions is obligatory on the day prior to surgery. If necessary, appropriate therapy should be initiated, such as a vaginal douche and/or antibiotics.

The following procedure is scheduled: first pelviscopy, possibly followed by laparotomy. This should also be discussed with the anesthesiologist in advance (see chapter 10).

The new technical procedure for gynecologic or general surgical operations must be clearly indicated on the operating schedule or on the blackboard in the operating room, in a manner that is clearly understood by the entire operating team—surgeons, assistants, anesthesiologists, and nursing staff. The type of procedure is indicated as pelviscopy/laparotomy, abbreviated as "pelv./lap." [This abbreviation is less confusing than the abbreviation "lap./lap." which is presently often used in the United States.—*Ed.*] With this designation the appropriate orders regarding instruments as well as personnel have been given, preventing, in case of an intraoperative emergency, complications arising from the remark: "Sorry, but that hadn't been scheduled!"

The endoscopic operative procedure is a major intra-abdominal operation with all its possible consequences.

In this regard, it should be emphasized again that optimum diagnostic and therapeutic benefits of endoscopic abdominal surgery can only be achieved if the patient has been convinced, by the appropriate preoperative psychological and physical preparation, of the high relative value of this modern endoscopic technique of abdominal surgery. Under no circumstances should the patient get the impression that, in these early days of the modern surgical era, success is guaranteed by the great endoscopic skills of the surgeon in combination with well-developed, conventional techniques, which may be expected by the patient in the case of a laparotomy.

6 _____ Medical Requirements for Endoscopic Abdominal Surgery

Endoscopic intra-abdominal operations require a high degree of surgical skill which can only be acquired after the abdomen has been opened by a laparotomy incision. The surgeon skilled in procedures in the open abdomen will experience three essential *restrictions* when he performs a procedure with an endoscope:

1. The endoscopic surgeon has only monocular vision; three-dimensional vision is impossible.

2. Changes in the distance between the objective lens and the object make the organs viewed appear to be of different size, so that the actual size can be estimated only by past experience or by comparing them to instruments or rulers introduced for this purpose.

3. Moving, grasping, cutting, or manipulating of sutures, for example, is limited, because every motion can only be performed through a fixed trocar sleeve, which allows mobility only around one central point.

These restrictions require of the surgeon:

1. Superior general surgical training.

2. Advanced endoscopic diagnostic capabilities.

3. Excellent manual dexterity.

In addition, it is of utmost importance that the endoscopic surgeon make the decision to purchase the entire spectrum of available endoscopic instruments and equipment in sufficient numbers, including backup instruments. Just as the quality and number of available instruments determine the success of Wertheim's operation, so do they determine the success of endoscopic abdominal surgery. In this case, for instance, the operative fields must be continuously maintained by the technical expediency of the pneumoperitoneum: it does not remain free once it has been established, as it does with a laparotomy.

As during a laparotomy, the endoscopic surgeon operates with assistance (Fig 22). Next to the instrument nurse, the surgical assistant observes the operative procedure through a flexible optical attachment, often referred to as a "spy" (Fig 23). The surgical assistant holds the eyepiece and adjusts the endoscope for the surgeon, resting his elbow on the surgeon's shoulder support (see chapter 13.3.) to prevent disturbing movements of the en-

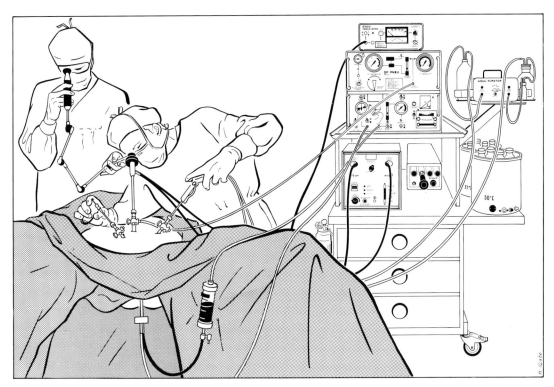

FIG 22.
A flexible optical attachment allows the surgical assistant to view the endoscopic procedure.

doscope. During more difficult steps in the operation, the assistant will hold instruments, remove forceps, and so on, as is routinely done during a laparotomy. In spite of only monocular vision, it is possible to use several hands to operate with the endoscope.

The *requirements* for endoscopic abdominal surgery can be summarized as follows:

- Diagnostic pelviscopies and tubal sterilizations may be performed by a gynecologist who is still in residency training. To perform intra-abdominal operative procedures, the surgeon must have had excellent gynecologic specialty training in operative gynecology or surgery. After extensive practice on the Pelvi-Trainer (see chapter 22) and with the experience of several hundred diagnostic pelviscopies, the surgeon must feel just as comfortable in the monocular evaluation of the internal genitalia as he does during a laparotomy with the familiar binocular, or stereoscopic, view.
- There should be a good probability that the patient's anatomical findings are suited for pelviscopic intervention.

FIG 23.
The articulated optical attachment ("spy").

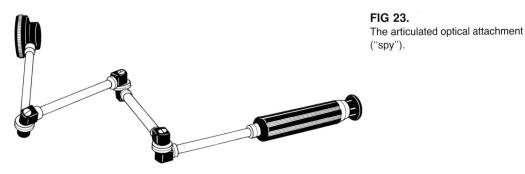

The patient should be completely prepared for a laparotomy, including positioning and anesthesia, so that the endoscopic surgeon, if necessary, can immediately proceed to a classic laparotomy. If the surgeon is a resident in training, a fully trained gynecologic surgeon must be available to assist him. [This statement bears reemphasis. It is very unfair to the patient if a surgeon with inadequate training in operative endoscopic procedures performs a diagnostic pelviscopy, finds pathologic conditions amenable to endoscopic intervention, but, lacking the skills or instruments, or the assistance and supervision of an experienced endoscopic surgeon, is forced to abandon the procedure or to subject the patient to a laparotomy.—*Ed.*]

7 _____ The Operating Team for Endoscopic Abdominal Surgery

As briefly touched on in chapter 6, the endoscopic surgeon, as opposed to the endoscopic diagnostician, always works with a surgical assistant. While a pneumoperitoneum is being established, they may save time by dividing their duties. The assistant may prepare the vagina with an antiseptic, introduce the vacuum intrauterine manipulator for mobilization of the uterus during the procedure (for sterility operations and the like), attach the dye reservoir for chromopertubation, and prepare the necessary pertubation equipment (see chapter 14.2.4. ff.).

The endoscopic surgeon communicates with the anesthesiologist to adjust the degree of relaxation of the abdominal wall, to the planned operative manipulation.

The scrub nurse must be trained in endoscopic operations and familiar with the terminology and the preparation of the instruments.

Additionally, a circulating nurse is needed, as with any laparotomy. The circulating nurse will adjust and operate the insufflation apparatus, endocoagulator, or high-frequency generator and will also operate the Aquapurator (see chapter 12.4.1.) or other irrigation and aspiration equipment. She will exchange suction bottles and containers with irrigation fluid at a moment when the surgeon is not using the irrigation and suction cannula, so that the Aquapurator or comparable equipment is always available for emergency situations.

The operative team must be skilled and cooperative. The success of an endoscopic operation largely depends on this integrated teamwork. The "monocular surgeon" needs optimum assistance—a fundamental difference from "diagnostic laparoscopy"!

[Close collaboration and enthusiasm of every member of the operative team, as well as the patient, are absolute requirements for the success of the operation if it is performed partially or totally under local anesthesia (see chapter 10.1.1.) or "volonelgesia" (see chapter 10.1.2.).—Ed.]

8 _____ Indications for Endoscopic Abdominal Surgery

In some cases, the possibility of performing essential gynecologic and general surgical procedures with the endoscope combines specifically gynecologic operations with procedures of general abdominal surgery. An attempt is made first to establish strict indications to reduce the number of laparotomies. With this conservative attitude, pathologic conditions may occasionally be overlooked or may not be diagnosed at an early stage. Since an endoscopic procedure constitutes only a minor physical insult to the patient, we are more inclined to expand the indication for inspection of the peritoneal cavity to conditions with a lower index of suspicion. Today, the endoscopic diagnostic exploration allows us to make a specific diagnosis and, in certain cases (see catalog of operations later in this chapter), to proceed immediately with its therapeutic correction. This option, conversely, has a substantial influence on the indications for surgery.

We are just entering the era of endoscopic abdominal surgery, and the catalog of indications presented below will certainly stimulate further discussion and possibly revision. The following aspects have been considered.

8.1. CATALOG OF INDICATIONS FOR ENDOSCOPIC ABDOMINAL SURGERY BASED ON DIAGNOSTIC PELVISCOPY

The first group of indications for a surgical exploration in gynecology consists of diagnostic questions:

1. Differential diagnosis: Normal or pathologic female genitalia?
2. Primary sterility.*
3. Secondary sterility or infertility.*
4. Previously diagnosed (e.g., by insufflation, hysterosalpingography, etc.) tubal factor in sterility.*
5. Follow-up after previous operation to correct sterility.*
6. Acute lower abdominal complaints during early pregnancy.
7. Suspicion of endometriosis.*
8. Second-look pelviscopy after hormonal treatment of endometriosis.*
9. Second-look pelviscopy after operative and/or cytostatic treatment of ovarian carcinoma, etc.
10. Therapy-resistant bladder irritability (e.g., endometriosis of the dome of the bladder?).*
11. Chronic lower abdominal complaints (e.g., with endometriosis or chronic appendicitis).*
12. Suspicion of pelvic varicosities or congestion.
13. Suspicion of chronic pelvic inflammatory disease (PID).*
14. Acute or subacute lower abdominal dis-

*Denotes indications which, if pathologic conditions are confirmed, may be corrected endoscopically subsequent to the diagnostic procedure and under the same anesthesia, provided that the patient has been properly prepared (see chapters 3 and 5).

eases: Differential diagnosis: PID vs. appendicitis.*

15. Differential diagnosis: Intrauterine or extrauterine pregnancy?*
16. Chronic pelvic neuralgia, spastic pelveopathy?
17. Bleeding corpus luteum?*
18. Differential diagnosis between ovarian or adnexal conglomerate tumors or myomas.*
19. Differential diagnosis: Double uterus or ovarian tumor.
20. Postmenopausal bleeding (e.g., granulosa cell tumor).
21. Pathologic amenorrhea.
22. Differential diagnosis: PID or parametritis and appendicitis, particularly in the postpartum period.*
23. Substitute for exploratory laparotomy for primary or second-look operation for ovarian carcinoma.
24. Suspicion of genital anomalies.
25. Vaginal aplasia with or without internal anomalies.
26. Uterine hypoplasia.
27. Search for and retrieval of a "lost IUD."*
28. Therapy-resistant abdominal complaints.*
29. Suspicion of perforation of the uterus.*
30. Pelviscopic monitoring during or after hysteroscopic intrauterine manipulation or operation.
31. Conventional or suction curettage under endoscopic control after perforation of the uterus.*
32. Acute intra-abdominal bleeding after trauma (see chapter 8.3.)?
33. General abdominal complaints after previous gynecologic laparotomy.*
34. Preoperative diagnosis with adhesiolysis after previous tubal sterilization operation in preparation for future microsurgical reanastomosis by laparotomy.*
35. Preoperative exploration of pelvic anatomy for indicated vaginal operations (e.g., total hysterectomy), to exclude intra-abdominal conditions which may be considered contraindications (see also chapters 14.2.2.5. and 14.2.8.1.) for vaginal surgery but amenable to incidental therapy, e.g., adhesiolysis of the omentum, bowel, etc. (see chapters 15.1. and 15.2.).*

36. Diagnosis of ovarian function for in vitro fertilization.*
37. Simultaneous pelviscopic diagnosis and monitoring of the progress of an operation to construct a neovagina, e.g., with Rokitansky-Küster-Mayer-Hauser syndrome.
38. Confirmation of sonographic findings.

Specific gynecologic indications for endoscopic operative procedures that have been successfully managed by pelviscopic operative methods:

8.1.1. Indications for Endoscopic Operative Procedures on the Uterine Corpus

Due to the availability of effective methods for complete hemostasis (see chapters 12.5.6. and 12.6.), the following *transabdominal* endoscopic procedures on the *uterine corpus* are feasible:

a. Excision of pedunculated subserous myomas.
b. Enucleation of intramural subserous myomas.
c. Management of perforation wounds caused by a probe, dilator, and curette.
d. Transmural extraction of partially perforated IUDs.
e. Adhesiolysis of omentum and bowel from the uterine corpus, or of retrocervical attachments after previous operations or in cases of superficial pelvic endometriosis.

8.1.2. Indications for Endoscopic Operative Procedures on the Adnexa

Among 10,000 pelviscopies performed in Kiel from October 1970 to the end of 1983 (see Fig 361), the following *operations on the adnexa, i.e., the tube, ovary, and parovarium,* have been clinically successful and can be recommended as the method of choice:

8.1.2.1. Endoscopic Operation on the Oviduct

a. Exploration (machine-monitored) of tubal patency with ascending blue dye solution and/or CO_2 gas in cases of sterility.
b. Fimbrioplasty and/or salpingostomy for peripheral tubal occlusion.
c. Salpingolysis.
d. Correction of adnexal pathology after sterility operations or conservative opera-

tions for tubal pregnancy in conjunction with chromopertubation.

e. Coagulation of endometriotic implants.

f. Resection of pedunculated hydatid cysts of Morgagni (see also chapters 8.1.2.3. and 14.2.12.).

g. Instillation of medications into the tubes (e.g., for pyosalpinges).

h. Biopsy of tubes because of suspected genital or abdominal tuberculosis, tubal carcinoma, and so forth.

i. Conservative operation for tubal pregnancy.

j. Radical therapy of tubal pregnancy (partial salpingectomy).

k. Salpingectomy (usually in conjunction with oophorectomy [salpingo-oophorectomy]).

l. Salpingectomy for hydrosalpinx.

m. Interval tubal sterilization by coagulation and transection.

n. Tubal sterilization by coagulation and transection in the postpartum and post-abortal patient.

o. Tubal sterilization by ligation.

p. Tubal sterilization by ring or plastic clip application.

q. Reversal after tubal sterilization by end-to-end reanastomosis.

8.1.2.2. Endoscopic Operations on the Ovaries

The following pelviscopic procedures have been very successful and have completely replaced the indications for a laparotomy:

a. Follicle puncture (e.g., for aspiration of mature oocytes for in vitro fertilization).

b. Gonadal biopsy with uterine aplasia for sex determination.

c. Gonadal biopsy for diagnosis of ovarian function.

d. Gonadal biopsy for suspicion of ovarian carcinoma.

e. Puncture of ovarian cysts with resection of the cyst wall in pediatric patients.

f. Puncture of ovarian cysts with subsequent excision of the ovarian cyst or oophorectomy.

g. Puncture and enucleation of chocolate cysts.

h. Puncture and enucleation of dermoids.

i. Ovariolysis in conjunction with sterility operations and in the presence of abdomi-

nal adhesions after gynecologic operations in preparations of follicle puncture for subsequent in vitro fertilization.

j. Cyst puncture and aspiration of ascitic fluid after hyperstimulation from hMG/hCG therapy.

k. Oophorectomy or salpingo-oophorectomy in combination with partial tubal resection.

l. Partial ovarian resection for Stein-Leventhal syndrome.

8.1.2.3. Endoscopic Operations on the Mesovarium/Mesosalpinx

Tumors in the area of the *mesovarium/Mesosalpinx* are easily accessible to pelviscopic operations. Usually they are easily resected and hemostasis is never a problem.

a. Resection of pedunculated hydatid cysts of Morgagni.

b. Enucleation of paraovarian cysts.

c. Enucleation of larger sessile hydatid cysts of Morgagni.

d. Coagulation of endometriotic implants.

e. Peritoneal closure by suture in the area of the mesosalpinx after extensive ovariolysis.

8.1.2.4. Endoscopic Operations on Other Structures in the Pelvis

Controlling the risk of hemorrhage opened up a wide spectrum for operative intervention for *pathologic conditions in the true pelvis of women:*

a. Biopsy and coagulation of endometriotic implants in the cul-de-sac and dome of the bladder.

b. Omental and intestinal adhesiolysis with partial resection of the omentum in the true pelvis.

c. Closure of gaping peritoneal wounds by suture after extensive ovarian, tubal, omental, and intestinal adhesiolysis.

d. General prophylaxis of adhesions after extensive endoscopic operative procedures by instillation of medications into the abdominal cavity (e.g., cortisone or Dextran for prophylaxis of adhesions or antibiotics for prophylaxis of inflammation).

e. Enucleation of subperitoneal myomas.

f. Peritoneal biopsy for suspicion of metastatic processes or after operative and/or cytostatic therapy for carcinoma.

g. Correction of chronic, usually postoperative peritoneal adhesions (nongynecologic).
h. Postoperative correction of chronic peritoneal adhesions (gynecologic).
i. Endoscopic suture of the intestinal wall after injury during *b* (see above).

8.1.3. Indications for Endoscopic Surgery for Correction of Sterility

From the gynecologist's view, there is a new catalog of indications related to tubal factors of sterility. Although pelviscopy has been predominantly and almost exclusively a method for the diagnosis of tubal sterility, used to evaluate the chances of the correction of tubal defects by a laparotomy at a later date, important progress has been made with the introduction of operative endoscopy. Ampullary defects can be corrected, with a success rate of 80%, with a combination of low-power magnification with the loupe (see chapter 12.2.4.) and blunt fimbriolysis (see chapter 14.2.4.2.), or by endoscopic salpingostomy (see chapter 14.2.4.3.).

Today, every laparotomy, including those performed under microsurgical conditions for the correction of tubal factor sterility, should, as a rule, be preceded by operative endoscopy. During operative pelviscopy the following procedures can be performed in an almost perfect manner:

General adhesiolysis; salpingolysis and ovariolysis; fimbrioplasty (e.g., blunt dilatation) and salpingostomy, both with eversion of the ampullary funnel and fixation by suture; and clip and ring removal after previous sterilization.

In the case of end-to-end reanastomosis—if this cannot be accomplished endoscopically—or implantation after a waiting period of 3–4 months from the endoscopic procedure, a laparotomy will be necessary only for the microsurgical correction of the tubal factor. Extensive peritoneal adhesions, which have a very detrimental effect during the postoperative healing phase after every microsurgical procedure on the tubal ampulla, are usually absent. This greatly raises the success rate of the microsurgical effort in operations to reestablish fertility.

Today, particularly in the presence of endometriosis, one should rely primarily on pelviscopic operative measures, at least until the endometriosis has been controlled partially by surgery (coagulation) and partially by endocrinologic measures (antigonadotropin or progestogen treatment). If a microsurgical operation is performed in the presence of adenomyosis or superficial pelvic endometriosis, postoperative adhesions, which diminish the chances of success of the operation, are unavoidable. In the United States, West presented statistical data showing that end-to-end anastomosis or tubal reimplantation for tubal obstruction due to intramural endometriosis yielded no pregnancy in a group of 33 cases.

After previous sterilization operations by electrocoagulation, ligation (Madlener, Pomeroy, and others), or clip application, it is also advisable to first perform an operative pelviscopy for:

1. The evaluation of the pelvic anatomy after previous operations
2. The removal of ligature material and clips
3. Extensive salpingolysis and ovariolysis and
4. Evaluation of the chances of success of a laparotomy with a tubal reversal operation

The microsurgical procedure for end-to-end reanastomosis, which is scheduled 2–3 months later, can then concentrate exclusively on the correction of the tubal defect.

The combination of operative pelviscopy with a microsurgical procedure performed at a later date has been very successful in this field.

8.1.4. Indications for Endoscopic Abdominal Surgery in the Adolescent and Infant

With the trend of changes in general gynecology, one field of special interest is dedicated to the adolescent and the infant (adolescent and pediatric gynecology). From the first few days of the infant's life onward, new fields and indications in both diagnosis and therapy have been opened to the activity of the endoscopic surgeon. These methods have been particularly beneficial to young patients. Until recently, the usual technique of exploratory laparotomy was a physically very distressing intervention that burdened the child for life with cosmetically distorting scars. On the other hand, because of these secondary effects, the decision to operate was often delayed, i.e., not made at the appropriate age and, therefore, caused irreparable, late sequelae.

Since the pneumoperitoneum can be monitored electronically at every pressure and volume level (see chapter 12.3.2.), and since the procedures and instruments have been miniaturized (see chapter 12.8.), almost all diagnostic and therapeutic procedures in combination with operative measures can be performed in the infant. It is particularly appreciated in this subspecialty, that the indications have been expanded to include salpingo-oophorectomy (see chapter 14.2.8.), such as for ovarian dysgenesis; they are now quite comparable to the catalog of indication for adults, given above.

8.2. ENDOSCOPIC ABDOMINAL OPERATIVE POSSIBILITIES APPLICABLE TO GENERAL SURGERY

For the first time, endoscopic operative techniques and operative experiences that were developed in the field of operative gynecology can also be applied to general surgery. Formerly the laparotomy was the only technique to gain access to the internal organs when they required surgical treatment. Although the present spectrum of indications is not yet extensive, the option for endoscopic operations in the abdominal cavity is an important and welcome addition to abdominal surgery, particularly in an area where chronic postoperative abdominal complaints (i.e., symptoms due to adhesions) may otherwise require a repeat laparotomy. The success of a repeat laparotomy, however, is very questionable because of the risk of recurrent adhesions, which have already been the indication for the present repeat operation. In such cases, endoscopic diagnosis with subsequent adhesiolysis (see chapters 14.2.2.1. and 15.1. ff.) and the possibility of endoscopic suture of the intestinal wall have brought about a dramatic change in classic surgical instruction. After endoscopic adhesiolysis in the abdominal cavity, particularly after transection of adhesive bands, most patients remain asymptomatic.

The newly developed possibilities of intra-abdominal endoscopic sutures, with either external or internal tying of knots (see chapters 12.6.1.–12.6.3.), allows the surgeon for the first time to add the classic technique for *appendectomy* with purse string and Z-sutures to the routine procedures of endoscopic operative techniques. For the microscopic surgeon, endoscopic suturing and tying presents no major difficulty. Since the endoscopic appendectomy is carried out under practically microsurgical conditions (see chapter 15.3. ff.), it allows, depending on the indication for surgery, primary healing of the operative field without post-

operative intestinal adhesions, which are unavoidable in up to 70% of classic appendectomies performed through a laparotomy.

Furthermore, there is the question of how to proceed in the future when suspected appendicitis is diagnosed. At present, such a diagnosis is an indication for a laparotomy. Even though the suspicion is not confirmed, the healthy organ, the appendix, is removed. For the time being, it remains an open question whether or not this practice can be continued, either endoscopically or in a classic manner, if the preoperative suspicion of appendicitis cannot be confirmed by endoscopic inspection. In other words, the direct question is, if the diagnosis of appendicitis is not confirmed, can we still justify the removal of a healthy organ? This new constellation will probably stimulate heated discussion as soon as general surgeons begin to use the endoscope first, if they suspect appendicitis, and cease doing a primary laparotomy, their usual practice.

Indications for the endoscopic removal of an appendix with endoscopically diagnosed changes presently include:

- therapeutic appendectomy for:
- sterility patients whose appendix is adherent to the adnexa after a previous laparotomy,
- "long" appendix extending into the true pelvis,
- appendix with extragenital endometriosis,
- appendix with a "familial disposition" (strong family history of appendectomies),
- chronic complaints in the right adnexal area without pelviscopic evidence of pathologic anatomical changes,
- subacute and/or chronic appendicitis with perityphlic adhesions, either considered as a differential diagnosis . . .
- or incidentally diagnosed during pelviscopy or laparoscopy for other indications.

An acute, highly inflamed appendix, perforation of the appendix, and so forth will certainly be discovered earlier by laparoscopy. Although in an acute state such conditions cannot be managed through the endoscope, an earlier diagnosis establishes the indication for a more timely intervention by laparotomy. This should significantly reduce the mortality rate, which is still quite high after perforation of the appendix (i.e., laparotomy delayed).

In summary, in the field of general abdominal surgery, the following catalog of indications may presently be considered for primary endoscopic intervention.

8.2.1. Catalog of Indications for Endoscopic Abdominal Surgery

a. Vague abdominal complaints, particularly after previous laparotomies
b. Omental and intestinal adhesions
c. Postoperative complaints due to adhesions after cholecystectomy
d. Symptoms compatible with partial intestinal obstruction
e. Suspicion of appendicitis
f. Postoperative suspicion of insufficiency of sutures or postoperative bleeding
g. Second look after surgery
h. Second look for postoperative metastases
i. Second look to monitor the success of cytostatic treatment after surgery for intestinal carcinoma
j. Preoperative endoscopic evaluation to determine the probability of success of a major operation (to avoid an exploratory laparotomy), and other indications

8.3. EMERGENCY PELVISCOPY IN GYNECOLOGY AND GENERAL SURGERY

In gynecology (e.g., suspicion of uterine perforation or tubal rupture) as well as in general surgery (e.g., after an automobile accident), there are questions of differential diagnosis which can be decided by the immediate inspection of internal organs. If such questions arise, one would be more inclined to consider an endoscopic diagnostic procedure, which has only a minor physical effect on the patient, rather than an exploratory laparotomy.

Since the diagnosis is made at an early stage, the endoscopic correction of the condition will frequently still be possible [e.g., an ectopic pregnancy (see chapter 14.2.11. ff.) or subacute appendicitis (see chapter 15.3. ff.)]. With the exception of the purely gynecologic indications, some of which have already been mentioned above (e.g., profuse bleeding from a ruptured follicle), other *indications apply to both men and women:*

a. Exclusion of hemorrhage after blunt abdominal trauma, e.g., automobile accident. However, as a rule, the diagnostic procedure should be considered as long as there is only a suspicion that has not yet been confirmed. Under no circumstances should valuable time be lost for the sake of an endoscopic inspection. In case of doubt, the exploratory laparotomy is principally preferred.
b. Suspicion of postoperative bleeding. In such a case, pooled blood can be aspirated and then the bleeding vessel in the area of the omentum or peritoneal surfaces can often be detected more easily with the endoscope than by a repeat laparotomy. Complete hemostasis is quickly accomplished with Roeder's endoloop, endoligature, or endosuture (see chapters 12.6.1.–12.6.3.).

Here again, a clear decision must be made rapidly as to whether or not the postoperative bleeding constitutes an acute threat to the patient's life. If not, an attempt of endoscopic management is indicated. In the presence of impending or acute shock, a laparotomy is preferred.

In an institution with an active endoscopic service, postoperative bleeding can be diagnosed at a much earlier phase, before excessive hemorrhage would cause fibrinogenemia and possibly death. In case of doubt, when postoperative bleeding is suspected, a laparoscopic exploration should be considered early, so that the appropriate corrective surgical measures can be taken.

A postoperative endoscopic intra-abdominal exploration for suspected bleeding does not constitute any substantial risk to the patient. The more typical wait-and-see attitude of the surgeon, until the signs of hemorrhage are so severe that the repeat laparotomy becomes mandatory, occasionally progresses beyond acceptable limits.

The rapid exploration of suspicious intra-abdominal signs is beneficial for both patient and physician. Whereas the temporizing attitude of classic surgery extended over hours, days, or weeks, and sometimes required prolonged hospitalization of the patient, early endoscopic exploration and correction will help to reduce the hospitalization time to a minimum and accelerate the patient's recovery time.

In summary, it should be emphasized that the expansion of the list of indications for the endoscopic inspection of the abdomen has brought about real changes in conservative and operative surgery. These changes are most impressive in comparative statistics of occupancy rates, hospitalization times, and the average duration of patient's confinement to bed before and after the introduction of endoscopic abdominal surgery.

In 1981, a total of 63,020 patient days were registered in the Departments of Gynecology, Obstetrics, and Oncology of the University Women's Hospital in Kiel. This calculates to an average hospital stay of 8.21 days of bed occupancy per patient, which is far below the average in the Federal Republic of Germany.

[For comparison, the statistical data for the year 1985 at Barnes Hospital, Washington University, St. Louis, Missouri, are:

	Patient Days	Length of Stay
Obstetrics	14,757	4.2
Gynecology/Oncology	13,076	5.79

These data do not include more than 1,400 ambulatory operations for which the patients were not admitted overnight.—*Ed.*]

9   Contraindications to Endoscopic Abdominal Surgery

There are *absolute* and *relative* contraindications to endoscopic abdominal surgery.

9.1. ABSOLUTE CONTRAINDICATIONS TO ENDOSCOPIC ABDOMINAL SURGERY

An absolute contraindication to endoscopic abdominal surgery is *any condition in which the patient cannot tolerate anesthesia*. If the anesthesiologist determines that the patient would not tolerate anesthesia, then the sum of all individual data on which his judgment was based will also be a contraindication to endoscopic abdominal surgery.

Furthermore, *severe bleeding disorders* are absolute contraindications if other procedures by laparotomy are also contraindicated.

Another contraindication, at the present time, is *acute peritonitis of the upper abdomen* with severe distention, because it would not permit the safe establishment of a pneumoperitoneum.

Regarding the absolute anesthesia intolerance, one must distinguish between endotracheal intubation anesthesia and conduction anesthesia, for example peridural anesthesia, as will be discussed further in chapter 10.

9.2. RELATIVE CONTRAINDICATIONS TO ENDOSCOPIC ABDOMINAL SURGERY

In the case of *tumors larger than fist size,* endoscopic abdominal surgery is usually not indicated. Exceptions are borderline cases in which the patient, for a variety of personal reasons, cannot undergo a major operation or, for medical indications, should not be operated on. In such cases it may be possible to determine by laparoscopy whether postponement of the definitive operation for vital or personal reasons is medically justifiable, or whether such postponement would be a greater risk to the patient's life than an operation at the present time.

The limitation to fist size does not necessarily apply to *ovarian tumors* which, in cases such as simple ovarian cysts, can often be easily aspirated, and then the remaining cyst sac can be ligated (see chapter 14.2.7.), excised, and removed through the 11-mm trocar sleeve.

Nor does the limitation to fist size apply to an *ovarian carcinoma,* even one exceeding 10–15 cm in diameter. In such a case, pelviscopy/laparoscopy could substitute for primary exploratory laparotomy, which imposes a much greater stress on the patient. With the endoscope, the diagnosis can be established and it can be determined if a debulking laparotomy would be possible in the same sitting, or whether at least sufficient biopsy material can be obtained to establish a histologic diagnosis. After appropriate cytostatic therapy, a second-look pelviscopy or, if necessary, a laparotomy should be considered. The primary exploratory laparotomy, which was required in the past, is avoided in such cases. This spares the patient considerable distress because the former second major operation, the second-look operation, will then become the first major surgical abdominal procedure that causes physical stress to the patient.

A *hiatal hernia* is only a relative contraindication, provided that the Trendelenburg position is limited to 15°, the intra-abdominal pressure is limited to a maximum of 10 mm Hg, and the operation is performed under endotracheal anesthesia. It is recommended that the abdomen be insufflated only to pressures of 8–10 mm Hg, which can be accomplished and monitored electronically with the OP-PNEU automatic apparatus (see chapter 12.3. ff.).

Contrary to past teaching, acute pelvic peritonitis in women is no longer considered an absolute contraindication to an endoscopic abdominal operation. Small bowels that are covered with a fibrinous exudate and obstruct the true pelvis can be easily pushed aside. Then pus can be aspirated and the pelvis irrigated with copious amounts of fluid. Culture and sensitivity tests of the pus are ordered. After pelvic irrigation and possibly puncture and aspiration of pyosalpinges, a highly active antibiotic that is well tolerated by peritoneal surfaces (e.g., Reverin™) is instilled into the pelvis. Postoperatively the patient is treated with appropriate antibiotics (including those for anaerobes, and possibly antifungal agents). After the results of the sensitivity tests become available, necessary changes in the antibiotic regimen will have to be made. The early utilization of endoscopic methods results in a much more favorable course of adnexitis and peritonitis, a drastic reduction in the hospitalization time, and shorter recovery time.

This more aggressive operative approach in pelvic peritonitis, which had not been recommended in the past but is generally accepted today, has yielded particularly favorable results in the preservation of fertility.

It is remarkable that the conditions formerly considered primary risks for medical laparoscopy, i.e., respiratory and cardiac insufficiency, coronary heart disease, impending hepatic decompensation, severe portal venous collapse, external hernias, and goiter, as described by Rettenmaier (1969), have hardly any clinical significance in surgical laparoscopy. This difference in risk factors is another reason why endoscopic abdominal surgery should be separated by distinct terminology from laparoscopy of the upper abdomen.

In my first atlas I still postulated that it would be a disservice to pelviscopy if its application were stretched too far, that is, if it were utilized instead of exploratory laparotomy or even surgical laparotomy. This admonition can no longer be substantiated today. *Particularly* in those cases, endoscopic abdominal surgery, with the simultaneous preparedness for a laparotomy, can, indeed, replace a great number of laparotomies. What used to be considered an overextension of the method (due to lack of hemostatic facilities) today constitutes a special catalog of indications for endoscopic abdominal surgery.

10 _____ Anesthesia for Endoscopic Abdominal Surgery

There is no single method of inducing anesthesia that is applicable to all patients. Therefore, the options that will be discussed by both the author and editor are:

1. Methods of inducing anesthesia that may be administered by surgeons: *local anesthesia* and *volonelgesia* (Friedrich et al., 1978), and
2. Methods that require an anesthesiologist or anesthetist for administration: *regional anesthesia* (i.e., caudal, epidural, and spinal anesthesia), as well as *general inhalation anesthesia* (i.e., the anesthetic is delivered by mask or endotracheal intubation).

Two or more individuals are directly affected by the type of anesthesia administered, the patient and the surgeon, and possibly the anesthesiologist, internist, psychiatrist, and others. Assuming that all these individuals are reasonable, they will agree preoperatively on a method that is acceptable, although not always optimal in every respect. It would be extremely rare for a patient to have contraindications to every type of analgesia and/or anesthesia. In the vast majority of cases, it is a matter of choice.

All patients have fears, and so do some surgeons. Most patients are fearful of pain and "do not want to feel, see, hear, or remember anything"—ideal working conditions for the surgeons and anesthesiologist, in most operations. Other patients are fearful of general anesthesia and the loss of consciousness; they "want to know what's going on" or "be in control of things," which may frighten some surgeons. Since our surgical infancy, we have been trained to "be in control, no questions asked, until all is done." Having patients "looking over our shoulders" through a flexible teaching attachment attached to the endoscope and expecting to be taken on a "guided tour" of the peritoneal and pelvic cavity is a new experience that at least the older ones of us have not been trained to cope with. But we can learn to cope, cooperate, and communicate, provided that we want to. Haven't we accepted conscious patients under regional anesthesia for cesarean sections who are holding their husbands' hands? Twenty-five-plus years ago we were not trained for such routines, either.

Since the editor perceives the need for more practical information on the subject of local anesthesia, this chapter will be expanded beyond the mere translation of the German text.

10.1. ANESTHESIA FOR ENDOSCOPIC ABDOMINAL SURGERY THAT MAY BE ADMINISTERED BY THE SURGEON

Notwithstanding the great advantages of good general anesthesia for endoscopic intra-abdominal operations, there is a substantial number of both di-

agnostic and operative endoscopic operations that
could or should be performed under local analgesia
or, preferably, "volonelgesia." These methods
may be selected for a number of reasons:

1. The patient may prefer one of these methods, accepting the fact that she may possibly experience some discomfort or pain during brief
phases of the operation, perhaps comparable to un-
pleasant experiences in the past, such as the den-
tist's drilling, menstrual cramps, or even labor
"pain."

2. Contraindications to other forms of anesthesia may leave local methods as the only option.

3. The surgeon may prefer local methods because he is skilled and comfortable in using them,
he knows that the procedure will, most likely, be
very short (e.g., tubal sterilization) and that a local
method is safer than general anesthesia and major
regional block anesthesia.

4. The operation may be scheduled to identify
the source of the patient's lower abdominal or pelvic pain. Since the surgeon cannot feel, see, hear,
or measure pain without communication with the
patient, local anesthetic methods are recommended, at least for the initial, diagnostic phase of
the endoscopic intra-abdominal procedure. General
anesthesia may then be administered during the
therapeutic, operative phase.

5. The anesthesiologist will rarely be the one
recommending local methods of analgesia, but
may resent being relegated to "standby" status
only. Comforting patients vocally is rarely considered an essential part of the training program in
anesthesiology.

6. The unavailability of an anesthesiologist/
anesthetist, mainly in developing countries, or due
to logistic and/or physical circumstances (e.g., office surgery, outpatient facilities, very active surgical service, etc.) may be the main reason for
scheduling certain types of endoscopic operations
(e.g., tubal sterilizations) without the benefit of
general anesthesia coverage. Under those circumstances, all aspects discussed under "volonelgesia" (see section 10.1.2.) become very essential.

10.1.1. Local Anesthesia

Many surgeons assume that operative manipulation
of the peritoneum is always painful so that local

anesthesia is indicated only for very specific operations, such as tubal sterilization. If additional procedures are indicated, they are not possible. If, for
instance, the patient is also suffering from superficial pelvic endometriosis that remains untreated at
the time of sterilization, coitus may continue to be
painful postoperatively. This is one reason why local anesthesia generally has no advantages in operative abdominal surgery.

10.1.2. "Volonelgesia"

The concept is an old one: Who can administer and
work under local anesthesia without much vocal
communication? The term "volonelgesia" (Friedrich et al., 1978) includes all essential phases of
this method of anesthesia:

> VOcal: communication before, during, and
>   after surgery
> LOcal: anesthesia (e.g., lidocaine 0.5%)
> VOLO: (*lat.*) I wish, want, prefer, am will-
>   ing
> NEuroLeptanalGESIA: diazepam, meperi-
>   dine, etc.

In the editor's outpatient facility, volonelgesia
has been used in over 3,500 endoscopic intra-abdominal procedures, primarily tubal sterilizations
by cauterization, Falope ring application, or Hulka
clip application, but more than 25% of them in
combination with, or for the purpose of, other endoscopic operations. Although most procedures
were completed within 5–20 minutes, several required over 2 hours' operating time for extensive
adhesiolysis, cyst resections, etc.

Vocal communication is essential in every
phase. Before the patient is scheduled for surgery,
she is shown a 15-minute film which explains to
her the pelvic anatomy, reproductive function, and
interruption of this function by various tubal sterilization methods. Some instruments are shown
and alternatives to the operation and possible complications are discussed, as are the consent forms
to be signed by the patient before surgery. Then
actual operating room scenes are shown, including
an endoscopic "guided tour" of the pelvic anatomy during the operation, as well as the patient's
postoperative condition. If the patient requests further information, it is usually given by the nurses
or counselors, rarely requiring any of the surgeon's
time. Any anxieties are usually dispelled when
these patients talk to our head nurse, the "star"
patient in the film they have just seen. Her enthu-

siasm, based on practical experience and satisfaction, is contagious. Her motto is: "If I can do it, you can do it!" It sows the seed for the "volo" aspect of volonelgesia. If patients accept it and prefer it, enthusiastic, cooperative nurses and surgeons will have the patient as a cooperative member of the team during the actual surgery.

During the operation, the patient's physical and psychological needs have to be met. The patient must be positioned on the table as comfortably as the surgical requirements permit. Warm antiseptic solutions are used for preparation of the patient's abdomen, perineum, and vagina. The patient's face is not screened off, so that she is not afraid to look around and see and converse with the nurses and the surgeon. She is also given the opportunity to use a flexible teaching attachment on the endoscope for a "guided tour" through her abdominal and pelvic cavity, if she so desires. If not, she will be distracted by conversations about her favorite subject, be it family, vacation, television, work, or another pleasant subject. She may hold the circulating nurse's hand for reassurance and comfort. She will be forewarned of possible "discomfort"—not pain. She will not be constantly alerted by inquiring whether or not anything hurts, unless it is for the purpose of identifying specific painful anatomical structures, if pain of unknown etiology was the indication for the endoscopic exploration. During and after the operation, the patient is congratulated on her excellent cooperation and tolerance. Then two nurses escort her on a short walk down the hallway to the recovery room, where she may rest in a reclining chair, is given light refreshments, and reads or converses with other postoperative patients or, sometimes, with visiting relatives. Thirty minutes to several hours later, most patients are alert and eager to go home escorted by a relative or friend.

Local anesthesia is safe and very effective if the tissues are well infiltrated with 10–20 ml of a 0.5% solution of lidocaine (Xylocaine) or similar analgesic. Higher concentrations are not necessary for local blocks but are preferable for nerve trunk blocks, i.e., pudendal and paracervical blocks. The local anesthetic is rapidly injected with a 21-gauge needle, about 4 cm (1.5 in.) long, on a 10-ml syringe. A small wheel is set below the umbilicus and the periumbilical subcutaneous tissues are injected in a radial fashion, some six to eight tracks. If the needle is advanced constantly during the injection, precautionary aspiration is not necessary. After the subcutaneous tissues have been infil-

trated, the needle is turned about 90° for the injection of the abdominal wall down to the peritoneum in a pyramidal pattern, all from the same original puncture site. If more than 10 ml is needed, the needle is left in the abdominal wall and only the syringe is refilled. Additional puncture sites, if needed, are infiltrated in the same fashion. In very obese patients, the deepest layers may be infiltrated during the introduction of the Veress needle.

If desired, a paracervical block may be given before the vacuum uterine manipulator-cannula is inserted. However, it will rarely be necessary because the discomfort caused by the introduction of this instrument rarely lasts more than a few moments.

Some surgeons prefer to inject a local anesthetic solution through the uterine manipulator into the fallopian tubes. Others spray or instill a topical anesthetic onto the surface of the tubes or other pelvic organs, or they inject these structures with local anesthetic solutions. We prefer to cover Hulka clips or grasping forceps with a 3% lidocaine jelly, which is spread onto the tubes before they are manipulated and the clips or rings are applied. Since one rarely waits long for the local anesthetic to become effective, its beneficial effect, if any, may consist of some analgesia during the first hour postoperatively.

Neuroleptanalgesia is essential to relieve anxiety and for generalized analgesic/sedative effect. For safety reasons, we prefer to start intravenous (IV) fluids in a large vein, usually forearm or antecubital vein, infusing 5% Dextrose in lactated Ringer's solution at a rapid rate, while very slowly injecting diazepam (Valium) at a rate of less than 5 mg/min. This technique prevents the pain and phlebitis which would result from rapid injection of this hyperosmotic solution. After the first 30–60 seconds, the patient usually indicates that it "gets to her head" or reports dizziness, double vision, or a sensation as if the ceiling or the lights were moving. Sometimes a total preoperative dose of 2.5 mg is required, usually about 5 mg, rarely more.

After the desired diazepam effect has been achieved, meperidine (Demerol) is injected IV in doses of 25–50 mg. If necessary during the operation, these doses may be doubled; however, since we do not have an anesthesiologist standing by in our outpatient facility, we do not exceed—not even during very long procedures—the maximum dosages of 10 mg for diazepam and 100 mg for meperidine.

If we anticipate that the endoscopic intra-abdominal procedure will be long or that a laparotomy might become necessary, we schedule the procedure in the hospital operating room under local anesthesia or volonelgesia, with general anesthesia standby. It has been our experience that anesthesiologists have a tendency to use these drugs in higher dosages or to administer other narcotics, such as fentanyl, either alone or in combination with a tranquilizer (droperidol, etc.), which may have more profound effects. Closer monitoring is necessary, and sometimes the use of oxygen by mask, which by itself raises the anxiety level of some patients. The use of morphine is discouraged because of its greater tendency to cause respiratory depression, particularly at high altitudes, as we have observed in La Paz, Bolivia.

During the operation, we prefer a very slow IV infusion rate of the electrolyte solution to prolong the drug effects and reduce the need for catheterization of the bladder. A very rapid postoperative infusion rate will increase the metabolism and wash out the medications so that the patient's recovery will be accelerated. Other factors contributing to the patient's rapid recovery are early physical activity (ambulation) and mental stimulation, so we encourage conversation, reading, watching television, and the like. Surgeons who operate in private offices or under camp situations in developing countries and do not utilize IV infusions during and after the surgical procedure but have the patient's family assist in postoperative care have also reported rapid recovery times.

Whenever endoscopic intra-abdominal surgery is performed under other than full-service hospital conditions, it is still mandatory to monitor the patient's vital signs, maintain emergency drugs and equipment for the management of adverse reactions and resuscitative measures, and have a prearranged agreement for the emergency transfer of patients to the nearest local hospital, if this should become necessary.

10.2. ANESTHESIA FOR ENDOSCOPIC ABDOMINAL SURGERY THAT REQUIRES AN ANESTHESIOLOGIST

Although it would be desirable always to have a trained anesthesiologist or anesthetist available, under the above-mentioned conditions and precautions, hundreds of thousands, if not millions, of tubal sterilizations and other operative endoscopic

procedures have been performed without the benefit of a person trained in anesthesia. However, more extensive operative procedures will require regional block anesthesia or general inhalation anesthesia, for which a specialist with experience in these methods is mandatory. The preferred method is general anesthesia (endotracheal intubation) because it affords maximal relaxation of the abdominal wall, well-controlled respiration, and an opportunity to progress to a laparotomy without any loss of time.

10.2.1. Regional Anesthesia

Regional anesthesia—caudal, epidural, or spinal block anesthesia—may be chosen because general inhalation anesthesia is contraindicated for medical reasons, because of the patient's fear of general anesthesia, or because it is the patient's or the surgeon's choice for other reasons. Regional blocks have a tendency to cause vasodilation and hypotension, which may be prevented or managed by generous IV infusion of electrolyte solutions and by the Trendelenburg position, which is usually required for endoscopic abdominal surgery. Because of vasodilation, the risk of intra-abdominal hemorrhage must be considered. Because of the Trendelenburg position, the patient must be monitored carefully to prevent or recognize the undesirable rise of the anesthetic level above T-10, which would require respiratory assistance.

Regional block anesthesia would allow the immediate transition from an endoscopic operation to a laparotomy.

10.2.2. General Anesthesia

The vast majority of diagnostic and operative endoscopic intra-abdominal procedures are performed under general inhalation anesthesia, preferably by intubation. For more than 20 years, at the Women's Hospital of the University of Kiel, at the request of the department of anesthesiology, *all operative pelviscopic procedures* have been performed under *general anesthesia* unless there were medical contraindications to general anesthesia. Under those circumstances, the anesthesiologist has recommended performing a certain operation (e.g., oophorectomy) under lumbar spinal anesthesia, which did not limit the surgical possibilities.

In the case of endotracheal anesthesia, a nasogastric tube should be inserted before the abdominal wall is punctured by the Veress needle. This technique prevents distention of the stomach, which could occur during the brief period of hyperventilation at the beginning of anesthesia and could otherwise be responsible for accidental puncture of the stomach, particularly in the case of gastric ptosis.

If it is necessary to raise the intra-abdominal pressure temporarily above the 12 mm Hg (1,596 Pa) level, as is sometimes the case in dissection of intestinal and omental adhesions, the anesthesiologist should be advised in advance. Such pressures cause an elevation of the diaphragm, which automatically reduces the respiratory volume. This must be compensated by assisted respiration, because it could produce acidosis in the patient's blood.

At this point, it should be reemphasized that the type and sequence of the procedure must be discussed with the anesthesiologist before the operation begins. The anesthesiologist must induce and maintain anesthesia in a manner that permits the immediate transition from an endoscopic operation to a laparotomy.

The anesthesiologist should be well acquainted with the course of anesthesia in patients in whom a CO_2 gas pneumoperitoneum must be maintained over prolonged periods of time. During long-lasting anesthesia, he must assure a sufficient tidal volume so that the absorbed volume of CO_2 gas, which varies from patient to patient, can be readily exchanged in the pulmonary alveolae. If the volume is too small, it may lead to mild acidosis if the CO_2 pneumoperitoneum is maintained for a longer period of time. An early indication is acceleration of the pulse rate. Disregarding this phenomenon may cause complications such as cardiac arrest (see also chapter 12.3.1.).

Establishing a pneumoperitoneum with N_2O gas is not recommended. During longer procedures, the unknown absorption rate may impose an unpredictable risk for the anesthesia.

11 ———————— Patient Position for Endoscopic Abdominal Surgery

Whether the patient should be positioned for a gynecologic or for a general surgical procedure depends on the intended surgery. The operating table must permit use of the Trendelenburg position, with the head end lowered to 25° (as a rule, 15° is sufficient) and lateral tilt positions to the left and right sides. Depending on the intended operation, the positions discussed in this chapter are possible.

11.1. PATIENT POSITION FOR ENDOSCOPIC ABDOMINAL SURGERY FOR GYNECOLOGIC INDICATIONS

For operative pelviscopy, the optimum position for the patient is a typical gynecologic position (Fig 24) as, for instance, required for a dilatation and curettage, with the patient's legs in knee-calf stirrups. It is important that the patient's buttocks extend beyond the edge of the table so that the vacuum intrauterine cannula can be moved freely as far posteriorly as possible to allow mobilization of the uterus as far anteriorly as possible, that is, toward the symphysis pubis (Fig 25). If the rubber padding extends beyond the buttocks, it will restrict the mobility of the uterine probe or cannula. The uterus cannot be elevated maximally to the

posterior aspect of the symphysis pubis, which will considerably restrict the surgical possibilities within the cul-de-sac (Fig 26).

During the preparation phase—abdominal, perineal, and vaginal antisepsis and introduction of the vacuum intrauterine cannula (see Fig 150 ff.)—the patient is positioned horizontally. At the beginning of gas insufflation, at the latest, the patient is brought into Trendelenburg position with her head lowered to approximately 15°. This usually allows the patient's bowels to slide automatically into the upper abdomen as the insufflation progresses (Fig 27).

11.2. PATIENT POSITION FOR GENERAL SURGICAL INDICATIONS

If endoscopic operative procedures are scheduled that do not require manipulation of the female genitalia, and in male patients, it is unnecessary to position the patient's legs in a modified lithotomy position. Occasionally the abduction and spreading of the patient's legs may be too restrictive for adhesiolysis in the middle and upper abdomen because the thighs will interfere with mobility of the instruments. In such cases, it is recommended that the gynecologic position be changed, at least tempo-

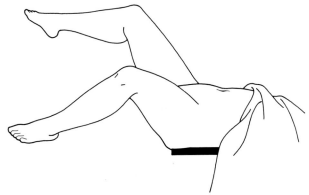

FIG 24.
The best patient position for operative pelviscopy is a typical gynecological position.

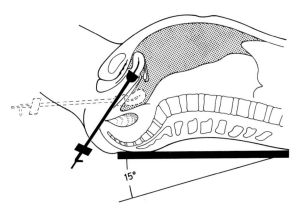

FIG 25.
Position of the patient's buttocks should allow mobilization of the uterus as far anteriorly as possible.

FIG 26.
Rubber padding that extends beyond the buttocks will restrict mobility of the uterine probe.

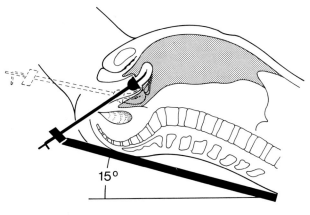

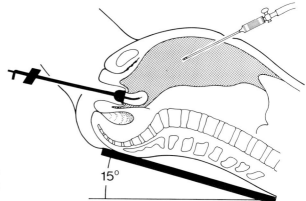

FIG 27.
A 15° Trendelenburg position allows the patient's bowels to slide into the upper abdomen during gas insufflation.

FIG 28.
A temporary change to a normal supine position may facilitate adhesiolysis.

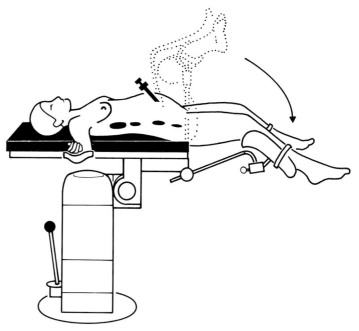

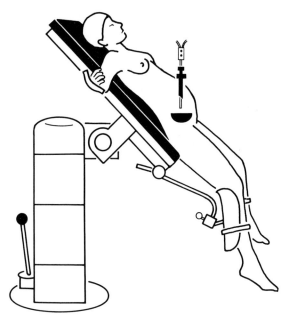

FIG 29.
Brief reversal of the patient's position allows fluid to drain from upper abdomen into small pelvis, for aspiration.

rarily, to a normal supine position with outstretched legs. The modern operating tables presently in use accommodate such changes without much effort (Fig 28).

——————

Comments on sections 11.1. and 11.2.:

If extensive irrigation of the pelvis was required during a major endoscopic operation (see chapter 12.4.1.), or if there was a large volume of blood in the abdomen (e.g., in a ruptured ectopic pregnancy), these fluids must, at the end of the procedures, be aspirated from the upper abdomen.

Since aspiration of fluid cannot be accomplished satisfactorily in the area of the diaphragm, after consultation with the anesthesiologist, the patient's Trendelenburg position will briefly be reversed by lowering the pelvis up to 45° (Fig 29). This will allow the fluids to drain from the upper abdomen into the small pelvis, from which they can easily be aspirated, possibly after the table has been returned to the horizontal position.

Positioning the patient properly will considerably facilitate endoscopic intra-abdominal operations. Always take full advantage of gravity!

12

Instruments and Equipment for Endoscopic Abdominal Surgery

Until the beginning of the 1970s, the technical development of instruments and equipment was influenced almost exclusively by the diagnostic requirements of laparoscopy. With indications for laparoscopy in gynecology expanded to include tubal sterilizations there came an increasing demand for reliable methods of achieving intra-abdominal hemostasis endoscopically. High-frequency current proved to be completely unsatisfactory for intra-abdominal coagulation (see section 12.5.1.). For this reason, we developed new hemostatic methods suitable for endoscopy (for example, endocoagulation, endoloop ligation, endoligature with external tying of slipknots, and endosuture with external and/or internal tying of knots) as well as a large number of new instruments and equipment. These new developments enable us today to perform a broad spectrum of operations in gynecologic and general surgery.

As mentioned initially, the present text focuses on instruments and pelviscopic/laparoscopic techniques, as well as on their practical application in endoscopic intra-abdominal surgery. An extensive description of the historical development, physical properties, and functions of instruments may be found in the first color atlas and textbook, *Gynecological Laparoscopy and Hysteroscopy*. Material from the earlier volume will be repeated here only if it is necessary for the understanding of operative pelviscopy.

To learn how to perform endoscopic intra-abdominal operations successfully, the reader is advised to study the first color atlas and textbook, which deals primarily with diagnostic procedures. The present atlas is specifically designed to teach operative techniques, not pelviscopy or laparoscopy in general. The present level of our knowledge can only be fully appreciated when both atlases are used in combination.

12.1. ENDOSCOPIC LIGHT SOURCE

A prerequisite for intra-abdominal endoscopic operations is the illumination of the pneumoperitoneum with clear, bright light. Since an incandescent light bulb transforms 97% of the electrical energy into heat and only 2% into visible light, presently only external light sources (Fig 30) are useful and acceptable for endoscopic purposes.

12.1.1. External Light for Diagnostic and Operative Procedures

Since 1965, modern endoscopic light sources (Fig 31) have been equipped with "cold light" (see Fig 30). The light source is mounted approximately 1.5 m (about 5 feet) from the objective lens of the endoscope. The light bulb contains an incandescent tungsten element in an iodine vapor milieu, and

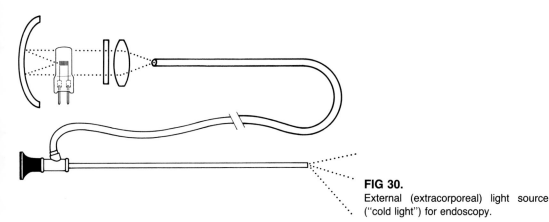

FIG 30.
External (extracorporeal) light source ("cold light") for endoscopy.

has an output of 75–250 W. Light sources with an output of less than 150 W should not be used for intra-abdominal operations because an articulated or flexible optical attachment ("spy," see Fig 23), used routinely by assistants and for teaching purposes, and loupes with magnifying powers of 2–6 X (see chapter 12.2.4.) reduce the light intensity at the eyepiece by 50% or more.

Modern light sources (Fig 32) are equipped

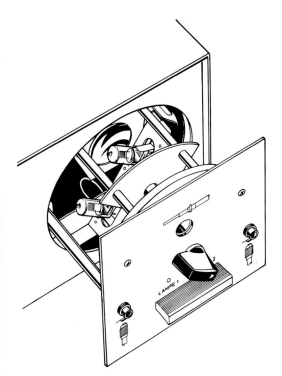

FIG 31.
Modern endoscopic light source.

with two halogen lamps to allow switching to a spare bulb if the first light fails. This precaution is absolutely necessary for operative endoscopy because the sudden loss of light (for instance, during a hemostatic procedure) could constitute an enormous risk. Therefore, it is advisable to ascertain *preoperatively* that both lamps are working properly.

12.1.2. Transmission of the Endoscopic Light

The physical phenomenon of so-called total internal reflection of a light beam in a quartz rod permits the transmission of light with almost no loss of intensity (Fig 33). If a quartz rod is extremely thin (e.g., 10–70 μm), optically isolated by an outside coating with a layer of quartz with a low index of refraction, and if many of these fibers are combined into a nonoriented, or incoherent, bundle, we have a flexible fiber optic light cable with almost no reduction in the light intensity it conducts (Fig 34). If a heat shield is inserted between the light source and the bundle of such nonoriented light-conducting fibers,* the light that exits the light cable will have a high intensity of illumination ("lux") but without its heat component. Hence the term "cold light." Utilizing extremely clear types of glass keeps loss to absorption to a minimum. This is particularly important for endos-

---

*Oriented or coherent fiberglass cables have an identical arrangement of the original glass fibers on the surfaces of both ends of the cable. Such glass fiber bundles permit the transmission of a "true image" and are utilized in medicine as flexible gastroscopes, etc. The image obtained is not homogeneous, like that transmitted through optical lenses, but is composed of many point images, comparable to the image obtained through an insect's eye (Fig 35).

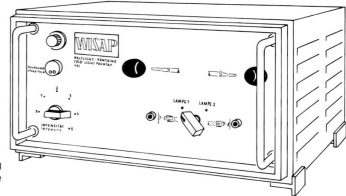

FIG 32.
Two halogen lamps allow switching to a spare bulb should the first one fail.

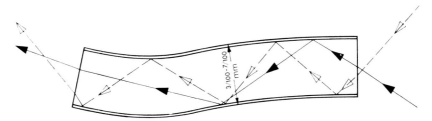

FIG 33.
Total internal reflection of a light beam in a quartz rod permits transmission of light with minimal loss of intensity.

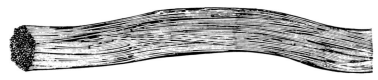

FIG 34.
A bundle of nonoriented quartz rods: a flexible fiber optic light cable.

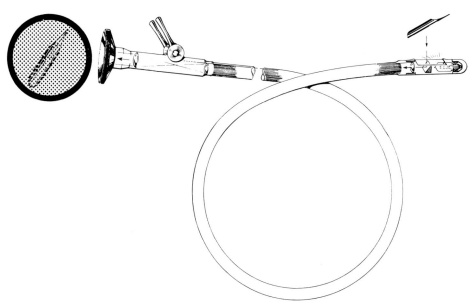

FIG 35.
The image obtained with oriented or coherent fiberglass cables, as are used in flexible gastroscopes, consists of many point images.

copy, because a color-correct reflection of the light is essential for the diagnostic evaluation of internal organs.

The quality of the light-conducting cable is based on the law of total internal reflection (see Fig 33) and depends on its light conductivity, that is, the numerical aperture of the glass, and the index of refraction of the core and the coat of the fibers. For purely technical purposes (control modules responding to light impulses), light-conducting cables are commercially available at a reasonable price. However, they are not suited for endoscopic purposes. They conduct only fractions of the light necessary for diagnosis, i.e., the light spectrum perceived by the human eye, and they favor the conduction of light in the ultraviolet or red ranges. This causes severe color distortions.

For routine endoscopy, the flexible light-transmitting cable is separate from the endoscope; the two are first joined just before the endoscope is introduced into the patient. In the connection (Fig 36) between the light-transmitting cable and the endoscope, about 50% of the light output is lost (see chapter 12.1.3.).

The quality of the light-transmitting cable should be checked before the operation is begun. If one end of the cable is held in the direction of a light source (window, operating room light, etc.)

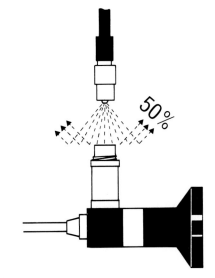

FIG 36.
Loss of light intensity in the connection of cable to endoscope.

the other end will light up. If a substantial number of glass fibers are broken, black spots will be seen (Fig 37) that resemble sun spots. If more than 15%–20% of the optical surface is black, the cable must be replaced.

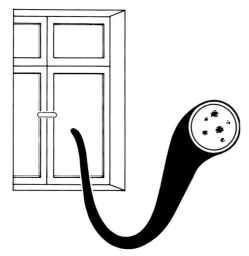

FIG 37.
Black spots indicate broken glass fibers.

12.1.3. External Light for Photographic Documentation

Although photographs of the body's cavities could be taken through endoscopes designed by Desormeaux and Stein, meaningful photo documentation began with the introduction of the electronic flash tube. The gynecologist Thomsen in 1951 was the first to take photographs in the cul-de-sac with an internal flash bulb (Fig 38).

After a period of development of three decades, a satisfactory external light source for photography became available to endoscopic surgeons in 1981. The electronic flash is emitted by a spherical flashtube (Fig 39) and transmitted to an integrated fiber light cable (Fig 40), permitting frame-filling 24 × 36-mm color slides of panoramic views of the small pelvis.

To prevent the 50% loss of light intensity that occurs in the connection between the light-transmitting cable and the endoscope, for photographic purposes it is necessary to use a special endoscope of 11 mm diameter with two integrated fiber light cables, which transmit the light and flash without interruption from the light source to the objective lens of the endoscope (see Fig 40).

It is always advisable—at least for the beginner—to use an endoscope of 11 mm diameter and with a visual angle of 30° for endoscopic abdominal surgery. This may require dilatation of the primary puncture site, made for the 7-mm endoscope routinely used, to 11 mm (see chapter 12.8.8.); however, the larger endoscopes afford a better pan-

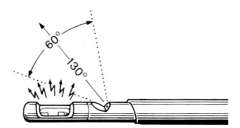

FIG 38.
Endoscope with built-in flash bulb for taking internal photographs.

oramic view of the organs operated on. Larger endoscopes are also required for operative procedures such as lysis of intestinal adhesions. Furthermore, their light output is sufficiently strong to transmit a bright image for two observers, even with a flexible teaching device or a loupe attached to the eyepiece. Since the endoscopic surgeon usually wants to document his operation photographically (see

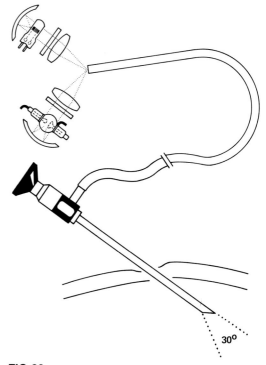

FIG 39.
Contemporary external light source supplies cold light and electronic flash, which are transmitted without interruption through an endoscope with integrated light cable for intracavitary illumination and endoscopic photography.

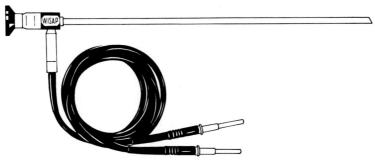

FIG 40.
Endoscope with two integrated fiber light cables for transmission of light and the electronic flash.

chapter 12.2.5.), for abdominal surgical procedures it is advisable to purchase an 11-mm endoscope with an integrated fiber light cable instead of an endoscope with a detachable light cable.

The combination light source, shown in Figure 41, was developed by Müller-Hermann, Weerda, and Pedersen (1982); it incorporates an autodynamically controlled through-the-lens computer flash system and is the most sophisticated light source today. It satisfies all requirements for diagnostic work with the routinely used 6.8-mm endoscope as well as those for surgery and photographic documentation with frame-filling color slides through the 11-mm endoscope with integrated fiber light bundle (see chapter 20, Figs 382 and 383).

12.1.4. Endoscopic Light Source for Cinematographic and Videotape Recording

The light sources that are satisfactory for diagnostic and operative procedures (see Fig 41) are unsatisfactory for movie and videotape recording. For cinematographic documentation, high-pressure vapor lamps (e.g., xenon-vapor lamps) are necessary to provide sufficient illumination for the exposure of 16-mm color film, because much light is absorbed by the red color of the pelvic organs.

The 16-mm movie camera must be attached directly to the eyepiece of the endoscope. Cinematographic documentation through an articulated optical attachment is presently not possible because the reversing prisms absorb too much light.

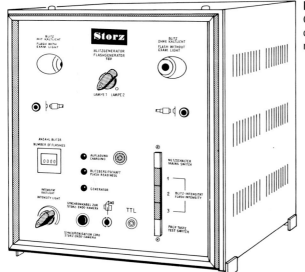

FIG 41.
Combination light source which can be used for diagnostic, operative, and photographic documentation purposes.

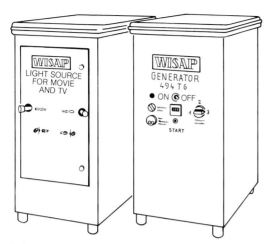

FIG 42.
Light source for cinematographic documentation.

FIG 43.
Halogen lamps, used in this instrument, will suffice for video documentation.

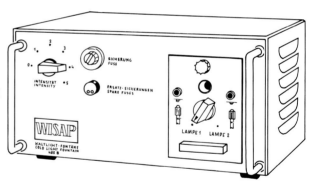

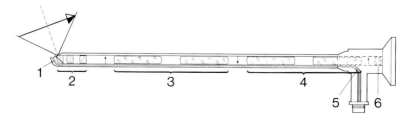

FIG 44.
A rod lens system: *1* and *5*, light-transmitting glass fibers; *2*, objective lens; *3* and *4*, rod lenses and reversal system; *6*, eyepiece.

Due to the greater sensitivity inherent in a television camera, an expensive light source with high-pressure vapor lamps (Fig 42) is not necessary. A 250-W halogen lamp (Fig 43) will suffice. Since the developments in the field of electronics are presently changing so rapidly, firm recommendations cannot be made at the present time.

Due to the high sensitivity of television cameras, the endoscopic image can be televised through the articulated optical attachment (see Fig 23). This is a necessity, because the surgeon usually cannot perform his operation using the unsharp image on the television screen.

12.2. ENDOSCOPIC OPTICAL SYSTEMS

Endoscopes are optical systems that are distinguished by type-specific characteristics. They are neither telescopes nor microscopes nor objective lenses. The basic optical calculations were made at the end of the nineteenth century by Ringleb (1910), von Rohe, Lange, and Kolmorgen, among others. Considerable improvements in the classic endoscopes were initiated by the English physicist Hopkins. In place of a succession of glass lenses separated by air spaces, as was previously used, he designed and calculated the requirements of a rod lens system in which the light is transmitted through quartz rods and refracted by "air lenses." A *rod lens system* (Fig 44) consists of light-transmitting glass fibers, an objective lens, rod lenses and reversal system, and an eyepiece.

The large aperture of the rod lens system con-

siderably increases the brightness of the image, so that the diameters of endoscopes can be reduced without loss of light efficiency and brilliance, that is, they can be made in smaller calibers yet still maintain the same excellent optical properties. Franke in 1968 succeeded in improving even the earlier conventional endoscopes through the use of electronic computers and the incorporation of new facts established by the experimental use of a Hopkins endoscope.

Hence, the endoscopes that are available to the endoscopic abdominal surgeon today produce exceedingly bright images that are almost free of optical distortion. Physically and mechanically, they have reached the culmination point presently achievable in the optical field with current manufacturing technology.

12.2.1. Endoscopes for Intra-abdominal Diagnosis

For primarily diagnostic purposes, endoscopes with an outer diameter of 7 mm are preferable, because the primary puncture for an endoscope of 11 mm diameter may constitute a greater risk. This risk may be reduced by techniques of "open laparoscopy" (see chapter 12.3.1.3.).

Multiple brands of endoscopes are in use worldwide. Two different systems are used to designate their optical angles (Fig 45). The 30° (or 150°) optical deflection of the pelviscope, as modified by Semm (Fig 46), affords straight-ahead and oblique viewing, particularly important for orientation if extensive adhesions are present. This deflection of the visual axis by 30° is also advanta-

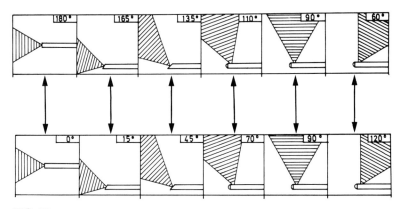

FIG 45.
Different systems of designation for optical angles afforded by a variety of endoscopes.

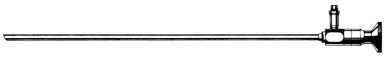

FIG 46.
Pelviscope modified by Semm with optical angle of 30°
or 150°, respectively.

geous for a panoramic view, particularly in the adnexal area and for the dissection of intestinal adhesions. A greater degree of deflection of the visual axis is not suited for intra-abdominal endoscopic operations, nor should it be used for diagnostic purposes, because it increases the risk of mistakes in orientation. Sheaths for rigid endoscopes are discussed in chapter 12.8.1.

Flexible endoscopy, which has become indispensable in gastrointestinal diagnostic and surgical procedures, is not expected to attain much importance in abdominal surgery. Especially in the presence of extensive adhesions in the abdomen, there have been difficulties in orientation, which may increase the risk of complications during sharp dissection. The existence of blind areas, particularly in extremely obese patients or those with extensive adhesions in the abdomen, may tempt the surgeon to work with flexible endoscopes; however, since orientation is severely restricted with these instruments, they offer no real diagnostic advantage.

12.2.2. Endoscopes for Intra-abdominal Surgery

If the diagnostic evaluation reveals a condition that appears to be correctable by pelviscopic surgery, the surgeon must determine whether surgery can be accomplished with the diagnostic endoscope or whether the diagnostic endoscope should be replaced by an 11-mm-diameter endoscope with a 30° angled view, which would afford a larger visual field and better possibilities for magnification (see chapter 12.2.4.). The 30° deflection of the visual axis offers a real advantage in operations on the adnexa and in the dissection of loops of bowel that adhere to the anterior abdominal wall. This decision depends primarily on the expected difficulty of the operative procedure and on the level of experience of the endoscopic surgeon.

Basically, it is recommended that the 11-mm endoscope be used for:

1. Operations on the tubal ampullae, when

the surgeon must work under low-power magnification with loupes (which absorb much light).

2. Intestinal adhesiolyses, when the cleavage lines between peritoneal surfaces and intestinal walls must be divided under considerable magnification.

3. All major procedures that require assistance, i.e., the use of an articulated or flexible optical attachment, "spy" (see Fig 23). Such procedures include radical and conservative operations for tubal pregnancy, oophorectomy or salpingo-oophorectomy, appendectomy, etc.

Semm does *not* recommend the use of the Palmer-Jacobs type of operating endoscopes for abdominal surgery (Fig 47) because the operating instruments are introduced through a channel that is parallel to the optical axis. Since all endoscopes afford only monocular vision instead of a three-dimensional image, depth perception may be misjudged and could result in unintentional injury of other structures, with serious sequelae.

[I have a more positive attitude regarding the use of operating endoscopes. Since monocular vision and consequently inadequate depth perception are handicaps inherent in the use of all endoscopes, every endoscopic surgeon must first learn to compensate for these handicaps and, with increasing experience, will become quite proficient. With the experience of several thousand cases, I am convinced that the advantages of an operating endoscope far outweigh the disadvantages. My preference is an operating laparoscope with a straight channel for ancillary instruments and a 45° angulation of the optical system (see Fig 47,B) because it does not require as much lateral contortion of the surgeon's spine as a straight or a doubly offset (see Fig 47,A) endoscope.

Many procedures (tubal sterilizations, adhesiolysis, etc.) can be performed through the operating channel of the endoscope and do not require a second puncture. However, if necessary, second, third, or more punctures for ancillary instruments

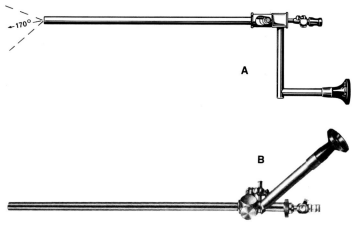

FIG 47.
In the Palmer-Jacobs type of operating endoscopes, illustrated here, operating instruments are introduced
through a straight channel parallel to the optical axis.

should be made in the same manner as done with
a straight endoscope. If there are wall-to-wall
adhesions in the lower abdomen and pelvis, it may
not be possible to find a suitable site for a second
puncture until partial adhesiolysis has been performed through the operating channel of the endoscope.

In extremely difficult cases, such as those with
adhesions extending into the middle and upper abdomen, we have found it very helpful to use a *second operating laparoscope* in place of one of the
ancillary suprapubic instruments. This allows the
surgeon to work from below to gain a better view
and approach for the operation in the middle and
upper abdomen, and at the same time it affords the
assistant the luxury of an independent view and
mobility. Experience with an operating laparo-
scope/pelviscope is also a tremendous asset for the
surgeon operating through a hysteroscope. If a
large submucous myoma has to be morcellated before it can be removed from the endometrial cavity
or for incision of a large septum, an operating lap-
aroscope/pelviscope with serrated scissors and biopsy forceps are preferable to hysteroscopic instruments. —*Ed.*]

Semm, in contrast, developed bimanual operative techniques which also require an assistant for
part of the procedure (Fig 48). Although handi-
capped by the inherent monocular vision, this technique permits operating with two or three instruments which, for cosmetic reasons, have been
introduced through two additional incisions within

the pubic escutcheon, about 10–15 cm apart, and,
if necessary, through a fourth puncture. The use of
two to three instruments improves the three-dimensional perception of position and mobility as well
as the size of pelvic organs.

Semm *never begins* with the blind insertion of
the operating endoscope—with the exception of
"open laparoscopy." Instead, he uses a 7-mm endoscope for diagnosis, then dilates the trocar
wound with a dilatation set (see chapter 12.8.8.)
so that it will accommodate the 11-mm trocar
sheath (see chapter 14.1.6.).

12.2.3. Support of the Endoscope for Bimanual Operation

For a bimanual endoscopic operation, it is necessary that the endoscope, which is introduced
through the umbilicus, be fixed at the surgeon's
eye level. There are four different possibilities:

1. *Mounting the eyepiece of the endoscope to
a headband*. This is particularly suitable if the endoscopic abdominal surgeon works without assistance. Attached to the headband (Fig 49) is a ball
joint with a bracket and a hinged quick-mount
adapter for the ocular of the endoscope. For operations on the tubal ampullae and intestinal adhesions, even the laparoscope with a loupe attached
(see Fig 51 and chapter 12.2.4.) can be mounted
in this manner as an optimum aid to the surgeon.

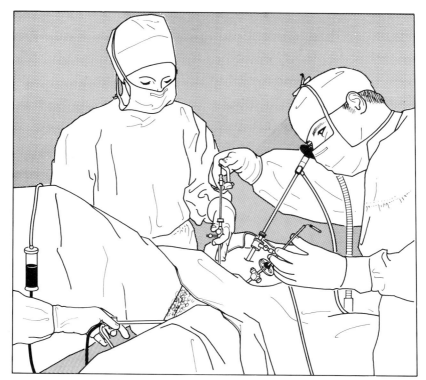

FIG 48.
Bimanual operating technique developed by Semm as an alternative to the use of Palmer-Jacobs operating endoscopes.

If, however, the operation is expected to take longer, the following technique is recommended:

2. *Support of the endoscope by a flexible arm.* A flexible gooseneck device designed by Semm (Fig 50) can be attached to the lateral rail of the operating table and arrested in any position. At-

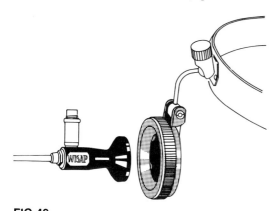

FIG 49.
Eyepiece of endoscope can be mounted to a headband.

tached to the free end of this device is a quick-mount adapter to which the ocular of the endoscope can be attached. Unlike the headband arrangement, this support device allows the operator complete mobility of his head and hands, facilitating his work greatly. Moreover, the endoscope is maintained in a fixed position relative to the operative field, which is not always guaranteed with the methods mentioned in (3) and (4). The coupling device is interchangeable to accommodate the pelviscopes, the articulated teaching attachment, still cameras, and so forth.

3. *Manual support by an assistant.* Since the endoscopic procedure is usually also a teaching experience, the use of a "spy"—an articulated and/or flexible teaching attachment (see Fig 23)—is recommended. In this case, the assistant observes the operative procedure and corrects the visual field of the endoscope, which has been introduced through the umbilicus, so that the surgeon can always perform the operative procedure in the center of the visual field. The assistant, who is holding the teaching attachment in one hand, is also in a

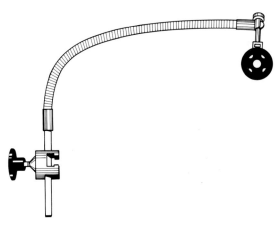

FIG 50.
Flexible gooseneck device, designed by
Semm.

position to assist the surgeon by holding and operating an instrument with the other hand (see Figs
22 and 377).

To reduce unintended movement of the endoscope, the assistant must support his elbow on the
shoulder brace for the surgeon (see chapter 13.3.).

4. If options 1–3 are not available, the surgeon may ask the scrub nurse or another person to
hold the endoscope in a position determined by the
surgeon. However, it is again recommended that
this person's elbow be supported on the shoulder
brace for the surgeon (see chapter 13.3.). Without
visual control by the assisting person, the endoscope can be held firmly only if it is fixed to a
solid support, i.e., an armrest.

12.2.4. Low-Power Loupe Magnification of the Endoscopic Image (Endoscopic Microsurgery)

In the past, endoscopic evaluation of internal organs for diagnostic purposes relied exclusively on
the image in the eyepiece of the endoscope. Approaching the organs with the objective lens of the
endoscope achieved a magnification of 1–2 X or
even 4 X. To succeed in operations on the tubal
ampullae, dissection of intestinal adhesions, and so
forth, however, magnifications of at least 2–6 X,
the customary range in microsurgery, are necessary. This can also be achieved for endoscopic surgery by attaching a loupe (Fig 51) to the eyepiece
of the endoscope. The articulated or flexible teaching attachment can even be mounted to the eyepiece of this loupe (see Fig 23). With this arrangement, the assistant is able to follow the operative
procedure under the same magnification.

12.2.5. Endoscope for Intra-abdominal Documentation by Photography, Cinematography, and Videotape Recording

As mentioned in chapter 12.1.2., approximately
50% of the light is lost by interrupting the light
conductor, that is, by attaching the fiber light cable
to the endoscope. Therefore, an endoscope with an
integrated fiber optic light cable (see Fig 40) must
be considered the optimum equipment for documentation of endoscopic findings. If it is not essential to produce frame-filling photographs, i.e., if
one is satisfied with circular photographs, regular
11-mm endoscopes with detachable fiber light cables and a remote external flash unit or one attached to the endoscope (Fig 52) may be used.

With endoscopes of only 6–7-mm diameter or
11-mm endoscopes with operating channels, only
small-sized photographs are possible, i.e., small
circular images on 24 × 36-mm color film or al-

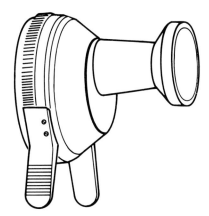

FIG 51.
Loupe which can be attached to eyepiece of endoscope
allows higher magnification.

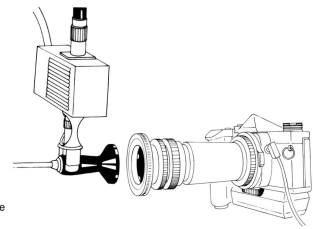

FIG 52.
For some documentation purposes, a detachable fiber light cable and remote external electronic flash or one attached to the endoscope may be satisfactory.

most frame-filling small images on 16-mm film in a miniature camera.

In regard to photographic documentation of endoscopic findings, it is of critical importance to consider the purpose of photography: small photographs will suffice to document findings in the patient's chart. Pictures for teaching, scientific, and investigational purposes require optimum light and flash techniques, as already described in chapter 12.1.3.

If the endoscopic operation is observed through a reflex camera (see Fig 378), the use of a loupe is unnecessary. The telephoto zoom lens with 70–140-mm focal length (Fig 53) and a 25-mm extension tube attached to the 11-mm endoscope results in a magnification of 4–6 X and, at the same time, format-filling 24 × 36-mm color slides.

If the findings are to be documented only for the patient's chart, an instant photograph (Polaroid) would suffice but no claim could be made that it is a precise document giving detailed information.

For cinematographic and videotape recording, only the 11-mm endoscope with a straight optical axis and integrated fiber light bundle is recommended. The 30° (150°) deflected endoscopes lose too much light within their deflecting prisms. The designs of light sources (see Figs 39 and 41) have been pushed to their extreme limits, which is expressed in their short life expectancy. In regard to the heat intensity, too, which is produced by the external production and focusing of the light on the proximal surface of the fiberglass light cable within the projector, the physical limits of present production techniques have been reached.

It is a well-known fact that only a fraction of the light transmitted into the abdominal cavity will be reflected back through the endoscope to expose and blacken the film or reach the sensor in the television camera; much of the light will not be reflected by the red color of the peritoneum, blood, etc. Light transmission is also restricted by the small diameter of the optical system in the endoscope, only 2–2.5 mm, and a length of 300 mm. With the telephoto lens attached, the length of the total system is 350–450 mm.

Finally, it should be mentioned that the technical design of endoscopes has reached the physically attainable limits. Optically, and in the area of light technology, one could not expect further improvements of the systems in the future (see also chapter 20).

12.2.6. Preparation of the Endoscope for the Intra-abdominal Procedure

Since the space of the pneumoperitoneum is maximally saturated with water vapor, this water vapor will immediately condense on cold objects intro-

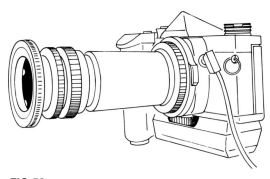

FIG 53.
Telephoto zoom lens on an SLR camera.

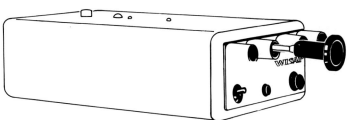

FIG 54.
Apparatus for prewarming the endoscopes.

duced into the abdomen. A cold objective lens of the endoscope, one with a temperature of below 37° C, will fog immediately after introduction into the abdominal cavity. Therefore, the endoscope should be prewarmed to 40°–45° C. This can be achieved in a warming apparatus (Fig 54). However, endoscopes must be warmed within the tubes of this device at least 1–2 hours before they reach the desired temperature, because heat conduction in air is very slow.

It is impossible to avoid contaminating the front lens and blinding it with blood or irrigation fluid during endoscopic intra-abdominal operations, particularly when irrigation is required. Simply wiping it off on the peritoneum, as was possible during diagnostic pelviscopy, is unsatisfactory, because the peritoneum of the intestinal tract is often also contaminated with blood. Therefore, the endoscope is withdrawn through the trocar sleeve and immersed in a bottle filled with physiologic saline or sterile water (Fig 55). This bottle is kept in a water bath that is thermostatically controlled at 50° C. For practical purposes, this water bath may be kept on a WISAP or other instrument cart (Fig 56) behind the surgeon, who can rapidly immerse the endoscope and clean it. The endoscope will be reheated and protected against fogging in the process.

Application of an antifog medium to the front

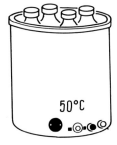

50°C

FIG 55.
Warm water bath holds bottles of physiologic saline solution or sterile water, into which endoscope is placed for cleaning.

lens, which was recommended in the past, has not been satisfactory in operative endoscopy.

For *each* operative abdominal procedure there should be two to three diagnostic 7-mm endoscopes and two 11-mm endoscopes—optimally with integrated fiber light cables—available in the warming apparatus (see Fig 54). With this precaution, there should never be a risk from the sudden loss of an endoscope due to mechanical problems or destruction (dropping), which could otherwise increase the operative risk and make a laparotomy necessary.

12.2.7. Sterilization and Maintenance of the Endoscope

The manufacturers of endoscopes provide specific instructions for the maintenance and sterilization of their endoscopic instruments. For optical instruments, the following *basic rules* should be adhered to. The optical instruments are thoroughly but gently cleansed mechanically, rinsed in water, and then sterilized in clear plastic (Fig 57) or metal trays. The use of Formalin tablets for this purpose is, without a doubt, the most gentle form of sterilization. The main disadvantage is that this sterilization requires approximately 24 hours.

The next best method is gas sterilization. However, one should request a guarantee from the instrument manufacturer stating which pressure differences the instruments can tolerate during gas sterilization, ranging from a vacuum to pressures of several atmospheres at 60° C. This should be compared to the data and the operation manual of the gas sterilization apparatus. A pressure increase from -1 Kp/cm^2 to approximately 6 Kp/cm^2 ($= 7$ Kp/cm^2) in a steam-saturated nitrous oxide environment will allow water to enter and will cause internal fogging of the lens system.

Some manufacturers also recommend autoclaving of the endoscope. The rapid heating of the inhomogeneous materials of which the endoscopes are constructed (glass, metal, synthetics) from 20° C to 120° C without doubt imposes a tremen-

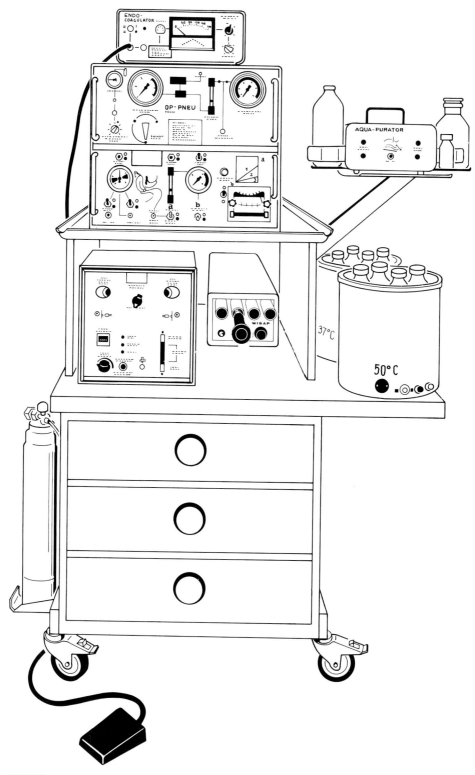

FIG 56.
WISAP instrument cart for endoscopic abdominal surgery.

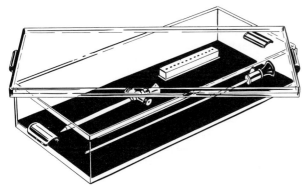

FIG 57.
Sterilization tray of clear plastic material for dry sterilization with formaldehyde tablets.

dous stress on the optical system that cannot be expected to have a beneficial effect on the life expectancy of the instruments.

By immersing the endoscopes, after careful mechanical cleansing, in antiseptic solutions (e.g., Cidex), a high degree of antisepsis can be obtained, but not total sterilization.

In summary, it should be emphasized that the sterilization of endoscopes is not yet without problems. The best method of circumventing this problem is to own a sufficient number of endoscopes so that there is no need for quick sterilization.

12.3. INSUFFLATION EQUIPMENT TO ESTABLISH A PNEUMOPERITONEUM

Laparoscopy became accepted in gynecologic procedures in the mid-1960s, when operative risks were reduced by improvements in this surgical method, i.e., the introduction of cold light optical systems and the automatically controlled pneumoperitoneum with CO_2 gas. The CO_2-PNEU device, which was developed in the early 1960s by Eisenburg and Semm (1965), originally for laparoscopy in internal medicine, followed in its technical design exclusively the requirements for insufflation of the abdomen for diagnostic inspection. This development terminated a decades-long era in which, in internal medicine, the pneumoperitoneum was established with air (Fig 58). In gynecology, it initiated the era of the controlled establishment of the pneumoperitoneum in the anesthetized patient (Fig 59). The CO_2-PNEU device (Fig 60) is in worldwide use as WISAP's CO_2-PNEU Automatic and its numerous copies; it controls CO_2 insufflation by mechanical means, monitoring time, volume, and pressure. The most important instrument, the ma-

nometer *(3)* "body cavity CO_2 filling pressure" shows the kinetic insufflation pressure as well as the actual intra-abdominal static pressure quite precisely between 0 and 60 mm Hg (0–7,980 Pa). Another manometer *(2)* indicates the gas volume insufflated into the abdomen. This is particularly important for the estimation of the relationship between the intra-abdominal (static) pressure and the size of the intra-abdominal accumulation of gas. From this relationship it can be recognized early whether the abdominal cavity is free or if a preperitoneal emphysema or omental emphysema is being produced.

The free flow of gas into the abdomen is indicated by the gentle and constant floating of the small ball in the visual gas flow control *(4)*. Erratic floating or bouncing of this ball is an instant indication of faulty position of the insufflation needle.

After the pneumoperitoneum has reached in-

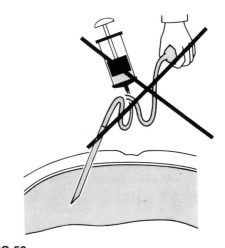

FIG 58.
Previously the pneumoperitoneum was established with air.

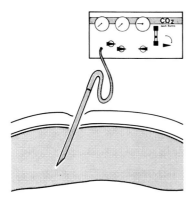

FIG 59.
CO$_2$-PNEU Automatic Insufflator allows controlled establishment of pneumoperitoneum with CO$_2$ gas.

An essential function of the CO$_2$-PNEU Automatic is its use as an indicator for a faulty position of the Veress needle. Figures 61–63 indicate how the direction of the pointer in combination with the gas flow indicator ball can be used to immediately recognize insufflation problems:

In Figure 61, the insufflation needle has entered a sealed pocket between adhesions: The manometer needle rises to a maximum value (40 mm Hg in the red area on its face) and the floating ball drops to the bottom.

In Figure 62, the insufflation needle is partially in the free abdominal cavity, but it touches strands of adhesions: the manometer needle oscillates between maximal pressures and 10 mm Hg; the floating ball in the flow indicator is bobbing up and down.

In Figure 63, the insufflation needle is placed optimally in the free peritoneal cavity: after elevation of the abdominal wall and movement of the needle to allow the omentum to drop off the needle tip in case it had been punctured, the manometer needle drops to a value that equals the internal flow resistance of the insufflation channels (approximately 5–8 mm Hg if tested before insufflation: needle test—see chapter 14.1.3.1.). The floating

tra-abdominal static pressures of 12–14 mm Hg, the insufflation switch lever is turned from the "hand" to the "automatic" position *(6)*, which will activate a mechanical regulating system to maintain a constant intra-abdominal pressure of 12–14 mm Hg. This automatic refill system will replenish the gas that has been absorbed or lost through loose fittings in the instruments.

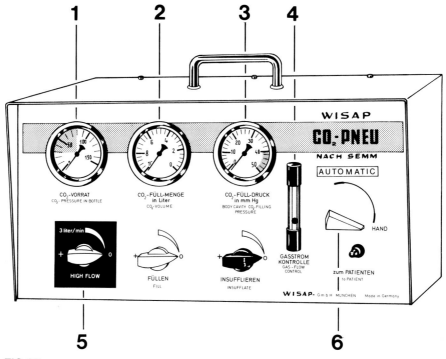

FIG 60.
The WISAP CO$_2$-PNEU Automatic Insufflator.

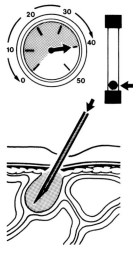

FIG 61.
See text.

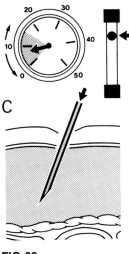

FIG 63.
See text.

ball remains at a constant level in the upper region of the indicator tube. This indicates that CO_2 gas is insufflated unencumbered at 1 L/min.

In developing the celiotonometer (Fig 64), the two functions previously performed by the manometer *(3)* in Figure 60—reading of the kinetic insufflation pressure and of the static intra-abdominal pressure—have been assigned to two manometers (Fig 65), and the safety level during insufflation of the pneumoperitoneum has been boosted considerably. The modified Veress needle (Fig 66) with Y-shaped Luer-lock adapters (Veress/Semm) affords the operator the opportunity to switch during the

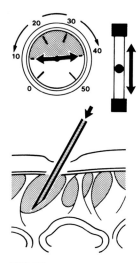

FIG 62.
See text.

insufflation procedure from the insufflation manometer (which indicates the kinetic—i.e., insufflation—pressure) to the static pressure in the abdomen and, in so doing, monitor the correct insufflation of the abdomen (see also chapter 12.3.1.1.).

With this new instrument, which combines the celiotonometer with the CO_2-PNEU Automatic according to Semm (see Fig 65), endoscopic abdominal surgery began a rapid development a few years ago. However, it became more and more apparent that a purely mechanical insufflation apparatus *cannot* produce the constant pneumoperitoneum conditions needed for a smooth and uninterrupted endoscopic operation. Mechanical pressure and insufflation regulators and monitors are not sufficient to maintain intra-abdominal pressure within the acceptable small tolerances and to replace the loss of large volumes of gas within a reasonable time and with the required technical accuracy. Equipped with only a mechanical device, the endoscopic surgeon fights a constant battle in trying to maintain or reestablish the field of view he requires for his operation. The insufflator I developed 20 years ago for diagnostic laparoscopy proved to be insufficient for more demanding endoscopic intra-abdominal operations. It is not suited for operative procedures that go beyond a simple tubal sterilization, ovarian biopsy, minor adhesiolysis, fimbriolysis, and the like—such as salpingo-oophorectomy and operations for tubal pregnancy.

Therefore, we developed a modern, electronic-pneumatically controlled insufflation appa-

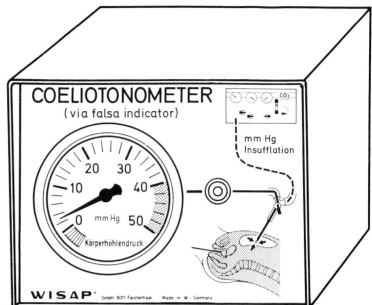

FIG 64.
The coeliotonometer.

ratus (see Fig 84), the OP-PNEU Electronic (according to Semm). It guarantees a maximal, electronically controlled refill speed up to 4.5 L/min, ideal for the production and maintenance of a pneumoperitoneum during endoscopic abdominal surgery. This apparatus will be described further in chapters 12.3.2. and 12.3.3.

12.3.1. Expansion Media to Establish the Pneumoperitoneum (Selection of Gas)

The characteristics of the gaseous media used in laparoscopy were discussed in depth on page 36 of the *Atlas of Gynecologic Laparoscopy and Hysteroscopy* and will be summarized as follows:

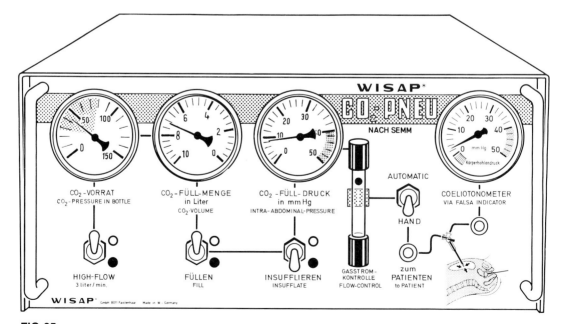

FIG 65.
Kinetic insufflation pressure and static intra-abdominal   pressure are now read by two different manometers.

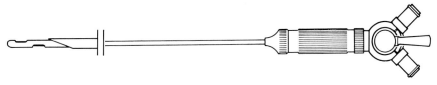

FIG 66.
Modified Veress needle with Y-shaped Luer-lock adapters (Veress/Semm).

Since operative procedures may take considerable time, *air* and *oxygen* are *not useful,* because they would increase the risk of embolism. Although *nitrous oxide* is physically and chemically soluble to the same degree, it constitutes an additional unpredictable risk to the patient. The abdominal cavity is distended with 3–6 L of nitrous oxide gas, which is a multiple of the lethal gas volume, in case it should be absorbed (see also chapter 10).

Other gases (e.g., argon, helium) so far have received only theoretical consideration (indifferent toward water vapor, optical lenses do not fog!). They are not yet on the market for routine use. Therefore, CO_2 gas is presently the best choice. Its solubility in blood and tissues exceeds that of oxygen by a factor of 10. It is a normal metabolic end product that is easily exhaled through the pulmonary alveoli.

Carbon dioxide gas can be insufflated directly into a human blood vessel, either intravenously or intra-arterially, in amounts of 100 ml/min without any noticeable long-range disturbances of the P_{CO_2}

metabolism in men (Lindemann, 1980). Only insufflation volumes of 150–250 ml/min may result in tachycardia and circulatory disturbances. In the case of an open foramen ovale (about 40% of all foramina ovalia are functionally open for gas) even intravascular CO_2 insufflation presents the risk of embolism. Figure 67 (from Lindemann, 1980) shows the experimental data regarding those facts, which were derived from dog experiments. Kastendiek (1973), who studied human subjects, could also show that even during a prolonged pelviscopy, the CO_2 gas that was absorbed from the peritoneum did not cause a significant acidosis in the circulating blood. This requires that the accumulating (i.e., absorbed or insufflated) gas be constantly exhaled through the alveoli, i.e., by normal respiration. However, a decrease in respiratory volume could result from excessive intra-abdominal pressure and, consequently, uncontrolled elevation of the diaphragm. Should the anesthesiologist (see chapter 10) fail to recognize that there is a reduction in the respiratory exchange of CO_2, this in-

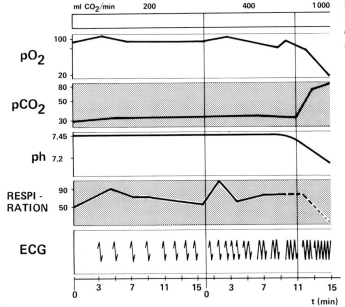

FIG 67.
Effects of intravascular CO_2 insufflation on blood gas tension, pH, respiration, and ECG (in dogs).

creases the risk of cardiac arrest with cerebral sequelae. Such an accident happened to one patient
in the United States who first underwent a hysteroscopy (a 10-minute procedure) followed by a
pneumoperitoneum and laparoscopic tubal sterility
operation with high-frequency current. Since her
respiration apparently was not adequately monitored or controlled, cardiac arrest occurred 35 minutes after the beginning of the surgery and resulted
in severe impairment of her cerebral function.

A beginning acidosis of the blood is always
preceded by an increase in the pulse rate. In com-
pliance with modern requirements for continuous
monitoring of the patient's cardiac function during
anesthesia, such tachycardia will be recognized immediately, and corrective measures will be initiated: hyperventilation, reduction of the intra-abdominal pneumoperitoneal pressure, appropriate
medication, checking of the equipment, and so
forth.

In the field of internal medicine, in many cen-
ters, laparoscopy is routinely performed under local anesthesia and the pneumoperitoneum is established with nitrous oxide. If a diagnostic or small
operative endoscopic abdominal procedure (e.g.,
tubal sterilization) is performed under local anesthesia, the anesthetic effect of nitrous oxide may
contribute to the patient's comfort. However, the
absorption rate and volume of nitrous oxide gas
cannot be estimated correctly. The fact that the patient has a multiple of the lethal dose of this gas in
her abdomen, therefore, constitutes an unpredictable risk to her safety under general anesthesia (see
also chapter 10).

In gynecology, three *sites* are *well suited
for insufflation.* The umbilicus (see chapter
12.3.1.1.), the posterior vaginal fornix (see chapter 12.3.1.2.), and minilaparotomy or ''open laparoscopy'' (see chapter 12.3.1.3.).

12.3.1.1. Transabdominal Insufflation of the Pneumoperitoneum by Blind Puncture and Veress Needle (see also chapters 14.1.3. to 14.1.3.2)

In general laparoscopy, several sites are recommended for the introduction of the Veress needle into the abdomen to induce a pneumoperitio-
neum (Fig 68) (see also chapters 14.1.2. to
14.1.3.2.). For gynecologic laparoscopy, i.e., pelviscopy, the *inferior umbilical area* is the most
common puncture site.

Umbilical puncture is achieved by introducing
the Veress needle with the right hand in a perpen-

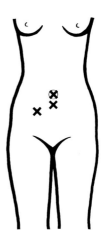

FIG 68.
Possible sites for introduction of Veress needle to create a pneumoperitoneum.

dicular direction into the caudal area of the umbilicus. The bifurcation of the aorta should have been
palpated before (see chapter 14.1.3.1.2.). The fifth
finger is spread to brace the hand against unintended excessive downward pressure. The Veress
needle is held only between the thumb and index
finger and is advanced through the skin and umbilical fascia. At the same time, the left hand elevates
the abdominal wall as high as possible (Fig 69).
During the slow insertion of the needle *with pressure exerted from the wrist joint,* one can count the
layers of the abdominal wall as they are individually perforated by the snaps of the spring mechanism of the needle.

[If the abdominal skin is tough or scarred, or
for any beginner, it may be safer to estimate the
diameter of the abdominal wall and then hold the
shaft of the Veress needle between the thumb and
index finger at a distance from the needle tip that
is shorter than the estimated diameter of the abdominal wall. Then the lateral aspect of the hand
or fist is braced against the surface of the abdominal wall to prevent the sudden, uncontrolled perforation of the entire abdominal wall. After the
first advance, the shaft of the needle can be
grasped higher and higher until all layers of the
abdominal wall have been penetrated with the
greatest caution, monitored by the repeated snaps
of the spring mechanism of the needle.—Ed.]

A sudden penetration of the tip of the needle
down to the large trunk vessels is possible only if
the needle is advanced from the shoulder and with
the full power of the arm. The needle should be

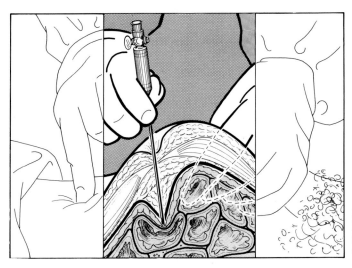

FIG 69.
Position of surgeon's hands and fingers during blind umbilical puncture with Veress needle.

introduced almost perpendicularly (Fig 70), because it is only the abdominal skin which is being elevated. The peritoneum remains in its almost horizontal direction. If the needle is introduced at a shallow angle, it will not perforate the peritoneum (Fig 71). It slides extraperitoneally in a caudal direction, which could only result in preperitoneal emphysema (Fig 72). Such preperitoneal sliding of an instrument can be observed experimentally through the endoscope when the second trocar is introduced, as shown in Plates 1, 95, and 268.

During this ''blind puncture'' in the caudal region of the umbilicus, one must constantly be aware of the anatomical position of the abdominal aorta, which was palpated before (Fig 73), and of the inferior vena cava and their bifurcation sites, as well as of the anterior projection of the sacral promontory.

The umbilicus is usually 1–2 cm below the bifurcation of these large trunk vessels, as shown in the aortogram in Figure 74. The umbilicus is identified by contrast material. If this topographic relationship is remembered, the aorta and the common iliac arteries can be palpated in almost all patients. At least the pulsation of the aorta and the left common iliac artery are palpable.

The distance between the large trunk vessels and the parietal peritoneum may be less than 1 cm in slender patients. If the umbilical plate is elevated manually, and if the needle tip is introduced vertically in the caudal area of the umbilicus, the probability of perforation of the thick-walled aortic vessels is extremely low. However, if the puncture is flat, i.e., tangential to the blood vessels, it is more likely that a larger area of the vessels may be injured by slitting them. This has been documented by a few medical-legal cases in which the patients died.

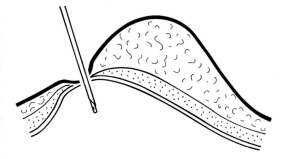

FIG 70.
The insufflation needle is introduced almost perpendicularly while only the abdominal skin is elevated.

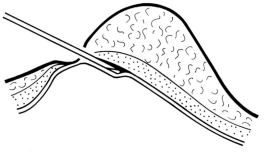

FIG 71.
A needle introduced at a shallow angle will not perforate the peritoneum.

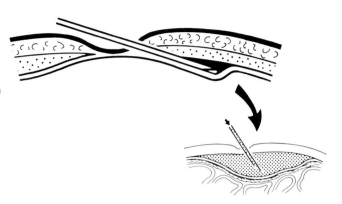

FIG 72.
A needle advanced at too shallow an angle will slide caudally in the extraperitoneal space, resulting in a preperitoneal emphysema.

Figure 75 shows the theoretical and practical possibilities of the placement of the tip of the Veress needle in a vertical direction to the umbilicus and their consequences:

1: preperitoneal location → preperitoneal emphysema
2: subperitoneal → pneumoperitoneum
3: large omentum → omental emphysema
4: intestines → distention of bowel or stomach
5: retroperitoneal → puncture of vessel with gas embolism (Fig 76) or → mediastinal emphysema (Fig 77)

Figure 78 demonstrates the short periumbilical distance to the common iliac arteries and veins in a horizontal direction through the abdomen of a slender patient.

Götze (1918) developed a safety snap mechanism, used in establishing a pneumothorax and to insufflate the abdomen with oxygen for pneumoroentgenography of the female pelvic organs. The principle of protecting organs from the needle tip, which was later adopted and modified by Veress (1938), is shown in Figure 79. Immediately after perforation of the parietal peritoneum by the sharp needle tip, the blunt insufflation cannula is pushed forward by the built-in spring mechanism, and it protects the peritoneal organs (i.e., the intestinal peritoneum) from injury by the cutting edge of the needle tip.

A positive sign for the accomplished perforation of the abdominal wall is a soft hissing sound after the insertion of the needle, provided that the abdominal wall is elevated manually. It occurs immediately after the perforation of the parietal peritoneum when the blunt inner cannula springs forward and, because of the negative pressure produced in the abdominal cavity by the maximal elevation of the abdominal wall with the left hand,

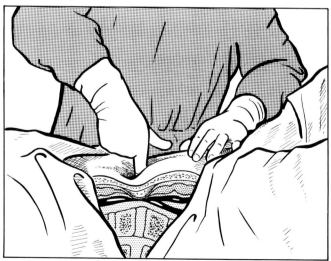

FIG 73.
Palpation of the abdominal aorta and the sacral promontory *before* introduction of the insufflation needle.

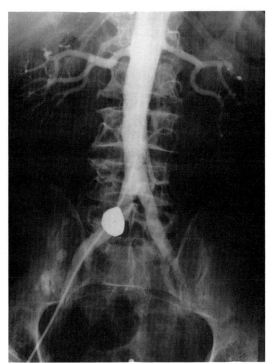

FIG 74.
Aortogram showing location of umbilicus about 1–2 cm below bifurcation. The umbilicus is filled with contrast material.

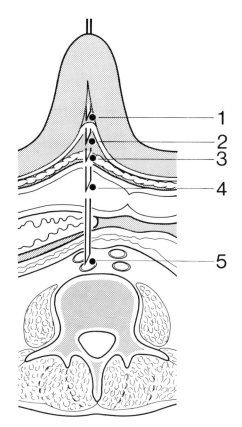

FIG 75.
Different placements of insufflation needle (in vertical direction to umbilicus) have different consequences; see text.

air is immediately aspirated. This phenomenon should always be observed or, as an alternative, an open barrel of a syringe containing some saline may be attached to the Veress needle (Fig 80); as soon as the needle tip reaches the free abdominal cavity, the sterile saline solution will be aspirated.

Other safety tests that should be done after the insertion of the Veress needle are described in chapter 14.1.3. ff.

12.3.1.2. Transvaginal Insufflation of the Pneumoperitoneum Through the Posterior Vaginal Fornix (Insufflation of the Cul-de-Sac of Douglas)

If it is not possible or safe to introduce the Veress needle through the umbilicus into the free abdominal cavity (see also safety tests in chapters 14.1.3.1. to 14.1.3.1.7.), the pneumoperitoneum may be established through the posterior vaginal fornix. For this purpose the posterior cervical lip is grasped with a tenaculum forceps to demonstrate the posterior vaginal fornix and the Veress needle is then introduced parallel to the cervix into the

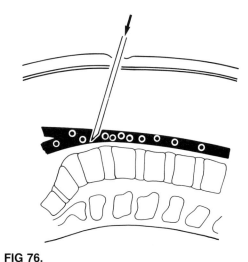

FIG 76.
Retroperitoneal needle placement may puncture vessels, leading to gas embolism.

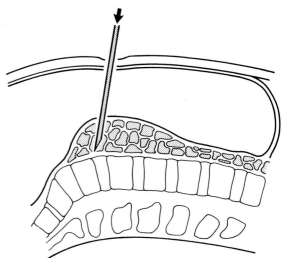

FIG 77.
Retroperitoneal needle placement may lead to
mediastinal emphysema.

cul-de-sac of Douglas (Fig 81). For this approach,
the rectovaginal examination must have revealed
no abnormalities (no large endometriotic implants).
The patient should not have a history of pelvic peritonitis, because this would increase the risk of rectal perforation. Plates 2 and 3 show the Veress
needle in situ from the perspective of the umbili-

cus, demonstrating the risk of puncturing bowel or
epiploic appendices.

12.3.1.3. Insufflation of the Pneumoperitoneum by "Open Laparoscopy"

Today, chronic, therapy-resistant lower abdominal complaints, as they occur with abdominal

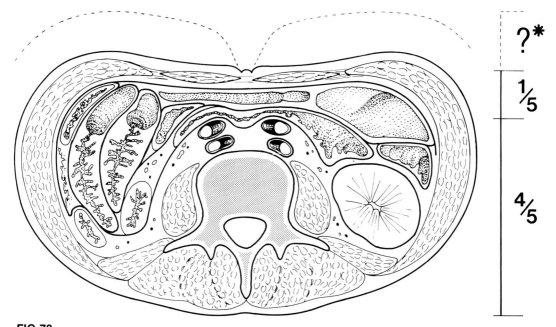

FIG 78.
The horizontal periumbilical distance to the common iliac arteries and veins in a thin patient is short. ?* =
subcutaneous adipose tissue.

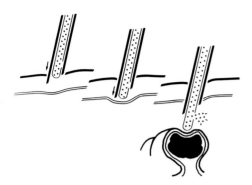

FIG 79.
Safety snap mechanism of the Veress needle protects organs from injury by the needle tip.

adhesions after previous gynecologic or general surgical laparotomies, are the domain of endoscopic abdominal surgery. Originally these abdominal conditions were considered contraindications for laparoscopy or, in gynecology, pelviscopy.

Due to improvements in instruments, techniques to establish a pneumoperitoneum, and operative methods, an abdomen that previously has been operated upon is no longer a contraindication to laparoscopy or pelviscopy.

In the majority of cases it is possible to safely gain access to the free abdominal cavity through the caudal area of the umbilicus, provided that the safety tests have been observed (see chapter 14.1.3. ff.). If, however, the patient has a history of multiple laparotomies with lysis of extensive

adhesions or a previous diffuse peritonitis, one must assume with a high degree of probability that, even with careful attempts to sound the peritoneal cavity, a loop of small bowel may be broadly attached to the parietal peritoneum and may be injured. For such cases, the "open laparoscopy" technique as recommended by Hasson is preferable. Hasson proposed this method in the United States in 1974, and it was modified by Koenig in Germany in 1979, to reduce the risk of the primary blind puncture by replacing it with a "minilaparotomy."

As shown in Figure 82, the abdomen is opened in the subumbilical area through a 2- to 3-cm midline incision made in the classic manner. After the omentum and bowels have dropped back after the opening of the parietal peritoneum, or after they have been pushed aside bluntly, a blunt trocar specially developed for this purpose (Fig 83) is introduced into the abdominal cavity under direct vision. Two guide sutures that have been placed into the peritoneal and fascial edges are pulled outward to produce a gas-tight seal between the operative incision and the cone of the instrument sleeve (see Fig 82).

For the active endoscopic abdominal surgeon, "open laparoscopy" is certainly a substantial improvement. Even in patients with a history of extensive abdominal adhesions, which often severely affect the quality of their lives, renewed attempts can be made to correct these adhesions endoscopically.

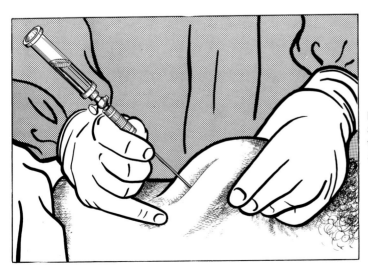

FIG 80.
Sterile saline solution may be used to verify perforation of the abdominal wall.

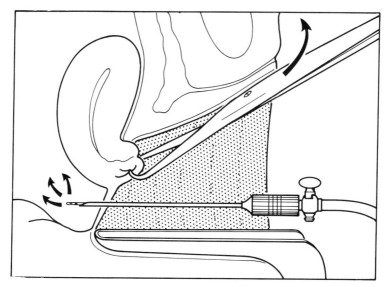

FIG 81.
Establishing a pneumoperitoneum through the posterior vaginal fornix.

12.3.2. Electronic and Mechanical Control of the Pneumoperitoneum for Intra-abdominal Diagnosis

As already discussed in chapter 12.3., the CO_2-PNEU Automatic apparatus, which I developed in the 1960s, is no longer satisfactory for endoscopic abdominal surgery. Therefore, the OP-PNEU Electronic insufflator (according to Semm) had to be developed. The essential characteristics of its construction are diagrammed in Figure 84. The parts labeled are as follows:

1: control manometer for CO_2 tank
2: main switch, illuminated
3: selection switch for static intra-abdominal pressure from 5 to 25 mm Hg
4: digital manometer for kinetic insufflation pressure
5: digital indicator for gas volume used, in liters
6: digital indicator for current gas flow, in liters/min
7: button to reset digital indicator to 00.0
8: flow meter (floating ball)

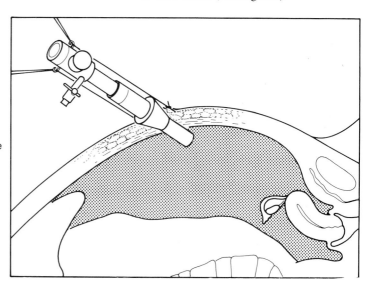

FIG 82.
"Open laparoscopy" technique (Hasson and Koenig).

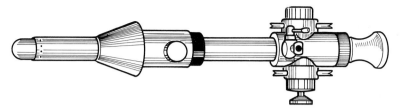

FIG 83.
Blunt trocar developed for use in "open laparoscopy."

9: electronic flow control (lights)
10: indicator light for determination of static intra-abdominal pressure
10a: indicator light for intra-abdominal pressure too low
10b: indicator light for intra-abdominal pressure too high, with acoustical warning signal
11: digital manometer for static intra-abdominal pressure
12: selection switch for gas flow of 1 L/min

and approximately 6 (Hi-Flo) L/min
13: operating instructions
14: gas outlet to patient

One of the requirements for the construction of the OP-PNEU Electronic was the development of the single-channel/dual-purpose insufflation system (Fig 85). Whereas in the past the surgeon had to operate the hand valve in the Y-connection of the Veress needle, this function has been incorporated into the celiotonometer (see Fig 64), where it

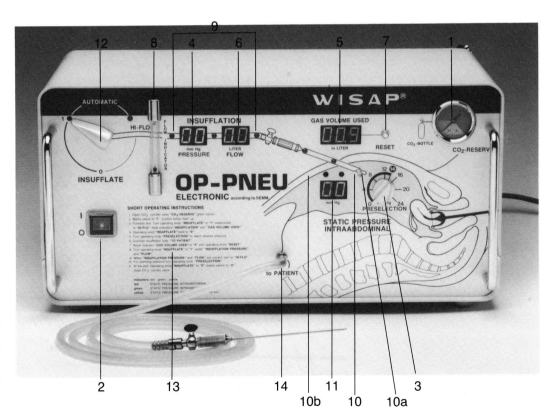

FIG 84.
The OP-PNEU Electronic insufflator for endoscopic abdominal surgery. See text for identification of labeled parts.

FIG 85.
Single-channel/dual purpose system
(according to Semm).

Insufflation Pressure   Static Pressure

is done by electronic circuitry. The single-channel/
dual-purpose insufflation system operates according to the following *principle:*

The regular, single-channel Veress needle is
used and connected by a tube to the gas outlet (*14*
in Fig 84). The actual intra-abdominal (static) pressure is measured intermittently through the same
system by an electronic sensor. An electronic program compares the gas flow pressure to the built-
in upper limit (40 mm Hg for the insufflation pressure), and regulates the maximum gas flow according to the determined pressures until the preselected *(switch 3)* maximum static intra-abdominal
pressure has been reached. At that point, the insufflation procedure is interrupted electronically.

Both insufflation pressure and intra-abdominal
static pressure are monitored alternately by quartz
sensors and displayed on digital indicators (*4* and
11). This allows the surgeon and his team to monitor the actual pressure conditions at all times.

In combination with the mechanical flow meter *(8),* this electronic insufflator incorporates all
control and safety devices of the mechanical CO_2-
PNEU Automatic apparatus. In addition, one large
digital indicator *(5),* displays information about the
actual volume of the pneumoperitoneum or, later
on, about the total volume of CO_2 gas used, and
another one *(6)* displays information about the volume of gas that flows through the Veress cannula
or, later on, the trocar sleeve.

For the primary insufflation procedure, the
flow volume of gas is limited to 1 L/min *(12)* so
that the insufflation pressure during the blind insufflation through the Veress cannula does not exceed
6–10 mm Hg.

The insufflation pressure and the static intra-
abdominal pressure (i.e., the current pressure) are
monitored as shown in Figure 86. If after insufflation of approximately 1 L of gas there is no indication for abnormal placement of the needle, the
gas flow regulator *(12)* can be switched to "high
flow" (see also Fig 227). For safety reasons, this
will be indicated by a red light. The maximal insufflation pressure is limited to 40 mm Hg, and the
electronic circuitry regulates the insufflation volume of gas up to this maximum pressure. The
maximum flow is automatically limited to 6 L/min.
It is reached only when the gas flows freely against
atmospheric pressure. If a Veress needle functions
very well, its flow resistance corresponds to 6 mm
Hg (798 Pa) when the gas flows at a rate of 1 L/
min; at a flow rate of 2.5 L/min, the resistance
already reaches the limit of 40 mm Hg.

This intermittent insufflation procedure will be
noticed by the surgeon both visually and acousti-
cally, because of the soft noises made by the
switching of the magnetic valves. Utilizing the
same orifice for insufflation and monitoring is the
only technical way to automate the insufflation
procedure.

FIG 86.
Manometers on OP-PNEU Electronic instrument for
measuring insufflation and actual intra-abdominal static
pressures.

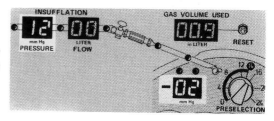

Since the insufflation of gas always prevents obstruction of the orifice, the static pressure can be determined immediately after the gas flow has been stopped. This measured value controls the succeeding gas flow by pressure and time, and therefore guarantees optimum safety.

Frangenheim (1976) and Steptoe (1976) measured the static pressure via a third channel in a Veress cannula which they modified. This method entails a great danger: since the diameter of the insufflation cannula should not exceed 3 mm, the channel for monitoring must be kept very narrow. The commercially available Veress needle measures only 2 mm in diameter. If the monitoring channel is contaminated by fluids (law of capillary attraction), or if the orifice is obstructed, the electronic sensor will read a static pressure of "0 mm Hg" and it automatically switches to "maximum insufflation." This erroneous determination may lead to a life-threatening overinflation of the abdomen. The single-channel/dual-purpose monitoring technique prevents such erroneous determinations with certainty.

12.3.3. Electronic and Mechanical Control of the Pneumoperitoneum for Endoscopic Abdominal Surgery

A diagnostic evaluation (see chapter 14.1. ff.) is done at the beginning of any endoscopic abdominal surgery. The endoscopes are changed (see chapter 14.1.6.) for the operative phase (see chapter 14.2.). For this the CO_2-PNEU Electronic (see Figs 84 and 85) is principally set to "high flow." In a routine case, an intraperitoneal pressure of 12 mm Hg is sufficient. If the patient has a very relaxed abdominal wall (e.g., postpartum), the pressure can be reduced to 8–10 mm Hg (1,064 Pa).

If bowels and omentum have to be dissected off the parietal peritoneum, the intra-abdominal pressure may have to be increased for a short period to 14–16 mm Hg for better visualization of lines of cleavage between layers, and to facilitate dissection. However, the anesthesiologist should always be notified *before* the pressure is increased, because this also increases the resistance to blood flow in the vena cava and elevates the diaphragm (Fig 87). Since this, in turn, decreases the tidal volume, the anesthesiologist must take compensatory measures that will increase the ventilation effort by a corresponding degree (as discussed in chapter 12.3.1.) to permit the uninterrupted exchange of CO_2 gas.

The Veress needle and the trocar for the endoscope—through which, in most cases, the gas is insufflated during the operative procedure—should be tested before they are used to determine their flow resistance at 1 L and 6 L of gas per minute ("high flow"). Occasionally the endoscope and its trocar fit so tightly that there is little free move-

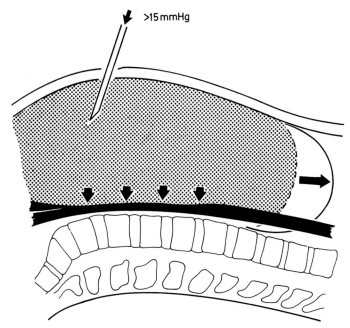

>15 mmHg

FIG 87.
An increase in intra-abdominal pressure increases resistance to blood flow in the vena cava and elevates the diaphragm.

ment of the endoscope inside the trocar sleeve and the large capillary space is too narrow to permit the flow of sufficient volumes of gas between the outer wall of the endoscope and the trocar sleeve. In such cases, the replacement gas must be insufflated through one of the trocars for ancillary instruments. If new trocar sleeves have to be purchased, one must be sure that the outer diameter of the endoscope and the inner diameter of the trocar sleeve are properly matched to allow sufficient space for adequate gas insufflation. As a rule of thumb, 4 L of gas per minute should flow through the trocar sleeve with a maximum insufflation pressure of 20 mm Hg when the endoscope is introduced.

If it should be necessary to utilize the OP-PNEU Electronic to its full capacity of 6 L/min, the endoscope may have to be withdrawn from the trocar sleeve. This reduces the insufflation resistance to the actual intra-abdominal pressure, the maximal capacity of the insufflator is utilized, and the abdomen can be reinsufflated in 1 minute with approximately 6 L of CO_2 gas.

12.4. TECHNICAL EQUIPMENT FOR INTRA-ABDOMINAL IRRIGATION

In gynecologic operative procedures there are two reasons for irrigation:

1. Irrigation and aspiration of the operative field, as is also done during a laparotomy.
2. Pertubation of tubes with gas or fluid to check their patency.

12.4.1. Equipment for Endoscopic Abdominal or Pelvic Irrigation

Every operative procedure causes some bleeding. Suction and irrigation cannulas are the instruments normally used with a laparotomy to maintain a clear view in the operative field. Although this requirement is easily realized during a laparotomy, it is difficult to transfer this technique to endoscopy when the abdominal cavity is accessible only via two or three trocar sleeves of 5 mm diameter. If the CO_2-PNEU Automatic or similar mechanically controlled insufflation apparatus were used, suction would deflate the pneumoperitoneum in seconds. On the other hand, the frequent exchange between the aspiration cannula and the instillation cannula was cumbersome and time-consuming. Most of these problems have been overcome by the newly developed combined single-channel/dual-purpose irrigation/aspiration cannula (Fig 88), which is used in conjunction with its companion Aquapurator (Fig 89).

This single-channel cannula, introduced through a 5-mm trocar sleeve, can be used alternatively for instillation of irrigation fluids and for aspiration of fluids and blood; the direction of flow of liquid is easily controlled by pushing the appropriate control buttons. If bowel or an epiploic appendix is sucked against the distal orifice of the cannula, it can be easily released by briefly applying finger pressure to the irrigation button. The buttons for irrigation and aspiration activate simple, spring-operated hose clamps. These appear to be primitive; however, they are mechanically far superior to valves, which can easily be obstructed by the aspirated material (blood, tissue, hair, and other particles). This will rarely happen with hose clamps.

On the one side of the Aquapurator is an aspiration flask of approximately 1 L capacity. To prevent contamination of the pump, an overflow vessel is mounted between the 1-L aspiration flask and the pump. On the other side, one of the commercially available bottles of sterile saline or Ringer's solution (see chapter 13.2.), prewarmed to 37° C, is attached. A sterile, sharpened, double-barreled cannula is introduced through its rubber stopper or through a built-in ventilation port, respectively. The irrigation fluid is instilled at a pressure of approximately 200 mm Hg and aspirated at a negative pressure of approximately 300 mm Hg.

[Alternatively, one of the soft, compressible

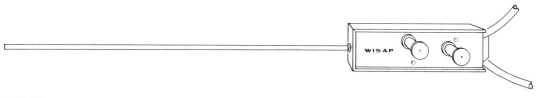

FIG 88.
Single-channel/dual-purpose irrigation aspiration/cannula.

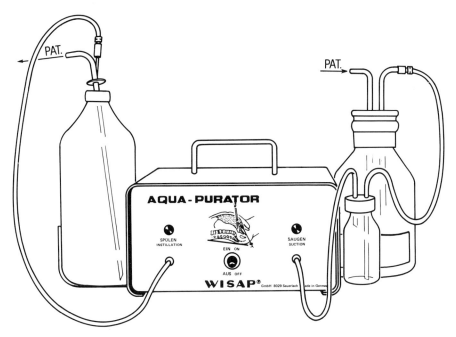

FIG 89.
The Aquapurator.

bags of sterile saline or Ringer's solution, which are routinely used in the United States, may be warmed up to 37° C and mounted inside a blood pressure cuff or a comparable device used for blood transfusions, so that irrigation can be done under the same pressure as with the Aquapurator. For aspiration, the regular operating room suction devices are equally effective.—*Ed.*]

The electronically controlled OP-PNEU Electronic apparatus will replenish quickly and without problems the gas that has been aspirated with the irrigation procedures; this is true even if 30–90 L of gas are used in, for instance, the operative pelviscopic management of an ectopic pregnancy. Such a large volume of gas is utilized because blood and clots must first be aspirated from the pelvis. Doing this through a 4-mm cannula frequently takes considerable time and often requires "dilution" of blood clots with saline or Ringer's solution.

12.4.2. Equipment for Tubal or Transuterine Irrigation

In the diagnosis and operative correction of sterility caused by pathologic conditions of the distal tube (see chapter 14.2.4.2. ff.), the continuous, pressure-controlled insufflation or pertubation of the oviducts is an absolute requirement for the success of the operation. At the beginning of the pelviscopic procedure, the cervix is occluded by the vacuum intrauterine cannula (Fig 90) that is connected by a tube to a reservoir containing the chromopertubation solution (Fig 91). It is connected to the universal pertubation apparatus according to Fikentscher and Semm, which delivers pressure in the range of 100–300 mm Hg required for the pertubation of the tubes, while at the same time recording the pressures on graph paper (Fig 92).

The common practice of inflating a sactosalpinx *manually* just before it is opened surgically is inadequate. For the careful microsurgical dissection of the original ampullary funnel, it is essential that the occluded ampullary bulb be kept under continuous pressure to assure the success of the operation (see chapters 14.2.4.2. and 14.2.4.3.1.). The insufflation of the occluded ampullary funnel, shown in Plates 73, 77, 88, and 97, succeeds only if the pressures are automatically controlled and maintained in the range of 150–300 mm Hg. This cannot be accomplished by hand.

Pressures are simultaneously monitored and graphically recorded during and after the operative

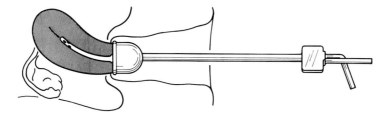

FIG 90.

In procedures to correct infertility of tube-related causes, the cervix is occluded by the vacuum intrauterine cannula at the beginning of the procedure.

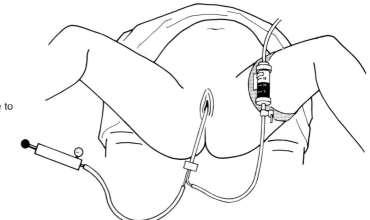

FIG 91.

The cannula is connected by tube to a reservoir containing the chromopertubation solution.

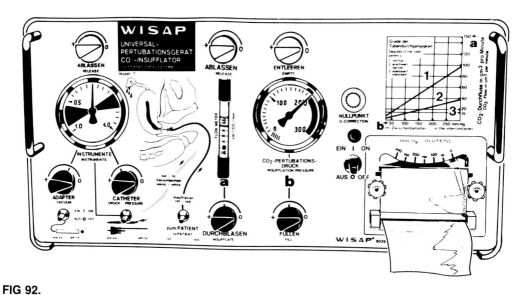

FIG 92.

The Universal Pertubation Apparatus monitors and records pressures during CO_2 or dye pertubation.

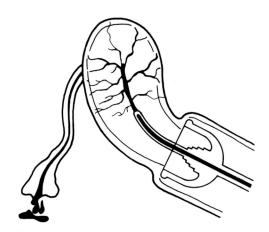

FIG 93.
During chromosalpingoscopy, blue dye may enter uterine blood vessels.

procedure. These basic data are used for comparison with data obtained at hydropertubation during the postoperative phase (see chapter 17.3.).

During chromosalpingoscopy, particularly if the instillation pressure is too high, blue solution (methylene blue or indigo carmine) may enter the uterine blood vessels and cause a blue discoloration of the uterus and the mesosalpinx (Fig 93). If this infiltration is noted mainly in the uterine fundus (see Plate 47) or in the area of the tubal cornu, also in the area of the lymphatic vessels (see Plate 48), it is less likely to be caused by a direct perforation of the cannula into the myometrium but more likely due to extensive adenomyosis deep within the myometrium. The endometrial tissue has grown from the cavity into the myometrium and provides conduits for trans-

mural and intravascular infiltration of dye solution.

A helpful variant for the mobilization of the uterus is the "uterus mobilizer" (Fig 94) developed by Valtchev and Papsin (1977). A cone is pressed into the cervix and seals it. It provides an opportunity to instill fluids and dye into the uterus and, at the same time, to move and tilt the uterus by a hinge device incorporated into the cone. This is particularly useful when the patient is in an unfavorable position (see Fig 26)—unlike the ones depicted in Figures 24, 25, and 27.

12.4.3. Equipment for Ovum Aspiration for In Vitro Fertilization

The instruments for aspiration of a mature ovum for in vitro fertilization (described in chapter 12.8.10.) and the technical procedure (described in chapter 14.2.14.) require a negative pressure, which is optimally produced by the Aquapurator (see Fig 89). If the ovum aspiration system (Fig 95) is connected and the Aquapurator is switched on, a negative pressure of approximately 2–3 mm Hg (266–399 Pa) is produced at the tip of the needle (A in Fig 95), it can be further regulated by a foot switch. This negative pressure will prevent follicular fluid from squirting out alongside the needle when the needle first perforates the thecal layer of the follicle. Intermittent suction is then applied to aspirate the follicular fluid under visual control (B and E). Negative suction pressure is induced whenever the small cannula, which is attached to the suction system and held by a finger ring (D), is closed with a fingertip. If no ovum is aspirated on the first attempt, the follicle is again

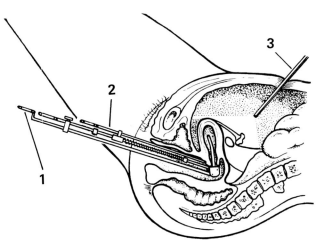

FIG 94.
The uterus mobilizer (Valtchev and Papsin): *1,* guide rods; *2,* tilt mechanism; *3,* endoscope.

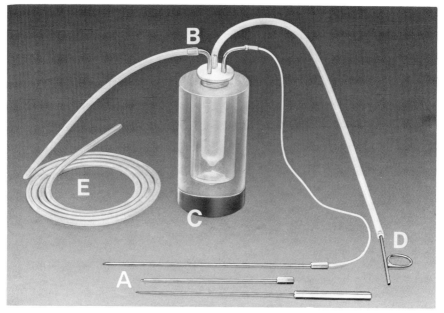

FIG 95.
Ovum aspiration system. See text for description of labeled elements.

filled with a transfer medium and reaspirated a second time.

The Plexiglas cylinder *(C)* provides an isothermic environment of 37° C for the collection tube. The glass cylinders and collection tube are preheated in an incubator.

For details concerning the aspiration needle, see chapter 12.8.10.

12.5. TECHNICAL EQUIPMENT FOR THERMAL HEMOSTASIS

The utilization of destructive heat results in an acceleration of the coagulation mechanism, primarily by heat-induced coagulation of protein. The first instrument for hemostasis was Paquelin's cautery. Since the 1920s, modern surgery utilizes heat that is induced in the body's tissues when high-frequency current travels through the human organism. The electrical current is introduced and concentrated on a specific active electrode, e.g., the electric knife, and dispersed through a large neutral plate attached to the patient's buttocks or thigh (Fig 96). Due to the skin effect, high-frequency current can induce fields of high current density, which can occur erratically and simultaneously at several areas in the abdominal cavity (Fig 97).

Consequently, accidents began occurring after the introduction of high-frequency current into operative pelviscopy for hemostasis and tubal sterilization. They occurred because the characteristics of high-frequency currents in their intra-abdominal endoscopic application were not clearly understood. For better comprehension of the basic reasons why high-frequency current cannot be used safely and effectively for endoscopic procedures in

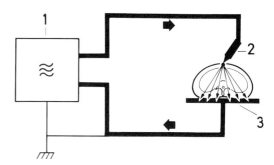

FIG 96.
In thermal hemostasis by high-frequency current, electrical energy *(1)* is concentrated on a specific active electrode *(2)* and is dispersed through a large plate *(3)* attached to the patient.

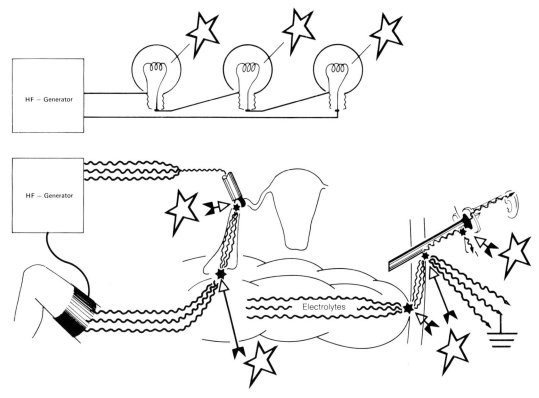

FIG 97.
High-frequency current induces erratic fields of high current density.

the abdominal cavity, its physical properties will again be summarized in the following section. For a comprehensive discussion, refer to pages 50–63 of the *Atlas of Gynecologic Laparoscopy and Hysteroscopy*.

12.5.1. Comments Regarding the Difference Between Hemostasis by High-Frequency Current in General Surgery and in Endoscopic Abdominal Surgery

The utilization of high-frequency current for hemostasis and cutting of animal and human tissues today is a generally accepted, widely used, and safe procedure in surgery, provided that isolation and explosion precautions are heeded. In the closed abdomen, however, the field of utilization is restricted (Semm, 1983). The experimental developments can best be followed by a historical survey, given below.

12.5.2. Historical Survey of the Utilization of Destructive Heat for Blood Coagulation

The first tubal sterilization by coagulation was done by Kocks in Bonn, Germany, in 1887; Kocks used galvanic current (a heated wire). Next, Werner in 1934 carried out high-frequency coagulation of the tubes by laparotomy, and Bösch in 1936 did the same in Switzerland by laparoscopy. In the 1960s it was primarily Frangenheim who recommended tubal sterilization by high-frequency current through the laparoscope. At the Second University Women's Hospital in Munich, Germany, all methods of tubal ligation by cutting and ligating, either by laparotomy or pelviscopy, were abandoned in 1964 in favor of the high-frequency current coagulation technique. We utilized only high-frequency generators with low energy output for this procedure. The Siemens high-frequency generator was most frequently used in Germany; its maximum output was 100 W. In most of our work we used only settings 1 and 2 (of a total of 10), i.e., approximately 10–30 W.

Gynecologic endoscopy had adopted high-frequency coagulation from general surgery, where it was used mainly on body surfaces (this also applied to the open abdomen!). Without much thought, this technique was transferred by the gynecologic endoscopists into the closed abdominal cavity. Although this method was used in only a few cases in Europe, since 1970, it spread like wildfire in the United States, particularly for tubal sterilization. In papers published in Europe, "coagulation of the tubes with high-frequency current, coagulation time at least 10–20 seconds" was recommended, but without any further data regarding the type of generator, current, or wattage.

In retrospect, this recommendation was scientifically incorrect. The inadequate information was based on the fact that high-frequency current could not be defined more accurately because the surgeons lacked sufficient experience with its intra-abdominal use at that time.

A comprehensive and meritorious discussion of the use of high-frequency current in medicine was first presented by Reidenbach (1983).

The danger of the use of high-frequency current in the closed abdominal cavity was first recognized in the United States. Why? In the United States, the surgeon also utilized high-frequency current from the generator that was the national standard, the Bovie high-frequency generator. This, however, had a maximum output of 350 W. At its lowest setting—position 1—this generator already had an output of 100 W. The destructive power of a 100-W electric heat output can be easily demonstrated (Fig 98): Try holding onto a burning 100-W light bulb—[Don't! But have you tried

to unscrew a 100-W light bulb that has just burned out?—*Ed.*] Now imagine prolonging this exposure for 10–20 seconds in the area of the adnexa in the closed abdomen!

Reports from the United States of the first accidents stimulated me at first to coagulate the tubes with the "bipolar forceps" of my tube set which, in 1962, we had assembled for tubal surgery under colposcopic/microscopic conditions. However, even in this form, the intra-abdominal use of high-frequency current is uncontrollable. Therefore, I recommended at the first Congress of the American Association of Gynecologic Laparoscopists (AAGL) in New Orleans, in 1972, that the use of high-frequency current for tubal sterilization in women be abandoned. As a useful substitute I offered a newly developed endocoagulation technique. With this method the human body has no direct contact with electrical current. In the decade that followed, it was shown that the endocoagulation technique has considerable advantages over high-frequency current.

12.5.3. Biophysical Reasons Not To Use High-Frequency Currents in the Closed Abdominal Cavity

Man uses electromagnetic waves in medicine within a broad range of frequencies, e.g., long wave to short wave radio, television, diathermy, röentgen rays, laser, to name just a few frequency ranges or areas of utilization. The high-frequency current within the range of 100 kHz to 300 MHz is used in surgery to produce destructive heat, to cut, and to make blood coagulate.

For conduction of electromagnetic waves, primarily conductors of the first order (i.e., metals)

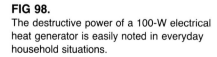

FIG 98.
The destructive power of a 100-W electrical heat generator is easily noted in everyday household situations.

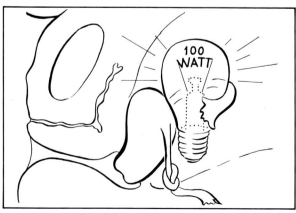

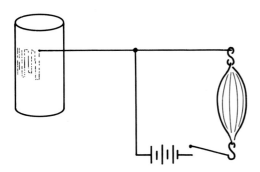

FIG 99.
Schematic of Luigi Galvani's experimental apparatus for his discovery of "animal electricity," Nov. 6, 1789.

are used. In the human body there are conductors of the second order (i.e., electrolytes), which conduct the electrical current in nerves, blood vessels, intestinal contents, muscles, and so forth. A brief historical survey will be given to define the physical properties of high-frequency current.

In 1789, Galvani was experimenting on frog legs when he discovered "animal electricity" (Fig 99). In 1831, Faraday discovered magnetic inductance (Fig 100) and laid the foundation for the introduction of alternating currents, and with it, high-frequency current. In 1860, Pflüger's law on muscle contractions in response to electrical stimulation was published. Hertz discovered electromagnetic waves in 1891, and Tesla, in the same year, the high-frequency transformer. In 1899, Nernst formulated the law which is named after him: $D = \sqrt{F/n}$, i.e., the electrical current required to stimulate muscle action (D) in the human body is inversely proportional to the square root of its frequency (n); in other words, the higher the frequency, the lower the stimulating effect.

This phenomenon has been further investigated in physics, and we refer to the *skin effect* when we talk about the effect of high-frequency current. What is the skin effect?

Figure 101 demonstrates Faraday's law: flux of current induces a magnetic field around the conductor that is directed according to the right-hand rule. Figure 102 also shows the negative feedback named after Lenz: the effect tends to oppose its source. In our case, this means that the eddy currents induced by the change in the magnetic field are counter-rotating with respect to the direction of the induced current. This will force the electrical current—as shown in Figure 103—to migrate out of the conductor onto its surface as the frequency increases. This is the skin effect. Figure 104 shows the same in the form of a mathematical formula that the skin effect increases with rising frequency. The effects of the direction of eddy currents—low and high frequency—are again shown in graphic form in Figure 105.

Transferred to medical application, this means that electrical current is conducted in nerves, and triggers contractions of muscle cells. In higher concentrations it induces electrolysis in animal cells, i.e., breakdown of water into hydrogen and oxygen. With increasing frequency, however, the electrical current no longer travels within or through the cell (i.e., animal tissues) but only on its surface. Stimulation of nerves, polarization of cell membranes, electrolysis, and the like do not occur, i.e., the body no longer reacts biologically but serves only as a conductor for the current. As such, it is subject to physical laws, i.e., it becomes warmer according to the field density of the electrical current.

If these physical data are combined, it is plausible that this current is not harmful to humans as long as it can migrate on the body's surface dependent on its surface characteristics. This phenomenon is frequently demonstrated at county fairs (Fig 106): a light bulb is held to the tip of the nose of one of the spectators and lights up, without, as one might have expected, electrocuting him.

However, if we force this current (see Figs 1, 96, and 97) to travel through the human body, we make it behave schizophrenically: as "current" it necessarily takes the route of least resistance and flows in tissues with a high electrolyte content (nerves, blood vessels, intestinal contents, etc.), while in accordance with the skin effect, it travels only on the surface of these structures.

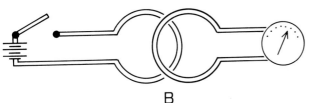

B

FIG 100.
Schematic of Michael Faraday's experimental apparatus for his discovery of magnetic inductance, Aug. 29, 1831; switching current on and off changes magnetic field *(B)*, inducing current pulse on secondary side.

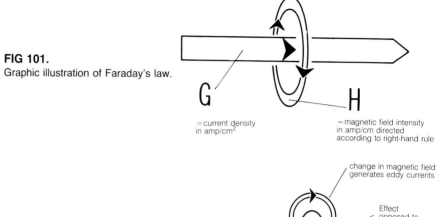

FIG 101.
Graphic illustration of Faraday's law.

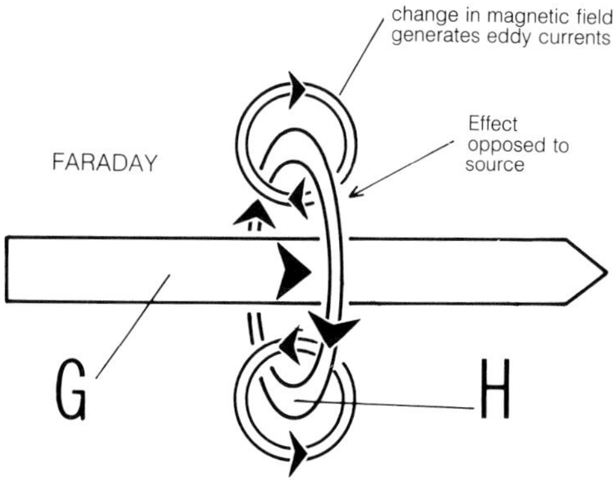

G
= current density
in amp/cm²

H
= magnetic field intensity
in amp/cm directed
according to right-hand rule

change in magnetic field
generates eddy currents

Effect
opposed to
source

FARADAY

FIG 102.
Cause of skin effect (Lenz's law).

G   H

FIG 103.
High-frequency current—skin effect.

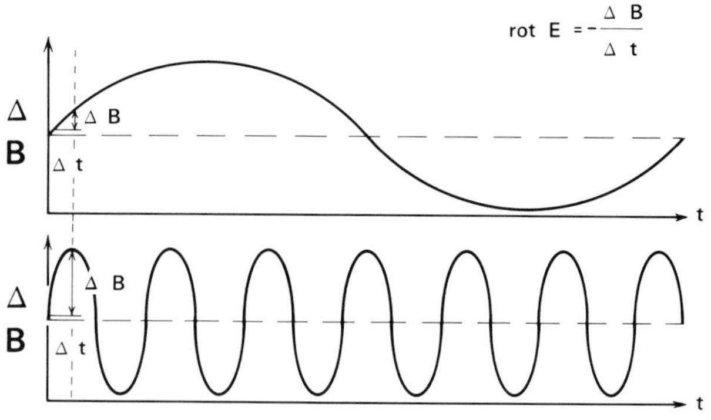

Direct current
≈ 100 kHz
Alternating current
> 100 MHz

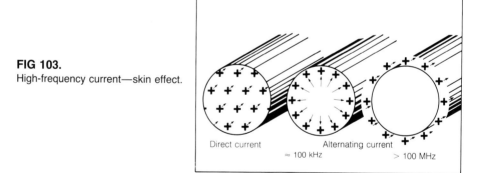

$$rot\ E = -\frac{\Delta B}{\Delta t}$$

Δ
B
ΔB
Δt

FIG 104.
Increasing skin effect with rising frequency.

Δ
B
ΔB
Δt

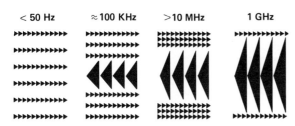

FIG 105.
Effects of the direction of eddy currents.

Migration of electrical current to the surface of the conductor according to

▶▶▶▶▶▶▶ = Current $\left\{ = rot\ E = -\dfrac{\Delta\ B}{\Delta\ t} \right.$

Since a seemingly bizarre network of conductors exists in a living organism, it is easily understandable that the high-frequency current reaches the return electrode via completely unpredictable pathways. Additionally, the electrolyte content changes constantly in one and the same organism, even with every heartbeat and the passage of current: i.e., pathways for the current also fluctuate.

In essence, in medicine, we distinguish between three different possibilities of producing destructive heat by high frequency:

Fulguration (Fig 107): In this case, electromagnetic waves induce spark discharge between the tip of the electrode and the surface of the organ across a bridge of air, i.e., without direct contact between the two. In this case, the development of heat is limited to tissue surface—the optically visible area of spark dispersion.

Coagulation (Fig 108): This denotes heating of the tissue until it actually cooks (see Fig 111) under the influence of the increasing electrical field density of the high-frequency current.

Electrotomy (Fig 109): This is the term for severing tissues with the so-called "electric knife" or the "electric loop." The type of cut—clean or crusty margin—depends on the type of current or the design of the high-frequency generator. Smooth electrotomy cuts are produced by an interrupted undamped or rectified undamped high-frequency current generated by tube-type or transistor-type generators (*1* in Fig 109). If a damped wave form, one that is used exclusively for fulguration, is superimposed on an undamped current (*2* in Fig 109), it causes a severe heating effect in the tissue to the point of boiling and, with that, an ex-

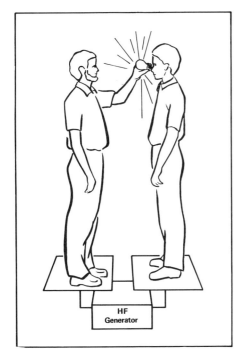

FIG 106.
A migrating current need not be harmful to man.

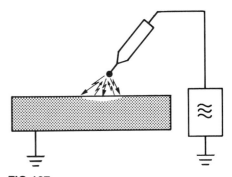

FIG 107.
Fulguration.

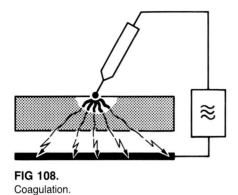

FIG 108.
Coagulation.

plosion of the cells, leaving a crust on the cut surface.

The electrolyte content of nerves, bowel contents, blood vessels, muscles, fatty tissue, tendons, and bones varies by several orders of magnitude. Therefore, the magnitude of destructive heat which the high-frequency current produces in the organism as a function of voltage and amperage can neither be predicted nor measured. Figure 110 shows in graphic form the effect produced by high-frequency current when it travels from the neutral

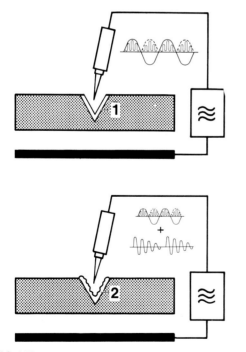

FIG 109.
Electrotomotomy (cutting): *1*, clean margin of cut; *2*, crusty margin of cut.

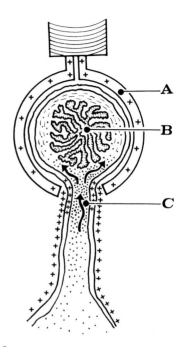

FIG 110.
Effect of heat produced by high-frequency current when it travels from the neutral electrode to the specific active electrode (A). The peritubal peritoneum (C) is rapidly heated; the tubal lumen (B) is heated less.

electrode (e.g., on the thigh) to the specific active electrode (*A* in Fig 110) on the tube: the highest degree of destructive heat develops at the point of highest current density (*C* in Fig 110). It first causes boiling of the water in tissues, followed by the explosion of cells by the evaporation of the water in the tissue (Fig 111). Due to the skin effect, only the peritubal peritoneum (*C* in Fig 110) is very rapidly heated to the boiling point, exsiccated, and possibly carbonized by spark formation (i.e., by temperatures up to 800° C). This will gradually decrease the coagulation current until, finally, a point of complete insulation is reached, i.e., the termination of the current flow and coagulation process. The tubal lumen (*B* in Fig 110) will certainly not reach the boiling point during the first intensive boiling process of the peritubal peritoneum.

Destructive heat will reach the tubal lumen only during the second phase by convection of heat from the metallic jaws of the coagulation forceps, which had been heated at the same time (*A* in Fig 110).

Therefore, the paradoxical recommendation to coagulate for 10–20 seconds has evolved empiri-

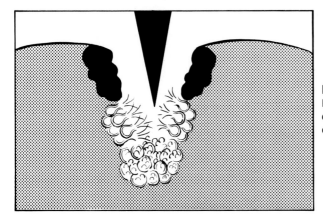

FIG 111.
Destructive heat at point of highest current density causes tissue water to boil and cells to explode.

cally and not from theoretical considerations. The fact that, in spite of this, the tubal lumen is not completely denatured is shown in Plates 310 and 311, which document a gravid uterus of 2–3 months' gestational size, although both tubes were almost completely absent.

If this exsiccation or carbonization effect, i.e., the insulation effect, occurs relatively late due to low electrolyte content within the tube, the adjacent tissues (adnexa, ureter, bowel, etc.) may sustain invisible heat effects when the *critical temperature of 57° C (135° F)* is exceeded. This temperature denatures thermolabile enzymes and induces thermal necrosis. As shown in Figures 1 and 97, this is possible at multiple unpredictable sites between the neutral and active electrodes.

Since the conductance (electrolyte content) of adnexal tissue and intestinal content is not predictable, even the most meticulous surgeon cannot estimate by visual inspection alone and with reasonable certainty the site and degree of coagulation.

A Practical Example:

During an emergency repeat cesarean section in Kiel, both tubes were lifted from the abdomen and coagulated for 10 seconds each with unipolar high-frequency current of approximately 40 W intensity. After the tubes had cooled, they were replaced into the abdomen and the cesarean section was completed. Two days postoperatively two defects had to be removed: one area of coagulation necrosis with a hole of more than 3 cm diameter on the transverse colon, and one of about 2.5 cm diameter in the ilium.

Reconstruction of the case:

The patient had to undergo a cesarean section for a prolapse of the umbilical cord at 4:30 A.M.

and without preparation. After the abdomen was opened, her bowels were displaced cranially with packs saturated with physiologic saline solution. The high-frequency current was conducted through bowels filled with material with a high content of electrolytes, across the packs saturated with saline solution, to the tubes positioned outside the abdominal walls. At the exit site from the bowel, heating above the critical temperature of 57° C occurred. This initiated the thermal necrosis of the intestinal wall. The patient survived.

The application of so-called bipolar high-frequency currents (Fig 112) prevents necrosis distant from the tube. If very low energy levels are used and coagulation is extended over a long time, the current may be forced to coagulate the tubes completely. If higher energy levels are used, the skin effect dominates again: the current coagulates beyond the immediate contact with the metal forceps. Aberration of the high-frequency current over 1–3 cm beyond the contact area between the jaws of the forceps and tissue has been reported, including

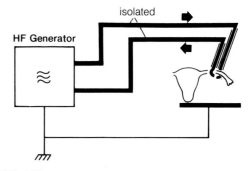

FIG 112.
Use of bipolar high-frequency current prevents distant necroses.

coagulation of the ureter ("law of least resistance").

During the coagulation, uncontrollable temperatures of over 140° C may occur between the prongs of the metal forceps. This heat transforms proteins into glue, and tissues adhere to the forceps. If they are forcefully removed, they tear primarily in the area which has barely been coagulated, i.e., in viable tissue. There is some bleeding from the torn vessels, which have not yet been completely coagulated. Hence, bipolar coagulation is an insufficient method. It may accomplish sterilization of the tubes if one is willing to accept destruction of the vascular and nervous supply to the ovaries (see also chapter 14.2.15. ff. and Figs 113–115).

12.5.4. Biologic Changes in the Area of the Adnexa After Utilization of High-Frequency Coagulation: Follow-up of 1,003 Sterilized Patients

In fear of legal consequences due to poststerilization pregnancies, we recommended, as early as the beginning of the 1960s, that high-frequency current be applied long enough to completely coagulate the tubes. The results of these measures are shown in Plates 302 and 303: the tubes have been transformed into a filiform strand of fibrous scar tissue except for the ampullary end. As we (Semm and Philipp, 1980) could prove experimentally with the electron microscope, even this apparently almost complete coagulation of the tubes does not result in 100% sterility (skin effect). The photographs show clearly that even the ovarian vasculature has been damaged severely. The extent of damage that can be caused in this area by tubal sterilization with unipolar high-frequency current is shown schematically in Figure 113.

The *arterial network that supplies the tube and ovary* is shown in Figure 114. The segments labeled in the diagram are as follows: *1*, uterine artery; *2*, ovarian artery; *3*, tubal branch of uterine artery; *4*, ovarian branch of uterine artery; *5*, arcade of subovarian anastomoses; *6*, lateral tubal branch of ovarian artery; *7*, arteries to the lateral pole of ovary; *8*, anastomoses between the lateral tubal artery and the subtubal arcade; *9*, middle tubal branch of ovarian artery; *10*, subtubal arcade; *11*, ampullary distribution of distal tubal artery (according to Palmer et al., 1981).

If the passage of "unipolar" high-frequency current through the body is avoided and, instead,

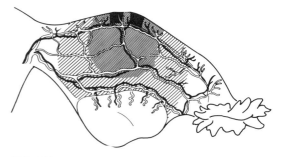

FIG 113.
Extent of damage caused by tubal sterilization with unipolar high-frequency current.

the "bipolar" variation is used (Fig 115), the areas of tissue that are destroyed by heat are reduced considerably, as shown in Figure 115 and Plate 306.

In any case, the utilization of high-frequency current unnecessarily damages additional adnexal tissues, which are of considerable importance for the arterial and venous blood supply (Fig 116) and the nervous supply of the ovaries. This has serious consequences for the future endocrine function of sterilized women, as clearly shown in cases of "poststerilization syndrome."

The effects of two different techniques of tubal sterilization—the unipolar high-frequency method and the endocoagulation method according to Semm—which were performed at the University

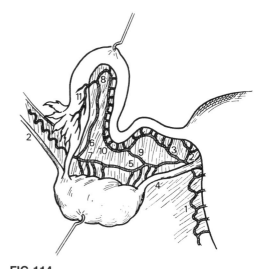

FIG 114.
Arterial network supplying the tube and ovary. See text for description of labeled segments.

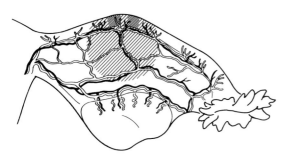

FIG 115.
Extent of damage caused by bipolar high-frequency current.

Women's Hospital in Kiel, Germany, during the period 1970–1978 were evaluated by follow-up questionnaires (Riedel and Semm, 1981). The main concern was the registration of late postoperative complications.

Of 1,136 questionnaires mailed out, 644 could be evaluated. Of these respondents, 258 had been sterilized by the unipolar high-frequency technique and 386 by the endocoagulation method. It should be emphasized that in the beginning, i.e., since 1973, the year the change occurred at the University Women's Hospital in Kiel, from the high-frequency technique to the endocoagulation method, the tubes were also coagulated very "radically" at multiple sites to prevent recanalization. This was done both as a precautionary measure, to prevent future pregnancies, and because the effectiveness of the endocoagulation method was not yet known. The results of a postoperative follow-up, if done today, would probably be even more favorable be-

cause, since 1978, we have limited coagulation to the muscular tubal wall and avoided damage to the mesosalpinx (Fig 117), as shown in Plate 308.

After high-frequency current sterilization ($n = 258$), 23 women (8.9%) had to have a hysterectomy within 3.1 years; in the endocoagulation group ($n = 386$) only 9 women (2.3%) needed one, although we had continued until 1977—even with endocoagulation—our usual, very "radical" practice of coagulating to the point of macroscopically visible effects, as we had done with the high-frequency method (Table 5).

Of 258 patients sterilized by the high-frequency unipolar method, 7.8% required one to three D&C procedures during the succeeding years, whereas a D&C was necessary in only 2.6% of women sterilized by the endocoagulation method.

Seventy-nine (30.6%) of patients who had been sterilized by unipolar high-frequency current reported menstrual disturbances during the following years. In the group sterilized by Semm's endocoagulation technique, there were only 45 (11.7%) with such complaints.

The combination of changes in the frequency of menstrual periods and premature onset of menopausal symptoms (Table 6) was found in 4.7% of the group sterilized by high-frequency current. In the endocoagulation group, this combination occurred in only 3.4% of women (Table 7). Menopausal symptoms alone, i.e., without simultaneous disturbances in the frequency of menstrual periods, were found in 7.4% and 2.8% of sterilized women, respectively.

In summary, 85.5% (330) of women who had

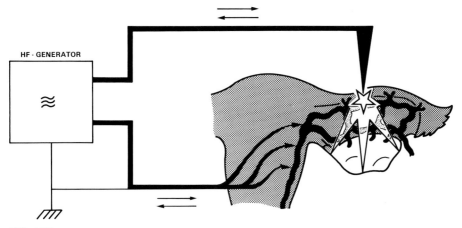

HF - GENERATOR

FIG 116.
High-frequency current unnecessarily damages additional adnexal tissues.

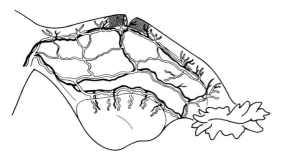

FIG 117.
Since 1978, Semm's group has limited coagulation to the muscular tubal wall.

been sterilized by the endocoagulation method experienced no disturbances in menstrual frequency and no menopausal symptoms during the follow-up. In the group sterilized by high-frequency current, such sequelae did *not* occur during the follow-up years in only 160 women (62% of women sterilized).

12.5.5. Compelling Medical Reasons Not To Use High-Frequency Current in the Closed Abdomen (in Pelviscopy/Laparoscopy)

From a biophysical point of view, the above discussions seem compelling enough to draw the following medical conclusions:

1. Modern technology to measure energy is now available and should be applied in medicine. In the case of tissue coagulation, the application of heat should no longer be estimated subjectively by the surgeons's eye (e.g., according to the discoloration of the tissue) but should be measured ex-

actly, as shown in Figure 118. However, the transformation of high-frequency current into thermal energy in the human body, which was discussed at length, cannot be measured.

2. The skin effect impedes the penetration of high-frequency current into the tubal lumen; the endosalpinx frequently is not coagulated by the effect of the electrical current but only secondarily by heat conduction (see Fig 110). If such heat conduction does not occur, recanalization is possible.

3. High-frequency current, particularly the unipolar type, may cause serious disturbances of the reproductive and hormonal function of the ovarian metabolism by the destruction of the ovarian blood vessels and their nervous supply.

4. Inherent in the use of high-frequency current is the risk of burn injuries to bowel, ureter, abdominal wall, etc., which, in spite of most careful adherence to meticulous technique, cannot be controlled by the surgeon.

5. Since high-frequency current cannot be controlled or measured accurately, it is not very useful for endoscopic intra-abdominal hemostasis.

If all these points are summarized, there are compelling biophysical and medical considerations why the therapeutic use of high-frequency current can no longer be considered safe in the closed abdominal cavity.

Today, it is no longer the method of choice to utilize human tissues as electrical resistance to produce destructive heat from the electrical current for hemostasis during an endoscopic procedure. With the availability of the endocoagulation technique

TABLE 5.

Postoperative Follow-up: High-Frequency Sterilization vs. Endocoagulation*

	POSTOPERATIVE			
	HYSTERECTOMY†		FRACTIONAL D&C‡	
STERILIZATION GROUP	NO. OF PTS.	(%)	NO. OF PTS.	(%)
Unipolar high-frequency coagulation (*n* = 258)	22	(8.9)	20	(7.8)
Endocoagulation (*n* = 386)	9	(2.3)	10	(2.6)
	P<.004		*P*<.005	

*Division of Gynecology, University of Kiel, Germany.
†Follow-up (mean): after HF coagulation, 3.1 years; after endocoagulation, 2.8 years.
‡Follow-up (mean): after HF coagulation, 2.9 years; after endocoagulation, 2.6 years.

TABLE 6.
Postoperative Follow-up After High-Frequency Sterilization*

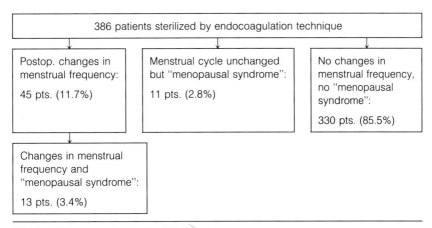

*Division of Gynecology, University of Kiel, Germany.

described below, the use of high-frequency current to produce heat for hemostasis would no longer be needed.

[Although I agree with Semm in principle, it is more realistic to assume that both bipolar and unipolar high-frequency techniques will not vanish suddenly from the endoscopic scene. It is more likely that they will never be replaced completely. Therefore, I consider it my editorial duty to append a few precautionary comments and warnings similar to those recommended by the Ob-Gyn Advisory Panel to the FDA and distributed by manufacturers

of instruments and technical equipment for high-frequency coagulation.

The metal trocar sleeve for insertion of 7-mm and larger laparoscopes should be used with an electrosurgical unit of 600 volts peak, 100 W of power at 200–500 ohms nonreactive resistance.

If an electrosurgical unit of high output rating is used, then a nonconductive trocar sleeve should be used for the primary puncture.

Under no circumstances should laparoscopy be performed with a spark-gap unit. High peak voltages of such units may result in excessive tis-

TABLE 7.
Postoperative Follow-up After Sterilization by Endocoagulation*

(258 patients sterilized by HF technique — see Table 6)

386 patients sterilized by endocoagulation technique

Postop. changes in menstrual frequency: 45 pts. (11.7%)

Menstrual cycle unchanged but "menopausal syndrome": 11 pts. (2.8%)

No changes in menstrual frequency, no "menopausal syndrome": 330 pts. (85.5%)

Changes in menstrual frequency and "menopausal syndrome": 13 pts. (3.4%)

*Division of Gynecology, University of Kiel, Germany.

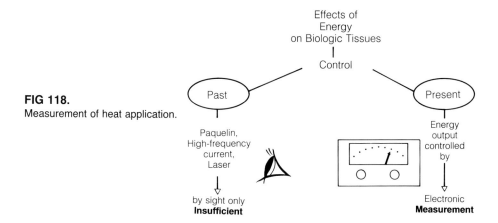

FIG 118.
Measurement of heat application.

sue destruction and possible bowel perforation and other electrical injuries.

For secondary punctures of less than 7 mm outer diameter, a nonconductive trocar sleeve should be used.

Do not use kinked or bent patient plates. Affix the plate (or disposable grounding pad) firmly to the patient's thigh to ensure a large skin contact area.

Connecting cables for the patient plate and the active electrodes must be checked before each use to ensure their faultlessness.

Insulated instruments must be checked before each use. Any breaks in insulation make an instrument potentially dangerous.

Use a power setting on the electrosurgical unit only as high as required by the surgical procedure. Consult the manufacturer of the electrosurgical unit for suggested setting. If desired effects are not achieved within the suggested setting range, *do not increase the setting* before verifying the following:

   a. the patient plate is properly fastened;
   b. all insulation is faultless;
   c. all cables and plugs are faultless;
   d. instrument tips are free of encrusted tissue.

Unwanted coagulation may be avoided by observing the following rules:

   a. apply high-frequency current only after the active electrode is in complete contact with the tissue to be coagulated;
   b. do not allow the active electrode to come into contact with any metal portion of any other instrument;

   c. do not allow the tissue to be coagulated to come into contact with any other tissue;
   d. coagulate tubular tissue (e.g., fallopian tubes) at the thinnest portion.

Follow the recommendations and instructions of the manufacturer of the high-frequency electrical surgical unit and contact that manufacturer if you have any questions about your electrosurgical unit.

Do not mix and match instruments and equipment of different manufacturers without proof that they are compatible.—*Ed.*]

12.5.6. Equipment for Controlled Endocoagulation

The experience gathered from several million tubal sterilizations by high-frequency current, particularly in the United States, were analyzed for accidents that have occurred with this method. We felt compelled to look for new ways and developed new instruments and equipment. Although they also utilize destructive heat for hemostatic purposes, they increase the temperature in the body's tissues only by convection. The human body has no contact with the electrical current, eliminating the electrical risk.

During a 10-year period of development of these devices and instruments, different systems were developed for control of the energy output at the site of coagulation. After experimental testing they were utilized in man.

12.5.6.1. Instruments for Endocoagulation

Today Semm's endocoagulation method entails the use of a well-designed and proven set of coagulation instruments for intra-abdominal endoscopic use.

The control device, the endocoagulator (Fig 119), is switched on and off by a pneumatic foot switch that does not use any electricity. The desired coagulation temperature can be preselected continuously in the range of 90°–120° C (total temperature range that can be regulated is 20°–160° C); the coagulation time, which is coupled to an acoustic signal, can also be preselected. The surgeon monitors only the screeching sound, which increases and decreases in pitch according to the temperature. It gives information about the coagulation temperature and the coagulation time. The screeching sound is switched off automatically when the temperature of the instrument, i.e., the tip of the coagulation probe, or the cutting edge of the myoma enucleator, or the heated jaw of the crocodile forceps, has cooled to a temperature below 60° C.

The important new feature in the construction of these coagulation instruments (crocodile forceps, point coagulator, myoma enucleator, see Fig 120) is that they have been miniaturized. The heated mass of metal has been reduced to a minimum. Therefore, the instrument cools down immediately after the heating cycle is switched off.

If any tissues are touched inadvertently, and provided that the heating cycle is turned off, no penetrating burn will result because the heated mass of the instrument is too small to release much heat by convection. The temperature rise which occurs in the tip of the therapeutic instrument can be monitored by the scrub nurse, who observes the pointer on the large scale thermometer. In addition, the built-in synchronous timer beeps every 5 seconds. The combination of acoustical and optical indicators for the heating cycle, which is triggered by a nonelectrical, pneumatic foot switch, is the optimum safety system for the patient that is technically achievable today.

The blind and uncontrolled burn by high-frequency current can now be replaced by the aimed and measured coagulation of protein: the coagulation effect can be very accurately confined to a small target area (see Fig 118).

If the temperature in the tissue is increased slowly by the radiation and convection of heat (Fig 121) (perhaps comparable to frying an egg in a skillet), the healing process is completely different from the healing that occurred after a burn with high-frequency current.

12.5.6.2. Histologic Changes After Heat-Induced Hemostasis

If animal tissue is heated above 120° C its protein is first transformed into a glue-like substance (soap boiler effect). If the temperature rises fur-

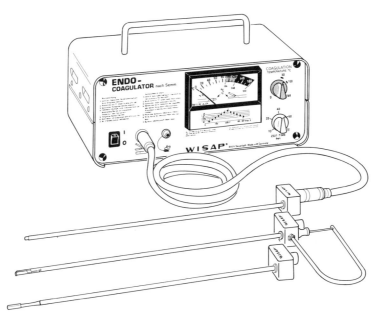

FIG 119.
The endocoagulator developed by Semm.

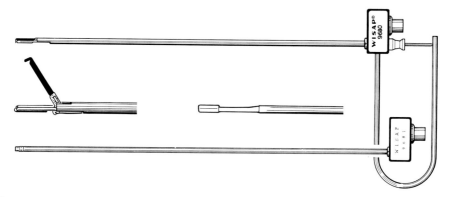

FIG 120.
The endocoagulation instruments developed by Semm: crocodile forceps, myoma enucleator, point coagulator.

ther, exsiccation and then carbonization occur, which can be clearly observed with tubal coagulation by high-frequency current (Plate 4). The tissue destroyed by such biologic measures sloughs off in a few days (Plate 5). An open wound results, which will be covered by a fibrinous exudate into which histiocytes and fibroblasts will migrate. Such an intra-abdominal wound is an ideal tissue for the formation of peritoneal adhesions.

Experiments have shown that protein that has been coagulated by the new endocoagulation method at the temperature of boiling water will not slough off (Plates 6 and 312 ff.). There is no exudation of fibrin, and histiocytes and fibroblasts migrate from the margin into this heat-coagulated protein.

Since such a tissue defect remains covered by dead tissue, which stimulates the regeneration process, the peritoneum cannot attach itself. The biologic requirements for the formation of adhesions are not present.

During the 10 years of our experience with this method, we demonstrated experimentally that coagulation of protein (comparable to the boiling

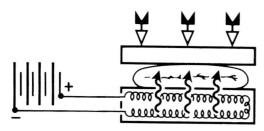

FIG 121.
Tissue temperature is increased slowly through radiating and convected heat.

of a breakfast egg) results, on the one hand, in absolute hemostasis but, on the other hand, such "wounds" have no tendency to form peritoneal adhesions. Experimental proof is particularly striking. This has been most clearly proved experimentally by enucleation of subserous myomas on the uterine corpus. Perfect hemostasis by endocoagulation causes coagulation changes up to 3 cm in diameter (see Plates 221–261); however, in multiple repeat pelviscopies (see Plates 223, 224, 237, and 243), no adhesions have yet been observed.

For this reason, we have introduced the endocoagulation technique for hemostatic purposes on the uterine corpus, even with laparotomies. It is well known that postoperative intestinal adhesions usually occur after myomectomies and closure of a uterine wound by single sutures, even if they are buried subserosally.

If the cervical coagulator (Fig 122) and the large coagulation probe are utilized, hemostasis is achieved even in large wounds on the uterine corpus. In contrast to wounds that are closed by sutures, those treated by endocoagulation remain free of adhesions.

In summary, it should be stated that the utilization of destructive heat for hemostatic purposes by endocoagulation works well. However, for intra-abdominal surgery it is only a substitute.

For decades, high-frequency coagulation was the only means of achieving hemostasis during endoscopic intra-abdominal surgery without resorting to laparotomy. A prerequisite for therapeutic success, however, was the presence of sufficient protein for coagulation in relation to the source of bleeding. Any bleeding in the omentum, for instance, is difficult to control by destructive heat.

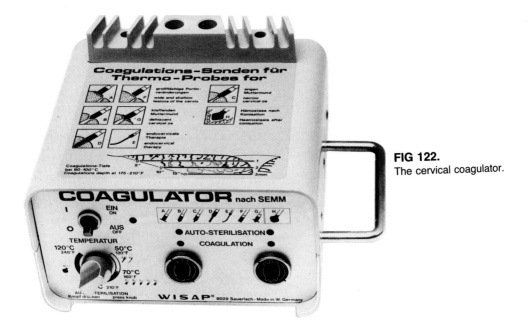

FIG 122.
The cervical coagulator.

Fat, which is present in large quantities, may at best fry the vascular wall, so that its curling and retraction may cause closure of the vessel. However, since no protein coagulation occurs, the risk of delayed hemorrhage is great.

After all thermotechnical possibilities had been exhausted experimentally, we developed additional methods for endoscopic abdominal surgery which are identical to the classic methods of hemostasis in surgery, i.e., endoscopic ligature and suture as described in chapter 12.6. ff.

12.6. INSTRUMENTS AND METHODS FOR CONVENTIONAL HEMOSTASIS BY LIGATURE AND SUTURE

Until recently, suturing endoscopically in the abdominal cavity was considered impossible. Endoscopic hemostasis by high-frequency current, how-

ever, had always been viewed as a substitute for classic suturing and ligating techniques. In abdominal surgery, hemorrhages are usually controlled with various suture materials. Since thermal methods were acceptable substitutes only in some areas, but were too dangerous in others, we developed suture material, applicators, and needleholders with which classic methods of hemostasis can also be applied endoscopically in the abdominal cavity.

12.6.1. Hemostasis by Loop Ligature

The loop with slipknot, which at the end of the last century was described by Roeder for tonsillectomy in children, is an important addition to the techniques employed in endoscopic intra-abdominal surgery. It is commercially available as "Endoloop" (Ethicon, Inc.); various catgut strengths are available in sterile packages. The endoloop is introduced into an applicator (Fig 123), which will fit through a 5-mm trocar sleeve for endoscopic

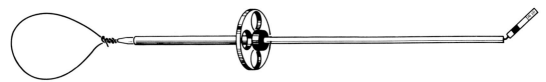

FIG 123.
Endoloop with its applicator.

work. The loop is introduced into the abdomen (Plate 7) and is used to control omental and adnexal hemorrhages. After ligation, its long end is cut (Plate 8) and the redundant tissue is resected (Plate 9). One requirement is that the tissue to be ligated can be grasped and pulled through the loop (Fig 124). The slipknot of this catgut suture material has proved to be very reliable for several decades. It has been used in thousands of applications, such as bleeding in the depth of the pelvis during Wertheim's operation and for the ligature of points of distant hemorrhage during vaginal procedures. After the catgut suture absorbs water and swells, the knot holds tightly. A knot in suture material that does not swell is insecure; in essence, Roeder's slipknot is only a modified throw knot, a reason why this knot should only be tied in catgut!

The endoloop (Fig 125) is commercially available in a sterile pack. The slipknot has already been tied and the long end is threaded through a plastic push rod and can be used as standard ligature for endoscopic oophorectomy (see chapter 14.2.7.) or salpingo-oophorectomy (see chapter 14.2.8.) and salpingectomy (see chapters 14.2.9. and 14.2.11.2.). For safety reasons, we always apply three endoloops when we resect these organs (ovary, adnexa, and tube).

We call this new type of gynecologic organ resection *endoscopic triple-loop technique*. It is also employed with appendectomy (see chapter 15.3. ff.) because it saves time.

After adhesiolysis, bleeding omental tissue is easily ligated (see Plates 7–9 and 19–22). However, it is preferable to ligate vascularized omental adhesions before their sharp transection, as is also

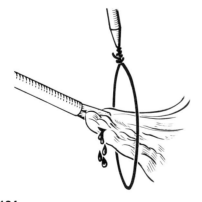

FIG 124.
The tissue to be ligated must be grasped and pulled through the loop.

customary in general abdominal surgery. This will be described in the next section.

12.6.2. Hemostasis by Endoligature and External Tying of Knots

Occasionally it is not possible to use the loop ligature described in chapter 12.6.1. for hemostasis. As in general surgery, it is necessary to ligate vascular bridges of adhesions, such as broad-based postoperative adhesions of the omentum to the anterior abdominal wall, prior to their transection. Due to contraction of the omentum after transection, the source of bleeding in the omentum is frequently very difficult to reidentify; this precludes pulling the bleeding area through the endoloop to control bleeding. It certainly pays off to ligate vascularized omental and intestinal adhesions before they are transected, because the search for a bleeding vessel is time-consuming and may be accompanied by considerable loss of blood. For such measures we developed the "open Roeder loop" as an endoligation technique. As material for the ligature we use the commercially available endosuture (Fig 126). This is a sterile catgut suture approximately 80 cm long that is supplied with a plastic push rod for the knot; it is armed with a straight, 3-cm-long needle of 0.8 mm diameter.

To be used as endoligature, the needle is cut off and the suture material is introduced into the abdominal cavity through a suture applicator (Fig 127), which fits inside a 5-mm trocar sleeve, as shown in Figures 136 and 137. The endoligature is applied and a slipknot is tied externally according to the technique demonstrated in Figures 128–134.

The catgut suture material (see Fig 126) is introduced into the abdomen (see Fig 128) with a 3-mm needleholder (see chapter 12.8.7.) through the same applicator (see Figs 123 and 127) which was designed for the introduction of the endoloop. In the abdominal cavity, the catgut is grasped with the 5-mm needleholder (see Fig 129), which guides it around the band of adhesions to be ligated. After the end of the suture has been regrasped with the 3-mm needleholder (see Fig 130) the catgut suture is withdrawn through the suture applicator out of the abdomen.

During this procedure, the conical seal attached to the shaft of the 3-mm needleholder (see Fig 141) has been pushed against the rubber seal of the suture applicator to further reduce the loss of gas. After the 3-mm needleholder has been

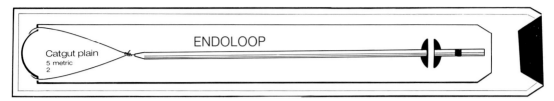

FIG 125.
Endoloop in sterile package.

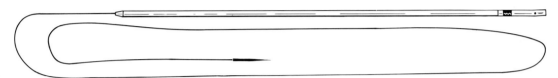

FIG 126.
Commercially available endosuture is made of catgut and comes supplied with a plastic push rod and a 3-cm long needle 0.8 mm in diameter.

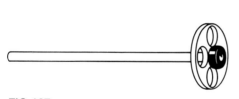

FIG 127.
Applicator for endoloop and endosuture.

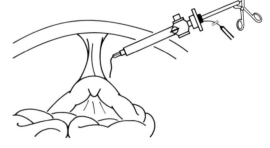

FIG 128.
Suture material is introduced into abdomen with a 3-mm needle holder.

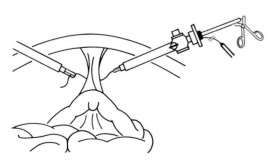

FIG 129.
End of suture material is grasped with a 5-mm needle-holder.

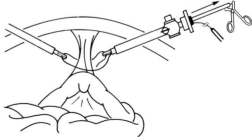

FIG 130.
Same end is guided around adhesion and regrasped with 3-mm needleholder; then the catgut is withdrawn out of the abdomen through the suture applicator.

withdrawn, the orifice in the rubber seal is closed with a finger, above which the slipknot is tied (see Fig 131). The applicator is then pulled upward so that the externally tied knot is fed into the plastic sleeve, which is then pushed back into the abdomen (see Fig 132). Under vision through the endoscope, the loop is tightened by the surgeon placing strong traction on the free end of the suture and simultaneously pressing with the plastic applicator rod against the knot. The long end is then cut with hook scissors (see Fig 133).

Occasionally, as is done with a laparotomy (see guiding principle on page 4), two loops are applied before the tissue is transected between them to avoid blood loss, as shown in Plates 31 and 353.

For safety reasons, the transected stump may be religated with an endoloop (see Plates 7–9). Figure 134, with schematic drawings 1–4, again demonstrates the four phases of the technique for tying an external slipknot.

12.6.3. Hemostasis by Endosuture With External or Internal Tying of Knots

The options for endoscopic procedures were extended considerably when we began to suture endoscopically. The endosuture (see Fig 126) is again used as suture material. It is available in two strengths. In principle, everything that can be grasped well with needleholders can be sutured. The possibility of low-power magnification with loupes (see chapter 12.2.4.) permits better placement of a needle than during a laparotomy.

Figures 135–145 demonstrate the use of the endosuture and external tying of the slipknot, using the example of an ovarian suture. A gaping ovarian wound resulted from the excision of an ovarian cyst (Fig 135). The catgut endosuture (Fig 136) is grasped with a 3-mm needleholder and is intro-

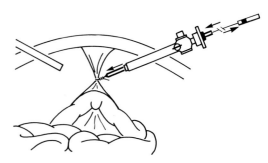

FIG 132.
The slipknot is fed into the applicator and then pushed back into the abdomen with the plastic pushrod while pulling on the external end of the suture.

duced through the applicator into the abdominal cavity. After the needle and suture have arrived in the abdominal cavity (Fig 137), the 5-mm needleholder first receives the needle and presents it in the proper position to the 3-mm needleholder, which grasps the needle so that it is aligned with one of the grooves and can be held securely at a right angle to the jaws of the needleholder. With the assistance of the 5-mm needleholder (Fig 138) the needle is pushed through the wound edge. After the needle is regrasped by the 3-mm needleholder, the needle is pushed through the opposite wound edge (Fig 139) and is pulled through by the 5-mm needleholder, then returned to the 3-mm needleholder that grasps the suture at a small distance from the needle and retracts both through the applicator (Fig 140). Before this is done, however, it is necessary that almost the entire length of the suture be pushed alongside the 3-mm needleholder into the abdomen. During suturing, the adjustable cone on the shaft of the 3-mm needleholder is closed up against the rubber sealing ring of the applicator (Fig 141) to prevent the loss of large quantities of gas.

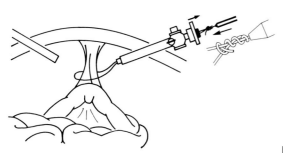

FIG 131.
A slipknot is tied externally.

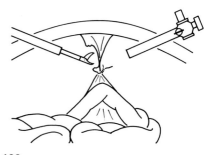

FIG 133.
The loop is tightened, its long end and adhesion are cut with hook scissors.

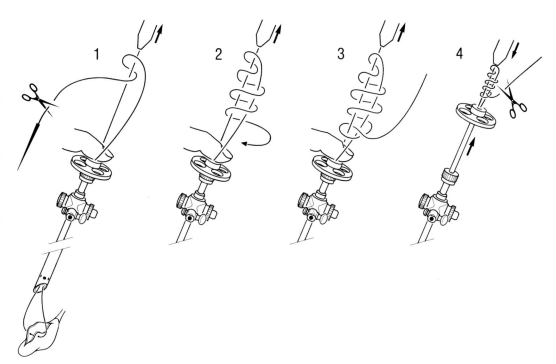

FIG 134.
Technique of tying the external slipknot. See text.

The slipknot is tied externally, as demonstrated in Figure 134, diagrams 1–4, and the end of the suture is cut about 1 cm from the knot (see Fig 134, 4). Now one breaks the plastic tube at the marked place (Fig 142), pushes it against the knot, puts tension on the suture by pulling on the broken-off end, and introduces the knot into the applicator sleeve by pulling the applicator sleeve outward (see Figs 134 and 143). After the full length of the applicator has been reintroduced into the 5-mm trocar sleeve, the knot is pushed with the plastic tube into the abdominal cavity (Fig 144). Under visual control, the loop is tightened and it adapts the wound edges on the ovary. Hook scissors (Fig

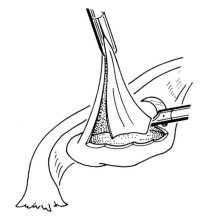

FIG 135.
Excision of ovarian cyst leaves gaping wound.

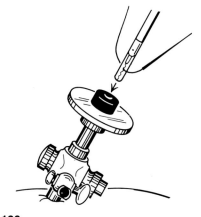

FIG 136.
Catgut suture is introduced into abdominal cavity through an applicator with 3-mm needleholder.

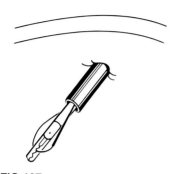

FIG 137.
Needle and thread in abdominal cavity.

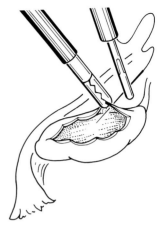

FIG 138.
The 5-mm needleholder receives the needle and presents it to 3-mm needleholder which pushes it through the first wound margin.

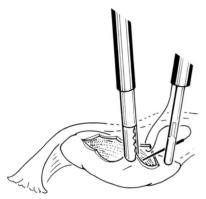

FIG 139.
Needle is pushed through opposite wound edge and will be regrasped by 5-mm needleholder.

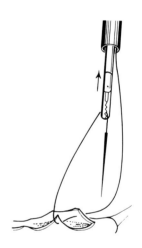

FIG 140.
Suture has been returned to 3-mm needleholder, and will be retracted through applicator.

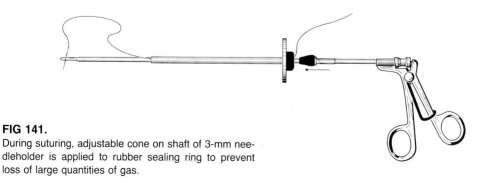

FIG 141.
During suturing, adjustable cone on shaft of 3-mm needleholder is applied to rubber sealing ring to prevent loss of large quantities of gas.

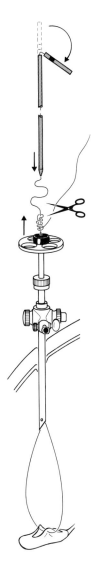

FIG 142.
After knot is tied and free end of suture is cut, plastic tube is broken.

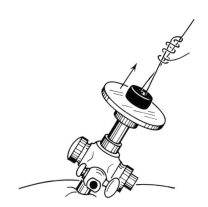

FIG 143.
Knot is introduced into the applicator sleeve.

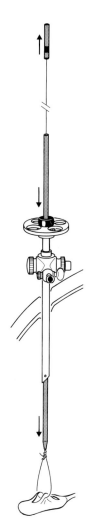

FIG 144.
Knot and plastic tube are pushed into abdominal cavity.

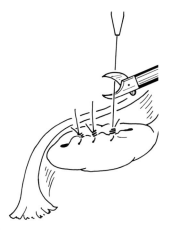

FIG 145.
Loop is tightened to adapt ovarian wound edges; then suture is cut with hook scissors, introduced in place of the 5-mm needleholder.

145), which have been introduced in place of the 5-mm needleholder, cut the suture.

This type of external tying of knots is accomplished very quickly; however, it requires that the full length of the suture can be pulled through the two wound channels produced by the needle. In an appendectomy (see Plates 361–377) and fimbrial suture after evagination (see Plates 87, 92, and 99) (see chapter 15.3.) this is not possible when the suture tract is too complex, such as a purse-string suture or a Z-suture. In such cases, the usual knot tying techniques used in microsurgery under microscopic conditions are utilized, which are demonstrated in six phases in Figure 146. This type, i.e., the internal tying of knots, requires some practice on the Pelvi-Trainer (see chapter 22); it should be a matter of routine for a microsurgeon.

It should be emphasized that endoscopic suturing does not require nearly as much careful attention as it usually gets with a laparotomy when the abdominal cavity is open. A laparotomy provokes both vascular and intestinal paralysis. The former causes a fibrinous exudate on wounds, the latter is responsible for the intestinal serosa remaining in the same place for a prolonged period, adjacent to peritoneal wounds. Because of fibrin deposition

and migration of histiocytes and fibroblasts, this later on leads to adhesions.

Even after prolonged pelviscopic procedures, full intestinal peristalsis begins within a short time; the patients move about and in the evening they receive a small meal. These facts are probably the main reason why, even after extensive adhesiolysis by endoscopy, recurrences are rarely observed. The same is true for sutures in the region of the ovaries. The explanation may lie in the fact that rupture of even larger ovarian cysts is the most common type of spontaneous healing of ovarian cysts in nature, after which we rarely observe intestinal or omental adhesions to the ovaries.

Regarding the prophylaxis of adhesions after extensive adhesiolysis with instillation of cortisone preparations, refer to chapter 17.2.

12.6.4. Hemostasis by Clips (Absorbable)

The new suture material by Ethicon, "polydioxanon," marketed under the names Vicryl and PDS, which is absorbable by hydrolysis, is now also available in the form of clips (Fig 147). With an appropriate applicator (see chapter 12.8.6.), small vessels in the abdominal region can easily be

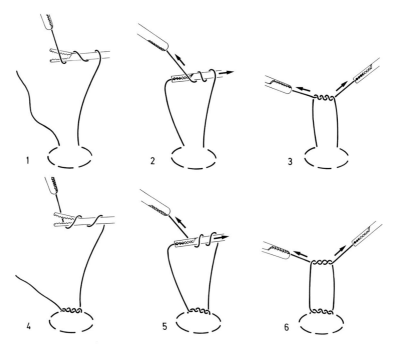

FIG 146.
When the external knot tying technique demonstrated in the preceding figures cannot be used, the usual knot tying techniques of microsurgery are used intraperitoneally.

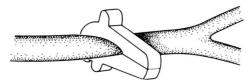

FIG 147.
Polydioxanon absorbable clips.

clamped with these clips. The clamps can also be substituted for quite a few time-consuming endo-sutures or endoligatures. After approximately 210 days, the clip will be broken down by hydrolysis and therefore will not remain as a permanent foreign body.

12.7. INSTRUMENTS FOR VAGINAL MOBILIZATION OF THE UTERUS

One of the most important requirements for successful gynecologic surgery in the pelvis is the optimal mobilization of the uterine corpus. After bimanual examination of the uterus (according to Schultze, Jena, Germany, 1827–1919; Fig 148) the endometrial cavity is sounded and measured (Fig 149). The vacuum intrauterine cannula (Fig 150; see also Fig 90) is then introduced into the endocervical canal and attached to the cervix uteri (see Fig 90) by negative pressure, which is produced by the electric vacuum pump built into the universal pertubation apparatus (Fikentscher and Semm) (see Fig 92) or by similar suction devices.

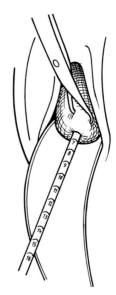

FIG 149.
Endometrial cavity is sounded and measured.

The functional parts of the vacuum intrauterine cannula are shown in Figure 151:

1. Intrauterine cannula with multiple perforations at its tip for the instillation of gas, blue dye solutions, etc.
2. Vacuum bell in three different sizes (see Fig 150).
3. Orientation plate (shows the direction into which the intrauterine tip of the cannula is bent and serves for the attachment of weights, Fig 152).
4. Connection for intrauterine instillation.
5. Connection for vacuum tube.

With one of the three sizes of vacuum intrauterine cannulas available, it is possible to move the uterus three-dimensionally in the pelvis. In the case of a retroflexed uterus, the cannula is first introduced with its curved tip pointing in the direction of the retroflexed uterine cavity, then it is rotated 180° in an anterior direction before the vacuum is applied. With this maneuver one achieves better elevation of the retroflexed uterine corpus (Fig 153).

The possibilities of perforating the uterus with the vacuum intrauterine cannula are demonstrated in Figure 154. The risk of uterine perforation is within the generally acceptable range of risks with any intrauterine procedure. However, with pelvis-

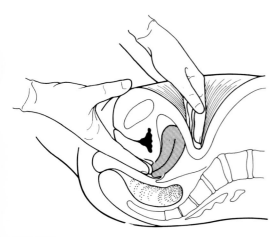

FIG 148.
Bimanual examination of the uterus.

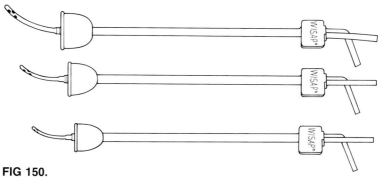

FIG 150.
Vacuum intrauterine cannulas, three sizes.

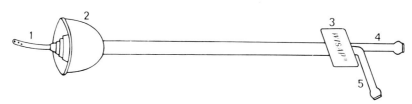

FIG 151.
Functional parts of the vacuum intrauterine cannula. See text for description of labeled parts.

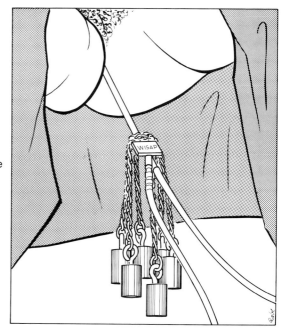

FIG 152.
Weights may be hung in front of the orientation plate to keep the uterus elevated anteriorly.

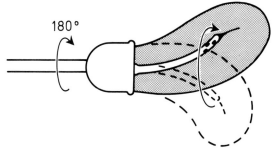

180°

FIG 153.
In the case of a retroflexed uterine corpus, the vacuum intrauterine cannula is first inserted in posterior direction, then rotated 180° to elevate the uterus anteriorly.

copy there is the added advantage that such perforation is recognized after the introduction of the endoscope and can then be corrected (see Plates 258–261).

Occasionally a vacuum intrauterine cannula is not applied optimally; the uterus cannot be elevated very satisfactorily. Another application of the vacuum intrauterine cannula should be tried under endoscopic control.

The vacuum intrauterine cannula is also used for the simultaneous instillation of dye solution for tubal diagnostic procedures, as discussed in chapter 12.4.2.

Another insufflation instrument that does not require vacuum but relies on mechanical traction, which pulls a conical seal against the uterine cervix, is the "Uterus Mobilizer" of Valtchev and Papsin (see Fig 94). The uterus is anteflexed by movements in a hinge close to the sealing cone.

[Additional comments regarding the introduction of Semm's vacuum intrauterine cannula are in order. Most surgeons use two vaginal specula to expose the cervix, grasp the anterior cervical lip with a tenaculum forceps, sound the uterus, and introduce the vacuum cannula. Because of the diameter of the vacuum bell, a regular Grave's vaginal speculum is difficult if not impossible to use; a Grave's speculum, which is hinged on only one side, may work satisfactorily in most cases.

However, I prefer to introduce Semm's vacuum intrauterine cannula without using any speculum if I have inspected the cervix during a recent preoperative office examination. After the patient has been prepared and draped in the operating room, I do a very careful bimanual examination to determine the size and position of the uterus, then I leave my left index finger in the vagina and press down on the posterior vaginal fourchette and perineum so that the vacuum intrauterine cannula can be introduced into the vagina until its bell has passed the introitus. Then I feel for the external cervical os with my left index finger and guide the tip of the cannula into the cervical canal, holding the shaft of the instrument between the right thumb and one or two fingertips, so that the cannula can be gently eased through the cervical canal into the endometrial cavity. Other surgeons may prefer to use their hands in reverse order.

This method has been used in more than 3,000 patients, most of them under local anesthesia or

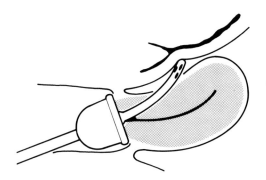

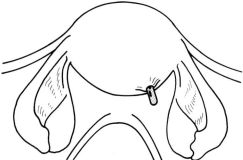

FIG 154.
Possibilities of perforation by the vacuum intrauterine cannula.

"volonelgesia." A uterine perforation was observed in only two cases, one immediately after a late first-trimester abortion, the other in a patient who had had a previous cesarean section. In both cases the tip of the cannula was seen through the vesicouterine peritoneal reflection. In the latter case the cannula was withdrawn and replaced properly, in the first case it was withdrawn and replaced by a large Pratt cervical dilator. Since that time I have never used a narrow-gauge uterine mobilizer in any postabortal patients but prefer to use as a uterine manipulator the largest dilator that had been used to dilate the cervix before the evacuation of the endometrial cavity.

Since the uterine sound is the instrument most likely to perforate the uterus, I do not sound the uterus before the introduction of a uterine manipulator for pelviscopy. Nor do I apply any cervical tenaculum, because it causes some bleeding and is not really needed for the method of introduction of the vacuum intrauterine cannula that I prefer, unless the vagina and/or the cervical canal are so narrow that they would not accommodate Semm's cannula. Then a Cohen cannula, a Ruben cannula, a Hasson cannula, a Humi cannula, or a Hulka tenaculum or a Sargis tenaculum is preferable.—*Ed.*]

12.8. ENDOSCOPIC INSTRUMENTS FOR ABDOMINAL SURGERY

Progress made within one decade in the field of intra-abdominal hemostasis under endoscopic conditions stimulated, at the same time, the development of appropriate and compatible instruments for grasping, cutting, aspiration, morcellation, and suturing to satisfy all needs. Thanks to the elimination of the high-frequency current risk, first-class metal instruments could be constructed; that require no restrictions in regard to sterilization and can be autoclaved. Insulating instruments with synthetic sheaths, which used to be bothersome (trocar sleeves!) and subject to damage, is no longer nec-

essary. Because no plastic parts are used, the life expectancy of instruments is increased considerably.

As discussed in chapter 12.2.2., endoscopic abdominal surgery is usually not performed with the so-called operating laparoscope (see Fig 47) but by the double or multiple perforation method or double or multiple entry technique. The diameter of the instruments depends on the working channels of the trocar sleeves and measures 5 or 11 mm in diameter. A special position is held by suture instruments, because they are introduced through a special applicator within the suprapubic trocar sleeves for operating instruments.

12.8.1. Sleeves for Endoscopes and Operative Instruments

Only trocar sleeves with trumpet valves are suited for the introduction of endoscopes and operative instruments. Valves that close automatically do not remain gas-tight when contaminated with small amounts of blood or tissue particles adhering to operating instruments. Since the lenses of endoscopes will also be soiled, they must be changed and cleaned frequently during operative procedures. Automatic valves, which in general are very practical, are not recommended for this purpose either.

[If they are used and become soiled or obstructed so that they are no longer gas-tight, they may have to be disassembled, cleaned, and reassembled during surgery. The pneumoperitoneum will have to be reestablished.—*Ed.*]

The trocar shown in Figure 155 with the previously customary blunt trocar sleeves must be available in sufficient numbers (see chapter 13) for instruments of 5 mm diameter and for 11-mm instruments for the photographic endoscope, as well as for the 6.8-mm diagnostic endoscope. In general, we recommend using trocars with conical tips. If the Z-puncture technique is used (see chapter 14.1.3.4.), a trocar with conical tip can be inserted through the muscular tissues with much less

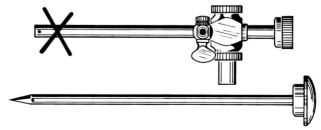

FIG 155.
Recommended conical trocar for endoscopes and operative instruments with blunt trocar sleeve.

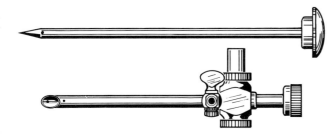

FIG 156.
Tip of new trocar sleeve with a beveled tip which facilitates its introduction.

risk and less effort than trocars with sharp, triple-edged pyramidal tips can be introduced through the linea alba. The sharp pyramidal trocar, however, is *completely* unsuited for the Z-puncture technique because of the risk of muscle lesions.

In addition, the trocar sleeve with a beveled tip (Fig 156) should be mentioned as an essential innovation. It considerably reduces the effort required to introduce this trocar sleeve. The elliptical profile gently dilates the wound made by the conical trocar tip. The blunt cylindrical trocar sleeves commonly used before (see Fig 155) function more like a punch and therefore have to overcome greater resistance during the perforation of the abdominal wall.

Use of the trocar with a conical tip requires that the Z-puncture technique be employed (see Fig 240). However, the conical tip can be pushed with ease only through muscle tissues. For the subumbilical perforation of the linea alba, on the other hand, only a triple-edged pyramidal trocar should be used. But this method of perforation leads to gaping fascial wounds into which the omentum may herniate postoperatively, as was documented in Plate 10. Particularly for the second to fourth punctures through the abdominal walls, trocars with sharp edges should *not* be used.

Before the introduction of the trocar sleeves, the trumpet valves should be checked to ensure that they are functioning flawlessly.

12.8.2. Instruments for Grasping and Holding

The most frequently used instruments in endoscopic abdominal surgery are atraumatic grasping tongs (Fig 157) and atraumatic grasping forceps (Fig 158). Both instruments are used for both grasping and dilating the tubal ampullae (see chapters 14.2.4.2. and 14.2.4.3.1.).

Other good grasping instruments are the bi-

opsy forceps (Fig 159) and the large claw forceps (Fig 160). The biopsy forceps must have a jaw at least 15 mm long and be armed with two teeth or spikes inside the jaws, for two reasons: (1) to grasp the ovarian tissue (see chapter 14.2.5.) and (2) in other cases, to grasp and adapt peritoneal edges by hooking the two spikes into them so that the defect can be closed with an endoloop (see Plates 166–168 and 270).

The large claw forceps serves to grasp the ovary or adnexa, for oophorectomy or salpingo-oophorectomy, and for enucleation of subserous myomas. With the biopsy forceps or the large claw forceps, large specimens are presented to the tissue punch, which will morcellate the tissues (see chapter 12.8.5. and Plates 157, 177 ff., 183, 189, 199, 209, 228, and others).

Occasionally the large spoon forceps (Fig 161) is very well suited for grasping and holding tissue, particularly if it is necessary to remove it through the 11-mm trocar sleeve. It is particularly well suited for removal of material from ovarian cysts and placental tissues, and contents of dermoid cysts or of an ectopic pregnancy (see Plates 140, 212, and 275).

It must be emphasized that neither the biopsy forceps nor the large spoon forceps can handle cutting functions. The small size of their joints and their mechanically thin-walled design do not tolerate much force. To take intra-abdominal biopsies or to cut, the beveled trocar sleeve is advanced inward and a tissue core is punched out by the rotating movement of the trocar sleeve, as will be described in more detail and with illustrations in chapter 14.2.5.

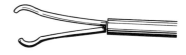

FIG 157.
Atraumatic grasping tongs.

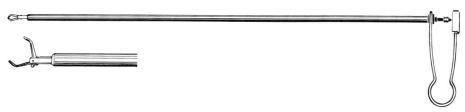

FIG 158.
Atraumatic grasping forceps.

12.8.3. Instruments for Aspiration

Among the aspiration instruments, we distinguish between the cannulas for needles for aspiration or puncture and those which are mainly used for irrigation and rinsing of the operative field. It is our routine in every pelviscopy to aspirate some fluid for cytologic as well as bacteriologic examinations. For this purpose, the atraumatic suction manipulator (Fig 162) is used. The fluid is automatically aspirated by spring action (Fig 163). Large volumes of fluid, e.g., ascitic fluids, are aspirated into the large aspiration bottle of the Aquapurator. If only small volumes of fluid are present, a small specimen bottle (Fig 164) is attached to the suction tube of the Aquapurator. The atraumatic suction manipulator is particularly well suited for atraumatic palpation and manipulation (Fig 165). It is available in diameters of 3 and 5 mm. If it becomes apparent at the beginning of a diagnostic laparoscopy that, with a high degree of probability, a suspicious preoperative diagnosis cannot be confirmed, the insertion of a secondary 5-mm trocar may not be necessary. The 3-mm atraumatic suction manipulator (see Fig 162, *1*) and its cone-tipped trocar (see Fig 162, *2*) can be introduced in its stead, and after the removal of the trocar the tubal ampullae can be held by light suction (Fig 166) and manipulated, the ovaries can be elevated, and so forth, so that all pelvic organs can be inspected without inserting the 5-mm trocar sleeve.

At the same time, the 3-mm atraumatic suction manipulator is utilized to aspirate fluid from the cul-de-sac for cytologic screening and bacteriologic cultures. If a 5-mm trocar sleeve has already been placed, the same manipulations are carried

out with the 5-mm atraumatic suction manipulator. For chromosalpingoscopy (Fig 167), for instance, the tubal ampulla can be sucked against the tip of this instrument without any trauma and then be brought directly into the visual field of the endoscope (see Plate 82).

The aspiration or puncture needle (Fig 168) has been ground at its end into a sharp needle tip with which ovarian cysts and the like can be punctured and the cyst contents can be aspirated for preliminary diagnostic evaluation. Negative suction pressure is created by the Aquapurator (see Fig 89) or similar apparatus and is controlled by finger pressure on the small hole close to the external end of the aspiration needle (Fig 169). After the needle tip is immersed in the fluid to be aspirated, this suction hole will be closed. This sequence avoids the unnecessary aspiration of gas from the pneumoperitoneum at the time the aspiration needle is introduced.

Irrigation and aspiration of larger volumes of fluid—also from ovarian tumors—is accomplished with the single-channel/dual-purpose irrigation/aspiration cannula (see Fig 88), the application and function of which were described in chapter 12.4. ff. Since the cannula or the tubing occasionally become obstructed, particularly when coagulated blood or chorionic tissue remnants from an extrauterine pregnancy are aspirated, there should always be two such cannulas available on the instrument table.

This single-channel/dual-purpose suction instrument (see Fig 88), when used in conjunction

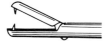

FIG 159.
Biopsy forceps.

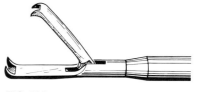

FIG 160.
Large claw forceps.

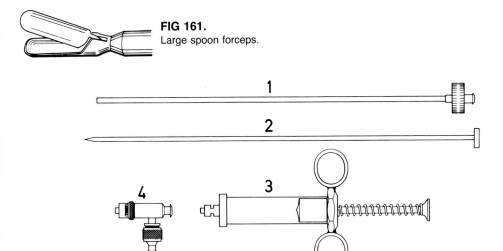

FIG 161.
Large spoon forceps.

FIG 162.
Atraumatic suction manipulator set. *1,* atraumatic suction manipulator cannula; *2,* trocar; *3,* aspirator syringe with spring-loaded plunger; *4,* 2-way automatic valve.

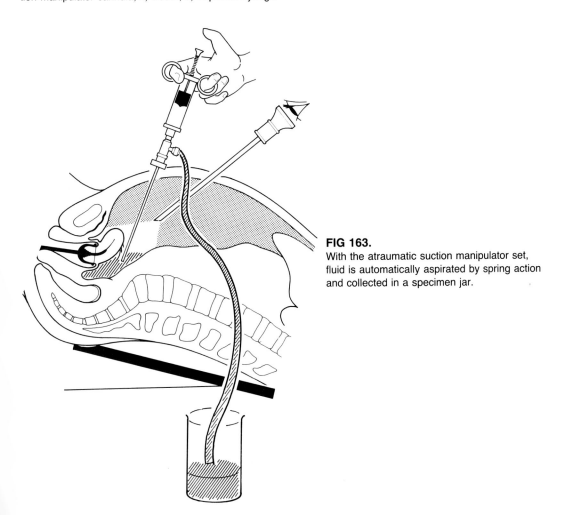

FIG 163.
With the atraumatic suction manipulator set, fluid is automatically aspirated by spring action and collected in a specimen jar.

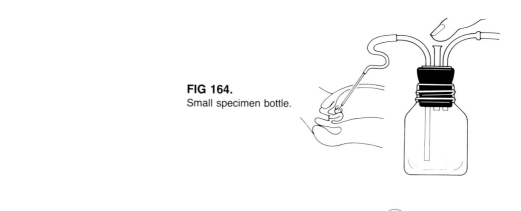

FIG 164.
Small specimen bottle.

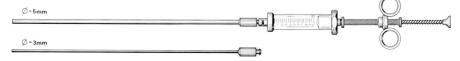

FIG 165.
Atraumatic suction manipulator with 2 cannula sizes: 5- mm and 3-mm diameter.

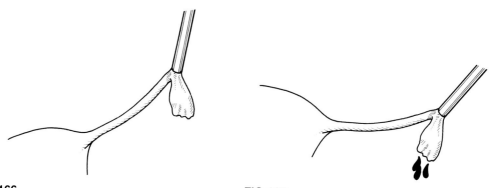

FIG 166.
Tubal ampulla can be held by light suction and manipulated.

FIG 167.
Use of atraumatic suction manipulator for chromosalpingoscopy.

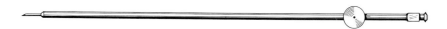

FIG 168.
Aspiration or puncture needle. The end has been ground into a sharp tip.

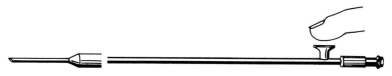

FIG 169.
Finger pressure controls negative suction pressure.

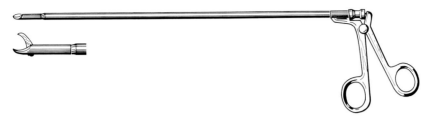

FIG 170.
Hook scissors for cutting of tissues and sutures.

with the Aquapurator (see Fig 89), is also very well suited for irrigation and rinsing of the operative field, aspiration of large ovarian cysts (e.g., chocolate or dermoid cysts), and aspiration of blood from a tubal pregnancy or postoperative bleeding. For a discussion of the operation and function of this instrument, see chapter 12.4.1.

12.8.4. Instruments for Cutting

Two cutting systems are available for intra-abdominal cutting: the 5-mm hook scissors (Fig 170) or 5- and 11-mm serrated scissors and microknives with exchangeable, disposable blades (Fig 171). The hook scissors are most frequently used because they allow safe and precise cutting. Tissues to be cut are grasped with the tip of the scissors blades (Fig 172, *1*), and pulled closer for a final determination of whether or not it really is the tissue to be cut (Fig 172, *2*) before it is transected (Fig 172, *3*). This technique obviates the blind cutting in obscured areas in which bowel wall or blood vessels are frequently hidden.

The straight serrated scissors, either in the 5-mm or 11-mm-diameter version, are used exclusively for the cutting of cyst walls (morcellation), so that the fragments can be withdrawn with the large claw forceps or large spoon forceps through the 11-mm trocar sleeve.

12.8.5. Instruments for Morcellation

After ovarian resection or enucleation of myomas, the solid tissue, depending on its size, may be re-

moved with either the large claw forceps (see Fig 160) or the large spoon forceps (see Fig 161) directly through the 11-mm trocar sleeve with a beveled end. If necessary, overhanging margins of tissue may be cut with scissors before the tissue is removed through the trocar sleeve. Larger and more solid tissues are more easily morcellated with the tissue punch (Fig 173). It is introduced through an 11-mm trocar sleeve—if necessary after dilatation of a 5-mm trocar channel (see chapter 12.8.8.). Depending on the size of the tissue to be morcellated, it is grasped either with a biopsy forceps or with the large claw forceps and pressed into the orifice of the tissue punch. The morcellation procedure is shown schematically in Figure 174 (see also Plates 172 and 196) and described below.

A. When the hand grips are operated, the sharp, obliquely ground orifice of the tissue punch cuts a piece of approximately 0.5–1 cm^3 off the tissue [e.g., ovary (*1*)] and transports the specimen into the "container" (*B*).

When the hand grips of the tissue punch are released, the pyramidal cutting head returns to its open position first. During this time, a retaining plate ensures retention of the tissue within the sheath. At the very end of the opening phase, the retaining plate snaps back into the pyramidal cutting head. This mechanism prevents the last tissue fragment in the shaft from dropping out through the open cutting orifice into the abdomen.

C. With the next cutting maneuver, the same procedure is repeated (*2*) and the tissue is stacked within the sheath of the tissue punch (*D2*).

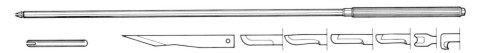

FIG 171.
Microknife handle and various styles of disposable blades.

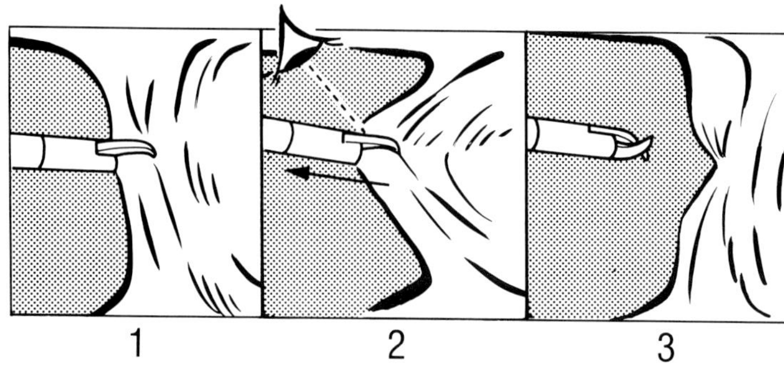

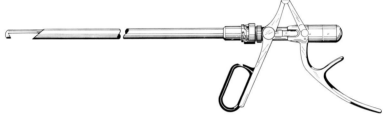

FIG 172.
Hook scissors used on tissue.
See text.

1   2   3

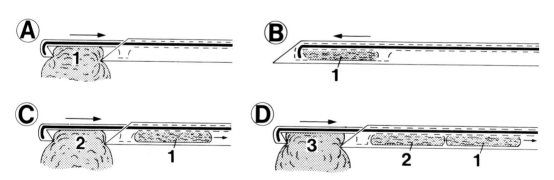

FIG 173.
Tissue punch for morcellation of large organs and tissues.

FIG 174.
Morcellation procedure. See text.

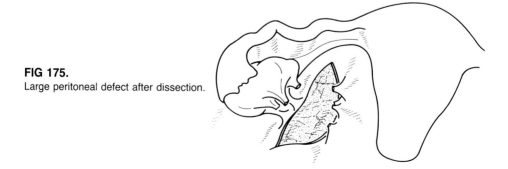

FIG 175.
Large peritoneal defect after dissection.

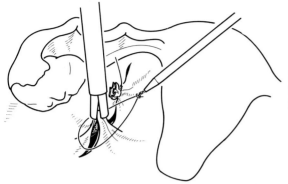

FIG 176.
Grasping of peritoneal wound edges with biopsy forceps and adaption by application of endoloops.

After approximately 15 to 20 "devouring movements" the tissue punch must be withdrawn and disassembled to remove approximately 15 cm^3 of tissue, which has been collected in its storage compartment.

12.8.6. Instruments for Ligation

The catgut loop, which was originally devised by Roeder at the end of the last century for tonsillectomies in children, has proved itself in conjunction with an applicator (see Fig 127) as an ideal technique for the ligation of squirting blood vessels in the omentum. This endoloop ligation is also a basic requirement for oophorectomy, salpingo-oophorectomy, or salpingectomy by the triple-loop technique (see chapters 14.2.7.–14.2.9.). Any bleeding or peritoneal defect resulting in the adnexal area after such procedures can be grasped with the two mouse teeth in the biopsy forceps, and hemostasis or adaptation can be ideally achieved by the application of this loop (Figs 175 and 176).

Roeder's loop is commercially available in a sterile package; it is made by Ethicon as Endoloop™ (see Fig 125). It can also be used with excellent results in a laparotomy to control hemorrhages in the depth of the pelvis or in vaginal operations for the control of hemorrhage in the adnexal area (see also chapter 12.6.1.).

If vascularized adhesions have to be ligated before they are transected, the suture material mentioned in chapter 12.8.7. is used. The ligating technique was described in chapter 12.6.2. If a sterile package of this suture material is not available, then normal, dry stiff catgut #1 or #2 can be used. A slipknot is tied externally and then pushed inside with a metal push rod (Fig 177). [In an emergency, a regular catgut suture may be removed from its sterile package containing conditioning fluid and allowed to dry on the instrument table until it is stiff enough to prepare a loop with slipknot. The knot will not slide as long as the catgut is wet and supple.—*Ed.*] Figure 178 shows an applicator for absorbable clips by Ethicon (see Fig 147). It is available in several sizes.

12.8.7. Instruments for Suturing

Occasionally the secondary puncture may result in heavier intra-abdominal bleeding from the parietal peritoneum. This may occur in approximately 5 of 1,000 pelviscopies, particularly in an area scarred by a previous laparotomy, but only very rarely directly from the periumbilical puncture site. To control such bleeding, a very large curved needle (Fig 179) has been used. It is introduced into the abdomen under visual control with the endoscope, as shown in Figure 180,A (Plate 14), to ligate the spurting vessel in the abdominal wall (Fig 180,B and Plate 15).

A new technique of controlling hemorrhage from an epiperitoneal artery with a straight ligature carrier is demonstrated in Figure 181, *1-4.*

1. The trocar that has traumatized the artery is withdrawn.

FIG 177.
Metal push rod for pushing catgut slipknot.

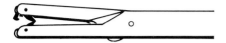

FIG 178.
Applicator for absorbable clips.

2. Under endoscopic vision, suture material is introduced with a straight ligature carrier, grasped with a needle holder, and pulled into the peritoneal cavity.

3. The straight ligature carrier is reintroduced on the opposite side of the bleeding vessel, the suture is threaded into its eye and then withdrawn.

4. Under endoscopic control, the ligature is tied across a gauze sponge by applying sufficient traction to achieve hemostasis.

If such needle or ligature carrier is not included in the instrument set, a laparotomy is the only alternative to achieve hemostasis.

Gaping wounds in an ovary after enucleation of an ovarian cyst (see Figs 135–145), in the tube after a tubal pregnancy (see Plates 264–266, 276, and 277), adhesions in intestinal walls after dissection, etc., and several operative steps for an appendectomy (see Plates 362–377) require an intra-abdominal suture with external and/or internal tying of knots. For this purpose, needleholders (Fig 182) with a 5-mm outer diameter for introduction through the 5-mm trocar sleeve and 3-mm outer diameter for the introduction through a suture applicator (see Fig 127) were developed. The 3-mm needleholder provides a movable rubber cone which is pressed into the hole of the rubber seal of the suture applicator (see Fig 127). It prevents the loss of gas during the suturing procedure.

The jaws of the needleholders are serrated so that the needle with the endosuture (see Fig 126), which is 0.8–1 mm in diameter, as well as the 0.4-mm needle on the 4-0 suture (Ethicon PDS, see

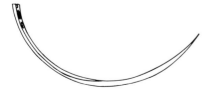

FIG 179.
Large curved needle for suturing bleeding vessels in the abdominal wall.

Fig 359, *9*) can be held securely. If a sterile package of *endosuture* with plastic push rod is not available and an external slipknot has been tied on a regular suture, the metal push rod is used to push the knot into the abdomen (see Fig 177). One must be sure to use only dry, quite stiff catgut #1 or #2 for this purpose. Soft catgut material does not permit the smooth introduction into the applicator and the slipknot does not slide well.

12.8.8. Instruments for Dilatation

Endoscopic abdominal operations are initiated with an endoscope of maximally 6.8 mm outer diameter, introduced through a 7-mm trocar sleeve. After diagnostic exploration it will be necessary to exchange the instruments for the large photoendoscope (see chapters 12.2.2. and 14.1.6.) and to introduce the 11-mm instruments for grasping and morcellation. This can be achieved by dilating the 6.8-mm laparoscopic channel or the 5-mm instrument channel to a diameter of 11 mm. To avoid the increased risk of bleeding with the new introduction of an 11-mm trocar, a dilatation set (Fig 183) was developed. In the order shown in Figures 184–187, the abdominal incision for the 5- or 6.8-mm trocar sleeves can be dilated to 11 mm diameter:

1. Removal of the endoscope (Fig 184).

2. Introduction of the guide rod (Fig 185).

3. Removal of the laparoscopic trocar sleeve and enlargment of the skin incision to 8–10 mm diameter using a scalpel (Fig 186).

4. Cautious introduction of the combined unit consisting of the 11-mm trocar sleeve and the threaded dilator (Fig 187). The threaded tip of the dilator is introduced into the skin incision and the guide rod is retracted by 10 cm to avoid injury to the dome of the bladder (Plate 12). The abdominal wall must be elevated to a maximum. The threaded dilating trocar is introduced with mild pressure and rotating movement (Plates 11 and 218).

After the guide rod and the threaded trocar have been removed, the 11-mm trocar sleeve is used to introduce the endoscope or the appropriate operating instruments.

Dilatation from a 5-mm to a 6.8-mm trocar sleeve is necessary when, for instance, there is

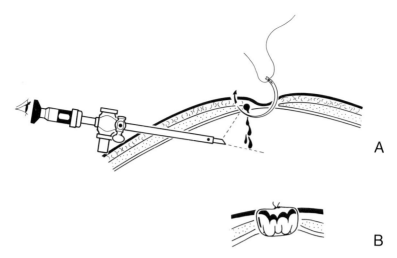

A

B

FIG 180.
The needle is inserted under visual (endoscopic) control and the spurting vessel is ligated.

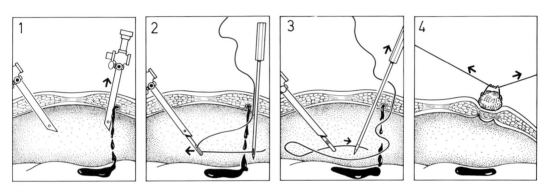

FIG 181.
Use of straight ligature carrier to control hemorrhage from epiperitoneal artery; see text.

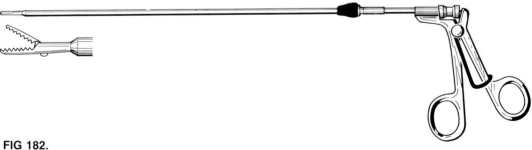

FIG 182.
Needleholder with serrated jaws for intra-abdominal suture and tying of knots.

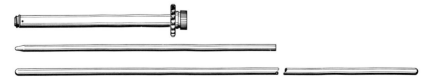

FIG 183.
Dilatation set.

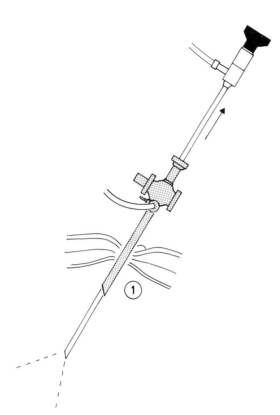

FIG 184.
Dilatation of abdominal incision: the endoscope is removed.

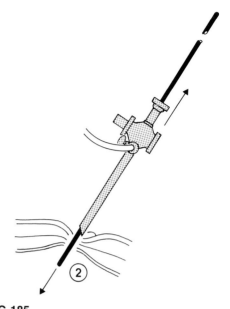

FIG 185.
Step 2: the guide rod is introduced and the trocar
sleeve is removed.

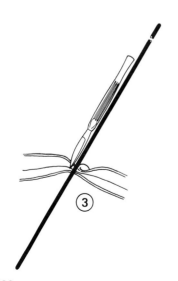

FIG 186.
Step 3: The skin incision is enlarged with a scalpel.

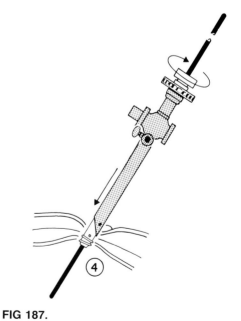

FIG 187.
Step 4: combined unit (11-mm trocar sleeve and
threaded dilator) is introduced by rotating it in a clock-
wise direction and with light pressure, while elevating
the abdominal wall.

some hemorrhage in the umbilical region or adhesions in that area must be dissected. This can be accomplished more safely by introducing the endoscope in the suprapubic area (see Figs 180 and 181) rather than by cutting adhesions immediately adjacent to the objective lens of an endoscope in the umbilical area. Dilatation of the suprapubic channel does not pose any problems, except that the appropriate guide rod and threaded dilator from 5 to 6.8 mm diameter must be available on the instrument table. In other words, the complete dilatation set consists of three threaded dilators of various diameters.

It is frequently difficult to identify an old agglutinated tubal orifice. Although the ampulla has been distended under a pressure of 150–250 mm Hg (see Fig 268), it is not possible to sound the orifice. In such cases, the conical tubal dilator is very helpful.

12.8.9. Instruments for Coagulation

Optimal hemostasis occurs when protein coagulates at 100° C (comparable to the coagulation of the white of an egg when it is boiled for breakfast). The endocoagulator apparatus (see chapter 12.5.6.) is used to electronically control the crocodile forceps, the point coagulator, and the myoma enucleator (see Fig 120), heating them, according to need, to a preselected temperature range between 90° and 120° C. With the crocodile forceps, which can be applied in one of two directions, any tissue can be easily grasped and properly clamped. Heating of the tissue occurs by the dissipation of heat (see Fig 121) from the lower jaw of the crocodile forceps or from the tip of the point coagulator.

If these coagulation instruments are not heated beyond 110°–120° C, the protein is coagulated but not transformed into glue (soap-boiler effect). The coagulated tissue will not adhere to the instrument, nor will it form a crust. If, however, the forceps is overheated, tissues will adhere to and encrust the forceps. This will also have a negative effect on the coagulation process.

The temperature in the tissues grasped by the crocodile forceps (Fig 188) will rise slowly. This can be recognized by the color change of the proteins grasped to a white color. The depth of the coagulation change is limited to 1–3 mm, even if the point coagulator or myoma enucleator is in contact with the tissue for a longer period of time.

If the instruments are heated to 120°–140° C, they may be used in the manner of a steam iron. They are rapidly moved in an ironing or painting motion across pathologic tissues such as extensive endometriotic implants.

The myoma enucleator (see Fig 120) is well suited for the bloodless resection of subserous myomatous nodules (see chapter 14.2.10.1.), the bloodless "peeling off" of the tubal ampulla, which is agglutinated to the ovary, and for superficial hemostasis in extended areas of the parietal peritoneum (see Plates, 225–232).

12.8.10. Instruments for Follicle Puncture

Puncturing follicles takes a certain amount of experience. One must avoid a sudden increase of the intrafollicular pressure when the needle punctures the follicle, which would allow follicular fluids to squirt out alongside the needle shaft. Presetting a negative pressure of 3–5 mm Hg on the Aquapurator (see chapter 12.4.3.) prevents such loss of follicular fluid and possibly of the ovum. The complete aspiration of the follicular fluid is monitored on the manometer and controlled with a finger or with a foot switch. The ovum aspiration set, shown in Figure 95, must be prepared for every follicular puncture.

The needle for follicle puncture is introduced through a trocar sleeve (see Fig 95, *A*) in the abdominal wall, which was inserted with a cone-tipped trocar.

A Teflon tube that corresponds to the inner diameter of the needle is threaded into the needle for follicle puncture (see Fig 95, *A*) and cut at the needle tip with a razor blade in an oblique direction. This Teflon tube, which is approximately 80 cm long, leads from the needle tip (*A*) through a connecting cuff into the ovum collection vessel (*B*),

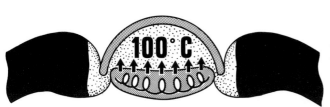

FIG 188.
Coagulation at 100° C: the temperature in the tissues grasped by the crocodile forceps rises slowly.

which is closed by a stopper traversed by three connection tubes: one for the introduction of a Teflon tube, the second for connection to the Aquapurator (*E*), and the third for a finger ring control tube (*D*). For follicle puncture, this latter tube is held in the surgeon's hand to control the force of suction with a finger, unless a foot control is preferred. The ovum collection tube is inside a transparent thermophore (*C*) which is preheated to 37° C and prevents the undercooling of the ovum during the aspiration procedure.

The transparent thermophore is preheated in an incubator which can accommodate two thermophores and six collection cylinders. This is sufficient for the collection of any number of aspirated ova, even after hormonal stimulation.

Lining the aspiration needle with a Teflon tube to allow the smooth, continuous transfer of the aspirated fluid without the induction of countercurrents is of fundamental importance. For this purpose, the Teflon tubes are cut flush with the needle tip and provided in sterile condition.

The embryo transfer set is shown in Figure 189. It consists of the transcervical applicator (*B*), which is introduced into the endometrial cavity with a blunt obturator (*A*). After the removal of the stylet, the transfer catheter, which has been marked with O-rings and into which the embryo has been aspirated, is then introduced through the transcervical applicator into the uterine cavity. The

embryo is released by turning the threaded axle (*C*). One revolution corresponds to approximately 0.01 ml of the 1-ml tuberculin syringe. The transcervical applicator is attached to the self-retaining vaginal speculum (according to Semm; Fig 190) to prevent any mechanical irritation of the uterine cavity. For reasons of sterility, it is recommended that only disposable materials be used for the transfer of the morula. Therefore, we constructed a mechanical device for use with the international version of disposable tuberculin syringes (Fig 191). The plastic syringe automatically snaps into this device in any desired position. The plunger of the disposable syringe moves 0.009 ml with every 360° revolution. We recommend that the embryo be instilled by 3½ revolutions (≈ 0.03 ml).

12.8.11. Instruments for Extraction of the Appendix

In classic surgical techniques, the lumen of the appendix is not allowed to come in contact with anything after the appendix has been severed. Therefore, we developed the appendix extractor (Fig 192). It has an inner diameter of 10.5 mm and its external end contains a 5-mm guide tube for operative instruments held by a gas-tight seal (Fig 193). It can easily accommodate the entire length of the appendix. Without contaminating any remaining organs or instruments, the appendix is re-

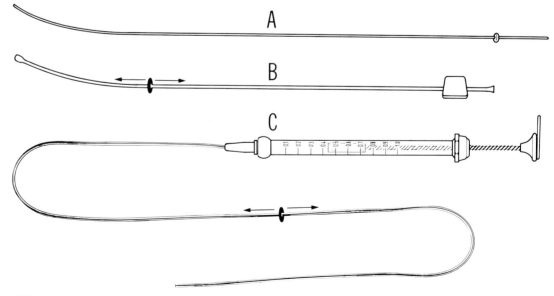

FIG 189.
Embryo transfer set. See text for description of labeled parts.

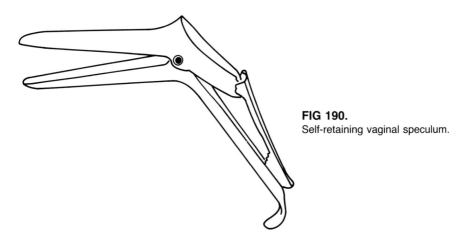

FIG 190.
Self-retaining vaginal speculum.

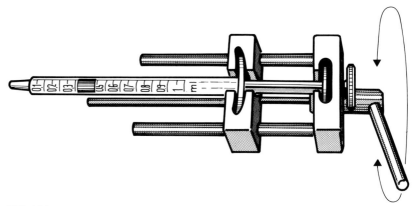

FIG 191.
Mechanical device for use with disposable tuberculin syringes: the plunger moves 0.009 ml with every 360° revolution.

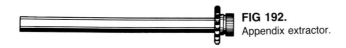

FIG 192.
Appendix extractor.

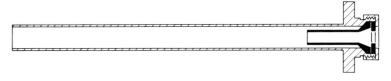

FIG 193.
The external end of the appendix extractor contains a tubular insert of 5-mm diameter to accommodate operating instruments.

moved from the abdomen inside the appendix extractor (Fig 194).

For every appendectomy there must be two appendix extractors available. Otherwise, there is no possibility of working with 5-mm instruments through an 11-mm trocar sleeve.

The appendix extractor has also been useful for other purposes. In all procedures in which it was necessary to introduce an 11-mm trocar sleeve, it can be used to introduce any 5-mm operating instrument through the sleeve without loss of gas. For this purpose, the appendix extractor is first pushed onto the 5-mm instruments and is then introduced as a unit into the 11-mm trocar sleeve. If this is done in reverse sequence, large volumes of gas are lost, because the appendix extractor does not contain a valve.

12.8.12. Instruments for Clamping of Large Vessels (Emergency Instrument Set)

If cutting instruments are used in surgery, there is an inherent danger that stabbing or cutting movements may extend beyond the therapeutically necessary limits. This may happen in spite of the best control of the movements of the body and meticulous techniques, but due to human inadequacies. This may even result in injury of the large trunk vessels. As a protective function, the organism immediately responds with a drop in blood pressure or even cardiac arrest. In modern anesthesiology, both can be brought under complete control, provided that the patient is intubated and the surgeon

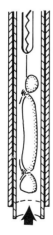

FIG 194.
Appendix may be removed without contaminating other organs, the abdominal wall or instruments.

is able to expose and clamp the injured vessel in the time available. Figure 195 shows a set of vascular clamps from the set of instruments for vascular surgery. It permits the atraumatic clamping of all vessels, including the aorta, without injury to the vascular wall or its intima, respectively. This is an *absolute* requirement for successful correction by a vascular surgeon.

Regular clamps from the gynecologic instrument tray must *not* be used for the clamping of vessels. They destroy the vascular wall, particularly the intima, by irreparably crushing them.

In all cases of fatal vascular injuries during laparoscopy which were brought to my attention for an expert opinion, the abdomen had not been opened immediately by a longitudinal incision as soon as cardiac arrest occurred and vascular clamps had not been applied. During my 10 years in Munich, Germany, vascular clamps were applied only once for an injury of the right common iliac vein (see *Atlas of Gynecologic Laparoscopy and Hysteroscopy,* 1977, page 22). In Kiel, these clamps had been life-saving in 1 out of 10,000 pelviscopies when the endoscope split open a finger-sized omphalomesenteric duct.

No endoscopic abdominal operation should be started unless a sterile pack with a set of vascular clamps is in the operating room.

12.8.13. Instruments for Closure of Skin Incisions for Trocar Insertion

The closure of 5-mm, 7-mm, or 11-mm trocar sleeve wounds in the umbilicus or the abdominal skin can be accomplished in different ways. For more than a decade we have been satisfied with the application of reusable, spring-loaded skin clips. The skin incision is put under tension with one or two towel clamps and a skin clip is firmly applied to the longitudinal incision in the umbilical region (Fig 196); it can also be applied to other incisions in the umbilical skin. It is removed after approximately 48 hours. After mechanical cleaning it can be reused frequently. After the application, the clip is covered with a gauze sponge which is taped to the skin (Fig 197).

More recently, we have used sterilizable or disposable staple guns (Fig 198) which result in wound closure that is hardly visible after complete healing. These atraumatic clips and metal staples, shown in Figures 196, 198, and 199, are removed

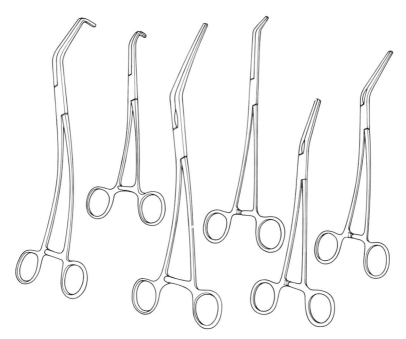

FIG 195.
Vascular clamps.

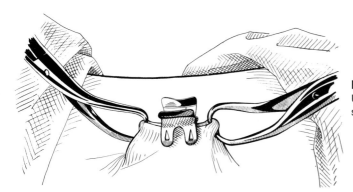

FIG 196.
Use of spring clip to close abdominal skin incision.

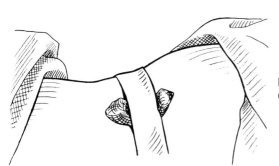

FIG 197.
Clip is covered with a gauze sponge, taped to the skin.

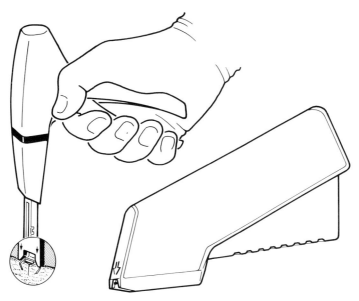

FIG 198.
Staple guns for closing skin incisions.

after 2 days and replaced by adhesive tapes; they leave no scars.

[There are three reasons why I prefer subcutaneous-subcuticular absorbable sutures rather than clips to close the skin:

1. Very few of my patients will be in the hospital 48 hours after endoscopic abdominal surgery.

2. Economy: Staple guns with magazines containing enough staples to close a long laparotomy incision are uneconomical when only two or three staples are needed. The time and effort required to place subcutaneous-subcuticular sutures

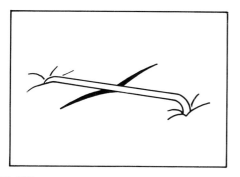

FIG 199.
Metal staple will be removed after 2 days and replaced by adhesive strips.

in the operating room is only a small fraction of the total time and effort required first to apply skin clips or staples and then to arrange for the patient's return for their removal.

3. If patients are given a choice between "hidden stitches" which do not have to be removed and clips that must be removed after they have returned home, their answer is unequivocally in favor of the sutures.

For more than 15 years, my patients and I have been very pleased with the following technique of closing endoscopic trocar wounds. Since very little strength is required for a very short period of time, 3–0 or 4–0 plain catgut with cutting needle X-1 (Ethicon) is very well suited. The needle enters at a deep, central point of the subcutaneous tissue on the surgeon's side of the wall of the wound. It exits 2–3 mm below the skin surface. On the opposite side it enters 2–3 mm below the skin surface and exits deep in the wound, where it is tied with a surgeon's knot. In very slender patients who had the trocar inserted in the midline, this first loop may also include the fascial margin or even the peritoneum. The ends of the suture are not cut, but are used for continuous subcuticular wound closure in the following order: center to the cranial apex on the opposite side, cranial apex to the center on the near side, center to the caudal apex on the opposite side, caudal apex to the center on the near side. Four to five knots are tied to anchor the long end to the original short tail at the depth of the wound. The knot is pulled above the surface of the skin and cut very short, so that the remaining tension will retract the knot below the skin surface. Transverse incisions are closed in a similar manner.

Unless there is slight bleeding from the wound edges, which would require a temporary pressure dressing with a gauze sponge taped to the abdominal skin, these wounds are left uncovered. Applying Band-aids, etc., would only create a bacteriologic moist culture chamber with a greater risk of promoting a wound infection. The patients are permitted to take a shower or bath as soon as they desire.—*Ed.*]

13

Establishing an Operating Room for Endoscopy

Operative pelviscopy has been developed over several decades. This is reflected in the arrangement of equipment in operating rooms in which endoscopy is performed: a light source here, an insufflator there, a coagulation apparatus in a third place, and so forth.

It is a prerequisite for successful, expeditious endoscopic abdominal surgery that all necessary equipment be concentrated in one area and the instruments be within easy reach. With a haphazard assemblage of operating instruments and equipment that have been collected over years, the endoscopic procedures presented in chapter 14 can frequently only be improvised; they cannot be performed at the level of modern technology available today.

13.1 PREPARATION OF INSTRUMENTS FOR DIAGNOSTIC PELVISCOPY/LAPAROSCOPY

Nurses familiar with the customary tray of operating instruments may feel overwhelmed by the completely unknown, apparently confusing array of instruments for endoscopy. In reality, it is quite simple to distinguish between endoscopes, fiber light cables, and instruments for vaginal manipulation and those for use through trocar sleeves, and to arrange them on the instrument table in a logical pattern.

A basic requirement today is that all necessary equipment be assembled on a special **endoscopy cart** (see Fig 56). Almost all electrical equipment is mounted on it:
- **OP-PNEU Electronic insufflator** (see chapter 12.3.2. ff.)
- **Light source,** optimally with endoscopic flash (see chapter 12.1. ff.)
- **Endocoagulator** (see chapter 12.5.6.1.)
- **Aquapurator** (see chapter 12.4.1.)
- **Universal pertubation apparatus** (WISAP) (see chapter 12.4.2.) [or comparable equipment— Ed.]
- **Two warm water baths** with thermostatic control, one set at a temperature of 37° C for the prewarming of bottles with physiologic saline solution and the like for intra-abdominal irrigation (see chapter 12.4.1.), the other set at a temperature of approximately 50° C and containing 1-liter bottles with sterile water for cleansing and warming of endoscopes (see chapter 12.2.6. and Figs 55 and 56).

Furthermore, a universal pertubation apparatus (such as that devised by Fikentscher and Semm) should be integrated with the endoscopy unit. It permits continuous tubal pertubation with gas or fluid (chromopertubation) and automatically controls and records pressure and time; it also provides the suction necessary to apply the vacuum intra-uterine cannula to the cervix or the pressure to inflate the cervical balloon catheter.

Finally, the warming device for endoscopes

should be integrated into the equipment cart.

This mobile unit is a fundamental requirement for operative abdominal endoscopy. If some piece of equipment is not available, it may in some cases be impossible to manage certain operative problems. In other cases, lack of a piece of equipment may give the impression that the endoscopic operation belongs to the realm of "artistic performance." In reality, operative abdominal endoscopy is primarily a question of having on hand a well-coordinated set of specific operative instruments and equipment.

The arrangement of an endoscopic operating room is shown in Figure 200. This figure also shows the integration of equipment for video recording of the intra-abdominal procedures. However, video recording is not essential in nonteaching institutions, because operation of the recording equipment is a considerable burden to the surgeon and the operating room personnel.

Since the diagnostic phase of endoscopy is not always followed by an operative phase, it makes sense to prepare the endoscopic instruments according to the field of application—much as the operating instruments for conventional procedures are arranged on the tray according to their use. A sterile set for pelviscopic/laparoscopic diagnostic procedures should contain the following instruments:

Diagnostic Set

NO.	DESCRIPTION OF ITEMS
2	Endoscopes, 30°, 6.5 mm diameter, with fiberglass light bundle
1	Magnifying loupe, attachable to eyepiece
1	Fiberglass light cable, 3.5 mm diameter
1	Injection needle (needle for probing/sounding test), 0.8 mm diameter, 120 mm long
1	Syringe, 10 ml

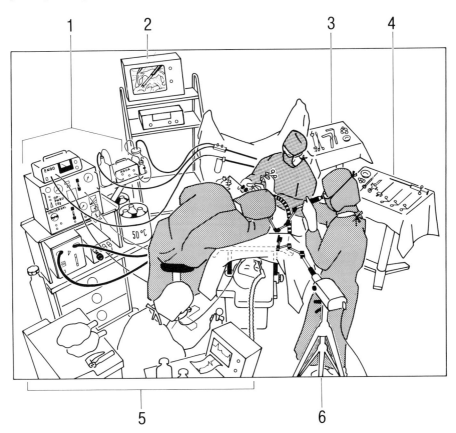

FIG 200.
Arrangement of equipment in an endoscopic operating room. *1,* endoscopy cart; *2,* video cart; *3,* vaginal instrument table; *4,* endoscopic instrument table; *5,* anesthesia; *6,* television camera with articulated optical attachment.

1	Veress insufflation needle for CO_2 insufflation
1	Trocar and sleeve, 7 mm diameter, with trumpet valve for endoscope
2	Trocars with sleeves with trumpet valves, 5.5 mm diameter, for second and third punctures
1	Dilatation set from 5.5-mm to 7-mm trocar sleeve size
2	Atraumatic grasping tongs
1	Atraumatic grasping forceps to dilate the tubal ampulla
1	Tubal dilator
1	Aspiration needle for cyst puncture
1	Crocodile forceps
1	Point coagulator
1	Myoma enucleator
1	Instrument cable for crocodile forceps or point coagulator or myoma enucleator
1	Suction manipulator with trocar, 3 mm diameter
1	Suction manipulator, 5 mm diameter
1	Spring-loaded vacuum syringe for suction manipulator
1	Hook scissors
1	Biopsy forceps with two grasping teeth and spring-loaded lock
1	Peritoneal scissors
1	Applicator for suture and ligature material
10	Endoloops
1	Single-channel/dual-purpose irrigation/aspiration cannula with two connecting tubes to the Aquapurator
1	Reservoir for chromosalpingoscopy
1	Set of vacuum intrauterine cannulas with two attached tubes or Luer locks (small, medium, large)
1	Large needle for hemostatic suture ligation in the abdominal wall
1	Chromosalpingoscopy solution, 100 ml, containing methylene blue [or indigo carmine—*Ed.*]
1	Specimen bottle for the collection of aspirated fluid
5	Skin clips for the closure of trocar wounds [or staples or suture material—*Ed.*]

Equipment (see Fig 56)

OP-PNEU Electronic insufflator; endocoagulator; Aquapurator; cold light source; universal pertubation apparatus; warming device for endoscopes; warm water bath set at 37° C for storage of bottles with physiologic saline solution; warm water bath set at 50° C for storage of bottles with sterile water for the cleaning of endoscopes during the operation.

13.2. PREPARATION OF INSTRUMENTS FOR ENDOSCOPIC ABDOMINAL SURGERY

For the smooth transition from the pelviscopic diagnostic phase to endoscopic abdominal surgery, it is necessary that the appropriate instruments be immediately available on a sterile tray. This applies to the prewarmed 11-mm endoscope (see chapter 12.2.2.) as well as to the following set of operating instruments:

Operative Set

NO.	DESCRIPTION OF ITEMS
1	Wide-field operating endoscope, 30°, 11 mm diameter, with two fiber light bundles
1	Dilatation set from 5.5-mm to 11-mm trocar sleeve size
1	Dilatation set from 7-mm to 11-mm trocar sleeve size
2	Operative trocars with sleeves, 11 mm diameter, with trumpet valves
1	Claw forceps with spring-loaded lock, 11 mm diameter
1	Large spoon forceps with spring-loaded lock, 11 mm diameter
1	Large operating scissors, serrated, 11 mm diameter
1	Tissue punch morcellator, 11 mm diameter
7	Microknives (exchangeable) with 5-mm handle
1	Needleholder, 3 mm diameter, with adjustable rubber cone
1	Needleholder, 3 mm diameter
1	Push rod for slipknots, 3.5 mm diameter
1	Applicator for endoloops and needleholder, 5 mm outer diameter
10	Endoloops
10	Endosuture sets

Equipment (see Fig 56): Same as for diagnostic set (see above).

Pelviscopic photographic set: Same as operative set, plus the following:

Endoscope: Large-field endoscope with forward view, 11 mm diameter, with integrated fiber optic bundles.

Light: WISAP/Storz combination light unit with flash generator with manually or electronically operated flash timer, electronic flash tube, as well as cold light source.

Camera: Mirror reflex camera with special variable-objective lens, f = 70–140 mm.

The instrument table must hold multiple sets of at least the most frequently used instruments, such as trocars and sleeves, atraumatic grasping forceps, scissors, etc., as is also customary for a laparotomy or, for example, Wertheim's hysterectomy operation. One would never attempt a laparotomy with only one pair of scissors or one forceps. In endoscopy, however, it has been quite common to have only one of each of these instruments on the instrument table. This tradition, which has developed over several decades, must be abandoned before one undertakes any endoscopic abdominal surgery.

The instruments to be used in the vaginal field (disinfection, speculum exposure of the cervix, cervical tenaculum forceps, uterine sound, dilators, vacuum intrauterine cannulas, reservoir for chromopertubation solution, hydropertubation solution and methylene blue, weights for the elevation of the uterus, etc.) are laid out on a separate instrument table (see Fig 200).

During an endoscopic procedure—much as during a laparotomy—an instrument will occasionally become inoperative or unsterile. Therefore, a small sterile supply of the most commonly used instruments should always be within easy reach.

It must be stated again that *easy access to multiple instruments will facilitate and accelerate the operative procedure,* just as it does during a laparotomy. Even before the induction of anesthesia, several bottles with sterile water and physiologic saline or Ringer's solution should be placed in the 50° C and 37° C water baths, respectively. Proper functioning of the OP-PNEU Electronic insufflator, the endocoagulator, and both light bulbs in the light source, as well as the mobility of the trumpet valves and all trocar sleeves, joints of instruments, and so forth, must be verified before the patient is anesthetized.

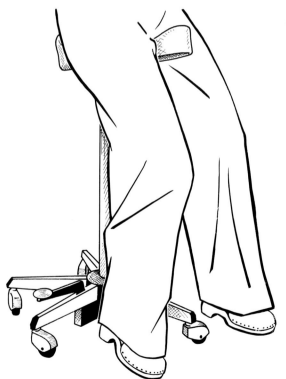

FIG 201.
The relaxing-seat. Height of the seat is adjustable.

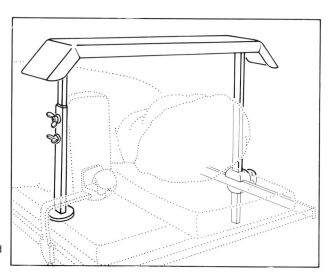

FIG 202.
Support device for surgeon's arm and shoulder.

13.3. Seating and Support Possibilities for the Endoscopic Surgeon During the Procedure

In the past it was customary to perform laparoscopic procedures in a standing position. For a smooth meticulous operating technique under microsurgical conditions, the surgeon must be seated comfortably. This applies to microsurgery by laparotomy as well as to endoscopic abdominal surgery.

Best suited for such purpose is the so-called relaxing-seat (Fig 201); the surgeon adjusts the height of the seat to a level that will allow him to sit as soon as he flexes his knees. In addition, a

support device for the endoscopic surgeon's arm and shoulder should be mounted on the operating table in front of the patient's head (Fig 202). Aided by the relaxing-seat and the shoulder support, the endoscopic surgeon assumes a half-sitting, half-lying position (Fig 203). It allows him to operate with two steady hands. A level built into the WISAP shoulder brace gives the endoscopic surgeon a visual indication that he begins his surgery in the optimum 15° Trendelenburg position. He can adjust this position up or down according to need.

For a bimanual operating technique the endoscope is held by an assistant, who follows the procedure through a "spy," an articulated or flexible

FIG 203.
Position of endoscopic surgeon, using relaxing-seat and support device.

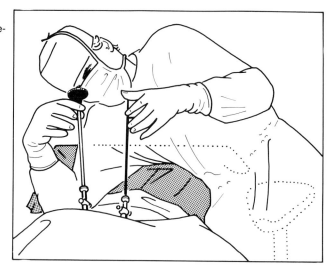

optical attachment (see Fig 23); or the endoscope may be held by an endoscopic adapter device attached to the surgeon's forehead (see Fig 49). The scrub nurse may also briefly hold the endoscope. Under optimum conditions, the endoscope is mounted in a flexible support arm which is attached to the operating table (see chapter 12.2.3. and Fig 50) and has interchangeable holding devices for the pelviscope, flexible teaching attachment, camera, and so on.

14

Course of Endoscopic Abdominal Surgery

The following guidelines may serve as preamble for this chapter (see also page 4 of the Introduction).

The techniques of endoscopic surgery are, in principle, not different from those taught and practiced in conventional surgery when the abdomen is open. Special "tricks" should be avoided, such as coagulating bleeding vessels in the omentum, or the simple clamping or ligating of the appendix, etc.

In this chapter, all presently feasible endoscopic operating techniques are described by a combination of narrative, line drawings, and original anatomical color photographs. The majority of these techniques were developed and clinically applied at the University Women's Hospital in Kiel, Germany, during the performance of more than 10,000 pelviscopies.

It should be reemphasized that the main purpose of this book is the demonstration of endoscopic abdominal surgery, for which a basic requirement is familiarity with the purely diagnostic techniques of laparoscopy or pelviscopy, previously described in the *Atlas of Gynecologic Laparoscopy and Hysteroscopy* (1977).

14.1. DIAGNOSTIC PHASE

On the following pages, an abridged account of diagnostic laparoscopic techniques will be presented,

more in the form of schematic sketches than by narrative discussion. A detailed description can be found in the *Atlas of Gynecologic Laparoscopy and Hysteroscopy*.

Each endoscopic abdominal operation begins with a diagnostic endoscopic inspection of the abdominal cavity to

1. confirm a diagnosis made by palpation and radiologic or ultrasonic examination and
2. make the decision whether the condition encountered can be managed endoscopically without undue risk, or if
3. the condition encountered requires primary intervention by laparotomy or
4. the surgical intervention should be terminated after diagnostic pelviscopy because the suspected diagnosis cannot be confirmed.

14.1.1. Preparation of the External Genitalia

Mobilization of the uterus is an absolute requirement for pelviscopy, except in cases when sounding the uterus is contraindicated, for example:
- differential diagnosis between intrauterine or extrauterine pregnancy
- follicle aspiration is undertaken for in vitro fertilization
- the patient is pregnant.

Before a uterine manipulator (see also chapter

12.7.) is introduced, the external genitalia and the vagina must be thoroughly prepared with an antiseptic.

Particularly in the evaluation of patients with sterility, in whom ascending chromosalpingoscopy will be required to test for tubal patency, any vaginal infection must be cleared up preoperatively to avoid an ascending infection.

After the uterus has been sounded (see Fig 149), the vacuum intrauterine cannula (see Figs 150, 151) is introduced for the manipulation of the uterus, even when no intrauterine instillation will be required (Fig 204).

During the endoscopic operation it is almost always necessary that the uterus be elevated from the cul-de-sac and pressed against the posterior surface of the symphysis pubis. Weights linked together by chains may be used for this purpose (see Fig 152). They can take the place of an assistant who, in most other cases, would be needed to elevate the uterus.

In principle, the uterus can also be elevated by means of other intrauterine cannulas (Fig 205; see also Fig 94); however, in most cases they fit only loosely into the cervix. Much of the mobility of the uterus is lost. This sometimes makes operating in the small pelvis quite difficult. The advantage of the vacuum intrauterine cannula is that the cervix is partially sucked into the suction cup, making it one unit with the cervix, thereby yielding optimum mobility.

For chromosalpingoscopy, the vacuum intra-

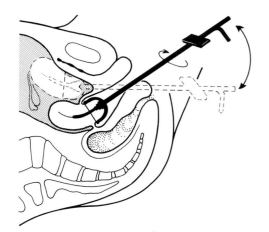

FIG 204.
The vacuum intrauterine cannula is used to elevate and manipulate the uterus regardless of whether or not chromopertubation will be necessary during the endoscopic operative procedure.

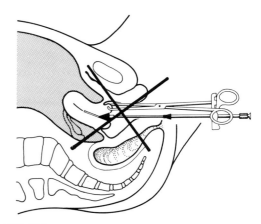

FIG 205.
The uterus can also be elevated by means of other intrauterine cannulas; however, in most cases they fit only loosely into the cervix.

uterine cannula is first filled with blue solution before it is applied to the cervix (see chapter 14.2.4.2.). This technique prevents insufflation of a sactosalpinx with air instead of blue solution, which otherwise might lead to a false diagnosis.

14.1.2. Preparation of the Abdominal Wall and Umbilicus

As the external genitalia are being prepared, the surgeon prepares the entire abdominal wall in the manner usual for a laparotomy. Particular attention is paid to the proper antiseptic treatment of the abdomen, because the umbilicus is considered by surgeons to be the most contaminated region of the human abdominal wall. Therefore, the umbilicus (Fig 206) is prepared with a sponge soaked in highly effective antiseptic solution and held in a sponge forceps, which is rotated ten times to the right. The sponge is changed and the procedure is repeated with rotation to the left. Any solid matter discovered is removed with a forceps.

This technique of antiseptic preparation of the umbilicus by rotation causes desquamation of the uppermost cornified squamous epithelial cells and therefore permits thorough cleansing of the umbilicus. This preparation method has not resulted in a single umbilical infection among more than 12,000 pelviscopies that I have supervised.

The pubic area is also carefully prepared with an antiseptic. Shaving or trimming of pubic hair is done only when a laparotomy is considered likely.

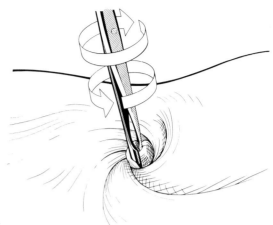

FIG 206.
Antiseptic cleaning of the umbilicus.

14.1.3. Limiting the Risk of Perforation

Most accidents during laparoscopy and pelviscopy occur during the primary puncture with the Veress needle or the trocar for the endoscope. After a period of development of laparoscopy in gynecology from the beginning of the 1960s until 1978, such fatal injuries declined from 1:100 to 1:100,000 (Semm, 1979; Phillips, 1979). In all these accidents, several factors coincided to cause the patient's death. Because of human inadequacies, errors are not completely avoidable in a surgical field. However, most errors should be avoidable if modern techniques are used with care. Therefore, we consider it essential to adhere strictly to the following safety tests, so that serious injuries can be reduced to a minimum.

14.1.3.1. Safety Tests With the Blind Puncture Method

The primary blind puncture through the lower umbilical fold by the Veress needle (Fig 207) requires basic knowledge of the topographic anatomy of the large vessels below the umbilicus and in the small pelvis. This is clearly shown in Figures 70 through 80.

With knowledge of these anatomical relationships, the blind puncture is carried out according to the following safety rules:

Test 1: Check the patency of the needle and its spring-loaded snap mechanism (needle test).

Test 2: Palpate the aorta.

FIG 207.
Primary blind puncture through the lower umbilical fold with the Veress needle.

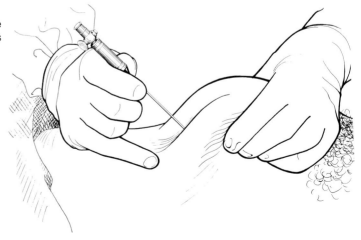

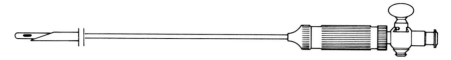

FIG 208.
Veress needle.

Test 3: Observe the spring-loaded snap mechanism of the needle.
Test 4: Hissing phenomenon.
Test 5: Aspiration test.
Test 6: Monitor insufflation pressure (manometer test).
Test 7: Volume test.

14.1.3.1.1. NEEDLE TEST

The Veress needle (Fig 208) is checked for unobstructed patency for gas flowing at 1 L/min. The manometer must not show a pressure higher than 6–8 mm Hg at 1 L/min gas flow (Fig 209). If the resistance of the needle against atmospheric air is greater, the needle is not clean and must be replaced.

At the same time, the insufflation cannula is pulled back and allowed to snap forward by spring pressure to check its smooth movement within the pointed outer needle.

14.1.3.1.2. AORTA PALPATION TEST

This test entails digital palpation of the position of the aorta to get an impression of how many millimeters distance there is between the aorta and the umbilical plate to be perforated (see Figs 73–78). One should also palpate the position of the bifurcation of the aorta. He who has palpated it will not puncture it.

14.1.3.1.3. SNAP TEST

During maximal elevation of the abdominal wall between the umbilicus and the symphysis pubis with the left hand (see Figs 69–72 and 75), the skin and umbilical fascial plate (see Fig 79) are perforated by the Veress needle, layer by layer (see chapter 12.3.1.1.). If necessary, an assistant may elevate the skin or, in the extreme case, the lower umbilical region may be grasped with towel clips. During this maneuver, the spring mechanism of the needle is watched (see Fig 79). The spring mechanism works best if skin, fascia, and the underlying peritoneum are perforated as close to the perpendicular axis as possible. If the needle traverses at a tangential angle to the parietal peritoneum (see Figs 70–72) the needle tip may be advanced extra-peritoneally for several centimeters before it perforates the peritoneum. This leads to some uncertainty in the evaluation of the puncture, because the spring mechanism does not work (see Plates 1, 13 and 268).

Only needle position 2 in Figure 75 is correct and will result in an optimum pneumoperitoneum, as shown in Figure 210.

If the needle remains in the preperitoneal position, a preperitoneal emphysema will be produced (Fig 211). If bowel is directly adherent to the umbilicus (history!), the gas will insufflate the intestinal tract (Fig 212).

If the stomach was distended by hyperventila-

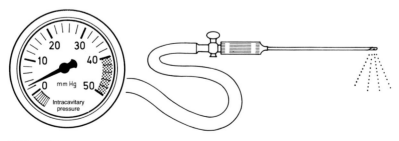

FIG 209.
In the needle test, the manometer should not indicate a pressure higher than 6–8 mm Hg with gas flow at 1 L/min.

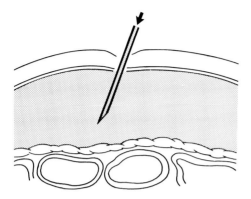

FIG 210.
Optimum pneumoperitoneum is created by a correct needle position.

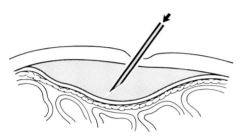

FIG 211.
Incorrect positioning of the needle may produce a preperitoneal emphysema.

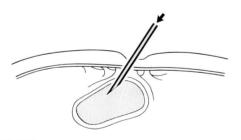

FIG 212.
When bowel adheres directly to the umbilicus, gas will insufflate the intestinal tract.

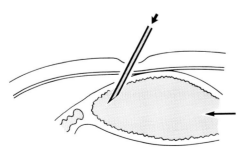

FIG 213.
Needle perforating the stomach.

tion before the endotracheal tube was introduced and no nasogastric tube has been used, ptosis of the stomach may result and the needle may be placed into the stomach (Fig 213). If the needle tip enters the large omentum (Fig 214) an omental emphysema will develop. If the needle is advanced too deeply (see Fig 77) a mediastinal emphysema may result. If the needle is advanced with greater force and too deeply and the results of the palpation test 2 are ignored, a vessel will be punctured (see Fig 76). However, this will be noted immediately during the aspiration test (test 5)—blood is aspirated (Fig 215).

14.1.3.1.4. HISSING PHENOMENON

The Veress needle is always introduced with an open valve. If the abdominal wall is elevated when the peritoneum is perforated by the needle and the blunt inner cannula snaps forward into the free abdominal cavity, some air will be aspirated immediately. This produces a hissing sound which is clearly audible. This hissing phenomenon can also be made visually evident by the aspiration of fluid (for this phenomenon see Fig 80).

14.1.3.1.5. ASPIRATION TEST

Another misplacement of the Veress needle that has not yet been illustrated can be diagnosed by the following aspiration tests:

After the single-channel Veress needle has been introduced, a Luer-Lock syringe filled with 10 ml of physiologic saline solution is attached to the needle (Figs 215 and 216). The aspiration test is positive if the needle tip has entered the lumen of a larger blood vessel (Fig 215; see also Fig 76). After instillation of 5 ml of saline solution (Figs 216 and 217), the reaspiration test must be negative. If the needle tip is in the correct position, the fluid will spread diffusely in the free abdominal cavity. It cannot be aspirated again (Fig 218). If

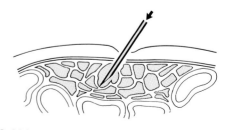

FIG 214.
Needle tip enters the large omentum; an omental emphysema will result.

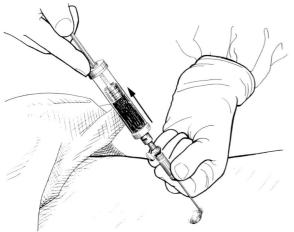

FIG 215.
The aspiration test will draw blood if a vessel has been punctured.

the needle tip has entered the intestinal lumen (Fig 219) the test is positive; intestinal contents are aspirated.

If the aspiration test is positive, insufflation should not be initiated under any circumstances; a decision must be made either to risk another blind attempt or to try transvaginal insufflation (see Fig 81), described in chapter 12.3.1.2., or to perform an "open laparoscopy" as described in chapter 12.3.1.3.

14.1.3.1.6. MANOMETER TEST

After a negative aspiration test, the gas insufflation tubing from the OP-PNEU Electronic insufflator is attached to the Veress needle (Fig 220) and the abdominal wall is elevated (Fig 221). The manometer for intra-abdominal pressure will first register in the negative pressure range, because elevation of the abdominal wall causes a negative

intra-abdominal pressure (Fig 222). At this point, the selection switch on the OP-PNEU instrument (Fig 223) is turned from 0 to 1 L/min and gas insufflation begins at a rate of 1 L/min. During intermittent gas insufflation, the insufflation pressure should not exceed 10 mm Hg (Fig 224).

Up to a filling volume of 1 L, the static pressure, which is continuously monitored on the OP-PNEU instrument, must not exceed 1–3 mm Hg (133–399 Pa) (Fig 225).

14.1.3.1.7. VOLUME TEST

As shown in Figure 226, the rise in intra-abdominal static pressure depends on the insufflated volume. After 1 L of gas has been insufflated (dig-

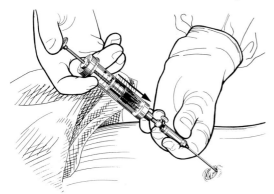

FIG 216.
Aspiration test. A Luer-lock syringe filled with 10 ml of physiologic saline solution is attached to a single-channel Veress needle.

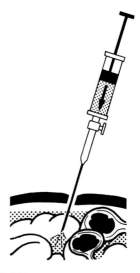

FIG 217.
Five milliliters of solution are instilled.

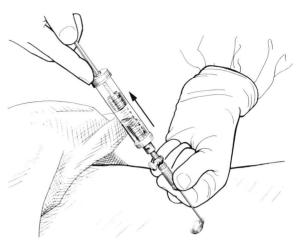

FIG 218.
A negative test: the fluid has spread in the free abdominal cavity and cannot be aspirated.

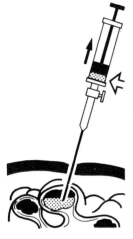

FIG 219.
A positive test: the needle has entered the intestinal lumen and intestinal contents are aspirated.

FIG 220.
Manometer test. The gas tube from the insufflator is connected.

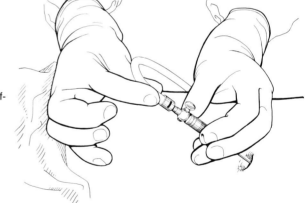

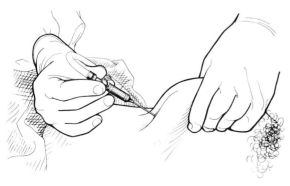

FIG 221.
The abdominal wall is elevated.

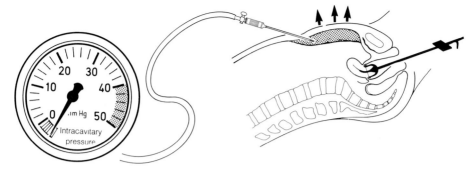

FIG 222.
Elevation of the abdominal wall causes a negative intra-
abdominal pressure.

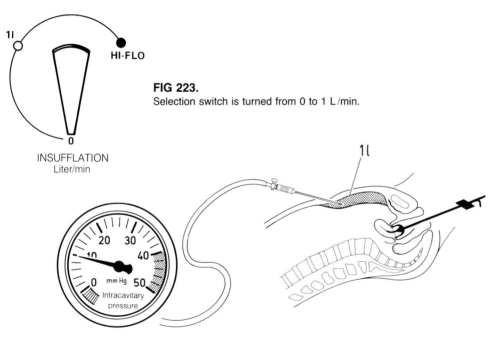

FIG 223.
Selection switch is turned from 0 to 1 L/min.

FIG 224.
During intermittent gas insufflation, filling pressure
should not exceed 10 mm Hg.

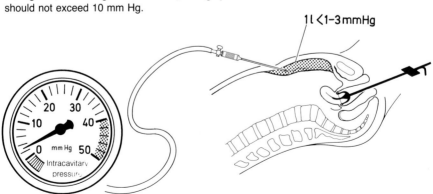

FIG 225.
Up to a filling volume of 1 L, the static pressure should not exceed 1–3 mm Hg except in very
obese patients → weight of abdominal wall.

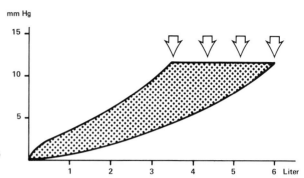

FIG 226.

The rise in intra-abdominal static pressure depends on the insufflated volume.

ital indicator), the static pressure of 1–3 mm Hg (see Fig 225) should not have been exceeded (exception: in a very obese patient, consider the weight of the abdominal wall). The manometers indicate different pressures (see Fig 86). For example, if the left manometer indicates less than 15 mm Hg insufflation pressure, and the right manometer indicates 2 mm Hg static intra-abdominal pressure, then, with a very high degree of probability, the needle outlet is in the abdominal cavity. One can switch to "high flow" provided that immediately after switching, the manometers show the following (Fig 227): an insufflation pressure of 40 mm Hg and an intra-abdominal pressure of 2 mm Hg. Further insufflation is monitored electronically.

14.1.3.2. Insufflation of the Pneumoperitoneum

The pneumoperitoneum is now established with maximum speed. The OP-PNEU instrument records the volume automatically. Although it could deliver maximally 6 L/min, only 2–2.5 L/min is flowing. *Reason:* Since the insufflation pressure is restricted to 40 mm Hg, the flow resistance from the insufflation tubing and the Veress needle allows only about 2.5 L/min of gas to flow. The

gas flow is reduced further by an increase of the intra-abdominal pressure—from 0 to 12 mm Hg, for instance—and, consequently, a falling pressure differential.

According to Poiseuille's law, the velocity of flow in the tube is proportional to the cross-sectional area of the tube:

$$D = \frac{(P_1 - P_2) \times r^4 \times l}{\eta \times t}$$

where D = volume of flow through a tube, $(P_1 - P_2)$ = pressure difference between pressure at origin (apparatus) and pressure at outlet (intra-abdominal pressure), r^4 = fourth power of the internal radius of the insufflation system (needle), l = length of the insufflation system (tube and needle), η = viscosity of the flowing medium, and t = time.

Thus, if one wanted to insufflate 6 L/min of gas through the Veress needle one would have to start with a pressure of more than 130 mm Hg. This could be life-threatening.

According to the pressure preset on the OP-PNEU insufflator (Fig 228), the pneumoperitoneum is established under constant electronic control of the static intra-abdominal pressure. When

FIG 227.

Relative positions on manometers immediately after switching to high flow.

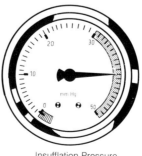

Insufflation Pressure
(mm Hg)

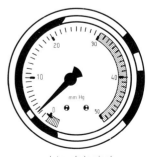

Intra-abdominal
Static Pressure
(mm Hg)

Preselection of
Static Pressure
Intra-abdominal
(mm Hg)

FIG 228.
The pneumoperitoneum is established under constant electronic control of the static intra-abdominal pressure after its upper limit has been preset on the Op-PNEU instrument.

the preset pressure is reached, the gas flow is stopped electronically.

14.1.3.3. Probing/Sounding Test: Safety Test Before Introduction of the Trocar for the Endoscope

Fortuitously or by skillful manipulation of the Veress needle, free access to the abdominal cavity is sometimes achieved despite the presence of massive adhesions in the abdomen, and a pneumoperitoneum can be established easily. However, with the subsequent insertion of the trocar it is possible to injure a loop of bowel adherent to the abdominal wall (see Plates 16, 331, and 337) or a vessel in the omentum. It must be stressed that omentum and intestines may be adherent to the abdominal wall *without* a history of a previous laparotomy!

To prevent such complications, we routinely do the probing/sounding test.

14.1.3.3.1. PROBING/SOUNDING TEST

In an effort to save time, this test is usually done at the end of insufflation, when the intra-ab-

dominal pressure is 8–10 mm Hg. After repeated disinfection of the abdominal wall (Fig 229), a spinal needle 12 cm long and 0.8 mm in diameter, is attached to a syringe containing 2–3 ml of physiologic saline (remaining from the aspiration test), and introduccd perpendicularly through the abdominal wall (Fig 230), approximately 2–3 cm below the umbilicus. As the needle point is advanced, CO_2 gas from the pneumoperitoneum is slowly aspirated (Fig 231) and continuous bubbling is observed in the syringe. This will stop suddenly when the visceral peritoneum is touched. The level at which the needle enters the abdominal wall is marked with fingers on the shaft of the needle, and bubbling of the gas is observed as the needle is withdrawn (Fig 232) until the bubbling stops again. The distance between the parietal and the visceral peritoneum—that is, omentum or bowel (see Fig 234)—can thus be estimated fairly accurately from the depth of the needle puncture.

After the peritoneal cavity has been sounded perpendicularly, the same procedure is repeated with the needle angled at 45° (Fig 233). For cosmetic reasons, the tip of the needle is retracted only into the fatty tissue of the abdominal wall, so that both muscles and peritoneum can be traversed at a 45° angle. Moving the needle tip in a circular pattern will again detect spaces without adhesions. However, if the tip of the needle comes in contact with velamentous adhesions or bowel (Fig 234), bubbling in the syringe will be temporarily or permanently interrupted before the maximal depth of the pneumoperitoneum cavity is reached. These probing/sounding tests give a clear indication in which area the trocar for the endoscope can be safely introduced.

[Essentially the same information can be obtained by moving the Veress needle during insuf-

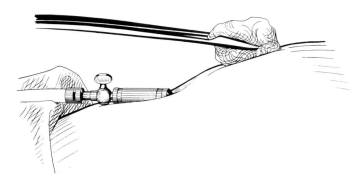

FIG 229.
Before the probing/sounding test, the abdominal wall is again disinfected.

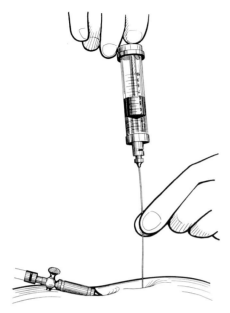

FIG 230.
A spinal needle is inserted perpendicularly.

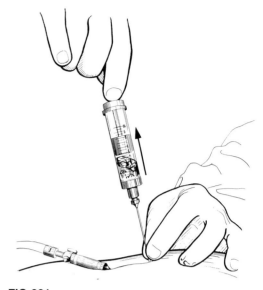

FIG 231.
CO_2 gas from the pneumoperitoneum is slowly aspirated.

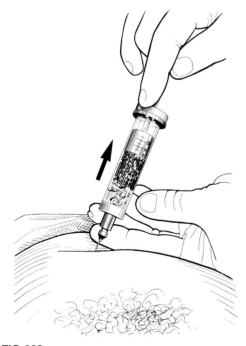

FIG 232.
The needle is withdrawn until bubbling stops.

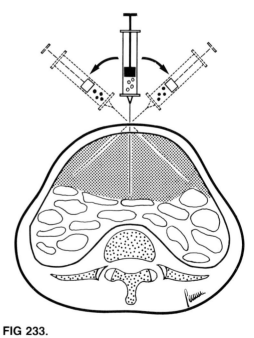

FIG 233.
The procedure is repeated with the needle angled at 45°.

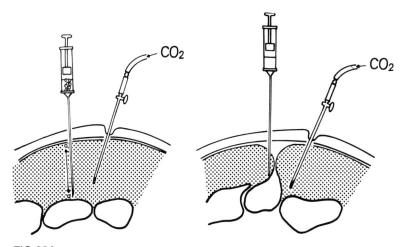

FIG 234.
Contact of needle tip with adhesions or bowel may interrupt bubbling prematurely.

flation with CO_2 gas at the rate of 1 L/min and observing the insufflation pressure. The pressure will suddenly rise whenever the lateral orifice above the needle tip is obstructed, i.e., touches bowel, omentum, parietal peritoneum, velamentous adhesions, etc.—*Ed.*]

It is our policy to insist that these eight safety tests be completed before blind insertion of the trocar can be justified.

If the probing/sounding test is equivocal or if the history raises the suspicion of massive intra-abdominal adhesions, one should refrain from blind insertion of the trocar for the laparoscope. The "open laparoscopy" technique is still feasible under these conditions (see chapter 12.3.1.3.).

14.1.3.4. Blind Introduction of the Trocar for the Endoscope

Before the insufflation of CO_2 gas begins, at the latest, the patient is brought into the 15° Trendelenburg position (Fig 235). In this position, the intestines will slide into the upper abdomen as the pneumoperitoneum develops. After an intra-abdominal static gas pressure of approximately 12 mm Hg has been reached (Fig 236) (for exceptions, see chapter 12.3.1.1.), and if the probing/sounding test was negative, the trocar for the laparoscope is introduced. For safety reasons, the diagnostic endoscope (7 mm diameter) should always be introduced first, even if subsequent operative procedures are planned.

After repeated disinfection of the umbilicus by

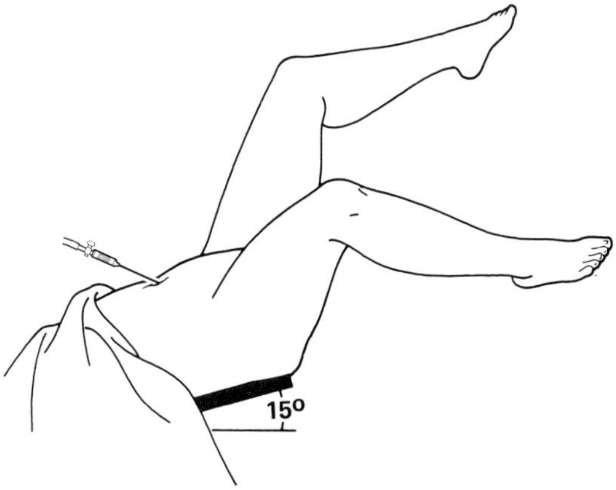

FIG 235.
Before insufflation with CO_2 gas is begun, the patient must be in the 15° Trendelenburg position.

15°

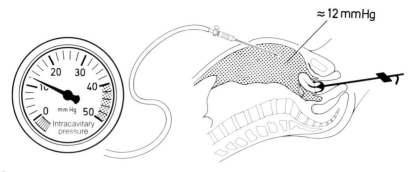

≈ 12 mmHg

FIG 236.
The intra-abdominal static gas pressure should be about 12 mm Hg before introduction of the trocar.

the rotation technique (Fig 237) a pointed 6-mm scalpel (No. 11 blade) is stabbed into the lower margin of the umbilicus in a direction almost parallel to the abdominal wall (Fig 238). The small puncture site from the Veress needle may be used as a point of entry for the scalpel (Fig 239). The horizontal (i.e., parallel) direction of the scalpel prevents incision of the fascia, particularly if the abdominal walls are thinned out postpartum.

Subsequently the trocar is advanced (not plunged!) through the abdominal wall according to the Z-insertion technique shown in Figure 240. This Z-insertion technique has four important advantages compared to perforation of the fascia in the linea alba:

1. The umbilical plate or the linea alba just caudal to it remains intact. If the peritoneum does not close completely after withdrawal of the trocar, a slit in the fascia may lead to entrapment of the omentum (see Plate 10) or even prolapse of the

omentum (see Figs 416 and 417 in *Atlas of Gynecologic Laparoscopy and Hysteroscopy,* 1977).

2. If the skin incision has been made large enough and if the dense fascial layer is avoided, not much force is required to advance the conical trocar through the muscle layers lateral to the umbilicus, particularly if a trocar sleeve with a beveled tip is used, as described in chapter 12.8.1.

3. The Z-track closes itself like a curtain as the trocar sleeve is withdrawn.

4. Due to the curtain-like closure, the wound does not have to be sutured in the area of the umbilicus. Closure of the skin with clips will suffice (see chapter 12.8.13. and Figs 196–199). The theoretical risk of bleeding from the muscle has never occurred in Kiel, where a conical trocar was used in more than 10,000 pelviscopies. The Z-track method should *not* be attempted with the triple-edged pyramidal trocar, since it could split the

FIG 237.
The umbilicus is again disinfected.

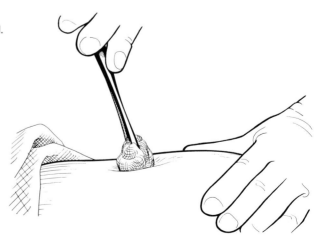

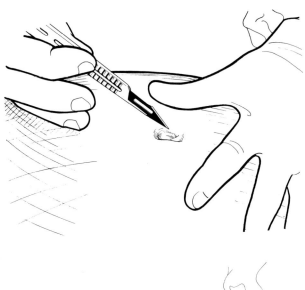

FIG 238.
A scalpel with a pointed blade is used to incise the lower margin of the umbilicus.

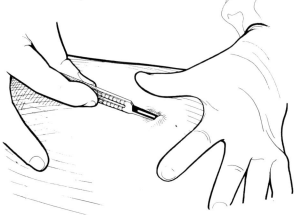

FIG 239.
The puncture site from the Veress needle may be used as the point of entry for the scalpel.

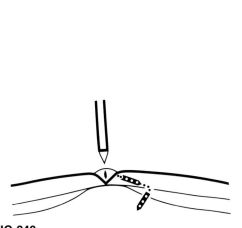

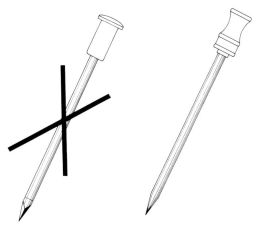

FIG 240.
The trocar is advanced using the Z-insertion technique.

FIG 241.
A sharpened triple-edged pyramidal trocar should not be used in place of a conical trocar.

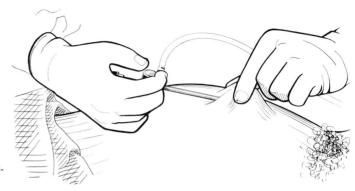

FIG 242.
The trocar is introduced and advanced 1 cm.

muscle instead of stretching it, leading to uncontrolled bleeding from the muscle (i.e., a hematoma).

Basic principle: The surgeon uses only wrist motion to advance the trocar through the abdominal wall (as was also described in chapter 12.3.1.1. for the introduction of the Veress needle, and demonstrated in Fig 69). As the conical trocar is pushed properly through the muscle layer, no force is required. Under no circumstances should a sharpened triple-edged pyramidal trocar (Fig 241) be used under the assumption that it would facilitate the Z-puncture.

After the insufflation tubing has been connected to the trocar sleeve (but the stopcock remains closed), the conical trocar is first introduced through the umbilical incision and advanced approximately 1 cm in the midline (Fig 242). Then the abdominal wall is elevated to a moderate degree and the trocar tip is pushed in a transverse direction about 2–3 cm to the right (Fig 243)—or to the left, depending on the results of the probing/sounding test. In this position, the trocar is elevated into a perpendicular direction and pushed slightly into the musculature. This maneuver prevents injuries due to splitting of the muscle during the Z-track technique when the angle of introduction of the trocar is changed toward the uterine fundus. When the trocar is pushed through the muscle layer and parietal peritoneum, the surgeon's little finger is used to prevent the trocar from perforating the abdominal wall too suddenly (Fig 244). The surgeon's left hand elevates the abdominal wall maximally.

After the trocar with the beveled trocar sleeve has been placed into the abdominal wall, the conical trocar is removed from its sleeve (Fig 245).

The trumpet valve automatically establishes a

gas-tight closure of the lumen. When the insufflation stopcock on the trocar sleeve is opened, the dial for intracavitary pressure on the OP-PNEU instrument shows the true intra-abdominal static pressure.

14.1.3.5. Introduction of the Endoscope and First Scan for Orientation

Immediately after the trocar is withdrawn, the endoscope is introduced. At first a 360° scan is done for orientation and to rule out injuries by the Veress needle and/or the trocar (Fig 246).

Particular attention must also be given to inspection of the retroperitoneal space in the area of the large pelvic blood vessels, because injuries to those vessels (Fig 247) at first cause only a retroperitoneal hematoma (Fig 248) and *not* bleeding

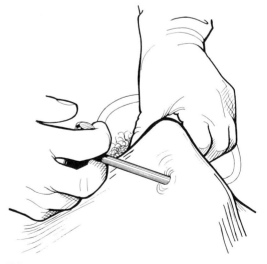

FIG 243.
The trocar tip is pushed transversely about 2–3 cm, to the right or left.

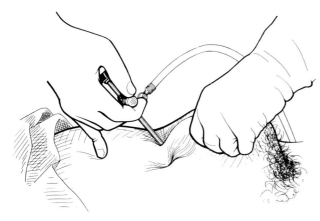

FIG 244.
The surgeon's little finger prevents sudden, uncontrolled insertion of the trocar. His left hand elevates the abdominal wall maximally.

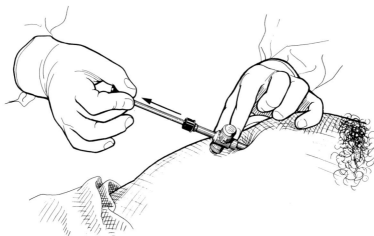

FIG 245.
The conical trocar is removed.

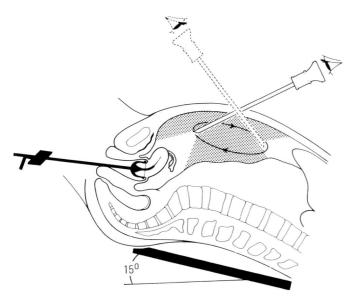

FIG 246.
The first 360° scanning of all surface areas to rule out injuries.

15⁰

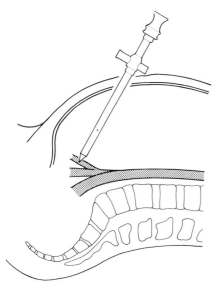

FIG 247.
Potential cause of injury to large pelvic blood vessels.

into the free abdominal cavity or the small pelvis.

In this context it should be emphasized that the entire abdominal cavity must immediately be searched with an endoscope if the anesthesiologists reports a drop in blood pressure. It must also be remembered that bleeding due to vascular injury rarely occurs into the free abdominal cavity first. Therefore, the cul-de-sac remains free of blood. Blood first spreads more or less profusely in the retroperitoneal space, sometimes up to the diaphragm (see Fig 248). All fatal accidents with laparoscopy that have been reported to me for an expert opinion in the recent past have occurred primarily because a drop in blood pressure or cardiac arrest was misinterpreted as anesthesia incident. The anesthesiologist reported asystole, and the surgeon failed to see—because of an inappropriate or inadequate search effort—blood in the free abdominal cavity (i.e., "massive hemorrhage"), which led to the cardiac arrest. Therefore, an incorrect diagnosis of anesthesia incident was made. Although cardiopulmonary resuscitation reestablished heartbeat, the patient exsanguinated.

Intra-abdominal vascular injury during a pelviscopy—either during the blind puncture with the insufflation needle or by introducing the trocar too deeply—is the most dangerous complication of endoscopy. However, it can be prevented if the safety tests and maneuvers described above are carried out routinely. They must remain routine, even if one considers oneself so skilled that one does not need to do them any longer.

When the anesthesiologist reports "anesthesia problem" or "cardiac arrest," one proceeds as follows:

1. Discontinue gas insufflation immediately.
2. Reduce intra-abdominal pressure to 8 mm Hg.
3. Do *not* remove the endoscope, but proceed with a 360° scan (Fig 249) to ascertain that a retroperitoneal hemorrhage can be ruled out. Waiting wastes precious minutes before the abdominal cavity can be opened and injured vessels can be clamped.

If retroperitoneal hemorrhage is discovered, one of the large trunk vessels (arterial or venous) has most probably been injured.

Since the patient has already been prepared for a laparotomy, a *longitudinal incision* is made without delay—without further scrubbing and disinfection. The injured vessel is immediately clamped with the vascular clamps (described in chapter 12.8.12.). Then one can calmly await the arrival of the vascular surgeon. A set of sterile vascular clamps must be ready for use for every pelviscopic procedure. Even if the clamps are not needed for many years, one should not abandon this routine precaution. The mortality rate from laparoscopic procedures has declined to 1:100,000. However, even these patients—as expert opinions have shown—could probably have been saved if the abdominal cavity had been opened and injured vessels clamped immediately.

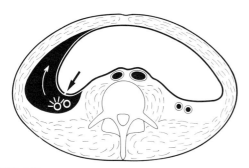

FIG 248.
Injury to blood vessels may cause an unsuspected retroperitoneal hematoma.

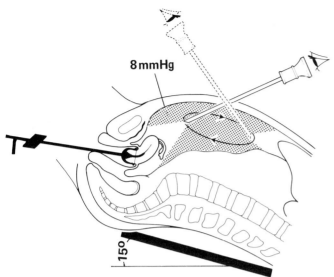

8 mmHg

150°

FIG 249.
If the anesthesiologist reports a problem, gas insufflation is discontinued, the intra-abdominal pressure is reduced to 8 mm Hg, and the surgeon undertakes a 360° scan of the area.

Once again, in abbreviated form:

1. In case of cardiac arrest, always think of vascular injury.
2. Search meticulously for retroperitoneal hemorrhage.
3. Hemorrhage almost never occurs in the abdominal cavity first.
4. No scrubbing, no prolonged disinfection.
5. *Immediate* laparotomy by longitudinal incision.
6. Compress the aorta or common iliac artery by hand.
7. Aspirate blood.
8. Clamp a generous segment of that vessel.
9. Calmly wait for the vascular surgeon.

A history of a previous abdominal operation used to be a contraindication to laparoscopy. Today, the postlaparotomy abdomen is the domain of endoscopic abdominal surgery. The rate of injuries from the blind puncture method, in the range of approximately 1%–3%, and a mortality rate of 0.001% (i.e., 1:100,000) can certainly be reduced further.

If patients have a suspicious history, the 11-mm trocar for endoscopic abdominal surgery should not be introduced through the abdominal wall by the blind puncture method. In such high-risk cases, the "open laparoscopy" technique proposed by Hasson (1974) is very helpful. With this technique, which was described in more detail in

chapter 12.3.1.3., it is highly unlikely that the large trunk vessels will be injured. However, an injury of a loop of bowel which is attached to the parietal peritoneum by broad-based adhesions cannot always be avoided, even when the abdomen is opened through a minilaparotomy and when the most meticulous dissection techniques are employed. In any case, the blunt trocar and sleeve developed by Hasson are valuable additions to the endoscopic instruments with which, in borderline cases, the risk from the primary puncture can be eliminated.

14.1.4. Second Diagnostic Scan

The first 360° scanning (see Fig 246) is done to rule out any injury caused by the puncture or insufflation procedure. The second diagnostic 360° scan (Fig 250) is undertaken to evaluate all visible organs before any additional manipulation is done, either by instruments inserted through a second and third puncture or by movement of the vacuum intrauterine cannula (i.e., the uterus). The organs inspected are the diaphragm, liver, gallbladder, omentum, bowel, anterior cul-de-sac, etc. This scan is also important with an "open laparoscopy," particularly as injuries to bowel and omentum could have occurred during the sharp entry into the peritoneal cavity with a scalpel.

During the pelviscopy, the uterus is then elevated against the posterior aspect of the symphysis

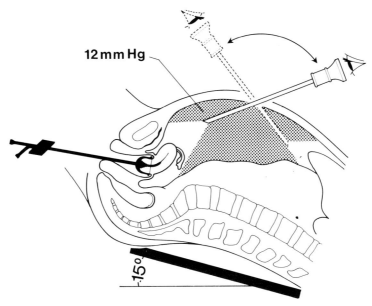

FIG 250.
The second 360° diagnostic scan.

pubis (Fig 251) and the cul-de-sac and adnexa are inspected. When the endoscope with a 30° optical angle is rotated (Fig 252), the entire small pelvis can be examined without undue contortions of the surgeon's cervical spine. In the presence of massive adhesions in the abdomen, this scan does not reveal very much; however, one should make an effort to understand as much of the pathologic anatomical relationships as possible.

A major mistake in orientation is made under the following circumstance: after a previous laparotomy the greater omentum adheres to the anterior abdominal wall (the parietal peritoneum). With the insertion of the trocar, one has perforated the omentum (Fig 253) and looks into a closed cavity formed by adhesions but cannot see the liver, diaphragm, and so forth. This situation is corrected by cautiously withdrawing the endoscope with the trocar sleeve until the omentum is released (Fig 254). Only after this maneuver has been performed is it possible to recognize the liver as a point of orientation and, consequently, to identify the omental adhesions correctly (Fig 255); then one decides what further action to take. In most cases, one will be able to remove omental adhesions that obscure one's view (see chapters 14.2.2.1., 15.1., and 15.2.).

FIG 251.
The uterus is elevated for inspection of
the cul-de-sac and adnexa.

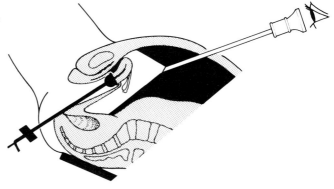

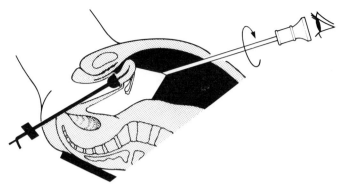

FIG 252.
Rotation of the endoscope allows inspection of the entire small pelvis.

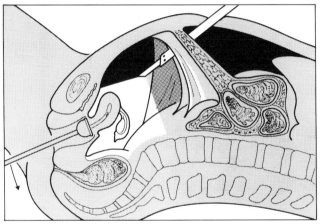

FIG 253.
View into a closed cavity without access to
liver and diaphragm indicates perforation of
the omentum or adhesions.

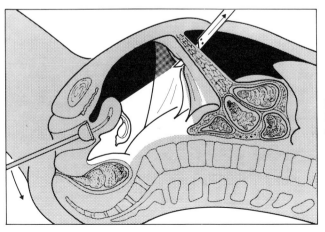

FIG 254.
Endoscope and trocar sleeve are withdrawn
carefully until omentum is released.

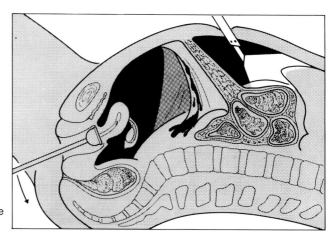

FIG 255.
The endoscopist can then recognize the liver as a landmark.

14.1.5. Second and Third Punctures To Establish a Diagnosis as an Indication for the Operative Phase

Mere inspection of the abdomen from the perspective of the umbilicus does not permit an accurate diagnosis to be made unless the uterus is elevated, the adnexa are viewed from all aspects, and the omentum and bowel are displaced out of the pelvis. At least one and possibly two additional 5-mm trocar sleeves must be introduced to properly evaluate all pelvic organs. Only after all pelvic and intra-abdominal structures have been clearly identified can an indication for further endoscopic procedures be established.

For cosmetic reasons, the trocar sleeves for the 5-mm operating instruments are always introduced in the pubic area (Fig 256). The lower abdominal wall is transilluminated so that larger subcutaneous vessels, usually veins, can be avoided and an avascular site can be selected; or the endoscopist may choose an old scar, such as one left by a Pfannenstiel procedure or appendectomy. A small transverse skin incision 4–5 mm long is made with a small, pointed scalpel.

The 5-mm trocars with conical tips for the second, third, and fourth puncture are always guided through the layers of the abdominal wall according to the Z-insertion technique (see Fig 240) until they reach the peritoneum. The peritoneum is punctured only under visual guidance (Fig 257). Visual control is absolutely necessary to prevent incidental injury of a subfascial arterial blood vessel (Plates 13–15).

If a vessel is injured despite this precaution— and a vessel may be injured in a scarred abdomen—bleeding is usually of the spurting type and

must be controlled, without a laparotomy, with a large curved needle according to the technique described in chapter 12.8.7. (see Plates 14 and 15).

Occasionally adhesions are present in the immediate vicinity of the umbilicus and cannot be diagnosed well from the vantage point of the umbilicus. In such cases the suprapubic puncture that was made for the introduction of the 5-mm operating instruments is dilated to accommodate a trocar sleeve for an endoscope (for technique see chapter 12.8.8.). Periumbilical adhesions can be inspected better (see Plate 10) and also be lysed from the lower abdomen (see chapter 14.2.2.1. ff.).

Occasionally it is necessary to dilate from the

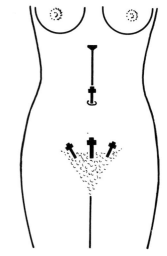

FIG 256.
The trocar sleeves for the operating instruments are introduced in the pubic area.

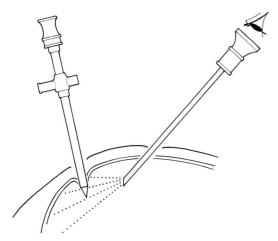

FIG 257.
The peritoneum is punctured under visual control.

5-mm trocar sleeve to an 11-mm trocar sleeve for the removal of larger tissue fragments (cyst wall, myomas) that have been resected from pelvic organs. This obviates the introduction of an additional 11-mm trocar. However, an 11-mm trocar sleeve is always necessary for appendectomy, salpingo-oophorectomy, and operations for an ectopic pregnancy. In such cases the 11-mm trocar is usually introduced under vision in the midline (see Fig 256). The intra-abdominal position of three suprapubic trocar sleeves can be seen in Plate 197.

Therefore, the second and third punctures, which were made to establish a final diagnosis or indication for the transition to endoscopic abdominal surgery, are, at the same time, preparatory measures for such intervention. However, the primary diameters of the channels for operative instruments are not always sufficient for some of these surgical procedures but may have to be replaced or augmented by instruments with larger diameters.

14.1.6. Transition to the Operative Phase: Exchange of Endoscopes

Pelviscopic diagnosis is principally carried out with an endoscope of maximally 7 mm diameter. Operative measures, however, should ·be carried out only with an 11-mm endoscope because it offers a larger and brighter field of view and the possibility for low-power magnification with a loupe and/or observation of the intra-abdominal operation by an assistant. At the same time, use of an 11-mm endoscope permits photographic documenta-

tion of specific findings or operative steps. Dilatation from the 7-mm trocar sleeve to 11-mm sleeve (discussed in chapter 12.2.2.) is accomplished with the dilatation sets (see chapter 12.8.8. and Plate 12).

Particularly at the beginning of his career, the endoscopic abdominal surgeon should not, for the sake of convenience, skip the step of dilatation, because monocular vision makes operative manipulations hard enough; they should not be restricted further by too small a field of view or poor illumination.

14.2. THE OPERATIVE PHASE

The decision for an operative endoscopic procedure is made:

- After careful consideration of all parameters.
- After comparing history and physical findings with the situation found by inspection.
- In consideration of the type and performance of the procedure agreed upon by the patient.
- In consideration of one's own capabilities.
- Under the condition that all technical requirements are met without exception, and all equipment and instruments are available.

The decision in favor of an endoscopic operation is strengthened by the facts that in the case at hand:

- By classic rules, a laparotomy is indicated.
- A laparotomy is possible at any time because the patient has been prepared for one.
- Ovaries, tubes, etc. bleed considerably less during the endoscopic operative procedure, in which there is no large abdominal incision to provoke vascular paralysis, as there is during a laparotomy.
- The operative correction of disease without a large abdominal incision will affect the patient's physical condition only for a few days.
- In regard to postoperative discomfort, the endoscopic procedure is far superior to a laparotomy.

14.2.1. Catalog of Abdominal Procedures Feasible With an Endoscope

For the remainder of this chapter, the endoscopic operations are first sketched as line drawings depicting the chronological sequence of operative steps, then, in the atlas of color plates at the end of the book, they are illustrated by life-sized color photographs taken during the operation. Explanatory line drawings with a comprehensive numbered index are printed adjacent to every original photograph. This combination of simplified artistic renderings of the operative procedure with original color photographs should enhance the reader's understanding of endoscopic operative activities.

Since endoscopic abdominal surgery was derived from the catalog of gynecologic operations, gynecologic procedures dominate in this text. The transition to extensive adhesiolysis, including suture of bowel (after perforation in an abdomen with massive adhesions), or to appendectomy no longer permits an absolute division to be made between purely gynecologic operative procedures and those of a general surgical nature. The latter endoscopic operations are no longer limited to women but are also possible in men.

However, according to the categories illustrated in Figures 7 through 18, we will be distinguishing between typical gynecologic endoscopic procedures and those that are more of a general surgical nature. In the cumulative total of approximately 10,000 pelviscopic procedures performed in Kiel between 1970 and 1983, the indication for operative pelviscopy was present in approximately 6,500–7,000 cases and the following classic gynecologic operative steps were performed successfully (see also Figs 7 through 18):

> Extensive adhesiolysis, occasionally with partial omentectomy
> Salpingolysis and ovariolysis
> Fimbrioplasty and salpingostomy
> Enucleation of pedunculated or prominent subserous myomas
> Conservative operation for ectopic pregnancy
> Radical operation for ectopic pregnancy by salpingectomy
> Ovarian biopsy
> Excision of ovarian cysts, ovarian suture
> Oophorectomy
> Salpingo-oophorectomy
> Coagulation of endometriotic implants in the pelvis
> Tubal sterilization

Beyond this list there are numerous other indications for surgery (e.g., excision of paraovarian cysts, excision of hydatid cysts) which were not included in this schematic sketch. They are essentially only technical variations of the major classic gynecologic interventions.

Of the abdominal operations that are not limited to gynecology, the following should be mentioned (see also Figs 19 through 21):

> Intestinal adhesiolysis, including intestinal suture.
> Omental adhesiolysis and resection after previous laparotomies.
> Appendectomy.

14.2.2. Typical Gynecologic Endoscopic Procedures

Operations specific to the field of gynecology can be performed only if the female genitalia are in direct view. However, if previous inflammation or surgery has caused intra-abdominal adhesions, the specific gynecologic procedures must be preceded by general surgical measures.

14.2.2.1. Omental Adhesiolysis in the Upper, Mid, and Lower Abdomen and Omental Resection

If a patient has had a previous abdominal operation it is often impossible to inspect the internal female genitalia with an endoscope. In the past one was satisfied with circumventing filamentous adhesions with the endoscope to gain access to the pelvic area. Often the adhesions were not even noticed! (See Figs 253 through 255, and chapter 15.1.)

Today, all omental adhesions and bands are dissected first to establish an unobstructed view into the pelvis. One should never begin to operate in the pelvis before the mid-abdominal cavity is completely free of adhesions. In a laparotomy, too, free access to the operative field is established first. Refer to the basic guidelines for endoscopic operations at the beginning of chapter 14.

Technically, the procedures described below are available for omental and intestinal adhesiolysis.

14.2.2.2. Adhesiolysis Without Prior Hemostasis (Bloody Adhesiolysis)

Poorly vascularized omental adhesions, usually in the midline in the area of the peritoneal suture from a previous laparotomy, are sharply dissected off the parietal peritoneum with hook scissors (Fig 258; see also Plates 35, 84 and 358). To accomplish this, the adherent omentum is grasped with atraumatic tongs and held under tension so that it can be dissected with scissors di-

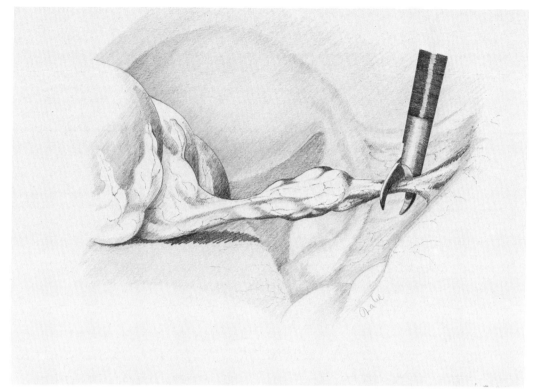

FIG 258.
Poorly vascularized omental adhesions are dissected off the parietal peritoneum using hook scissors.

rectly within the avascular layer of its attachment to the peritoneum.

Traction with atraumatic tongs is very helpful. It should never be omitted. The endoscopic surgeon should also keep in mind the rule: Do nothing else in a pelviscopic operation than in a laparotomy. In a laparotomy, tissues are kept under tension with a forceps to identify cleavage lines for the dissection of the omentum.

If it is certain that the adhesions are a great distance away from bowel, the omental tissue is coagulated for 20 seconds with the crocodile forceps (Plate 16), which is then rotated like a hair curler (Plate 17) before the tissues are cut with hook scissors (Plate 18). If this type of adhesiolysis is complicated by bleeding from an arterial or venous blood vessel, the vessel is grasped and ligated with an endoloop (see chapter 12.6.1.).

TECHNIQUE

As shown in Figure 259, the endoscopic surgeon introduces an endoloop through a second puncture into the abdomen, advances atraumatic tongs or a biopsy forceps through the loop (Plates 7, 19, and 20), grasps with it the bleeding vessel or the bleeding segment of omental tissue, pulls the vessel or segment through the endoloop (Plate 22), and ligates it by placing traction on the suture material while simultaneously pushing the plastic applicator tube down to apply the slipknot.

After the suture has been cut (Fig 260) the transected margin of the omentum is carefully checked for bleeding which, if necessary, is controlled by another endoloop. The ligature after sharp lysis of adhesions to the ovary (Plate 21) is shown in Plate 22. If a longer omental pedicle remains after dissection, a ligature is applied at the most appropriate level and the protruding omental tissue is resected. The removal of the omental specimen is accomplished after the 5-mm puncture has been dilated to accommodate an 11-mm trocar sleeve. The large spoon forceps is well suited to grasp the specimen (see chapter 12.8.2.). If necessary—if the size of the specimen is too large—

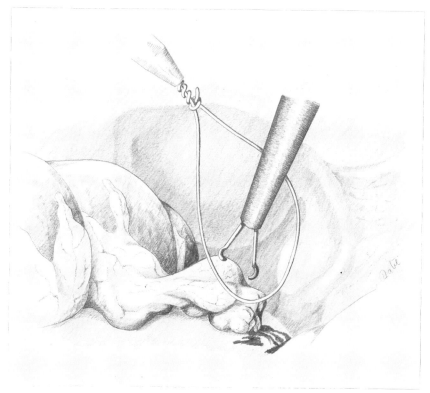

FIG 259.
Technique of ligating a bleeding vessel or bleeding segment of omental tissue.

the omentum is first cut into narrower strips either with hook scissors or with the large serrated scissors.

Occasionally, lysis of omental adhesions may be accomplished bluntly by traction with one or two atraumatic grasping forceps. With this technique, the risk of bleeding is decreased. If, however, bleeding does occur, it can usually be controlled by an endoloop. Broad-based vascular adhesions of the omentum to the anterior abdominal wall, however, should not be lysed without prior hemostatic measures. One should not even attempt lysis on such adhesions, for several reasons: If heavier bleeding occurs in the omentum, the bleeding site is difficult to find (as it is during a laparotomy), continuous omental bleeding obscures the anatomy, and suction of blood from the omental-intestinal area is difficult. The difficulties are caused by the fact that the suction tip always aspirates omentum, bowel, or fatty tissue of the epiploic appendices, respectively, which are quite mobile, before any substantial volume of blood is aspirated.

Since we have been able to apply intra-abdominal ligatures by tying slipknots externally, it is advisable to save time by lysing adhesions after prophylactic hemostasis has been achieved, as described in the following chapter. Our motto is: Prophylactic hemostasis usually saves more time than control of hemorrhage!

14.2.2.3. Adhesiolysis After Prophylactic Hemostasis (Bloodless Adhesiolysis)

In the bloodless technique of adhesiolysis, vascularized omental and intestinal adhesions are ligated before their sharp dissection. In principle, the technique is comparable to the application of Roeder's endoloop with slipknot, except that it is not supplied in a commercial package ready for use. Instead, a suture has to be passed around the tissue to be ligated and the slipknot has to be tied externally by hand. It is convenient to use the endosuture described in chapter 12.6.3. after its needle has been cut off. The sequence of illustrations shown in Figures 128–133 demonstrates graphically all steps of the operation.

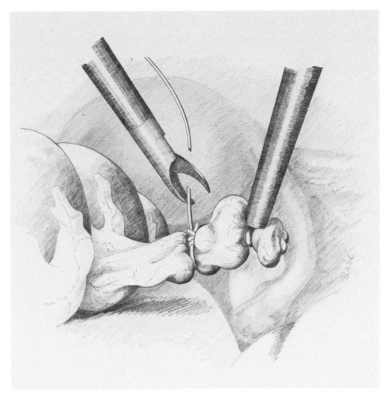

FIG 260.
The suture is cut and the transected margin of omentum is checked for bleeding.

At first the end of the suture is carried by the 3-mm needleholder through the applicator into the abdomen under direct vision through the endoscope (Plate 23). The 5-mm needleholder, which was introduced through a third puncture, grasps the end of the suture (see Plate 23) and carries it behind the omental segment to be ligated. There the 3-mm needleholder accepts the end of the suture again (Plate 24). The mobile sealing cone (see Fig 141) on the shaft of the 3-mm needleholder has, in the meantime, been pushed against the applicator seal to reduce loss of gas. After additional length of the 80-cm-long catgut suture has been introduced into the abdomen, under visual control, the end of the suture is slowly retracted through the applicator with the 3-mm needleholder.

The 5-mm needleholder may assist in this procedure. While the slipknot is being tied externally (refer to chapter 12.6.3. and Fig 134), the hole in the rubber seal on the applicator is closed off with a finger (see Fig 134, steps 1–3). Next, the plastic end piece is broken off at the blue marking (see Fig 142) and the plastic tube slides down to the slipknot. To facilitate the introduction of the slipknot, the applicator is pulled back from the trocar sleeve (see Fig 134, step 4) until the knot disappears in it. Then the applicator is pushed into the trocar sleeve until its collar touches the end of the trocar sleeve. The plastic rod is used to advance the knot into the abdomen (see Fig 144). There the loop is tightened (Plate 25), as soon as the loop has been placed properly with the 5-mm needleholder. Once again, one pulls on the end of the suture while pressing the plastic rod against the knot to ascertain that the ligature has been properly applied; then traction on the suture keeps the adhesions under tension, so that they can be transected sharply (see Plate 25).

If one is skilled in this technique it is feasible to lyse those very vascular bands which are frequently present in postoperative intestinal/omental adhesions. Plate 26 shows a broad-based attachment of the omentum to the ascending colon. This adhesion has formed after an abdominal hysterectomy with bilateral salpingo-oophorectomy. It had caused colicky pain and symptoms of partial intestinal obstruction. After this velamentous adhesion has been identified, the end of the suture is introduced with the 3-mm needleholder (Plate 27) according to the technique previously presented. Then the suture is passed behind the band of adhesions (Plate 28), tied externally, ligated at a safe distance from the bowel, and cut (Plate 29). This is followed by a second ligature (Plate 30), resulting in a bridge that can be transected. Under simultaneous traction on the second ligature, the bridge of tissue is transected with hook scissors (Plate 31). A second example of a bloodless adhesiolysis is shown in Plates 346–353. These two examples may suffice to demonstrate the variety of possible applications of the endoligature.

14.2.2.4. Omental Resection

Particularly in sterility patients who have undergone previous operations, the omentum extends deep into the pelvis, where it is usually partially fixed and may interfere with the function of the tubes. In general surgery it is customary to resect such long lobes of omentum. This can also be achieved by loop ligature, as described in chapters 12.6.1. and 14.2.2.1. (see Plates 7–9), or endoligature or endosuture, depending on the pathologic anatomical findings during the exploration. For the endosuture, the same procedure is used as is used for bloodless adhesiolysis, except that the needle is not cut off at the beginning but will be passed through the omentum according to the familiar Dechamps technique in the open abdomen. Sometimes the needle can be replaced by the conical jaws of the 3-mm needleholder. The omentum can then be easily removed through the 11-mm trocar sleeve by picking up small portions with the large spoon forceps, if necessary, after dividing the specimen with large scissors.

14.2.2.5. Pelviscopic Adhesiolysis in Preparation for a Laparotomy Either During the Same Operation or at Another Time

A strong suspicion of uterine, intestinal, or omental adhesions, particularly if they can be palpated in slender patients, are contraindications for a vaginal hysterectomy.

By combining endoscopic omental and intestinal adhesiolysis with a subsequent vaginal hysterectomy, the endoscopic surgeon can avoid a laparotomy in many cases. To explore this possibility, a diagnostic pelviscopy is performed to determine whether intestinal and omental adhesions to the uterine corpus or, more commonly, to the anterior uterine wall are so extensive that only the abdominal route is feasible, or if fundal adhesions could be lysed and the uterus removed vaginally without difficulties.

In numerous cases we have been able to lyse those omental adhesions from the uterine corpus (Plate 32) and subsequently to remove the uterus vaginally by routine techniques and without undue problems or risks. The pelviscopic transection of the suspensory ligaments of the ovaries may also be very worthwhile in potential problem cases in preparation for the vaginal operative technique (see also chapter 14.2.8.1.).

Occasionally the size of a myomatous uterus raises differential diagnostic questions as to whether the vaginal or abdominal route should be chosen in a specific patient. In these cases, too, preliminary pelviscopy helps the surgeon to decide whether or not the vaginal technique is prudent. One ascertains precisely the position and size of myomas that may have to be morcellated to make the vaginal procedure a safe, low-risk operation.

In the case of sterility due to tubal factors, the preliminary endoscopic inspection is necessary to make an exact diagnosis and to determine if the tubal defect can be corrected by pelviscopy or if a laparotomy is required. Follow-up findings after two sterility operations by laparotomy (bilateral salpingostomy), shown in Plate 33, are an excellent indication for operative pelviscopy: meticulous adhesiolysis, ovariolysis, and salpingolysis will reexpose the ovaries for pelviscopic follicle puncture for in vitro fertilization (see chapter 14.2.14.). Operations on severely damaged tubes, either by laparotomy or pelviscopy, may no longer be sensible.

Another indication for preoperative pelviscopic diagnostic evaluation is a woman's request for tubal reversal after a previous operative sterilization with tubal transection. One must determine whether an end-to-end anastomosis will have to be done under microsurgical conditions by laparotomy or if it can be attempted with the pelviscope. In favorable cases, end-to-end anastomosis can also be performed pelviscopically with microsuture.

In such cases or, as in the present case with bilateral intramural tubal occlusion (Plate 34), it is first determined whether a reconstructive operation will ever be feasible after previous operative trauma to the tubes, then it can immediately be followed by intra-abdominal adhesiolysis and salpingo-ovariolysis (Plate 35). Suture ligatures, plastic clips, or Silastic rings that had been applied to accomplish the tubal ligation are also removed at that time.

Peritoneal defects produced under pelviscopic conditions will heal during the following weeks almost without scar formation. The microsurgical reconstructive procedure, which is done 2–3 months later by laparotomy, can then be limited to end-to-end anastomosis or tubal implantation, because there are few if any adhesions in the pelvis, as shown in Plate 36. This obviates the need for repair of widespread peritoneal defects which are so detrimental to microsurgery, and the success rate will be increased by a considerable percentage. We could prove this from numerous reconstructive operations at the University Women's Hospital in Kiel. For example, a 34-year-old patient with secondary sterility after a right salpingectomy for tubal pregnancy was found to have extensive abdominal adhesions (Plate 37), which were cut, step by step, in each instance after hemostatic coagulation with a crocodile forceps (Plates 38, 39). Six months later, tubal reimplantation could be performed microsurgically in the absence of any adhesion (Plate 40).

In summary, pelviscopic adhesiolysis in combination with a laparotomy or vaginal operation, either during the same operation or subsequently, has considerably expanded the gynecologic operative options and resulted in a marked improvement in the live birth rate after such operations.

14.2.3. Endoscopic Operative Management of Superficial Pelvic Endometriosis

According to statistical data reported by Baly and Gossak (1956), superficial pelvic endometriosis is detected in 18% of general laparotomy cases, and according to Greenblatt (1982) in as many as 21.4% of cases. Among more than 10,000 pelviscopy procedures carried out for various indications in Kiel, endometriosis was found in 24% of cases.

In the selected group of pelviscopies done in Kiel for sterility (861 cases), pelvic endometriosis was diagnosed in 51%.

The surgical excision of endometriotic implants is still considered the optimal treatment of pelvic endometriosis. At least five theories on the development of this condition are worth discussing (Fig 261). However, in individual cases no theory can be correlated with specific anatomical findings or with specific events in the patient's history. Therefore, the etiology of endometriosis in a single case under investigation or under treatment remains unknown. The hormonal suppression of endometriotic implants by progestational agents and antigonadotropins is possible when corresponding receptors are present. According to Schweppe (1983), this applies to only 60% of cases. The remaining implants are not amenable to hormonal therapy. Therefore, hormonal therapy is much inferior to surgical therapy, as we confirmed during years of pelviscopic observations and repeated pelviscopies on the same patients.

A description of the extent of endometriosis is quite problematic. Acosta (1973) divides it into three groups. The revised classification of the American Fertility Society (1985) describes four stages or degrees of endometriosis according to a new scoring system that takes into account the site (peritoneum, ovary: right and left) and size (less than 1 cm, 1–3 cm, more than 3 cm), and depth (superficial vs. deep) of endometriotic implants, partial vs. complete posterior cul de sac obliteration, and the site (ovary, tube: right and left) and extent (less than ⅓ vs. ⅓-⅔ vs. more than ⅔ enclosure) and consistency (filmy vs. dense) of adhesions. The AFS scoring table is augmented further by diagrammatic sketches of the visual findings at diagnostic surgery (see Chart 1, p. 159).

For visual pelviscopic diagnosis, we found the comparison between verbal description and the visual image time-consuming and bewildering.

I.	Mesonephric theory (embryonal dissemination)	● von Recklinghausen (1896), Gebhardt
II.	Serosal epithelial aberration theory (persistent celomic epithelial metaplasia)	● Ivanoff (1898), Meyer (1907)
III.	Invasion theory (myohyperplasia) (tubal adenomyosis)	● Cullen (1908), Sampson (1921) ● Philipp and Huber (1939)
IV.	Lymphogenic metastases theory	● Halban (1924), Javert (1952)
V.	Implantation theory (tubal regurgitation, transmission)	● Sampson (1921)

FIG 261.
Theories on the development of endometriosis.

Therefore, considering previous proposals, we have prepared our own chart (see Chart 2, p. 160). This endoscopic endometriosis classification (EEC) visually distinguishes four grades of dissemination, including patency of the fallopian tubes. The regions of distribution, which can be quickly and correctly determined by pelviscopy, are translated into a simple, logical display, subdivided by grades corresponding to the following verbal descriptions:

EEC I: Discrete peritoneal endometriotic implants which are disseminated in the area of the cul-de-sac, smaller than 5 mm in diameter, and not forming nodules. Tubes are clearly patent. The ampullae are of normal shape and there are no peritubal or periovarian adhesions. Cervical implants.

EEC II: Endometriotic implants in the cul-de-sac of more than 5 mm in diameter and in the sacrouterine ligaments of less than 5 mm in diameter, which are forming nodules, and/or in the vesicouterine peritoneal reflection, small foci on or behind the ovaries, ampullary phimosis or stenosis, single- or double-sided minimal peritubal and/or ovarian adhesions.

EEC III: Extensive, confluent endometriotic implants in the vesicouterine reflection and/ or cul-de-sac, nodules more than 5 mm in diameter in the sacrouterine ligaments, chocolate cysts, adenomas in the tubal cornua, salpingitis isthmica nodosa, intramural adenomas, severe ampullary phimosis or stenosis, unilateral or bilateral hydrosalpinx/sactosalpinx, extensive peritubal and/or ovarian adhesions.

EEC IV: Extragenital distribution of endometriotic implants, e.g., on bowel, appendix, parietal peritoneum, and—endoscopically not detectable—umbilicus, lungs, etc.

Every individual focus detected contributes to the classification.

14.2.3.1. Excision of Endometriotic Implants

Large, confluent endometriotic implants in the dome of the bladder (Plate 41) and in the pelvis are scraped off with biopsy forceps or large spoon forceps in a manner comparable to curettage.

The remaining "basalis" is eradicated thermobiologically with a point coagulator sweeping across the entire area (Plate 42). The application of destructive heat is possible only with the endoco-agulation system, because it is only heat that radiates from the tip of the point coagulator (or the lower jaw of the crocodile forceps or the myoma enucleator), and not an electrical current. This heat penetrates to a maximum depth of 1–2 mm, leading to thermobiologic necrosis of the tissue.

In this context, it should again be emphasized that a similar coagulation with the use of high-frequency current is not without risk under any circumstances. The current is conducted through tissues that contain electrolytes, and its distribution cannot be controlled by the surgeon. Therefore, the heat that develops in tissues cannot be controlled by the surgeon, neither its intensity nor its distribution. Even tissues that during the endoscopic observation do not show a white discoloration due to an increase in the field density of the high-frequency current will be "invisibly" warmed up to more than 57° C in a wide marginal area surrounding the region of visible temperature changes. Still, these lower temperatures induce thermolabile metabolic enzymes to disintegrate, and therefore cause cell death. This significantly endangers not only the walls of the large blood vessels that traverse the pelvis, covered only by peritoneum, but also the ureter, which cannot always be identified in its course.

Endometriotic implants in the sacrouterine ligaments (Plate 43 and others) should first be endocoagulated with the point coagulator (Plates 42, 44) and then be removed by sharp biopsy (Plate 41) because such implants often grow deep into the paravaginal tissues. Their location is demonstrated in Figures 262–265.

Occasionally, large epithelial defects remain after excision of endometriotic implants. Such defects are closed by endosuture and external tying of knots, just as they would be closed during a laparotomy (see Plates 51–57).

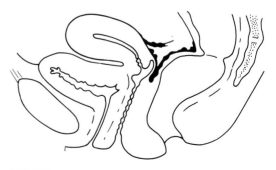

FIG 262.
Endometriosis in the area of the uterine ligaments.

THE AMERICAN FERTILITY SOCIETY
REVISED CLASSIFICATION OF ENDOMETRIOSIS
1985

Patient's Name _____ Date _____

Stage I   (Minimal) - 1-5
Stage II (Mild)   - 6-15
Stage III (Moderate) - 16-40
Stage IV (Severe)   - >40
Total _____

Laparoscopy _____ Laparotomy _____ Photography _____
Recommended Treatment _____
_____
Prognosis _____

	ENDOMETRIOSIS	<1cm	1-3cm	>3cm
PERITONEUM	Superficial	1	2	4
	Deep	2	4	6
OVARY	R Superficial	1	2	4
	Deep	4	16	20
	L Superficial	1	2	4
	Deep	4	16	20

	POSTERIOR CULDESAC OBLITERATION	Partial	Complete
		4	40

	ADHESIONS	<1/3 Enclosure	1/3-2/3 Enclosure	>2/3 Enclosure
OVARY	R Filmy	1	2	4
	Dense	4	8	16
	L Filmy	1	2	4
	Dense	4	8	16
TUBE	R Filmy	1	2	4
	Dense	4*	8*	16
	L Filmy	1	2	4
	Dense	4*	8*	16

*If the fimbriated end of the fallopian tube is completely enclosed, change the point assignment to 16.

Additional Endometriosis: _____
_____
_____
_____

Associated Pathology: _____
_____
_____
_____

To Be Used with Normal
Tubes and Ovaries

L   R

To Be Used with Abnormal
Tubes and/or Ovaries

L   R

CHART 1.
American Fertility Society Revised Classification of Endometriosis. (From *Fertil Steril* 1985; 43:351. Reproduced by permission.)

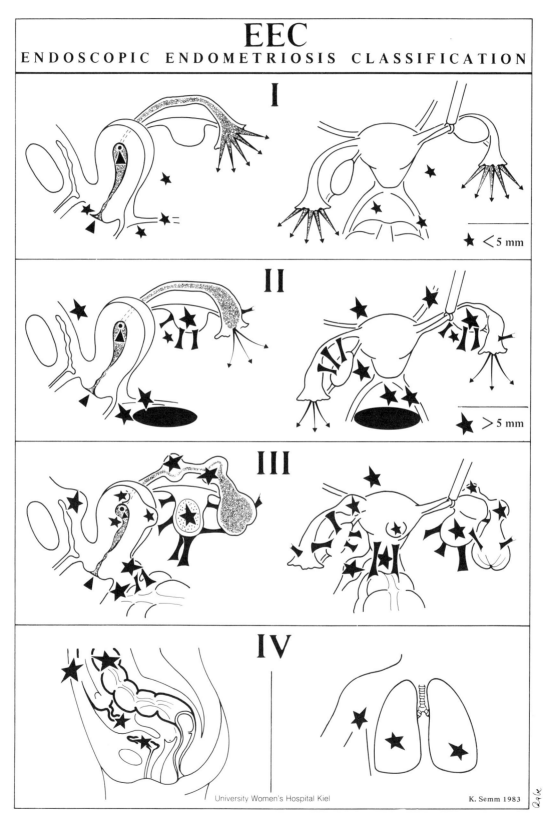

EEC
ENDOSCOPIC ENDOMETRIOSIS CLASSIFICATION

I

★ < 5 mm

II

★ > 5 mm

III

IV

University Women's Hospital Kiel

K. Semm 1983

CHART 2

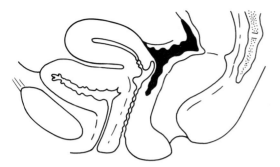

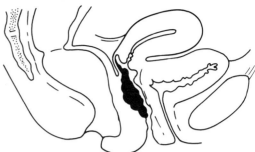

FIG 263.
Confluent endometrial implants in the cul-de-sac.

FIG 265.
Retrovaginal-pararectal endometriosis.

In the presence of paracervical and retrovaginal endometriosis which forms nodules, a combined approach is recommended (Fig 266): vaginal incision of these nodules under pelviscopic control. This can be accomplished by using the articulated or flexible teaching attachment (see also Fig 344).

With this technique it is highly unlikely that the rectal ampulla will be injured. However, the risk of injury to the rectal ampulla is always present if endometriotic nodules in the posterior vaginal fornix are opened blindly.

In all operations to remove endometriosis, one must be extremely cautious whenever the rectal ampulla is attached to the posterior wall of the cervix (see Plates 43, 44); the same is also true during a laparotomy. During preoperative counseling, the patient should routinely be advised of this risk and of the possible need for a colostomy.

The excision of endometriotic implants and chocolate cysts of the ovary is described in chapter 14.2.6.

Endometriotic implants on bowel cannot be coagulated. We have learned from histologic examinations (Plate 45) that endometriotic implants

may extend deep into the muscular layers. Therefore, caution is mandatory for the dissection of retrocervical-rectal implants. Such intestinal endometriotic implants are only diagnosed endoscopically. Their management, if indicated, requires a laparotomy and bowel resection.

If endometriosis is present in the appendix (Plate 46), an appendectomy is indicated (see chapter 15.3. ff.), which in this case is performed during the same operation.

Occasionally, pedunculated or subserous myomas (see Plates 221–247) can be enucleated and may then reveal histologic findings of adenomyomas. In retrospect, this may explain the patient's complaints.

However, adenomyosis within the uterine wall is ordinarily not amenable to pelviscopic surgery. This also applies to adenomyosis of the tubal cornu. Adenomyosis of the tubal cornu is suspected when the tubal cornu is bulging (Plate 47). Because of the infiltrating growth of endometrial tissues, it is sometimes also suspected from an intense blue discoloration of the adenoma and the tubal cornu during chromosalpingoscopy (Plates 47, 48). This is an absolute sign of adenomatous infiltration of the myometrium. Salpingitis isthmica nodosa, the so-called pearl string tube (Plate 49), likewise cannot be treated pelviscopically.

14.2.3.2. Coagulation of Endometriotic Implants

Endometriotic implants in the dome of the bladder (Plates 50, 61, 62) or the cul-de-sac, which generally resemble powder burns, are usually coagulated with the point coagulator. Depending on the size of the implants, the temperature is set between 100° and 120° C. If larger areas must be coagulated with the point coagulator or the myoma enucleator, temperatures between 120° and

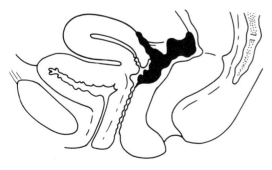

FIG 264.
Retrocervical and pararectal endometriosis.

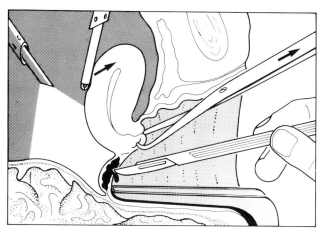

FIG 266.
Combined approach to paracervical and retrovaginal endometriosis: vaginal incision of
nodules under pelviscopic control.

130° C can be selected on the monitor. To prevent
the coagulator from adhering to the peritoneum, it
is moved across the surface to be coagulated as if
it were a steam iron, as described in chapters
12.8.9. and 14.2.3.1. Implants in the sacrouterine
ligaments, which are the most frequent ones (Fig
267), must be coagulated to greater depth. This
can usually be done only after blunt penetration of
the implants by the heated point coagulator, or after biopsy. This occasionally leaves larger serosal
defects; but there is no problem closing them with
one to three endosutures to prevent postoperative
adhesion of the ovary or even a loop of small
bowel (see Plates 51–57).

Small implants on the surfaces (EEC II) of the
ovaries (Plate 58) are also easily removed with biopsy forceps (Plate 59) and then completely eradicated with the point coagulator. Chocolate cysts
(see Plate 125 ff.), however, are coagulated only
after careful excision of the cyst sac (see chapter
14.2.6. ff.).

Coagulation of the bladder dome is usually
performed with the point coagulator (temperature
setting of 100° C). This is in contrast to the high-
frequency technique, in which energy flows from
the urine with a high electrolyte content to the active electrode, increasing the risk of perforating the
wall of the bladder dome.

Coagulation of bowel must be avoided, because the endometrial tissues often penetrate into
the muscle layers.

The coagulation of retro-ovarian endometriotic
implants is particularly important. To accomplish
this, the ovary must be carefully elevated with an

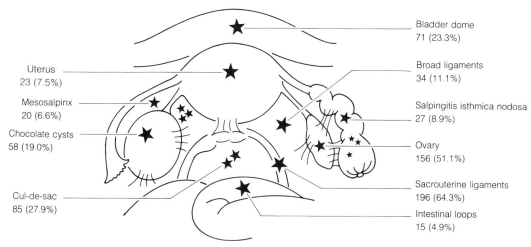

FIG 267.
Distribution of endometriotic implants in a series of 305 cases. Numbers indicate number of cases.

additional instrument introduced through a secondary incision so that the point coagulator (Plate 60) can be applied under optimal visual control. In this context, special consideration should also be given the thermocolor test to diagnose endometriotic implants.

As illustrated in Plate 61, without low-power magnification with a loupe, no endometriotic implant can be detected in the dome of the bladder during the early proliferative phase. If, however, the suspicious area is heated to 100° C, healthy peritoneum will show a white discoloration and endometriotic implants will turn brown (Plate 62) because of the hemosiderin effect.

Pelviscopy for the evaluation of a patient's sterility is usually performed during the follicular phase (see chapter 14.2.4.4.). At that time, peritoneal endometriotic implants have just discharged their blood and can be distinquished from normal peritoneum only by a barely detectable, more intense reddish color. This subtle color difference is indistinguishable in color prints (Plate 63). It can only be diagnosed by careful inspection of the pelvis under low-power magnification with a loupe. If there is any doubt, the thermocolor test is utilized. Fine black spots that show against the white background indicate the presence of endometriosis (Plate 64). This intensive search for endometriotic implants was indicated in this case because the pool of blood was highly suspicious for the presence of active endometriosis, although implants in the cul-de-sac were practically invisible.

The complete recovery from widespread endometriotic implants after coagulation (see Plate 149) is documented in Plate 151 on the occasion of a repeated pelviscopy 14 months later.

14.2.4. Pelviscopic Sterility Operations

The pelviscopic diagnosis of sterility and, more recently, its operative therapy as well, may be considered the father of endoscopic abdominal surgery. On the one hand, it was the forerunner of almost all endoscopic techniques in the abdominal cavity; on the other hand, it was the factor that stimulated the introduction of pelviscopy under low-power magnification with loupes (see chapter 12.2.4.).

14.2.4.1. Endoscopic Salpingo-Ovariolysis

Pelviscopic salpingolysis and ovariolysis, although on a small scale, has already been performed for decades in conjunction with diagnostic pelviscopy. The possibility of safely controlling any type of bleeding that could occur during these procedures now expands the endoscopic operative options to the level of classic laparotomy techniques.

If velamentous adhesions are present they are first coagulated with the crocodile forceps (Plate 65) so that they can be transected without bleeding (Plate 66). If bleeding occurs in spite of this, bleeding vessels are coagulated or, if necessary, controlled by applying an endoloop or endosuture. The advantage of endocoagulation is that coagulated, sharply transected tissue pedicles definitely will not form any postoperative adhesions.

The dissection of broad-based adhesions between the ovaries and the posterior wall of the broad ligament (see Plate 60), in most cases due to pelvic endometriosis, will usually result in large retro-ovarian defects in the peritoneum (see Fig 175). These are closed either by adapting the wound edges with the teeth of a biopsy forceps (see Fig 176) and applying an endoloop or, as is usually done by laparotomy, by endosuture (see Plates 51–57). Which technique is preferable will be decided by the local situation. The application of an endoloop saves time.

The dissection of a broad-based adhesion between a sactosalpinx and the ovary (Plates 67–70) should be done under low-power magnification with a loupe to prevent vascular injuries on the ampulla and fimbria as much as possible. Particularly if adhesions, even minor ones, involve the ampulla and fimbria, it is highly recommended that the crocodile forceps (Plate 71) or the point coagulator be utilized before cutting with hook scissors (Plate 72). The myoma enucleator is particularly well suited for bloodless "peeling off" of the ampulla. Here, too, the general rule applies: prophylactic hemostasis takes less time than control of hemorrhage.

14.2.4.2. Endoscopic Fimbrioplasty

Fimbrioplasty with an endoscope or by laparotomy is one of the most successful operative techniques for correcting infertility due to tubal factors. An apparatus should be used to monitor and control the pressure with which blue solution is instilled into the tube agglutinated at its ampullary end. When the pressure reaches a range of 150–200 mm Hg, the tube will be distended (Fig 268, Plate 73). Under low-power magnification with a loupe (see chapter 12.2.4.) the agglutinated ampullary end of the tube is located and bluntly

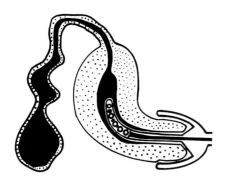

FIG 268.
Instillation of dye before endoscopic fimbrioplasty.

opened by gentle teasing and dilation (Plate 47) with atraumatic grasping tongs and atraumatic grasping forceps (see chapter 12.8.2.). Seepage of traces of blue solution indicates the spot of the old fimbrial orifice. It is first probed and, at the same time, dilated with a conical tubal probe. Then one prong of the atraumatic grasping tongs or the tip of the atraumatic grasping forceps is introduced into the ampulla and the ampulla is dilated until it admits the atraumatic grasping tongs to a depth of 2–3 cm (Plate 75).

The prongs are spread apart and in this position are withdrawn from the ampullary tubal end once or several times (Fig 269). This achieves blunt dilatation of the agglutinated ampulla. The preampullary and ampullary segments of the tube that previously were distended (see Plate 73) collapse, and a grade I tubal patency (Fig 270) will be indicated on the pertubation apparatus.

Particularly in the presence of superficial pel-

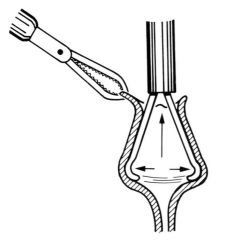

FIG 269.
Dilating the ampulla.

vic endometriosis and a pool of blood in the cul-de-sac (Plate 76), the tubal ampullae are not completely closed, but they show a high degree of fimbrial stenosis or phimosis (Plate 77).

If in such cases, despite widespread endometriotic implants, hysterosalpingography seems to indicate normal tubal patency, the pelviscopic diagnosis of disseminated endometriosis (Fig 271) may be delayed for years. The true condition which absolutely prevents conception can only be detected by diagnostic pelviscopy with chromosalpingoscopy. Pelviscopically, one can see that the tubes are distended, but usually only traces of the blue solution can escape (Plate 78). As just described, the narrow orifice is probed with two atraumatic grasping forceps or tongs (Plate 79) and opened by blunt dissection and dilatation (Plate 80). Occasionally this is possible only after searching for the fimbrial orifice and dilating it with the 5-mm ampullary probe (see chapter 12.8.8.).

During the subsequent chromosalpingoscopy and CO_2 gas insufflation, it is considered a definite sign of the elimination of the phimosis, i.e., the ampullary resistance or the fimbrial agglutination, when a preampullary tubal dilatation no longer occurs.

The ampullar tubal occlusion, which was shown in the hysterosalpingogram (Plate 81), is confirmed by pelviscopic examination. The ampulla is elevated by the atraumatic suction cannula (Plate 82). Two atraumatic grasping tongs are used to bluntly dilate and evert the ampulla (Plate 83).

If superficial pelvic endometriosis is present, additional intraoperative and postoperative measures are necessary (for these refer to chapters 14.2.3.ff, 14.2.4.4. and 17.3.1.).

14.2.4.3. Endoscopic Salpingostomy

According to the international nomenclature (Fig 272), established in 1980 by the International Federation of Fertility Societies (IFFS), we distinguish between a distal and an isthmic salpingostomy. Both can be accomplished by endoscopic operative techniques.

14.2.4.3.1. DISTAL SALPINGOSTOMY

Bilateral dense ampullary tubal occlusions are usually accompanied by perisalpingeal and periovarian adhesions and always require adhesiolysis first (Plate 84). After the closed tubal ampulla has been distended by chromosalpingoscopy under pressures monitored automatically up to 300 mm Hg, and then dissected out, the original left am-

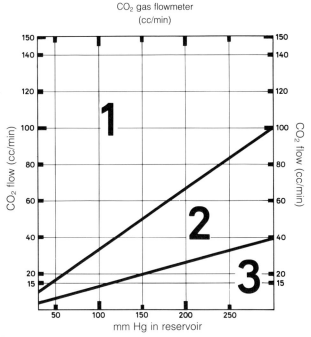

CO₂ gas flowmeter
(cc/min)

FIG 270.
Tubal patency grades as determined by flow and pressure ranges. *1* = normal, *2* = constricted, *3* = severely constricted.

pullary orifice can be recognized under low-power magnification. It allows traces of blue solution to escape (Plate 85).

After blunt dilatation, the entire ampulla is everted (Plate 86) and fixed in this position by an endosuture, which is tied externally (Plate 87).

Under a pressure of 250 mm Hg, the right ampulla is represented by a sactosalpinx (Plate 88).

Depending on the size of the sactosalpinx, a strip of its wall, about 1–2 cm long and 4 mm wide, is coagulated with the point coagulator in the area of the old dimple in the tubal ampulla (Plate 89). Subsequently the distended sactosalpinx is grasped and incised in the coagulated zone with hook scissors or, preferably, with microscissors (Plate 90). This causes the blue solution to emerge

FIG 271.
Hysterosalpingography may seem to indicate normal tubal patency; therefore the correct pelviscopic diagnosis of disseminated endometriosis may be delayed in some cases.

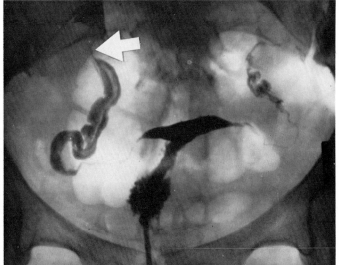

1. OVARIOLYSIS

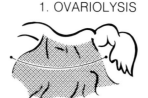
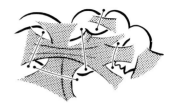

a. Transection of several bands

b. Resection of a periovarian capsule

c. Removal of dense periovarian adhesions

2. SALPINGOLYSIS

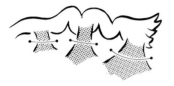
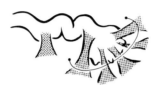
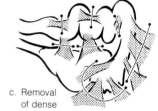

a. Transection of several bands

b. Resection of a periampullary capsule

c. Removal of dense peritubal adhesions

3. FIMBRIOPLASTY

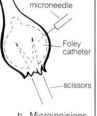

atraumatic grasping tongs

microneedle

Foley catheter

scissors

a. Blunt dilatation

b. Microincisions

4. SALPINGOSTOMY (Salpingoneostomy)

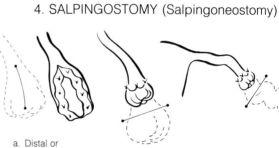
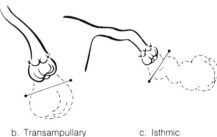

a. Distal or prefimbrial

b. Transampullary

c. Isthmic

5. TUBAL IMPLANTATION

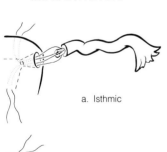

a. Isthmic

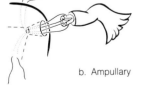

b. Ampullary

6. END-TO-END ANASTOMOSIS

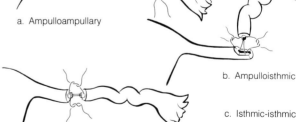

a. Ampulloampullary

b. Ampulloisthmic

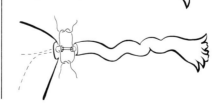

c. Isthmic-isthmic

d. Isthmic-uterine

FIG 272.
IFFS nomenclature for the operative correction of tubal factors in sterility.

under pressure. If any bleeding occurs, coagulation with the crocodile forceps is helpful.

After the wall of the sactosalpinx has been split, the closed atraumatic forceps is introduced into the tubal ampulla, and the forceps is opened and closed to evert the ampulla, as is usually done in laparotomy (Plate 91). The margins of the ampulla are attached to the tubal surface by endosutures after a new tubal ostium has been formed by splitting and eversion (Plate 92). The end result, in which both tubes are patent and stabilized by endosuture, is shown in Plate 93.

Operative steps of the opening of a sactosalpinx are graphically illustrated in Figures 273–278. First (Fig 273), a strip is coagulated with the endocoagulator, which has already been shown in Plates 89 and 97. The coagulation temperature is set at 110°–120° C to expedite this procedure, and the point coagulator is moved across the scarred area in the sactosalpinx much like a steam iron.

Then the tube is sharply incised with hook scissors or, preferably, microscissors, assisted by one or two atraumatic grasping tongs or forceps (Fig 274). After the eversion of the old tubal orifice has been completed, as shown in Plates 86 and 91 (Fig 275), the needle of the endosuture (Fig 276) is pushed through the wound edge and then— as during a laparotomy—the wound edge is sutured (Fig 277), with the assistance of a 5-mm needleholder, to the corresponding spot on the tubal serosa. After a slipknot has been tied externally, the wound edge is fixed to the tubal serosa and the suture is cut (Fig 278). About two to four sutures with externally tied slipknots (see chapter 12.6.) suffice to maintain the ostium in an everted condition (see Plates 87 and 91). For a surgeon skilled

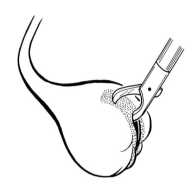

FIG 274.
Tubal incision.

in tying microsurgical instrument knots, it is recommended to use absorbable polydioxanon (PDS) or polyglyconate (Maxon) 4–0 monofilament absorbable suture material for all sutures and to tie the knots internally. This produces anatomical results almost identical to those achieved by microsurgery (for schematics pertaining to sutures and knots, see Fig 146). To tie knots internally, a fourth incision is necessary, through which the ampulla can be held in an appropriate anatomical position.

Plates 94–99 show the same phases during an actual operation in the presence of bilateral sactosalpinges, diagnosed by hysterosalpingography.

Whether or not this operation will be successful usually becomes obvious as soon as the everted ampullary ends of the tubes are inspected under low-power magnification with a loupe: in most cases of large sactosalpinges, only small islands of typical, folded endosalpinx are left, whereas major portions of the inner wall of the sactosalpinx are covered with smooth serosa (see Plates 92, 93, and 99). Such an appearance indicates with a high degree of probability that the endosalpinx, which is

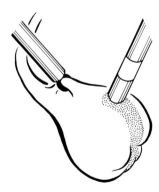

FIG 273.
Distal salpingostomy. A strip is coagulated with the endocoagulator.

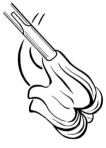

FIG 275.
Eversion of old tubal orifice.

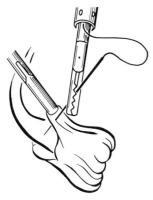

FIG 276.
Endosuture needle is pushed through wound edge.

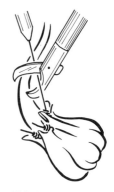

FIG 278.
Suture is cut.

normally covered with 500 cilia per mm^3, has been destroyed to a large extent by a previous inflammatory process, i.e., bacterial infection, reducing the chance for conception through the tube to almost zero.

Pelviscopic salpingostomy is in competition with microsurgical techniques under laparotomy conditions. The endoscopic approach in principle causes no major trauma to the tubal ampullae, as might be the case, for instance, during an unsuccessful salpingostomy by laparotomy—even under microsurgical conditions (Plate 100). Such postoperative sequelae would destroy all chances for future success. However, such postoperative adhesions have never been observed after pelviscopy. Our pregnancy rate is approximately 24%. Therefore, a primary endoscopic salpingostomy should always be given priority over one performed by laparotomy.

This recommendation is based essentially on

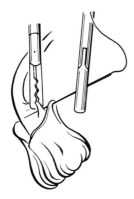

FIG 277.
Wound edge is sutured to adjacent tubal serosa.

the fact that the occluded ampulla is not simply opened and everted, as it was in the past, but is kept open by sutures, as is customary during a laparotomy.

The possible argument that, so far, heavy catgut has been used for endosutures and the knots must be tied externally, in contrast to the suture material used for tubal microsurgery, does not have much merit. The postoperative healing phase after pelviscopic procedures is completely different from the healing phase after a laparotomy. In the latter case, a postoperative intestinal paralysis has a very negative effect on the healing process in the area of the abdominal wound and on the ampullae that were operated on. The postoperative conditions after endoscopic salpingostomy are shown in Plates 101 and 102: There are no adhesions on the ampullae, which are clearly patent for blue solution and CO_2 gas. The absorption of the catgut suture did not leave any recognizable traces. This, naturally, applies particularly to the use of PDS 4-0 sutures tied internally, because polydioxan material is completely absorbed after approximately 260 days.

14.2.4.3.2. ISTHMIC SALPINGOSTOMY

After "conservative" surgery for tubal pregnancy by partial salpingectomy, a tubal stump remains. The stump is dissected out and its end (Plate 103) is coagulated with the crocodile forceps and opened with scissors (Plate 104). The chromosalpingoscopy solution emerges immediately. The chances for conception are the same as if the same procedure had been performed by laparotomy. The patient whose operation is illustrated in Plates 103 and 104 conceived through this fistula in the tube (Plate 105) 7 months after the operation and delivered a healthy child.

14.2.4.4. Endoscopic Tubal Surgery in the Presence of Endometriosis

The principal steps in operative pelviscopic therapy of superficial pelvic endometriosis were described in chapter 14.2.3. If pelvic endometriosis coexists with tubal factor sterility, then, according to the triple-phase therapy regimen (see chapter 17.3.1.) for genital endometriosis, the surgical measures on the tubal ampullae should be restricted to a minimum during the first pelviscopy. Depending on the extent of the endometriosis (Acosta I–III, AFS stages I–IV, see Chart 1, p. 159, or EEC I–IV [Semm, 1983], see Chart 2, p. 160) the blunt dilatation of an ampullary phimosis and a salpingostomy should be performed only in cases corresponding to the Acosta I–II, AFS I–II, or EEC I–II classification. Even with the most meticulous coagulation of all visible clusters of endometriosis, small implants remain that can only be eradicated hormonally during the second phase. However, such micro-implants bleed during the healing phase of the ampullary wounds. In combination with the healing processes in the coagulation wounds, the dilated or opened ampullae reagglutinate quickly. It is therefore advisable to refrain from major surgical manipulations on the tubal ampullae during the first pelviscopy for pelvic endometriosis in the Acosta III category (AFS stages III and IV, EEC II and III). The success rate is greater if the surgical correction of the tubal factor is carried out after hormonal treatment at the time of repeat pelviscopy (triple-phase therapy, see chapter 17.3.2. and Plate 106).

Often one may be surprised by the "good," even "juicy," or "picture of perfect health" appearance of the ampullae or fimbria in the presence of a large pool of blood in the cul-de-sac as well as pelvic endometriosis. These tubes are indeed patent, and one wonders why these patients are sterile.

Since we know about the difficulties in finding a suitable culture medium for the conjugation of male and female gametes during in vitro fertilization, there is a very plausible explanation for this fact:

The conjugation of female and male gametes takes place in the area of the tubal ampulla next to the ovary or, in other words, in the fluid collected in the cul-de-sac. If this is highly contaminated with "menstrual blood" and, therefore, saturated with phagocytes for the removal of this fluid (which, after all, must be considered detritus), spermatozoa as well fall prey to this absorption mechanism. On the other hand, this is not the usual milieu in which conjugation of the ovum and the sperm cell, as well as transport of the fertilized ovum, take place.

This fact, in combination with changes in the fimbrial apparatus, may be the explanation for the clinical experience that genital endometriosis is the most common cause of female sterility.

14.2.4.5. Pelviscopic Tubal Surgery in Preparation for Subsequent Microsurgical Measures to Reestablish Fertility by Laparotomy

As already indicated in chapter 14.2.2.5., adhesiolysis, salpingolysis, and ovariolysis are preparatory measures for the planned reversal of a tubal sterilization by laparotomy under microsurgical conditions. Adhesiolysis in conjunction with diagnostic pelviscopy is also very important if the decision is made at that time that a sactosalpinx or other condition should be operated on, at a later time, by laparotomy and microsurgical techniques. Large peritoneal wounds have an aggravating effect on the tubal ampulla during the healing process from microsurgical reconstruction. To improve the rate of success of microsurgical stomatoplasty or, for instance, isthmic end-to-end anastomosis or tubal reimplantation, respectively (see Fig 272), meticulous salpingo-ovariolysis (see Plate 33 ff.) 2–3 months before the reconstructive laparotomy is of fundamental importance. At the beginning of the microsurgical operation, performed 3 months after the adhesiolysis, shown in Plates 33–35 and 37–39, the abdomen was free of adhesions, particularly as far as the internal genitalia were concerned (see Plates 36 and 40). Therefore, combining a preliminary endoscopic operative removal of peritubal adhesions with a microsurgical procedure should be the method of choice today. For details, refer to chapter 14.2.2.5.

14.2.5. Pelviscopic Ovarian Biopsy

Ovarian biopsy is the oldest endoscopic surgical procedure in gynecology. However, the cutting force of all presently available biopsy forceps is very limited, because of the mechanical limits of 5-mm biopsy instruments. Therefore, they are not suited to punch a cylinder of tissue of sufficient size for histologic evaluation out of an ovary with a leather-like surface. To overcome this problem, Palmer designed a biopsy forceps, which allows the surgeon to grasp the ovary with 3.5-mm biopsy tongs and punch out a tissue cylinder with a sharp-edged sleeve which encases the tongs and is "drilled" into the tissue. However, this special instrument is not absolutely necessary if the ovary is grasped with the regular biopsy forceps (see chapter 12.8.2.) and the beveled trocar sleeve is used as a tissue punch. To get the best grasp on the ovary, it is recommended that the uterus be tilted into the cul-de-sac and behind the ovary to elevate the ovary along the pelvic wall and to hold it there. Then the ovary is grasped between the two jaws of the biopsy forceps, which should be at least 1.5 cm long and have two internal spikes to catch the tissue (Fig 279 and Plate 107). After the jaws of the biopsy forceps have been closed, the trocar sleeve, with its elliptical, beveled tip (Fig 280) is pushed downward under rotating movement (Fig 281), and it punches out a sufficiently large cylinder of tissue (Plates 108 and 111). If the grasp of the tissue was inadequate and the tissue cylinder was not large enough at the first attempt, one tries a second time by introducing the jaws of the forceps deep into the gaping wound. This usually results in a better grasp with the 15-mm-long spoons of the biopsy forceps so that a sufficiently large tissue cylinder for histologic examination can be obtained by advancing the trocar sleeve. Hemostasis is achieved (Fig 282) with the point coagulator by the endocoagulation method (Plate 109).

Plate 110 shows a biopsy from the suspended ovary on the opposite side at the moment that the trocar sleeve is advanced and rotated to punch out a tissue cylinder. Gentle hemostasis with the point coagulator heated to 100° C has just been completed in Plate 111.

Hemostasis by high-frequency current, as shown in Figure 283, is not limited to hemosta-

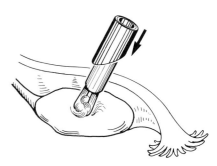

FIG 280.
Note elliptical beveled tip of the trocar which is pushed downward.

sis in the area of the biopsy wound of the ovary. Since high temperatures develop in the ovary and, in particular, also in the vessels and nerves leading to the ovary, which are the conductors for the current, such hemostasis also results in unintended thermobiologic disturbances of the ovarian function. Since biopsy specimens are usually taken from ovaries that are already at high risk, such measures—namely, high-frequency coagulation of the ovary—are no longer justifiable.

When a biopsy site is selected, the hilar region of the ovary should be avoided, because biopsy will always cause excessive bleeding in this area. It is difficult to control such hemorrhage by simple coagulation of the mesovarium, and control of hemorrhage results in major damage in the area of the vascular and nervous plexi, which are so important for the endocrine and exocrine functions of the ovary. In an emergency, such hemorrhage must be controlled by an endoloop or endosuture.

If the hemorrhage is not yet controlled, endoscopic oophorectomy (see chapter 14.2.7.) is the last resort. This is too high a price for a diagnostic biopsy.

The most meticulous technique is required for

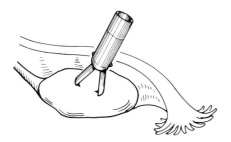

FIG 279.
Biopsy forceps to grasp ovarian tissue to be biopsied.

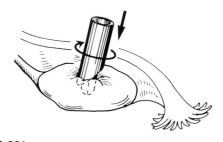

FIG 281.
Trocar is pushed downward in a rotating motion to punch out tissue cylinder.

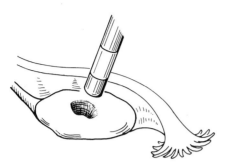

FIG 282.
Point coagulator is used for hemostasis.

ovarian biopsies in the pediatric age group (for histologic determination of ovarian function, etc.). This is particularly important for so-called streak ovaries to avoid sacrificing all of the ovarian tissue and its possible function to the biopsy.

14.2.6. Pelviscopic Puncture and Excision of Ovarian Cysts

The surgical options that will be described in the following sections are technically feasible with the endoscope, but they introduce a certain dilemma in the area of ovarian surgery. On the one hand, it is gratifying to the physician to spare the patient the physical stress of a laparotomy by performing the ovarian operation with the endoscope. On the other hand, this approach burdens the physician with the great responsibility not to perform this procedure on an inappropriate object, i.e., an ovarian malignancy. Endoscopic ovarian surgery must, therefore, only be performed by the most experienced gynecologic surgeon who adheres strictly to accepted indications.

It should be emphasized that according to our present teaching, the total ovary must be excised whenever there is the slightest doubt or suspicion of a malignancy.

Among the polymorphic pathologic ovarian changes for which the endoscopic surgical approach should become part of classic ovarian surgery are benign cysts, such as simple serous cystadenoma, theca-lutein cysts, chocolate cysts, and dermoid cysts. The surgeon must be thoroughly familiar with anatomy under low-power magnification with loupes and highly skilled in endoscopic techniques. At the end of the procedure the pelvis must be irrigated with 1–2 L of physiologic saline solution.

The following endoscopic operative procedures on the ovary are currently technically feasible and may be recommended as the method of choice:

1. Ovarian biopsy
2. Puncture of ovarian cysts (never be satisfied with aspiration alone!)
3. Puncture of follicle or aspiration of oocyte
4. Resection of ovarian cyst wall and suture
5. Enucleation of ovarian cyst (e.g., theca-lutein cyst, chocolate cyst, dermoid cyst) and suture
6. Partial resection of ovary (e.g., for Stein-Leventhal syndrome)
7. Oophorectomy

14.2.6.1. Puncture of Ovarian Cysts

The presence of an ovarian cyst that has been diagnosed by bimanual examination and ultrasound is confirmed by pelviscopy. The cyst is then dis-

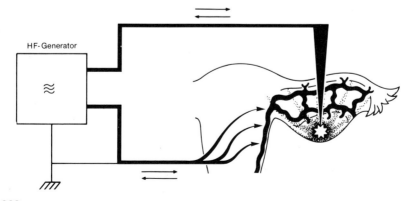

FIG 283.
Hemostasis by high-frequency current also results in thermobiologic damage to ovarian function.

172   *Chapter 14*

sected from the surrounding adhesions (Plate 112).
If the cyst wall is completely smooth, and a neoplastic lesion can be ruled out from the patient's
history (in the case shown in Plate 112, age of 28
years), the cyst is punctured with the aspiration
needle (see chapter 12.8.3.) to evaluate a sample
of its contents (in Plate 113 it is a clear serosan-
guineous fluid). If the cyst contains less then 10
ml, the contents are aspirated with the syringe (see
chapter 12.8.3.); if the volume is greater, the
Aquapurator is used (see chapter 12.4.1.). In any
case, the cyst contents, which have been aspirated
either into the 10-ml syringe or the specimen bottle
(see Fig 164; also refer to chapter 12.8.3.), or into
the aspiration flask of the Aquapurator (see chapter
12.4.1.), are submitted for further cytologic examination and possibly bacteriologic culture.

In the past, if only clear serous fluid was aspirated, this was the end of the treatment. Today,
the cyst wall should always be incised and the inner surfaces inspected under low-power magnification with a loupe. If it is not completely smooth
but contains papillomatous or solid structure, one
cannot be absolutely certain that the lesion is benign. Further definitive operative therapy by laparotomy is required. To prevent any contamination
by small droplets that may already have escaped,
the pelvis is carefully irrigated with 1 L of normal
saline solution.

However, if the inner wall is smooth (Plate
114) and the cyst is small, the exposed area of the
cyst wall is sharply resected by several bites with
the biopsy forceps: the cyst wall is grasped with
the biopsy forceps and pulled into the trocar sleeve
(Fig 284) so that the tissue can be resected by rotating the trocar sleeve. The remaining base of the
tissue is coagulated with the point coagulator or a
crocodile forceps (Fig 285), or the cyst wall,
shown in Plate 114, is wrapped around the biopsy
forceps (Plate 115) so that the actual cyst wall can

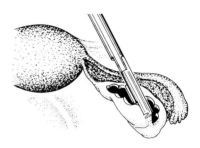

FIG 285.
The remaining base of the tissue is endocoagulated.

be separated from the healthy ovarian matrix before it is resected. The base of the cyst is then coagulated with the point coagulator, the ovarian
wound is closed by endosuture, and a slipknot is
tied externally (Plate 116; see also Figs 135–145).

If the cyst is larger, the base of the cyst is not
coagulated but, as described in chapter 14.2.6.2.,
carefully enucleated, as is customary during a laparotomy. This procedure is described in the following section.

14.2.6.2. Excision of Ovarian Cyst and Ovarian Suture

If aspiration of the ovarian cyst has revealed
that the cyst is most probably benign and so large
that the cyst sac has to be enucleated, we use the
following operative technique, with good success.

For practical purposes, the cyst is not completely opened, but after aspiration (Plate 117) and
splitting of the tunica albuginea (Plate 118) with
hook scissors (Fig 286), the cyst is grasped with
claw forceps and a biopsy forceps (Fig 287 and
Plate 119) and twisted off (Plate 120) with the
large claw forceps (Fig 288). Occasionally this requires assistance by hook scissors.

In the case of theca-lutein cysts, chocolate
cysts, and, in particular, dermoid cysts, there is
amazingly little bleeding during the enucleation,
which is relatively easy. The overhanging cyst wall
is resected (Plate 121), the pelvic cavity is thoroughly irrigated (Plate 122), and the ovarian
wound is closed with endosuture (Plate 123; see
also Figs 135–145). Plate 124 shows the end result
after bilateral excision of ovarian cysts.

Here is an example of the excision of a chocolate cyst:

First it is punctured to confirm the diagnosis
(Plate 125). Cysts up to 10 cm in diameter (Plate
126) are first aspirated until approximately two
thirds of the contents has been evacuated. Then the

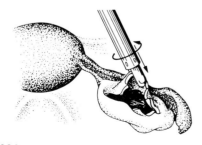

FIG 284.
Cyst wall is resected by rotating movements of the trocar sleeve.

tunica albuginea (Plate 127) is incised and the cyst walls are grasped with one to at most three (usually not necessary) biopsy forceps (Plate 128) and peeled off the underlying ovarian tissue by curling and twisting the biopsy forceps. The thinned-out cyst wall, which has no endocrine function, has been resected. The remaining ovarian tissue is reconstructed with two to three endosutures (see Plate 116 and Figs 135–145). The postoperative anatomical appearance 12 months after the endoscopic excision of this right chocolate cyst of 8 cm diameter is shown in Plate 225. Plate 129 shows the anatomical appearance 2 years after a laparotomy for suspected Stein-Leventhal syndrome and anterior suspension of the uterus (Baldy-Webster): ovaries and bowels form a conglomerate tumor. After dissection of a loop of small bowel and mobilization of both ovaries (Plate 130), a chocolate cyst is enucleated from the ovary (Plate 131) and the wound is closed with endosuture (Plate 132). This is followed by generous irrigation of the pelvic cavity (Plate 133).

The series of color photographs in Plates 134–141 shows the procedure in the presence of a dermoid cyst of approximately 9 cm diameter in which an alveolar process has already been identified radiographically (Fig 289). Grasping of the incisor in its alveolar process (Plate 134) with the large claw forceps is documented in Plate 135. Before this could be done, the cyst was diagnosed by puncture and aspiration (Plate 136), and after the tunica albuginea was split, the dermoid was enucleated (Plate 137). The cyst base is shown in Plate 138; enucleation of the cyst walls was accomplished without difficulties by twisting and curling in the manner of a hair curler (Plate 139). Tena-

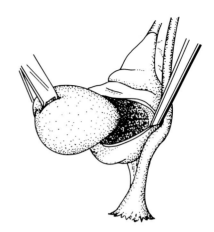

FIG 287.
The cyst is grasped with forceps and twisted off.

cious sebaceous material and hair were removed with the large spoon forceps (Plate 140) and the pelvic cavity was then thoroughly irrigated.

The wound in the remaining ovarian tissue was closed with two endoloops (Plate 141). The anatomical end result is shown in Plate 142 during the last irrigation cycle.

The 21-year-old patient was discharged with-

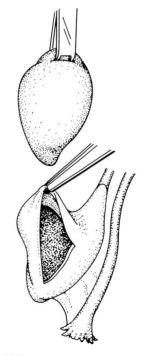

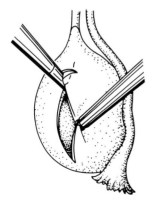

FIG 286.
The tunica albuginea is split with hook scissors.

FIG 288.
Cyst removed with the large claw forceps.

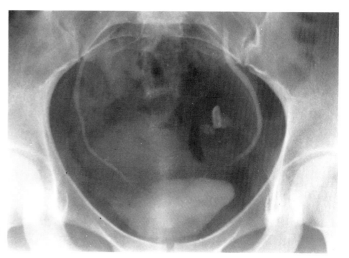

FIG 289.
Dermoid cyst. Alveolar process has been
identified radiographically.

out complaints on the fifth postoperative day. Findings were normal at the time of the postoperative bimanual gynecologic examination and on sonograms obtained 6 and 21 months after the operation.

Another excision of a dermoid cyst is shown in Plates 117–124.

During a laparotomy, a large ovarian wound must be controlled with a meticulous row of sutures, usually of the mattress type. It has even been proposed (Brosens, 1978) that such ovarian wounds be closed by microsurgical techniques, since it is well known that ovarian sutures have a great propensity to form adhesions to adjacent structures during the postoperative healing process.

Such propensity to form adhesions could not be confirmed after more than 400 pelviscopic operations on the ovaries, which were reevaluated by numerous repeat pelviscopies. This is again probably due to the same reasons that have already been mentioned with tubal surgery (see chapter 14.2.4. ff): absence of intestinal paralysis and mechanical irritation of the peritoneum.

It is a normal physiologic process of the ovarian function that even larger follicle cysts rupture and heal spontaneously without suture. Therefore, it is acceptable in pelviscopic ovarian surgery to approximate the edges of nonbleeding ovarian wounds with one to three endosutures. This will result in excellent, reconstructed ovaries that are usually completely free of postoperative adhesions (see chapter 12.6.3. and Figs 135–145).

To the novice, the procedure of tying exter-

nal slipknots, described in chapter 12.6.2. and 12.6.3., may seem complicated. To the surgeon familiar with microsurgical techniques, however, learning this suture technique is no real problem.

At the end of every operation on the ovary, the pelvic cavity is thoroughly irrigated with 1–2 L of normal saline solution, which is most conveniently performed with the Àquapurator (see chapter 12.4.1.), until (1) there is no sign of bleeding and (2) even the last small remnants of tissue have been removed from the pelvic cavity.

One must pay attention that the irrigation fluid does not rise above the level of the pelvic rim and drain toward the liver. If necessary, the patient's Trendelenburg position may have to be reversed by several degrees. Irrigation is facilitated by using atraumatic grasping forceps to keep epiploic appendices, bowels, tubal ampulla, and so forth away from the irrigation-aspiration cannula (see Fig 88). Aspiration without the benefit of the single-channel/dual-purpose irrigation-aspiration cannula is very time-consuming and extremely frustrating unless one has the facility to keep tissues that are floating in the pool of fluids away from the suction cannula with an additional instrument. [Sometimes I have reintroduced the Veress needle for this purpose, which obviates closure of the puncture site—*Ed.*]

If irrigation fluid inadvertently runs off into the upper abdomen, i.e., into the subphrenic space (see Fig 28), the pelvis must be temporarily lowered up to 45° (see Fig 29) so that the fluid can be easily and completely aspirated with the suction cannula.

14.2.6.3. Removal of Ovarian Cysts by Oophorectomy or Salpingo-Oophorectomy

After ovarian cyst puncture and aspiration (see chapter 14.2.6.1) or excision (see chapter 14.2.6.2.) it may occasionally not be prudent, for medical reasons, to preserve the remaining ovarian tissues or the patient's age may be an indication for oophorectomy or salpingo-oophorectomy. Depending on the indication and technical feasibility either oophorectomy or a salpingo-oophorectomy could be performed according to the "triple-loop technique" described in chapter 14.2.7. or 14.2.8.

Plate 143 shows an ovarian cyst with a smooth wall to be punctured in a 54-year-old patient with extensive endometriosis. After aspiration of the clear serous contents and inspection of the smooth inner cyst walls, the large claw forceps reaches through the endoloop (Plate 144), which has been introduced through another trocar sleeve, and grasps the tube and the entire collapsed cystic shell while the suture is applied to the very base of the mesosalpinx (Plate 145). With the surgeon pulling firmly on the claw forceps, the mesovarium and the tube are ligated. After the third ligature (Plate 146) has been applied, the tube and mesovarium are transected with hook scissors at a right angle to the tissue stalk (Plate 147). The ovarian cyst sac is removed in one piece through the 11-mm trocar sleeve. The ligated tissue stump is coagulated with the point coagulator (Plate 148) to prevent formation of adhesions. Endometriotic implants are also coagulated (Plate 149), and the pelvic cavity is irrigated with 1–2 L of saline solution at 37° C (Plate 150). The positive thermocolor test should also be noted.

Plate 151 shows pelvic organs completely free of adhesions 13 months after a right salpingo-oophorectomy performed because of an ovarian cyst, which was shown in Plates 143–150. There is no recurrence of endometriotic implants.

A benign cyst, shown in Plate 152, was found in a 69-year-old patient. After aspiration of the cyst contents, the entire adnexa is surrounded by an endoloop (Plate 153) and ligated by the triple-loop technique. After bloodless transection of the stalk with hook scissors (Plate 154), it is advisable to use the large spoon forceps to remove the tissue through the 11-mm trocar sleeve (Plate 155). The end result of the operation after irrigation of the pelvic cavity and coagulation of the tissue stump is shown in Plate 156.

14.2.7. Pelviscopic Oophorectomy

If the ovary is freely mobile or only moderately adherent to the broad ligament, oophorectomy by the endoscopic route after the triple-loop technique presents no particular technical difficulties. Provided that the appropriate instruments are available, it is certainly technically easier and can be performed anatomically more correctly than by the vaginal route. This procedure leaves no postoperative adhesions. The physical stress to the patient is identical to that of a tubal sterilization. The patient is free of discomfort within 4–5 days and fully recovered, that is, she can resume her normal activities and life-style.

In addition to the umbilical incision for the endoscope, three punctures are made in the suprapubic area: two lateral ones with the 5-mm trocar sleeves for the instruments and a median puncture for the 11-mm trocar sleeve (see Fig 256 and Plate 197).

Figures 290–296 illustrate schematically, along with Plates 157–165, the typical operative phases of the triple-loop technique.

The endoloop is introduced on the side from which the ovary is to be removed, the large claw forceps reaches through the loop (see chapter 12.8.2.) to grasp the ovary (Fig 290 and Plate 157), which may possibly have already been dissected off the broad ligament, and the utero-ovarian ligament and mesovarium are put under tension (Plate 158). If grasping of the ovary should be difficult for anatomical reasons, one reaches through the endoloop and pulls it up to the trocar sleeve through which the claw forceps was introduced (see Plate 104). Then it will no longer be damaged by further grasping attempts. The tube usually also slides into the loop. With the aid of atraumatic grasping tongs (Plate 159), which are introduced on the contralateral side, the tube is pushed aside so that the ligature can be applied in the proper position (Fig 291). The endoloop is tightened by pulling firmly on its long end (Plate 160 and Fig 292).

For safety's sake, the tissue pedicle is ligated three times (Fig 293). We refer to this as the triple-loop technique. In this technique, one attempts to apply every successive loop distally (Plate 161) to the previous loop and moving in the direction of the pelvic wall. This produces a long tissue stalk (see Fig 293).

The tissue stalk with its three ligatures is kept

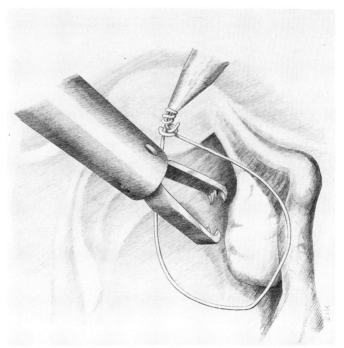

FIG 290.
Triple-loop technique for oophorectomy. The large claw forceps
reaches through the endoloop to
grasp the ovary.

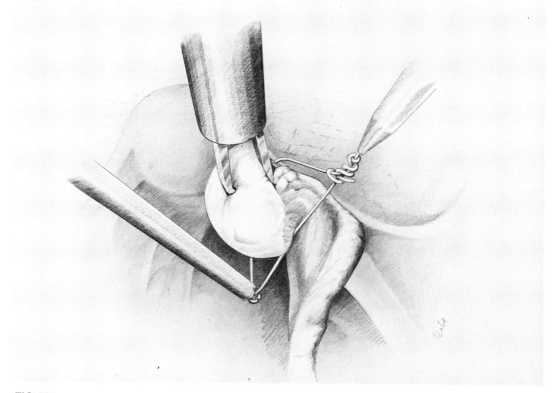

FIG 291.
The tube is pushed aside so that the ligature can be applied in the proper position on the mesovarium.

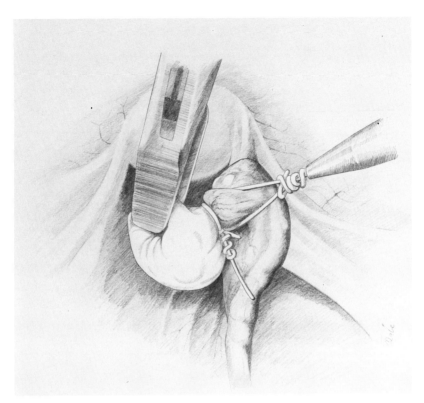

FIG 292.
The endoloop is tightened by pulling firmly on its long end while pushing the slipknot down with the plastic rod.

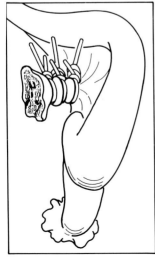

FIG 293.
The tissue pedicle is ligated three times.

under tension with the claw forceps (Fig 294), and scissors are introduced to transect the stalk at a right angle (Plate 162). For this purpose, scissors are introduced on the same side on which the oophorectomy is being performed to allow cutting at a right angle (Plate 163). To prevent adhesions after complete ovarian resection, the exposed surface of the ligated stump (Plate 164) is briefly coagulated with the point coagulator (see chapter 12.5.6.1. and Fig 295). One must avoid heating of the catgut sutures at the same time, because it could result in the knot's unraveling. The triple-loop technique is well suited for pelviscopic application because the mesosalpinx can be bunched together by a ligature just as well as during a vaginal salpingo-oophorectomy. This is not possible to the same extent during a laparotomy. In that case, the abdominal retractors prevent the tying together of the infundibulopelvic ligament and the utero-ovarian ligament, etc., without tension.

In the meantime, the ovary has been deposited in the cul-de-sac and can now be removed in one of two ways:

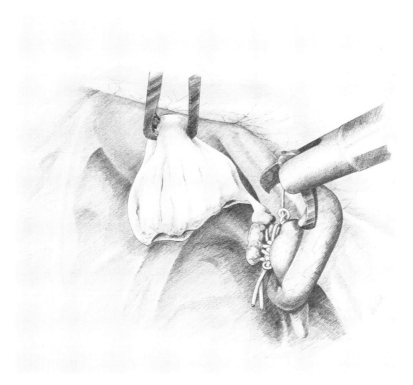

FIG 294.
The tissue stalk with its three ligatures is kept under tension with the claw forceps while being cut with hook scissors.

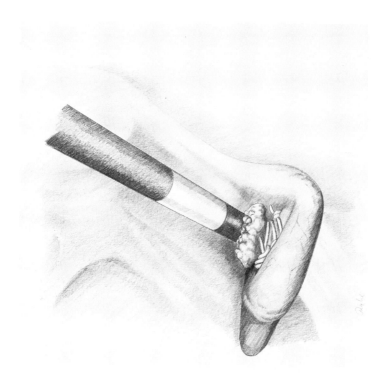

FIG 295.
The exposed surface of the ligated stump is briefly endocoagulated with the point coagulator.

The ovary can be grasped (see Plate 155) with the large spoon forceps (see chapter 12.8.2.) and, if it is not too large, removed in one piece through the 11-mm trocar sleeve. If it is too large to fit through the elliptical orifice of the 11-mm trocar sleeve, it often helps to partially incise the surface of the tissue with scissors to reduce its diameter and shape to make it fit through the sleeve. If simple removal of the ovarian tissue is not possible because of its size, the tissue punch (see chapter 12.8.5.) is introduced through the 11-mm trocar sleeve to morcellate the ovarian tissue with it (Plates 165 and 172). For this purpose the ovary is grasped with the 5-mm biopsy forceps and pushed into the cutting orifice of the morcellator (Fig 296). This particular procedure should be practiced first on some other tissue before the endoscopic procedure, such as on placental tissue or umbilical cord, perhaps utilizing the Pelvi-Trainer (see chapter 22). One must remember that a new cutting movement with the tissue punch can occur only after the cutting jaw has been completely opened and the elevator plate has snapped back into its usual start-

ing position inside the end of the instrument (see Fig 174). If this has been overlooked only once, the tissue punch must be removed from the trocar sleeve and emptied before morcellated pieces of tissue fall into the pelvic cavity.

If one or both ovaries have been morcellated, small pieces of tissue that may have fallen into the pelvic cavity must be removed with biopsy forceps or the large spoon forceps. Subsequently the pelvic cavity is carefully irrigated with 1–3 L of saline solution until the peritoneum is smooth and slick as a mirror. One must pay attention that none of the irrigating fluid runs off into the mid and upper abdomen. In case this does happen, the patient's 15° Trendelenburg position must be reversed and the head must be elevated to a maximum position, after previous consultation with the anesthesiologist, so that the fluid may run off from the subphrenic space through the midabdomen and collect in the cul-de-sac (refer also to chapter 12.4.1. and Figs 28 and 29).

Risk of complications: The mesosalpinx was not ligated tightly enough by the triple-loop tech-

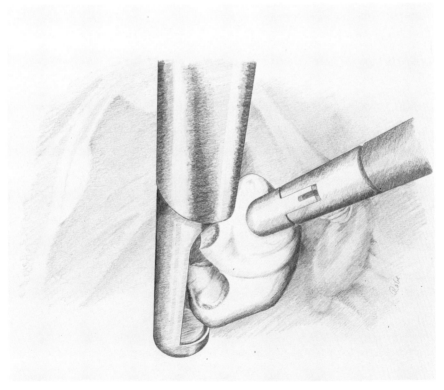

FIG 296.
Morcellation of large ovary. Ovary is grasped with 5-mm biopsy forceps.

nique or the ovarian pedicle was transected too close to the ligatures. When the ovarian pedicle is transected under those circumstances, the ligatures slip off and hemorrhage occurs from the ovarian artery and from the medial pole of the ovary, i.e., the ovarian branch of the uterine artery, as well as the corresponding veins. At the same time, the wound opens in a longitudinal direction.

Such a mishap, however, is no reason to panic. During pelviscopic operations, bleeding from the vessels named above is relatively mild. So far, we have always been able to regrasp the squirting vessels with the biopsy forceps (Plate 166) and to religate the ovarian artery with several additional endoloops (Plate 167). The ascending blood vessels in the mesosalpinx are controlled with a second ligature (Plate 168). Use of destructive heat to coagulate such hemorrhages from the parametrium is *not* recommended.

In the presence of fibrosis, such as after ovariolysis, it is not possible to apply an endoloop to the utero-ovarian ligament; in such cases, an endosuture is placed into the tubal cornu and always controls the hemorrhage.

The end result after bilateral oophorectomy is shown in Plate 164. The 34-year-old patient had recurrent carcinoma of her breasts and positive estrogen receptors and, therefore, an indication for ablative hormonal therapy.

For the same indication, a left oophorectomy was necessary in a 53-year-old patient who, 4 years before, had a myomatous uterus of 14–16 weeks' gestational size and was treated by total abdominal hysterectomy, right salpingo-oophorectomy, and left salpingectomy (Plate 169). The infundibulopelvic ligament was held under tension with a large claw forceps and ligated with an endoloop (Plate 170). After the third ligature (Plate 171), bloodless resection was carried out with hook scissors. Then the ovary was morcellated with the tissue punch (Plate 172), the stalk was coagulated with the point coagulator (Plate 173), and the pelvic cavity was irrigated (Plate 174).

It is obvious that such a clean anatomy at the end of the operation requires only a minimal healing effort.

At the end of the operation one must be careful that the vacuum adapter is not removed from the cervix with excessive force. If the patient has a moderate descensus of the uterus, the uterine corpus may be pulled down so far that the ligatures slip off because, after all, the infundibulopelvic ligament and the utero-ovarian ligament have been

tied together. Such uncontrolled "yanking off" of the uterine manipulator may just lead to such a complication.

The risk of retraction of the ovarian artery may be prevented by a suture ligature similar to the one applied during Wertheim's operation, as shown in chapter 14.2.8.1. and Plates 175 and 176.

This complication is not very serious, but it is time-consuming. With a more cautious technique it is easily avoided.

14.2.8. Pelviscopic Salpingo-oophorectomy

Technically simpler than the endoscopic oophorectomy just described is the triple-loop technique for pelviscopic salpingo-oophorectomy (see Figs 300–305). When a salpingo-oophorectomy is done, a thicker tissue stalk is formed by including the tubal tissue in the ligature. The risk of the ligature slipping off, which was mentioned above, rarely ever exists. The triple-loop technique is comparable to that performed during an oophorectomy (see Figs 290–296).

If the pelvic anatomy is such that the infundibulopelvic ligament and the utero-ovarian ligament can barely be approximated or only under strong traction, it is advisable that the infundibulopelvic ligament, i.e., the ovarian artery, be doubly ligated by itself and then transected, as described below.

14.2.8.1. Transection of the Infundibulopelvic Ligament

After discussion of endoscopic oophorectomy described above, the operative steps of salpingo-oophorectomy will be described in the following section. In 95% of cases it can be accomplished without problems by using the triple-loop technique, and without any risk that the ovarian artery may retract from the ligature. Under some anatomical conditions it is not possible to extend the infundibulopelvic ligament sufficiently to tie it to the utero-ovarian ligament. In such cases it is recommended that the infundibulopelvic ligament—as, for example, during a wide-cuff hysterectomy with salpingo-oophorectomy—be doubly suture-ligated and then transected. Plate 175 shows the infundibulopelvic ligament under traction as the needle of the endosuture is passed through its base (Fig 297). After the ligament has been doubly suture-ligated in a classic manner, it will be transected (Fig 298) and the cranial stump secured one more time with

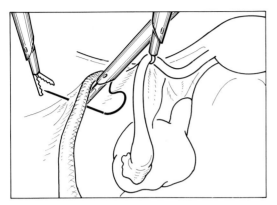

FIG 297.
Suture-ligation of the infundibulopelvic ligament.

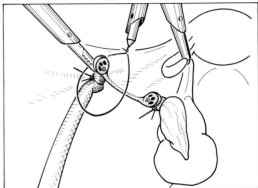

FIG 299.
The cranial stump is secured again with an endoloop.

an endoloop (Plate 176, Fig 299). The ovarian tumor (histology: ovarian fibroma, 6.5 cm diameter) was subsequently removed through the vagina while a total vaginal hysterectomy with anterior and posterior colporrhaphy was being performed.

Therefore, the operation shown in Plates 175 and 176 serves not only as an endoscopic operation on the adnexa, but also as a preparatory or supporting procedure for vaginal operations. A salpingo-oophorectomy, which may occasionally be difficult, can be simplified substantially if it is preceded by an endoscopic ligature of the infundibulopelvic ligament. This option expands the spectrum of the preparatory endoscopic adhesiolysis prior to a vaginal total hysterectomy, as discussed in chapter 14.2.2.5. and illustrated in Plates 32 and 38.

The endoscopic suture technique offers the possibility of separately ligating the infundibulo-

pelvic ligament, which in some cases makes it safer or makes the vaginal removal of adnexal tumors possible.

14.2.8.2. Salpingo-oophorectomy

The salpingo-oophorectomy begins—possibly after a preparatory operation, described in chapter 14.2.8.1.—much like the oophorectomy described in chapter 14.2.7.

After introduction of an endoloop on the corresponding side, the ovary and tube are grasped simultaneously with large claw forceps and pulled toward the center of the pelvis (Fig 300). The catgut loop (Fig 301) is guided under tension with an atraumatic grasping forceps into the cul-de-sac until it reaches the pelvic wall (Plate 177).

When the loop is closed, the ligature should be applied as close as possible to the pelvic wall or the uterus. This is repeated three times (Plate 178, Fig 302) before the tube and the vascular pedicles are transected (Plate 179, Fig 303). The raw surface of this triply ligated tissue stump will be coagulated with the point coagulator (Fig 304) to prevent the future development of adhesions in the intestinal area, as shown in Plates 148, 164, 169, and 213.

In numerous second-look pelviscopies (see Plate 151) we established that postoperative adhesions never occurred on these tissue pedicles. Coagulating cut surfaces prevents the transudation and deposition of fibrin and the emigration of histiocytes and fibroblasts. Therefore, healthy peritoneum does not come in contact with raw tissue to form adhesions. The adnexa are usually removed in two phases. First the resected adnexa are grasped with the large claw forceps and the tube is

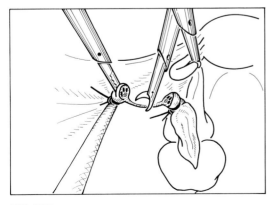

FIG 298.
Infundibulopelvic ligament is transected.

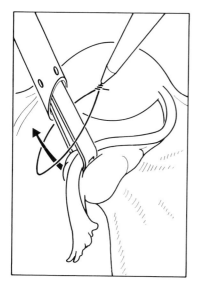

FIG 300.
Salpingo-oophorectomy. The endoloop is introduced, and the ovary and tube are grasped simultaneously with large claw forceps and pulled toward the center of the pelvis.

cut off (Plate 180, Fig 305). The tube is then extracted in one piece through the 11-mm trocar sleeve (Plate 181), whereas the ovarian tissue is morcellated (see Plates 165, 172, and 196).

Even after previous abdominal or vaginal total hysterectomy, salpingo-oophorectomy is feasible.

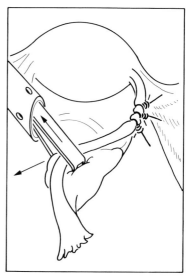

FIG 302.
Three ligatures are placed.

The anatomical findings with an ovarian cyst on the right side are shown in Plate 182. The aspiration needle is introduced. After aspiration and evaluation of the cyst, the claw forceps reaches through the endoloop (Plate 183) to grasp the tube and ovary. The atraumatic grasping forceps guides the catgut loop to the base of the mesosalpinx (Plate 184) before the loop (Plate 185) is pulled

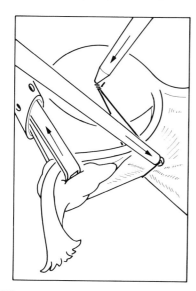

FIG 301.
Catgut loop is guided under tension into the cul-de-sac.

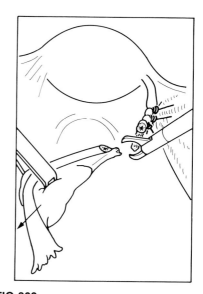

FIG 303.
The tube and vascular pedicles are transected.

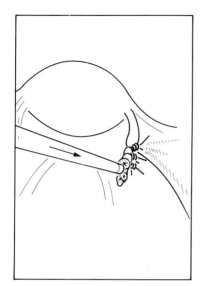

FIG 304.
Raw surface of tissue stump is coagulated with the point coagulator.

tight. The second loop is placed behind the first one (Plate 186). The entire adnexal pedicle can be transected without loss of blood (Plate 187) and removed in one piece through the 11-mm trocar sleeve. The final phase of the operation, coagulation of the stump with the point coagulator, is shown in Plate 188.

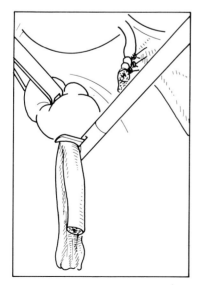

FIG 305.
Tube is cut off the resected adnexa.

If ovarian endometriosis (Plate 189) recurs or if it is resistant to hormonal therapy, a salpingo-oophorectomy may become necessary in rare cases. The atraumatic grasping tongs guide the endoloop around the adnexa because, as demonstrated in Plate 190, the loop does not spontaneously surround the tube (only occasionally will this be the case). The end result after coagulation and triple ligation of the stump is shown in Plate 191.

Occasionally the tube and ovary cannot be grasped together; then the large claw forceps reaches through the endoloop (Plate 192) and elevates only the tube to allow the atraumatic grasping tongs (Plate 193) to place the loop behind the ovary. This automatically results in the formation of an ovarian "stalk" (Plate 194) for further ligatures. If this first ligature does not reach far enough, it may now serve as a bridle and will be cut off at the time of ovarian resection.

Plates 195–197 show again: Grasping of the endoloop with atraumatic grasping tongs to be guided around the left adnexa, which has been grasped with the large claw forceps and pulled into the center of the pelvis (Plate 195), morcellation of the ovary (Plate 196), and anatomical results after bilateral salpingo-oophorectomy. In Plate 197 it is clearly visible that the adnexal pedicles have been securely ligated and coagulated; the optimum placement of the three trocar sleeves can be seen above the uterus.

14.2.9. Salpingectomy for Hydrosalpinx

If an adnexal tumor has been palpated by pelvic examination, the differential diagnosis may occasionally be narrowed down to a myomatous uterus and a hydrosalpinx. A hydrosalpinx is relatively common after vaginal hysterectomy and after tubal sterilization (see Plate 198 ff., and Plates 204 and 214).

Pelviscopic removal of a hydrosalpinx by the triple-loop ligature technique is relatively simple and can be accomplished without complications.

The banana-shaped hydrosalpinx of approximately 2–3 cm × 8–10 cm in largest dimensions is shown in Plate 198 after being detected in a 44-year-old patient about 6 years after a simple vaginal hysterectomy. The large claw forceps reaches through the endoloop (Plate 199) to grasp the hydrosalpinx and pull it toward the middle of the abdomen. While being kept under strong tension with the large claw forceps, the first loop ligature is applied (Plate 200). After all three endoloops have been applied, the hydrosalpinx and ovary are resected en bloc with hook scissors (Plate 201) and extracted from the abdomen through an 11-mm trocar sleeve. Plate 202 shows the coagulation of the adnexal pedicle, and Plate 203 shows the end result after irrigation of the pelvic cavity. The patient left the hospital 5 days after the operation and could immediately resume her usual activities. Follow-up over a period of 3½ years was uneventful. The adnexal tumor on the right side of the 50-year-old patient, which was palpated and then confirmed by ultrasound, turned out to be a hydrosalpinx (Plate 204) during the pelviscopy. While the adnexal conglomerate is grasped with the large claw forceps, the endoloop is placed with atraumatic grasping tongs (see Plate 204). It ligates the infundibulopelvic ligament, the utero-ovarian ligament, and four-fifths of the fallopian tube—in any case, the entire dilated segment of a tube (Plate 205). The adnexae are severed bloodlessly (Plate 206) and, after the shape of the specimen has been adjusted by a few incisions with scissors (Plate 207), it is extracted in one piece through the 11-mm beveled trocar sleeve with elliptical orifice.

A hematosalpinx (Plate 208) that results from torsion of the stalk of a hydrosalpinx can likewise be removed. The tube is grasped with the large claw forceps (Plate 209) and ligated by the triple-loop technique (Plate 210), severed (Plate 211), and the soft tubal tissue grasped with the large spoon forceps and removed (Plate 212). The pelvic anatomy at the end of this procedure is shown in Plate 213 during coagulation of the remaining tubal stump.

The hydrosalpinx shown in Plate 214 is a typical finding after tubal sterilization, in the present case, 6 years postoperatively. It is easy to place the endoloop properly (Plate 215).

A tightly ligated tissue pedicle (Plate 216) is formed before the hydrosalpinx of approximately 2.5 × 5.5 cm is amputated (Plate 217). Up to this point, the procedure has been performed through two suprapubic 5-mm trocar sleeves. For extraction of the hydrosalpinx sac, one of the 5-mm channels is dilated with the dilatation set (see chapter 12.8.8.) to 11 mm in diameter (Plate 218) and the sactosalpinx that had developed after a tubal sterilization is pulled from the abdomen (Plate 219). The end result is shown in Plate 220.

Eighteen cases of such hydrosalpinges after tubal sterilization that reached up to 10 cm in largest dimension have thus far been corrected by the triple-loop technique in the category of "minor pelviscopic operations."

14.2.10. Pelviscopic Operations on the Uterus

Before the development of endocoagulation techniques to achieve safe hemostasis, endoscopic procedures on the uterus were contraindicated. Hemorrhages from the surface of the uterus could not be controlled pelviscopically. With the aid of the new coagulation technique—the point coagulator, the myoma enucleator, and/or the crocodile forceps (see chapter 12.5.6.1.)—even bleeding from extensive wounds on the surface of the uterus can now be controlled without the risk of adhesion formation (Plates 221, 222). Plate 223 documents the operative result 17 months after enucleation of the myoma shown in Plates 221 and 222. It could be confirmed in numerous second-look pelviscopies that the endocoagulation technique affords excellent protection against postoperative adhesions: if a protein layer has been coagulated by destructive heat at the temperature level of boiling water, there is no deposition of fibrin, histiocytes, and fibroblasts, so that healthy peritoneal tissue cannot adhere to it.

As previously mentioned, we have also transferred this technique to laparotomies. We no longer use sutures to control bleeding from the uterine corpus, but use endocoagulation to completely eliminate postoperative adhesions (see chapter 12.5.6.2. and Fig 122), as smooth peritoneal scars after enucleation of myomas have shown (Plates 223, 224, and 237).

14.2.10.1. Pelviscopic Enucleation of Myomas

Small subserous leiomyomas are usually not indications for a laparotomy. If they are diagnosed during a pelviscopy, however, we remove them routinely. This eliminates the risk for the patient that she might need a laparotomy because of the subsequent growth of the myomas. We believe our routine is justified because the procedure itself is without risk and we are certain that postoperative adhesions will not be stimulated.

Even subserous intramural myomas up to 5 or 6 cm in diameter (Plate 225) (for details of the operation, see Plates 226–232) may be removed pelviscopically, although morcellation may be cumbersome. Alternatively, one can remove the enucleated myoma at the end of the pelviscopic procedure by a posterior colpotomy. One need only complete all operative measures first, including irrigation of the pelvic cavity. After the posterior vaginal fornix has been opened, the myoma must be removed quickly because the pneumoperitoneum deflates through the vagina.

The technical steps of the enucleation of pedunculated and intramural myomas are shown in Figures 306 through 316.

After all procedures for which the pelviscopic operation was indicated have been completed, a decision is made as to whether or not a myoma should be removed (Fig 306). Depending on the size of the myoma, it is grasped with the double-toothed biopsy forceps or the large claw forceps (see chapter 12.8.2.) and its stalk is stretched. The stalk is grasped with the crocodile forceps (Fig 307) and carefully coagulated from both sides. One must take sufficient time so that a)_ protein contained in the stalk is coagulated. This avoids the need for possible time-consuming hemostasis with a point coagulator. Subsequently the myoma is twisted off at its stalk (Fig 308), as is done by laparotomy, if necessary by using the myoma enucleator or cutting with scissors.

If the stalk was sufficiently coagulated there should not be any frank bleeding from the wound bed. Secondary oozing is controlled with the point coagulator (Fig 309). One need not be concerned about the extent of the white discolored tissue segments. It has been proved experimentally that tissue coagulated at 100° C will reperitonealize from the sides without sequestration or crater formation (see chapter 12.5.6.2.) and without adhering to other intraperitoneal structures (see Plates 5 and 6).

Depending on its size, the myoma is removed—as illustrated in chapter 14.2.7. for ovarian tissue—with large claw forceps directly

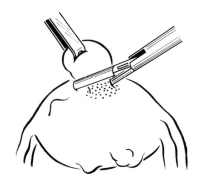

FIG 307.
Stalk of the myoma is grasped with the crocodile forceps and coagulated.

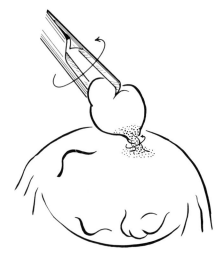

FIG 308.
The myoma is twisted off its stalk.

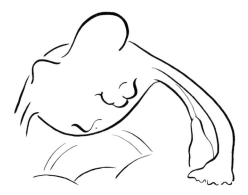

FIG 306.
Multiple myomata in uterine fundus.

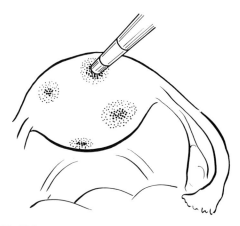

FIG 309.
Secondary oozing is controlled with the point coagulator.

through the 11-mm trocar sleeve, or it is morcellated with the tissue punch (Fig 310; see also chapter 12.8.5.). This is followed by careful irrigation
of the uterine corpus and the pelvic cavity.

Subserous intramural myomas (see Plate 225),
even the ones in the cervix, cannot primarily be
grasped with the claw forceps. In these cases, the
serosal capsule must first be coagulated (Fig 311)
with the crocodile forceps (Plate 226), the myoma
enucleator, or the point coagulator, depending on
the size of the myoma, in a band 4 mm wide. With
the assistance of a biopsy forceps, the capsule is
then incised with hook scissors (Fig 312, Plate
227). The capsule is stripped off the myoma as far
as possible, operating with a myoma enucleator
(Fig 313) heated to 120° C in the appropriate line
of cleavage. Depending on the size of the myoma,
it is grasped with biopsy or claw forceps, and with
rotating movements (Fig 314, Plate 228) it is
shelled out with the myoma enucleator, most of the
time with almost no blood loss (Plate 229).

Afterbleeding is controlled by the generous
use of the point coagulator or myoma enucleator
(Plate 230). If, on occasion, larger quantities of
protein have to be heated to 100° C, the temperature of the crocodile forceps or point coagulator
may briefly be increased to 120°–130° C. To keep
the forceps from sticking to the uterine tissue, the
instrument should be rotated during the coagulation. If larger craters remain after the coagulation,
endosutures are recommended (Fig 315 and Plate
231). One or two endosutures (Fig 316) with externally tied slipknots (Plate 232) will reapproximate the capsule walls, as has been described in
chapter 14.2.6.2. for ovarian suture.

The myoma shown in Plate 233 is more than
2 cm in diameter; its stalk is being coagulated with
a crocodile forceps and then twisted off without
loss of blood. For safety's sake the wound in the
uterine corpus is recoagulated with the point coagulator (Plate 234).

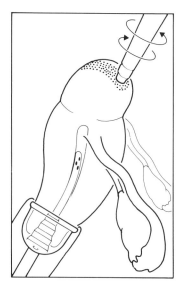

FIG 311.
For subserous intramural myomas, the serosal capsule
must first be coagulated.

The egg-sized pedunculated myoma, shown in
Plate 235, is generously coagulated at its broad
base with crocodile forceps; then the myoma is
twisted off with large claw forceps. After almost
bloodless enucleation, the wound crater is recoagulated adequately (Plate 236). The subsequent morcellation is performed with the tissue punch. If the
myoma contains calcium and therefore cannot be

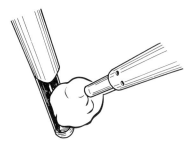

FIG 310.
Morcellation and removal of myoma.

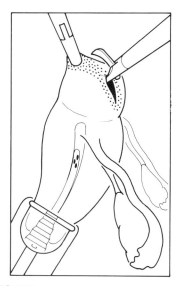

FIG 312.
The capsule is incised with hook scissors.

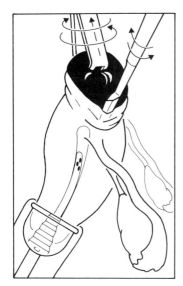

FIG 313.
The capsule is stripped off the myoma by pulling and twisting with claw forceps and simultaneous cutting, pushing and coagulating with the myoma enucleator.

morcellated, it will be removed through a posterior colpotomy. The anatomical findings at second-look pelviscopy 6 weeks after the original operation are shown in Plate 237: the coagulated wound areas have reepithelialized without adhesions.

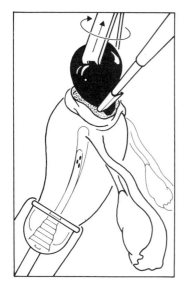

FIG 314.
The myoma is removed with rotating movements of the claw forceps.

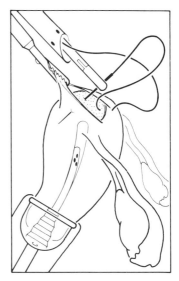

FIG 315.
Endosutures are placed in the capsule walls.

In the case of a cervical adenoma of approximately 2 × 3 cm diameter, a strip of uterine serosa and the myoma capsule of approximately 4 mm in width and 3–4 mm in length have been coagulated and bloodlessly split with hook scissors (Plate 238). The enucleation is also done bloodlessly by pulling and twisting with claw forceps and by thermocoagulation with the myoma enu-

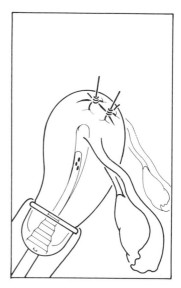

FIG 316.
Endosutures with slipknots have closed the defect.

cleator (Plate 239). After complete hemostasis has been achieved, the myoma crater is obliterated by applying two endosutures (Plate 240) and external tying of slipknots (see also Figs 315–316).

The postoperative anatomical findings 5 months after extensive omental and intestinal adhesiolysis (Plate 241) with myoma enucleation (Plate 242) are shown in Plate 243.

In sterility patients we remove by coagulation (Plate 244) and morcellation (Plate 245) essentially all myomas that are accessible without risk before we begin with the ascending chromopertubation and fimbrioplasty (Plate 246).

Plate 243 shows the anatomical findings 17 months after enucleation of the myoma shown in Plates 221 and 222; Plate 243 shows the pelvic anatomy 5 months after enucleation of the myoma shown in Plates 241–242. In the area of the scar, only an irregular structure in the serosa of the uterus can be recognized (see Plate 224).

Neither in other second-look pelviscopies (see Plate 237) nor in laparotomies done from 6 to 36 months postoperatively have we ever observed adhesions in the scarred areas on the uterine corpus, not even if the coagulated areas were more than 3 cm in diameter, as we could show in our motion pictures on gynecologic operations.

Supravesical myomas (fibroma of the bladder dome), which are occasionally encountered, can easily be enucleated after the parietal peritoneum has been incised (Plate 247); after morcellation they can be removed through the 11-mm trocar sleeve. The peritoneal wound is closed without complications either by suture or endoloop. Vascular band-like adhesions after cesarean section (Plate 248) can be endocoagulated with the crocodile forceps and severed without bleeding (Plate 249).

14.2.10.2. Pelviscopic Removal of a "Lost IUD"

The increased utilization of intrauterine contraceptive devices (IUDs) also led to an increase of cases in which the IUD was lost through the natural route of the cervical canal; sometimes, usually after incorrect application, the IUD may also perforate the myometrium into the free abdominal cavity. In combination with ultrasound, x-rays, hysteroscopy, and operative pelviscopy, it should no longer be necessary to search for and remove such "lost IUDs" by laparotomy.

As confirmed by x-ray and/or ultrasound, the "lost IUD" is located in the pelvic cavity. If, according to the sonogram, the IUD is expected to be in the uterine cavity, one first tries to probe for the IUD and extract it with a hook or grasping forceps or similar instrument. If this fails, hysteroscopy is indicated, combined with pelviscopy under general anesthesia. Often the IUD can be found in the uterine cavity (Plate 250) and extracted under direct vision.

In the following case, we found hysteroscopically only a short IUD string in the uterine cavity, which could not be removed when pulled. The patient, who had been prepared for a laparotomy, was repositioned for pelviscopy to search for the IUD pelviscopically. The CU-7 IUD, which 7 months earlier had been introduced immediately after termination of a pregnancy, had, in the meantime, partially perforated the myometrium. One arm of the IUD clearly elevated the serosa on the posterior wall of the uterus (Plate 251).

This serosa on the posterior wall of the uterine corpus, which was elevated by the arm of the CU-7 IUD, was first generously coagulated (Plate 252). After bloodless incision of the coagulation site, the IUD could be freed with atraumatic grasping tongs (Plate 253) and then grasped with a biopsy forceps and mobilized. With slow traction on the short arm (which was not enwrapped with copper wire), the IUD could be completely extracted from the myometrium (Plate 254), followed by extraction of the IUD string (Plate 255). Because of the risk of contamination with bacteria from the uterine cavity, the incision, although not bleeding, was carefully coagulated with the point coagulator, which was also introduced into the wound canal (Plate 256). This resulted in a satisfactory degree of thermal sterilization of the wound canal. The postoperative healing process was without complications; the physical stress for the patient was comparable to that of sterilization by pelviscopy. She left the hospital 3 days after the procedure free of discomfort and able to return to work. Three months later the patient requested the insertion of a new IUD.

In a similar case, an IUD had perforated transcervically and migrated up to the cecal area where, probably due to the reaction to copper, it caused an aseptic abscess. After the diagnosis was made pelviscopically, a laparotomy was performed during the same operation. Pelviscopic operative intervention is not suited for such cases because the manipulation of inflamed bowel should only be undertaken by a laparotomy.

If an IUD is found within the omentum (Plate 257), however, it can now be removed without complications by the pelviscopic route through an 11-mm trocar sleeve after the omentum has been partially resected (refer to chapter 15.1.).

A Copper-T IUD that had perforated the cervix and was lodged under the vesicouterine peritoneal reflection could be removed uneventfully by traction under pelviscopic vision.

[The "usual and customary" routines to remove an IUD are extremely wasteful: office exploration with inappropriate instruments, ultrasound, x-ray, hospitalization, general anesthesia, D&C, and possibly hysteroscopy, laparoscopy, or laparotomy. Many of the cases referred to me did not require any of these procedures. My routine is the following:

1. A careful history will often give a hint as to where one should search for the IUD.

2. A very thorough inspection of the vagina and cervix as well as bimanual examination may reveal abnormalities on the pelvic organs that are compatible with the extrauterine position of an IUD.

3. After exposure of the cervix with a Grave's speculum and disinfection with an antiseptic, a small, rigid, endoscopic grasping forceps of 3 mm diameter is cautiously and gently eased through the cervical canal into the endometrial cavity, where it is opened and used for palpation and usually grasping and withdrawal of the IUD. Only on rare occasions is it necessary to grasp the cervix with a tenaculum forceps, which decreases the tactile sensitivity of the gynecologist.

4. If the IUD is palpated but cannot be retrieved with the grasping forceps, exploration with a hysteroscope is appropriate. It may be done in the office or in an outpatient surgical facility under paracervical block analgesia, possibly in combination with "volonelgesia" (see chapter 10.1.2.); or

5. If an IUD cannot be palpated, consider ultrasound or x-rays after placing a metal probe, another IUD, a small catheter, or the like into the uterine cavity as a fixed reference point for the localization of the "lost IUD." Many of the images presented to me in consultation have been misleading or totally useless.

6. Laparoscopy/pelviscopy is indicated if bimanual pelvic examination is highly suspicious for an extrauterine position of the IUD or if the pre-

liminary workup outlined above confirms this suspicion.

If laparoscopy/pelviscopy is indicated, in most cases it can be performed on an outpatient basis, provided that all appropriate instruments and equipment are available and that the surgeon is experienced in endoscopic gynecologic surgery. Skills in endoscopic cutting, hemostasis, coagulation, morcellation, and endoligation are absolute requirements if both the patient and the surgeon intend to avoid a laparotomy if at all possible. If both the patient and the surgeon, as well as the operating room staff, are so inclined, this procedure can often be accomplished under "volonelgesia" (see chapter 10.1.2.), possibly augmented by intraperitoneal local or topical anesthesia. Only in rare cases, such as Semm's case mentioned above, will a laparotomy be required.—*Ed.*]

14.2.10.3. Suture of the Uterus After Perforation with a Curette

If the uterus was perforated with an instrument, probe, dilator, or curette (Plate 258), the internal genital organs are immediately evaluated by diagnostic pelviscopy. First the pelvic cavity is thoroughly irrigated to establish good visibility. If a bowel injury can be ruled out with certainty, bleeding from the uterus is controlled by coagulation of the perforation wound with the point coagulator (Plate 259). Subsequently the uterine wound is closed by endosuture (Plate 260). Usually one or two endosutures with external tying of slipknots will suffice to adapt the wound edges and at the same time achieve hemostasis (Plate 261). It is remarkable that there is hardly any bleeding from the needle tracts when the uterus is sutured endoscopically.

The postoperative course in all of our cases was uneventful. If a second-look pelviscopy was done, no adhesions were noted at the sites that had been sutured.

14.2.11. Pelviscopic Operations for Tubal Pregnancy

As recently as 30 years ago, it was generally held that a salpingectomy was the method of choice in the treatment of tubal ectopic pregnancy to avoid the risk of recurrence in the same tube. However, some cases were reported in which the first tubal pregnancy was treated by salpingectomy and the second and third tubal pregnancies on the other side were managed by conservative operations (all by laparotomy), followed by another one or two intrauterine pregnancies resulting in healthy children.

Therefore, this dictum can no longer be maintained.

By laparotomy, conservative operations for tubal pregnancy, i.e., those to preserve the tubes, are very time-consuming because hemorrhages are difficult to control. This applies in particular to microsurgical techniques that are presently under discussion. Bleeding during endoscopic intra-abdominal operations is much less serious than under laparotomy conditions, which provoke vascular paralysis. Encouraged by our good experiences with the endocoagulation method for hemostasis, in 1975 we began the conservative treatment of ectopic pregnancy by pelviscopy. Since we have also learned to control hemorrhage by endoloop and endoligature or endosuture, both the conservative as well as the radical operation of tubal pregnancy by laparoscopy has become the official method of choice in our hospital.

If the patient's history and pelvic examination raise the suspicion of an ectopic pregnancy, it is confirmed by ultrasound. On the other hand, the current high technical level of pelviscopy permits very early confirmation of a suspected tubal pregnancy, which can then be treated immediately. Due to modern technology, most cases of tubal pregnancy can now be discovered before they rupture or in the early phases of a tubal abortion, when the tube is dilated 2–4 cm. This early diagnosis prevents growth of the extrauterine pregnancy to a stage when it completely destroys the tube and sometimes also the ovary by forming a tubo-ovarian conglomerate tumor which, in an extreme case, even now may require a salpingectomy or even a salpingo-oophorectomy.

There is no doubt that a new era has begun with endoscopic abdominal surgery for the operative correction of tubal pregnancy. A laparotomy forced us to employ operative techniques with a very low risk of recurrence. This indeed was a salpingectomy. The risk that postoperative bleeding might require a repeat laparotomy was extremely low. Modern transfusion and anesthesia techniques permitted us to compromise between the safest operative techniques in regard to the risks of postoperative hemorrhage and recurrences, and conservative treatment of tubal pregnancy, which preserved the tube. The decision whether radical or conservative treatment was indicated depended on the anatomical findings at laparotomy.

With this laparotomy technique we had no way to observe the apparent reconstructive capabilities of the tubes during phases of the reconstructive process. After radical operations (salpingectomy) as well as after conservative procedures, we could usually observe only extensive adhesions in the pelvic cavity.

In the past 8 years, since the introduction of pelviscopic tube-preserving operations for tubal pregnancies, we have made the following observations:

1. With pelviscopic procedures, there is less bleeding than with a laparotomy.
2. Postoperatively, hardly any adhesions can be observed.
3. The postoperative tubal patency rate is approximately 80%.
4. The operative wound in the tube (see Plates 271 and 272) heals almost without visible scars.
5. If postoperative tubal obstruction occurs, it usually can be corrected microsurgically in an abdomen free of adhesions.
6. If hemorrhage did occur subsequent to pelvic conservative intervention, it could always be controlled pelviscopically, although only by ligation of the tube.
7. If the anatomical situation a priori was not suited for pelviscopic correction, the transition from a diagnostic or operative pelviscopy to a laparotomy caused no problems.

In summary, from the experience gained with numerous second-look pelviscopies, we established that the tube has regenerative capabilities of a magnitude completely unknown in the past. Even "tubal fragments" in tubes left in situ because they were not bleeding could regenerate to functioning tubes. These factors, which were unknown in the laparotomy era, have considerably changed our attitude regarding operations on fallopian tubes.

14.2.11.1. Conservative Management of Tubal Pregnancy

Depending on the localization of ectopic pregnancy, the following techniques are suited for operations on fallopian* tubes:

---

*Falloppio: Gabriele (Latin: Fallopius), Italian anatomist, 1523–1562, in Padua.

14.2.11.1.1. ECTOPIC PREGNANCY IN THE DISTAL TUBAL AMPULLA

If the tubal pregnancy is in the ampullary region, consequently a tubal abortion, three suprapubic punctures are made (two of 5 mm diameter each, one of 11 mm diameter) (see Fig 256 and Plate 197). After displacing loops of bowel, which are usually bloody, into the upper abdomen, blood is aspirated from the cul-de-sac with the single-channel/dual-purpose irrigation-aspiration system (see chapter 12.4.), followed by generous irrigation. The use of the single-channel/dual-purpose irrigation-aspiration system facilitates the dilution and evacuation of old blood coagula.

When the view is clear, the ampullary portion of the tube is dilated bluntly with two atraumatic grasping forceps and the products of conception are removed with the biopsy forceps or the large spoon forceps. Irrigation and suction of the ampullary portion of the tube expedite this activity. Merely aspirating the products of conception usually is not technically possible and is incomplete.

We have employed this technique since 1975 and have found that the complete removal of all chorionic tissues is the basic requirement for conservative pelviscopic treatment of tubal pregnancies. Bruhat, of Clermont Ferrand, France, is of the opinion that even partial aspiration of the ectopic pregnancy is sufficient to initiate the complete absorption of the chorionic tissues. This may indeed apply to many cases. However, we observed four cases out of approximately 100 ectopic pregnancies treated in this manner in which the chorionic tissues continued to grow after the incomplete evacuation of the products of conception from the tube. After 2 or 3 weeks, another repeat pelviscopy was necessary. In one case the tube had to be removed by laparotomy.

Therefore, we recommend the careful evacuation of all chorionic elements with the biopsy forceps or the large spoon forceps, as complete evacuation would also be the rule for termination of an intrauterine pregnancy.

The chorionic tissue is best removed from the cul-de-sac with large spoon forceps. Aspiration with the 4-mm cannula causes problems. The introduction of a suction cannula with a larger lumen is also problematic because the pneumoperitoneum will be deflated too rapidly. This loss cannot even be replaced by the OP-PNEU Electronic instrument with an insufflation rate of 6 L/min.

If uncontrollable hemorrhage occurs during the evacuation of the ampulla, the ampulla should be ligated with an endoloop. After 5–10 minutes, during which time one cleans out the cul-de-sac and the subphrenic space, the ligature is released again. In 90% of cases, the bleeding subsides. If not, one may try to control bleeding by selecting the most appropriate area for an endoligature in the mesosalpinx. If this too fails, another endoloop is applied permanently. Even with a laparotomy there would hardly be any other option.

14.2.11.1.2. ECTOPIC PREGNANCY IN THE MID-SEGMENT OF THE TUBE

If the pregnancy is in the middle segment of the tube (Fig 317), a strip 2–4 cm long and 4 mm wide is coagulated over the most convex area of the dilated tube (Fig 318), using the myoma enucleator or point coagulator in a similar manner as already shown with salpingostomy (see chapter 14.2.4.3.). One must allow 2–4 minutes for this procedure to produce complete hemostasis in this strip. Assisted by the atraumatic grasping tongs, the tubal wall is split longitudinally, completely within this coagulated strip (Fig 319). Radial incisions are also being discussed.

Depending on its size, the amniotic sac is removed with a biopsy forceps or large spoon forceps (Fig 320). The biopsy forceps is used to stabilize the wound edge.

Sometimes the tube contracts so vigorously af-

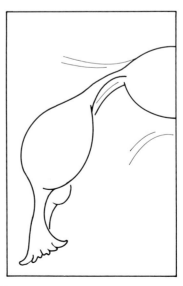

FIG 317.
Ectopic pregnancy in the mid-segment of the tube.

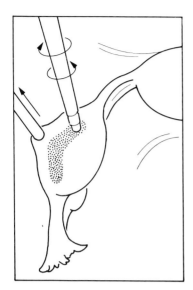

FIG 318.
A strip is coagulated over the most convex portion of the tube.

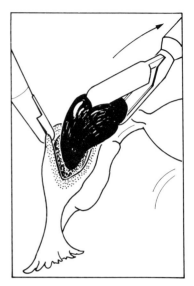

FIG 320.
The amniotic sac is removed.

ter it has been incised that the whole amnion and chorion are expelled spontaneously. During the several decades of my operative experience, I have never had an opportunity to observe such an event when the abdomen was open. It appears that thermal stimulation of the coagulation plays a role.

Assisted by irrigation and suction under vision

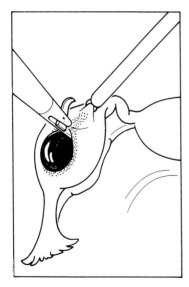

FIG 319.
The tubal wall is split longitudinally within the coagulated strip.

and by thermal stimulus, the empty tube contracts rapidly. Chorionic tissue elements must be completely removed; this can be accomplished quite well by constant irrigation, suction, and grasping with the biopsy forceps, if necessary, under low-power magnification with a loupe. Any bleeding is controlled with crocodile forceps or by ligation with endoloops.

Within the time frame of the operation of approximately 15–20 minutes, the tube usually retracts considerably. This controls minor bleeding, and also reconstructs the tube to its original shape. Smaller wounds in the tube may be left unattended after the evacuation of a tubal pregnancy; larger ones may be reapproximated by one or two endosutures (Fig 321). This adaptation by suture is recommended, because in one case we noted a tubal fistula at the time of a repeat pelviscopy whereas the remainder of the abdomen was completely free of adhesions. During chromosalpingoscopy, the blue dye solution escaped from the tubal ampulla as well as from the tubal fistula.

After such conservative, tube-sparing endoscopic management of 56 tubal pregnancies, we had an opportunity to perform 18 repeat pelviscopies; in 80% of them, chromosalpingoscopy revealed patent fallopian tubes.

Plate 262 shows a yet unruptured ectopic pregnancy in the middle segment of the tube in the ninth week of gestation which was diagnosed by palpation and ultrasound; it also shows a large ret-

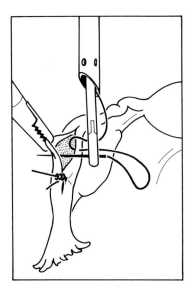

FIG 321.
Large wounds in the tube may be reapproximated with one or two endosutures.

rocervical myoma. As shown in Figure 318, a strip 4 cm long is coagulated with a point coagulator (Plate 263). This step is followed by longitudinal incision of the tube with hook scissors (Plate 264). The products of conception are removed with the spoon forceps (Plate 265). After generous irrigation and repeated biopsy, the wound is closed with endosutures (Plate 266) with external tying of slipknots. It is quite sufficient to only reapproximate the tubal peritoneum.

The following tube-conserving operations for ectopic pregnancy could be reexamined by second-look pelviscopy: the left tube with a pregnancy of 8 weeks' gestation is just beginning to rupture (Plate 267). When the 5-mm trocar is introduced, the peritoneum is pushed far ahead of the trocar before its conical tip perforates the peritoneum (Plate 268).

After aspiration of blood from the cul-de-sac and irrigation to improve visibility, the tubal wall is first coagulated in the thinnest area. Then, after longitudinal incision, the amniotic sac and all remnants of chorionic tissue are extracted (Plate 269), the cavity is thoroughly irrigated, and the tubal wound edges are reapproximated with an endoloop (Plate 270). Seventeen months after the endoscopic conservative operation for tubal pregnancy, the internal genital organs are completely normal and without adhesions (Plate 271).

The tube shows a grade I tubal patency for CO_2 gas (according to Fikentscher and Semm; see Fig 270) and the methylene blue solution emerges freely (Plate 272).

Since in another case the tubal pregnancy has already ruptured in the ninth week of gestation, generous irrigation (Plate 273) is required before the ruptured site (Plate 274) can be localized. After coagulation and longitudinal incision, the amniotic sac (Plate 275) is removed with a large spoon forceps and the wound cavity is irrigated with copious amounts of saline solution. It may be noted in Plate 276 that the tube has already contracted and almost returned to its normal shape. The wound edges are adapted by endosuture (Plate 277).

At the end of these surgical corrective measures, irrigation with saline solution should continue until the aspirated fluid is completely clear. This may require as much as 2–3 L. Then the upper abdomen is also inspected. If blood is noted in the subphrenic space, it is first aspirated with the single-channel/dual-purpose irrigation-aspiration cannula. Then, after consultation with the anesthesiologist, the head of the operating table is elevated (see Fig 29). With this maneuver it is also possible to aspirate the blood, which had been dispersed over the entire abdominal cavity before the operation began. This lavage of the entire abdominal cavity is essential to prevent adhesions and to shorten the recovery period.

In every attempt at endoscopic management of a tubal pregnancy, it must be clearly understood that in the case of failure or excessive hemorrhage, the procedure can be extended at any time to the classic form of therapy by laparotomy.

If it appears that hemorrhage cannot be controlled or if the patient is of an age at which the conservative (i.e., tube-preserving) management of a tubal pregnancy can no longer be justified from a medical point of view (i.e., is no longer indicated), the endoscopically much simpler salpingectomy is preferred. It obviates all bleeding problems, as will be discussed in the next section.

14.2.11.2. Salpingectomy for Tubal Pregnancy

If a tubal pregnancy occurs in an older patient who has completed her family or if the patient has stated explicitly that she does not care to have her fallopian tube preserved, endoscopic partial salpingectomy is indicated; it is explained schematically in Figures 322–325. In contrast to the tube-preserving operation, which even by laparotomy may sometimes be difficult because of almost uncontrollable hemorrhage, partial salpingectomy by the triple-loop technique and the removal of the products of conception is a relatively simple procedure.

The tube is grasped in the area of its largest diameter and the first endoloop is applied (Fig 322). The tubal segment with the products of conception is ligated by three endoloops (Fig 323), comparable to the technique for oophorectomy or salpingo-oophorectomy (see chapters 14.2.7. and 14.2.8.). The tube containing the products of conception is then severed with hook scissors at a 90° angle (Fig 324). The products of conception are then removed from the abdomen through the 11-mm trocar sleeve with a large spoon forceps, either in one piece or divided into smaller portions.

Then the pelvic cavity is thoroughly irrigated with 1–2 L of physiologic saline solution until the aspirated fluid is clear. The cut surface of the tissue pedicle is coagulated with the point coagulator (Fig 325)—as has already been mentioned repeatedly—for the prophylaxis of postoperative adhesions with intestinal peritoneum.

As was emphasized in chapter 14.2.11.1., irrigation of the pelvic cavity and the entire abdominal cavity up to the subphrenic space is mandatory. The postoperative absorption process is reduced by the complete elimination of blood from the abdomen, resulting in a shorter recovery period for the patient.

In the case of a 41-year-old patient with a 9-week tubal pregnancy (Plate 278), it was necessary

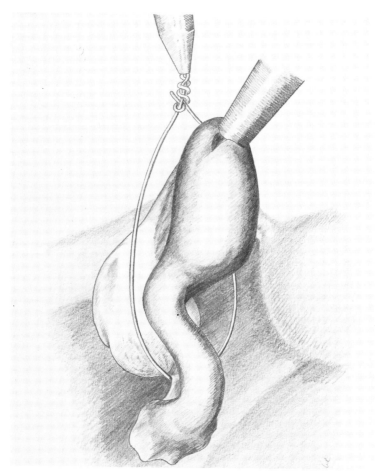

FIG 322.
Salpingectomy for tubal pregnancy. The tube is grasped at its largest diameter and the first endoloop is applied.

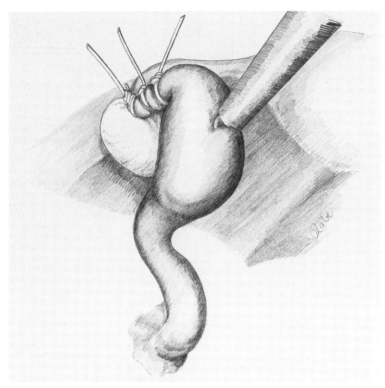

FIG 323.
Three endoloops are applied to tubal segment containing products of conception.

first to aspirate 810 ml of fresh and old blood before the left gravid tube (Plate 279) became visible. A primary salpingectomy was indicated in this case. Visibility improved after irrigation of the pelvic cavity. The large claw forceps is introduced through an endoloop to grasp and pull the tubal pregnancy through the loop (Plate 280), which is then tightened close to the products of conception. This is followed by placement of two more ligatures until the fallopian tube can be resected by cutting with scissors at a right angle. In preparation for the removal of the products of conception, the amniotic sac is first opened (Plate 281) and the fetus (Plate 282) is removed through the 11-mm trocar sleeve. After the tube has also been extracted, the abdominal cavity from the cul-de-sac to the subphrenic space is thoroughly irrigated. The operative result after this pelviscopic salpingectomy is shown in Plate 283.

Younger pregnancies can be managed by salpingectomy and the specimen can be removed en bloc through the 11-mm trocar sleeve (Plate 284).

14.2.11.3. Operation for an Abdominal Pregnancy

In rare cases, ovum nidation occurs outside the genital tract in the free abdominal cavity. Preferred sites are certainly endometriotic implants. After aspiration of 850 ml of blood, we found a nidation site of 4–5 cm diameter (8th week of gestation) in the pelvis attached to the sacrouterine ligament below the right ovary. The chorionic tissue with a fetus 2.6 cm long could be removed with large spoon forceps. The peritoneal bed had a tendency to bleed but could be coagulated with the point coagulator. After another irrigation of the entire abdominal cavity—with the pelvis lowered (see Fig 29)—the endoscopic surgeon noticed considerable hyperemia but otherwise normal internal genitalia.

14.2.12. Excision of Hydatid Cysts of Morgagni

Hydatid cysts of Morgagni are derived from the wolffian duct. Their rate of malignancy is low.

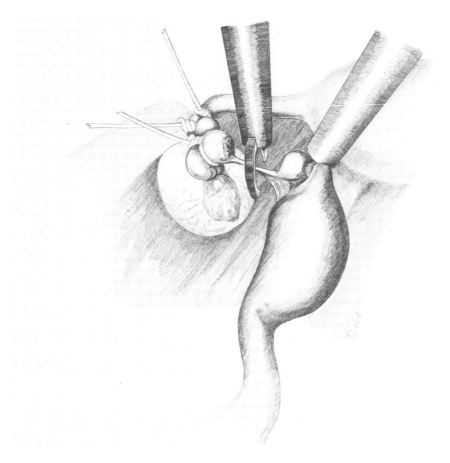

FIG 324.
The tube is severed with hook scissors at a 90° angle.

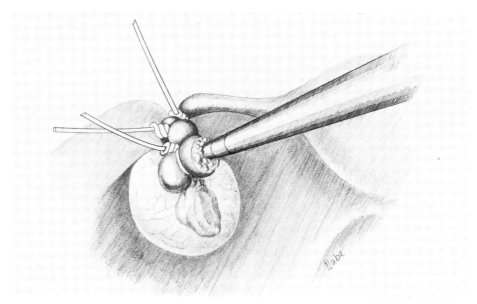

FIG 325.
The cut surface of the tissue pedicle is coagulated with the point coagulator.

They interfere with the mobility of the tubal ampullae, to which they are attached like weights. Therefore, we always remove such aberrant tumors during pelviscopic procedures. The stalk (Plate 285) is always very vascular (artery, vein). Therefore, simple transection always causes brisk bleeding. For this reason, it is necessary to begin with the coagulation of even small stalks with the crocodile forceps (see Plate 285) to permit bloodless transection with hook scissors (Plate 286). The extent of the vascularization of hydatids (derivatives of the wolffian ducts) is clearly shown in Plates 287 and 288. Avascular, so-called serosal cysts (Plate 289) may be severed without prior coagulation.

If coagulation is omitted before transection, the stalk of the hydatid cyst usually retracts into the area of its origin on the tubal ampulla. There it is difficult to find the artery of the hydatid; it can usually be coagulated only at the expense of considerable destruction of tissue in the ampullary area. Hydatid cysts without a stalk are coagulated first before their peritoneal envelope is incised, similar to parovarian cysts (see chapter 14.2.13.). After the covering peritoneal tissue has been incised, the cyst is mobilized and its vascular stalk, which is always present, is coagulated and then transected.

As a medical expert, I had to review a case in which high-frequency current was used for hemostasis after excision, causing thermal injury to the ureter. The patient died after nephrectomy, which was required after multiple operations for ureteral fistulas.

It should be reemphasized that high-frequency current is not suited to control hemorrhages from such stalks.

14.2.13. Pelviscopic Excision of Parovarian Cysts

Parovarian cysts, which usually have smooth walls and hardly any stalk, can easily be enucleated under laparotomy conditions after the peritoneum has been incised in the area of the broad ligament. If the anatomical relationships are well known, one should first try to perform this enucleation pelviscopically. This poses practically no risk of hemorrhage.

The parovarian cyst (Plate 290) of about 4–5 cm diameter is first inspected to find an area with few blood vessels, which is then broadly coagulated in a strip of approximately 6 cm long (Plate 291). The peritoneum is incised with hook scissors and the parovarian cyst can then be slowly enucleated by utilizing two biopsy forceps or tongs to strip the peritoneum off and ligate its stalk with an endoloop (Plate 292). One should avoid grasping the cyst itself, because this would cause it to rupture, making distinction of anatomical relationships difficult.

[If such a cyst ruptures, one should prevent the evacuation of all fluid by grasping the perforation site with a grasping forceps or needle-holder or by applying an endoloop. A partially deflated cyst is easier to manipulate and may even facilitate further dissection and access to the stalk.—*Ed.*]

After enucleation and transection of the stalk, the cyst fluid is aspirated. One of the suprapubic 5-mm trocar sleeves is dilated to 11 mm diameter so that the empty cyst sac can be grasped with large claw or spoon forceps (Plate 293) and removed in one piece.

[I have found it quite convenient to perform these procedures with the 11-mm operating laparoscope with a straight operating channel and a 45° deviation of the optical channel (see Fig 47,*B*) and only one suprapubic 5-mm trocar sleeve for ancillary operative instruments. This obviates in many cases the need for a second suprapubic incision and for the terminal dilatation of one of these channels to 11 mm diameter for the removal of the operative specimen.—*Ed.*]

At the end of the procedure it is again mandatory that the pelvic cavity be irrigated with 1–2 L of physiologic saline solution until the aspirated fluid is clear. After final inspection of the operative field, the peritoneal incision is closed, as shown in Figures 175 and 176, by adaptation of the wound edges with endoloops: the wound edges are grasped with the spikes within the large biopsy forceps and reapproximated. If this is not technically feasible because of too much tension or for some other reason, the gaping peritoneal defect is closed with one to three endosutures and external tying of slipknots, as shown in Plates 52–57 after the excision of a cluster of retrocervical endometriotic implants. With one of these techniques, the serosal defects can be closed in every case, because wound areas are not forcefully separated during pelviscopic procedures, as they are by abdominal retractors during a laparotomy.

14.2.14. Aspiration of Oocytes for In Vitro Fertilization

Since the recent introduction of new possibilities for the treatment of tubal factor sterility in women by in vitro fertilization by Steptoe and Edwards, pelviscopy has achieved a status of considerable importance in this field. The puncture and aspiration of mature follicles by pelviscopy imposes a minor physical insult compared to a laparotomy, while being almost equally effective. A particular advantage is the fact that pelviscopy can be repeated several times without undue physical stress to the patient. This does not apply to a laparotomy performed for the same purpose.

Patients who are presently awaiting in vitro fertilization are usually those who already have had one or more previous laparotomies in the past, either for tubal pregnancy or for other corrective procedures on their tubes. Usually there are extensive adhesions in the abdomen. Therefore, a primary procedure in conjunction with follicle puncture will consist of measures described in chapters 14.2.2.1.–14.2.2.5.

In a last effort to exhaust all possibilities available, fimbrioplasty or salpingostomy (see chapters 14.2.4.2. and 14.2.4.3.) or endoscopic salpingolysis and ovariolysis (see chapter 14.2.4.1.) are sometimes performed at the time the mature follicle is punctured and aspirated. One or two 5-mm trocar sleeves for operative instruments will be needed to bring the ovary into the proper position for aspiration. The aspiration needle, which is introduced through a 2.5-mm trocar sleeve (Plate 294), should not puncture the follicle perpendicularly (which causes the follicular fluid to squirt out and be lost) but the theca of the mature follicle should be perforated tangentially.

The mature follicle is punctured with either a single- or a double-lumen cannula (see chapter 12.8.10.) and the 2.5-mm trocar sleeve for the needle is introduced in the area of the linea alba.

It is the recommendation of the Australian group (Lopata, 1980) that the inside of the aspiration needle be coated with a Teflon tube, as described in chapter 12.8.10. It transfers the aspirated fluid uninterruptedly within a single smooth-walled tube all the way from the tip of the aspiration needle to the collection vessel (see Fig 95). This prevents disturbing countercurrents and, therefore, injury of the aspirated ovum: the zona pellucida, which is very important for the penetration mechanism of spermatozoa, should not be traumatized during transport. Nevertheless, transport of the ovum through the aspiration system can still be compared to a ride in a canoe over Niagara Falls!

After aspiration of the follicle (Plate 295), the ovum is caught in the isothermic trap (see Fig 95, B and C). If the egg is not found in this first aspiration specimen, it is recommended that the follicle be irrigated with 1–2 ml of incubation medium. Occasionally, two to ten follicles (Plates 296–299) can be aspirated successfully.

Further manipulations of the ovum should be done immediately adjacent to the operating room, because the ovum in its early stages of development is very sensitive to injuries caused by transportation.

The first perforation of the follicle by the tip of the aspiration needle should take place at a negative pressure of -3 to -5 mm Hg. This negative pressure is automatically obtained with the aspiration set (model Kiel) used with the Aquapurator. It prevents loss of the follicle at the time of the puncture and the loss of fluid, which often already contains the ovum.

Then the negative pressure is carefully adjusted under visual control by using a special tube with a holding ring which slips onto the surgeon's finger (see Fig 95, D). A negative pressure from 0 to -30 mm Hg is produced by intermittently opening and closing this finger control valve, resulting in the complete and slow aspiration of the follicular content. The finger control can also be connected to a foot control with a manometric safety device (water seal).

The best time for follicle aspiration is calculated on the basis of LH and E_2 determination and sonographic measurement of the size of the follicle.

In the beginning, it was believed that only spontaneously matured follicles of a normal ovarian cycle should be utilized. However, as experience in veterinarian medicine and that of the Australian group has shown, even oocytes resulting from hMG/hCG (superovulation) or clomiphene stimulation are suited for in vitro fertilization. These experiences have also been confirmed in Kiel, where pregnancies have resulted in healthy children.

In practical terms, it turned out that in many cases the first pelviscopy accomplished mainly adhesiolysis and ovariolysis, etc., so that repeat pelviscopies during the following cycles could be limited to the aspiration of follicles.

The moment of spontaneous follicle rupture is documented in Plate 300.

14.2.15. Pelviscopic Tubal Sterilization

As Naujoks provocatively enunciated as early as 1925 in his monograph describing 28 operative sterilization methods under the title, *The Problem of Temporary Sterilization of Women,* the strong desire of mankind for such surgical intervention has been ever-present for many decades. But the necessity of a laparotomy with its relatively serious physical effects on the patient severely limited the realization of this desire.

One of the first to use the laparoscope in combination with high-frequency current to sterilize women was Bösch, who published his first experiences as early as 1936. However, clinical utilization began after M. Cohen in the United States published his book on low-risk laparoscopic techniques in 1970. Stimulated by a meeting with me, he convinced himself that the risks inherent in this technique have been reduced in Europe by the introduction of fiber light optical systems, and, in particular, the CO_2-PNEU instrument. His endorsement helped to overcome the prejudices against gynecologic laparoscopy in the United States.

After that, since 1970, the introduction of laparoscopy in America reached almost explosive magnitude, with 95% indications for tubal sterilization. As early as 1971, it stimulated the foundation of the American Association of Gynecologic Laparoscopists, which had 4,000 members within 3 years. The number of gynecologic laparoscopies performed per year in Europe—primarily diagnostic laparoscopies for the evaluation of sterility—was exceeded in the United States, since 1971, by a factor of 100 with the operative utilization of this method for tubal sterilization. In the beginning, tubal sterilization was performed exclusively with high-frequency current, after Werner (1934) was the first to utilize the coagulation of fallopian tubes by high-frequency current in the open abdomen and Bösch (1936) was the first to utilize this technique under laparoscopic conditions. A level of clinical significance for this procedure in Europe is based on the meritorious work of Palmer (1946) and Frangenheim (1964).

The goal of operative tubal sterilization was and still is to create a barrier between the ascending spermatozoa and the ovum. Since Naujoks had reported numerous failures of operative steriliza-

tion procedures, it appeared to be desirable to destroy as much of the tube as possible by thermal necrobiosis produced by high-frequency current. With this single fixation of purpose, it was completely neglected for decades that the fallopian tube and the ovary share the same supply routes, both arterial and venous (see Fig 114), as well as the same nervous supply. The extensive coagulation of the tube by high-frequency current must, of necessity, also destroy the mesovarium with its vascular and nervous supply. As discussed in chapter 12.5. ff., the high-frequency current flows, according to the law of the conduction of electrical current, through routes of least resistance, primarily through nerves and blood vessels. When the electrical current flows from the neutral electrode attached to the patient's thigh or buttocks (see also Figs 1, 2, 96, 97, and 116) to the specific active electrode on the fallopian tube, it passes, of necessity, through many organs on the last segment of this route. According to the increasing field density in the area of the specific electrode (coagulation forceps), these organs are heated to temperatures above 57° C (beginning of thermal necrosis of thermolabile enzymes). This temperature is the upper limit of biologic life. Above 57° C, cell metabolism is biologically inactivated, i.e., killed.

In this context it should again be mentioned that two thirds of the arterial blood supply to the ovary is derived from the ascending branch of the uterine artery or the tubal branch, and that only one third of the arterial blood (i.e., oxygen) is supplied by the ovarian artery.

The tubal branch (see Fig 114) is always interrupted by the sterilization methods most frequently employed today. This applies to the coagulation methods with high-frequency current—unipolar or bipolar—as well as to mechanical techniques using suture, clip, or ring (see chapter 14.2.15.2).

In this regard, the papers of Riedel and Semm (1981) should again be mentioned. They examined in a follow-up study the phenomenon which, in the meantime, has been described as poststerilization syndrome. One thousand twenty-four women were contacted; one group had been sterilized by the original high-frequency current sterilization technique utilized at the University Women's Hospital in Kiel during the years 1970–1973, the other group had been sterilized by the new endocoagulation method (see chapter 14.2.15.1.3.) in use since 1973. There was a statistically significant difference in the severity of the poststerilization syndrome between the high-frequency current methods and the endocoagulation methods (see Tables 5–7). This is even more remarkable if one considers that immediately after the development of the endoco-agulation method, we were still unaware of the ex-tent of our destructive activity in regard to the physiology of the mesovarium, and therefore we continued to try to destroy as much of the tubal tissue as possible with the endocoagulation method. Only after we had gained a clearer under-standing of the biologically and operatively com-pletely unnecessary extent of tissue destruction, since 1977–1978, did we limit the coagulation only to the muscular portion of the tube. Even when we subsequently transect the tube (Fig 326; see also Fig 328), we avoid contact with the surrounding vascular and nervous system in the mesosalpinx (see Fig 117 and Plates 307–309).

After operative tubal sterilization, and re-gardless of which of the following methods is used, in addition to the instructions mentioned in chapter 3, the patient must be advised in particular of the possibility of tubal pregnancies after steril-ization.

14.2.15.1. Tubal Sterilization by Destructive Heat

Even after the monograph by Naujoks (1925) was published, no operative sterilization methods have proved entirely successful in preventing preg-nancy. Even a total vaginal hysterectomy may re-sult in vaginal-tubal fistulas and, consequently, tubal pregnancies. The vast experiences gathered from many millions of tubal sterilizations should actually lead to a change in the nomenclature. A 100% effective sterilization is only possible after removal of the gonads, i.e., by castration. All other methods result only in a reduction of the fer-tility rate (Semm, 1976).

If the patient is advised of these facts, subse-quent legal consequences for the physician should be forestalled. It is obvious that this type of infor-mation must be "with consent" and documented by signature. For the past 4 years, we have re-quested that the signature on the consent form be attested by a notary public. This is a cumbersome way of doing business, but it forces the patient to acknowledge the fact that she has been informed,

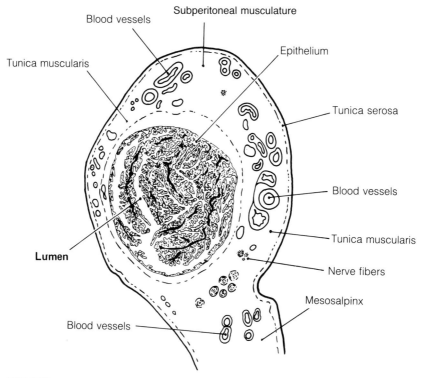

FIG 326.
Anatomy of the fallopian tube.

and relieves the physician of unjustified suits that try to claim that a method failure is actually negligence on the part of the physician.

In the monograph by Naujoks (1925), *The Problem of Temporary Sterilization of Women,* no mention was made of any technique for tubal sterilization by destructive heat. Attempts at sterilizing by destructive heat, however, date back to Kocks (Bonn, 1878). He attempted by the transvaginal-transuterine route to close the intracavitary tubal ostia by coagulation with galvanic current. This was followed by the same attempts by Mikulicz-Radecki (1927), but under hysteroscopic control. Special efforts were made by Lindemann (1971) to close the intrauterine tubal ostia through the hysteroscope by means of destructive heat from high-frequency current. Nor did the endocoagulation current which I proposed (1972) result in a safe sterilization method by the transuterine route. Therefore, hysteroscopic tubal sterilization by destructive heat is presently of no clinical importance (see also chapter 12.5. ff.).

Different results, however, were obtained in attempts by Werner (1934) in Aalen, Germany, who was the first to perform human tubal sterilizations by laparotomy utilizing high-frequency current for coagulation. He was followed by Bösch (1936) in Switzerland, who utilized the same technical procedure of coagulating tubes by high-frequency current but by laparoscopy. Independent of them, Power and Barnes (1941) of Ann Arbor, Michigan, rediscovered sterilization by fulguration of the tubes through the peritoneoscope for America. In Germany, it was mainly Frangenheim (1964) who introduced tubal sterilization by unipolar high-frequency current as a routine method in gynecology. Although the use of high-frequency current for this technique appeared to be the best surgical treatment, this was already extensively disputed in chapter 12.5.1.ff. and also in the *Atlas of Gynecologic Laparoscopy and Hysteroscopy* (published in 1976 in German, in 1977 in English).

Nevertheless, it is still held that the creation of a barrier between the ascending semen and the descending ovum by interrupting the fallopian tube by means of destructive heat is the method of choice. The thermal effect of high-frequency current, which cannot be controlled even by the most meticulous surgeon, can be completely substituted by the endocoagulation technique. With this method, the human body is no longer in direct contact with the electrical current.

Finally, it should be reemphasized that it was the possibility of tubal sterilization by coagulation of the tubes by means of high-frequency current which led, in the early 1970s, to the explosive introduction of laparoscopy in the United States. These experiences, gathered from millions of cases of operative pelviscopy or laparoscopy in America, were the stimulus for me to develop the endocoagulation method and, on another front, after eliminating the high-frequency risk in the abdominal cavity, to progress in developing endoscopic abdominal surgery.

In summary, it should be emphasized that the use of destructive heat to interrupt tubal continuity is probably the best method of tubal sterilization at this time. It can be accomplished rapidly and, moreover, has the lowest risk of unwanted pregnancies and does not cause a foreign body reaction in the patient, as is the case for the clip and ring method.

14.2.15.1.1. TUBAL STERILIZATION BY UNIPOLAR HIGH-FREQUENCY COAGULATION

As is clearly shown in Plate 4, heating of the fallopian tube by high-frequency current leads to the visible denaturation of proteins and, through exsiccation, even to carbonization. As shown in Plate 5 and discussed in chapter 12.5.6.2., this type of necrobiosis leads, later on, to sequestration of the destroyed tissue, which may cause fistulas in tubes coagulated by such means. This is probably the reason why some pregnancies have occurred with this method even if large segments of a fallopian tube have been destroyed. An experimental indication for these events is contained in statistics from America which were published by Phillips (1979): the additional transection of the tubes is more likely to lead to future pregnancies than not cutting the tubes.

When we refer to a tubal sterilization by unipolar high-frequency current, we generally distinguish between the following *techniques:*

1. Coagulation of the fallopian tube 2–3 cm distal to the uterine corpus without subsequent transection.
2. The same, but with subsequent transection.

The following *instruments* are used:

1. The insulated atraumatic grasping forceps, or
2. The insulated biopsy forceps.

The latter one is also suited for tubal biopsy. The tissue grasped by the biopsy forceps is not heated and is therefore suitable for histologic purposes, because the electrical current emanates from the surface of the biopsy forceps into the human tissue (skin effect).

Because the hemorrhage that resulted from tubal transection could not be controlled properly before the introduction of the endoloop or endoligature and, therefore, required a laparotomy, American gynecologists in particular recommended that cutting the tube with scissors after high-frequency current sterilization should be avoided.

Plates 301–304 show the typical postoperative anatomical changes 2–5 years after high-frequency sterilization (Plate 305; also see Fig 113) without transection: almost the entire length of the fallopian tubes has been destroyed. Only a small ampullary fimbrial remnant is seen. At the same time, it can be clearly recognized that the entire mesovarium, i.e., the endocrine and excretory functions of the ovary, has been severely damaged by the tubal sterilization (see Fig 116). In other words, the sterilization has also caused a partial castration of the patient, resulting in an earlier menopausal age or menstrual disturbances, which are responsible for a higher rate of D&Cs or hysterectomies (see chapter 12.5.4.; Riedel and Semm, 1981; Tables 5–7).

The area of destruction for sterilization by unipolar high-frequency current is shown in Figure 113.

It should be summarized once more that high-frequency current in its unipolar application travels through the human body from the neutral electrode to the specific, active one, as shown in Figure 96. According to the laws of electrical conductivity of electrolytes, it follows a route that cannot be predicted by the surgeon. The highest concentration of electrolytes is in nerves, blood, intestinal contents, and urine. In other tissues, the conductivity is less by a factor of 10 to 20. Variations in the electrolyte content of tissues and the skin effect (see Figs 100–106) influence the conduction of the current through the body and cause intermittent temperature peaks (see Figs 1 and 97).

The magnitude and site of the occurrence cannot be calculated in advance. Even though the operative field is meticulously controlled, burn injuries to bowel and ureter may not be detected by the surgeon. If the temperature in tissues is increased to 57°–90° C, the tissues may become necrotic because of the denaturation of thermolabile protein molecules, although color changes may not occur in this temperature range. Discoloration of proteins occurs only with temperatures above 94° C; only then the typical white color becomes apparent (a boiled egg with breakfast!). Conduction of the current takes place mainly through the vascular and nervous system of the ovary (see Figs 116 and 283). This causes severe impairment of the endocrine as well as the in- and excretory metabolism of the ovary due to partial damage of the mesovarium. This can be interpreted as partial castration.

These observations were confirmed experimentally in the late 1970s. Recognition of the "poststerilization syndrome" led to a statement at the annual meeting of the AAGL in Williamsburg in 1980 that lawsuits to compensate for damages caused by unipolar high-frequency currents could no longer be defended.

During the first Congress of the AAGL, held in 1973 in New Orleans, I made the recommendation (Semm, 1974) to completely avoid high-frequency current for tubal sterilization and, instead, to utilize heat only to coagulate the tube, which can then be transected without bleeding.

14.2.15.1.2. Tubal Sterilization by Bipolar High-frequency Coagulation

The course of bipolar high-frequency current shown in Figure 112 reduces the risk of the high-frequency current. It is no longer forced to travel through major portions of the human body in opposite directions to its physical description, the skin effect (see Figs 100–107 and chapter 12.5.3.). However, as was previously mentioned, even with bipolar high-frequency current, the human tissue offers electrical resistance, so that heat is induced by an increase in current density in the tissue (electrical conductor of the second order = electrolyte), which has been grasped between the branches of a grasping forceps (electrical conductor of the first order = metals) (see Fig 110). Due to the electrical resistance of tissues, which differs from case to case, and in spite of the controlled elements introduced by Wittmoser (1976) for use with bipolar coagulation forceps, neither the level of the coagulation temperature nor the extent of the coagulation zone can yet be exactly controlled.

Due to the skin effect, the bipolar application of high-frequency current will also cause thermal necrosis in an undeterminable area adjacent to the tissues grasped by the forceps (Plates 301–306). The coagulation of the fallopian tube with bipolar grasping instruments for the purpose of sterilization may still be tolerated from a technical point of view. However, its utilization for the coagulation of endometriotic implants, particularly in the dome of the bladder and adjacent to the ureter, may be problematic, because its depth effect cannot be calculated in advance: the depth of penetration of secondary currents induced in tissues surrounding the forceps depends both on the electrolyte content of these tissues and on the degree of exsiccation or carbonization of the tissues between the branches of the forceps.

In summary, after unipolar and bipolar currents have been utilized in millions of cases for tubal sterilization, we have learned that it is not an ideal way to produce the temperature necessary for hemostasis for intra-abdominal surgery in the closed abdomen.

14.2.15.1.3. Interval Tubal Sterilization by Coagulation (on the Nonpuerperal Uterus)

The technique of coagulating the fallopian tube at 100° C with subsequent bloodless transection by the endocoagulation technique (using the crocodile forceps) has been described in detail and its physical significance has been scientifically documented on pages 50–62 of the *Atlas of Gynecologic Laparoscopy and Hysteroscopy*. The following description is therefore limited to the technical procedure itself and the biologic changes related to it.

The jaws of the crocodile forceps were designed so that its two-dimensional hinge mechanism (Fig 327) would facilitate working with this instrument. The fallopian tube is grasped with the hooked jaw (Plate 307) between 1 cm to maximally 3 cm distal to the surface of the uterus without including the mesosalpinx, and then the tube is coagulated (Plate 308). For the subsequent bloodless transection (Plate 309) of the tube, it is extremely important to consider its anatomy, as illustrated in Figures 114 and 326. One must assure that the fallopian tube has been completely severed (Fig 328). When the tube is inadvertently grasped incorrectly it will be coagulated only partially, only in the area of its muscularis, as shown in the original sketch (Fig 329) accompanying the color photograph by Frangenheim: the tube was grasped only to the subperitoneal muscularis, which can be clearly recognized by the serrated pattern of the grasping forceps imprinted on the tissue (see also Fig 341). The muscularis itself (see Fig 326) ac-

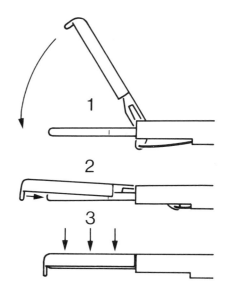

FIG 327.
Jaws and hinge mechanism of crocodile forceps.

tually escaped from the jaws of the forceps. Subsequently the tube is severed only partially, either with or without opening its lumen (Fig 330). Such inadequate technique may lead to an apparent "recanalization," as Frangenheim (1980) has clearly shown in his atlas. This, however, is not a real recanalization in the true sense of the word, but only healing and reconstruction of the tube, which has been injured by heating and cutting (identical to the failure of clip application, see Figs 340–342). The cut surfaces did not separate.

Traumatic injury of the tube, either by scalpel or temperature, induces much mitotic activity, as Philipp and Semm (1980) demonstrated electron

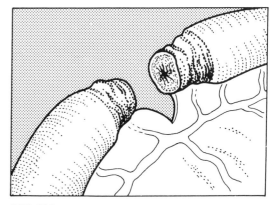

FIG 328.
Assure complete severance of the fallopian tube.

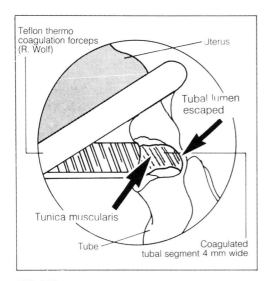

FIG 329.
Tube was grasped and coagulated incorrectly.

microscopically (Fig 331). Under this proliferative pressure, the tubal tissue has a very strong regenerative propensity.

If this mitotic activity is taken into account, it is easy to understand the recanalization of tubes which were severely damaged by high-frequency current, as shown in the two cases illustrated in Plates 310 and 311. The tubes on the right side appear to consist only of solid strands of fibrous tissue when reexamined 14 and 18 months, respec-

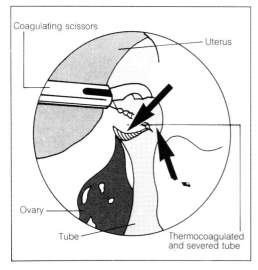

FIG 330.
Tube was severed only partially.

tively, after sterilization by unipolar high-frequency current; nevertheless both patients were 3 months pregnant.

If, however, the tube is carefully coagulated and transected, as shown in Figure 328 and Plate 309, the results are good. Our statistics from Kiel showed that the uncorrected pregnancy rate was 0.2% in 1,014 cases. In the two cases of pregnancy, histologic study revealed no evidence of morphological damage to the tubes. Either they had been only partially coagulated and cut, or they had not been coagulated at all because the anatomical structures had not been identified correctly.

The endocoagulation technique, if properly applied, does not involve or damage the mesosalpinx (see Figs 117 and 326). The procedure hardly affects the nutritional (i.e., incretory and excretory) system of the ovary. The anatomical findings in Plate 312, observed 38 days after sterilization by crocodile forceps (i.e., the endocoagulation method), show that

• the coagulation wound has healed without sloughing,
• the ends of the tube are separated far apart,
• the vascular system in the mesosalpinx is completely intact, and
• no adhesions have formed.

The anatomical relationships 3 years after tubal sterilization with crocodile forceps are shown in Plates 313 and 314. The cut ends of the tubes are

• well peritonealized,
• separated from one another,
• free of adhesions,
• well vascularized, and
• ideally suited for end-to-end anastomosis (even under endoscopic conditions).

In the cases presented, reanastomoses were successfully performed under microsurgical conditions followed by subsequent pregnancies.

An important advantage of the endocoagulation method for tubal sterilization is that all other endoscopic procedures for the control of pathologic conditions in the entire abdominal cavity which are described in this atlas can be performed during the same operation. As far as adhesions, endometriotic implants, and so forth are concerned, the patient is cured when she leaves the operating room. At the time of the sterilization procedure, other conditions that may have been present for years can be prophylactically eliminated, such as complaints related to endometriosis after unsuccessful conservative therapy and previously unrecognized risk

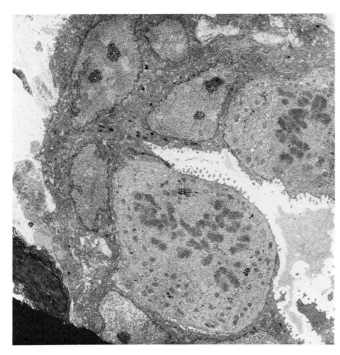

FIG 331.
Traumatic injury to the tube induces much mitotic activity, as shown in this electron micrograph.

factors (for instance, risk of intestinal obstruction in the presence of adhesions; see chapter 14.2.2.1.).

From a medical/ethical point of view, it should also be emphasized that the sterilization procedure relieves the patient not only of the fear of pregnancy; ancillary measures, such as coagulation of endometriotic implants in the sacrouterine ligaments, will relieve the patient of her dyspareunia. After the sterilization procedure she may find that intercourse can be a real pleasure without discomfort.

In summary, the operative sterilization method by endocoagulation in combination with a broad spectrum of other corrective measures in the entire abdominal cavity can be considered the method of choice for operative sterilization.

14.2.15.1.4. TUBAL STERILIZATION BY COAGULATION DURING THE POSTPARTUM OR POSTABORTAL PHASE

Tubal sterilization in the postpartum period differs from interval sterilization insofar as the surgeon must take into account certain technical requirements related to the postpartum size of the uterus. Postpartum sterilization by pelviscopy should be delayed until the uterus has retracted to approximately one handbreadth below the umbili-

cus. If it retracts even more, the tubal cornua are displaced deeper into the cul-de-sac, so that it becomes more difficult to find them and to displace bowels. Since the risk of infection is increased in the postpartum period, uterine elevators (e.g., vacuum intrauterine cannula) should not be introduced into the uterus. However, the three-puncture technique solves all of these problems. The uterus is elevated with an atraumatic grasping forceps and the tubal cornu is brought into position for the coagulation forceps, so that the tube is exposed and far away from bowels, etc. One should never coagulate in narrow spaces, to avoid the risk of inadvertent contact with bowels, etc.

In the postpartum period, the tube is extremely vascular. A thorough and prolonged coagulation (at least 20 seconds) is required. If the coagulation is inadequate, oozing or even hemorrhage from spurting vessels may occur after sharp transection with hook scissors. In the past, this used to be a serious risk and required laparotomy. Today, any such bleeding can be controlled by endocoagulation, loop ligature (see chapter 12.6.1.), or endosuture (see chapter 12.6.3.).

There is no doubt that these new methods will force us to reevaluate previous routine techniques for routine tubal sterilization. Our medical care should be not simply goal-oriented, but the patient's welfare should be our primary concern.

[I feel very strongly that pregnancy is the worst time for a woman to make such an important decision with far-reaching consequences; if anything, we should protect her from making a decision that she may regret in the future. Only under rare circumstances may I consent to a tubal sterilization at the time of a cesarean section. Under ordinary circumstances, she should observe the development of her infant for at least 6–12 weeks before submitting to a tubal sterilization which, at that time, is a simpler and safer procedure.—*Ed.*]

14.2.15.2. Tubal Sterilization by Ligation

As Naujoks stated in his 1925 monograph (see chapter 14.2.15.), the interruption of tubal patency with needle and thread used to be the method of choice. For several years this classic method lost much of its importance, because tubal ligation by unipolar or bipolar high-frequency current *seemed* to have many advantages. However, efforts continued to accomplish this classic operation under endoscopic conditions.

Now it is relatively simple to ligate the tube with an endoloop (see chapter 12.6.1.) similar to Madlener's technique (Plate 315) and then transect it (Plate 316). This endoscopic technique, which is a modification of the techniques described by Madlener (1919) and Irving (1950), among others, is shown schematically in Figures 332–334. The tube is grasped with atraumatic grasping tongs (Fig

332), pulled into an endoloop, ligated (Fig 333), and then cut with hook scissors (Fig 334) without any blood loss. Since this ligature method, which is simple and without risk, was already known to have a recanalization and pregnancy rate of 0.1%–5% when done by laparotomy, it never attained much clinical importance.

[Actually, in Madlener's technique the tubes were first crushed, then ligated with nonabsorbable suture. This could either prevent separation of the tubal ends or be responsible for fistula formation. This explains the high failure rate of up to 10%. In Irving's technique, the proximal tubal stump is buried in the myometrium of the uterus, whereas the severed distal tubal stump is buried in the mesosalpinx. In Pomeroy's technique, a loop of the midportion of the tube is elevated and ligated at its base with absorbable catgut suture and the loop is resected. The suture material is absorbed rapidly, reducing the chances of inflammation and formation of fistulas. The ends of the tubes separate as soon as the suture material is absorbed. The failure rate is in the same range as that with most endoscopic methods, between 1 and 5/1,000. Semm's endoloop technique could therefore be considered an endoscopic modification of the Pomeroy technique.—*Ed.*]

Instead of applying a ligature, surgeons tried to interrupt the continuity of tubes by clips or rings/bands. At first tantalum clips (Fig 335) were used, which had originally been introduced in

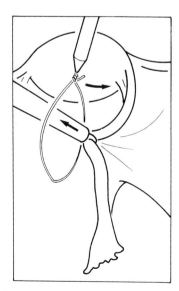

FIG 332.
Tubal ligation by endoloop. The tube is grasped with atraumatic grasping tongs and pulled into the endoloop.

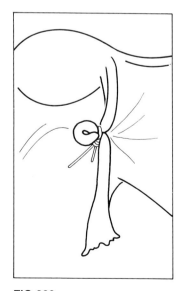

FIG 333.
Tube is ligated.

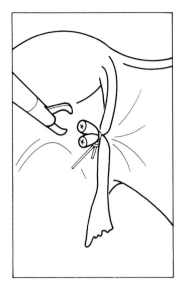

FIG 334.
Tube is cut with hook scissors. There is little or no blood loss.

America for hemostatic purposes in general surgery. It was simple to apply these clips to the tube with a special applicator designed for this purpose (Fig 336). With double clip application, this technique appeared to be absolutely safe. However, as shown in Figure 337, there is sufficient spring action in the metal clip to partially release the pressure from the lumen of the tube. A capillary slit remains, through which spermatozoa as well as the fertilized egg may pass—as proved by a pregnant

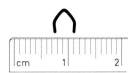

FIG 335.
The tantalum clip for tubal sterilization.

uterus 7 months after the application of four tantalum clips, shown in Figures 350 and 351 in the *Atlas of Gynecologic Laparoscopy and Hysteroscopy* (1977). The pregnancy rate after clamping tubes with tantalum clips is approximately 10%. Therefore, this method had to be abandoned.

Successful ligation of the tubes will be described in the following sections. The original expectation that these operative techniques might be reversible has not been borne out.

14.2.15.2.1. TUBAL STERILIZATION BY CLIP APPLICATION

Hulka (1973) was the first to disrupt tubal continuity by a combination of plastic material and a gold-plated stainless steel spring (Fig 338). The endoscopic application of a Hulka clip with the specially designed applicator (Fig 339) is not very difficult, provided that the tube has a normal configuration and is narrow.

The main problem with all clips is the closing of the hinged jaws. When the jaws are closed, the fallopian tube is squeezed from the area of the narrow angle of the hinged jaws so that the lumen of

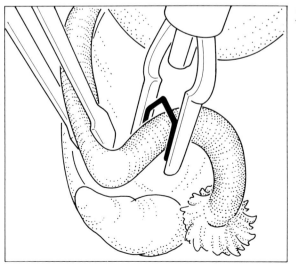

FIG 336.
The tantalum clip applied with a special applicator.

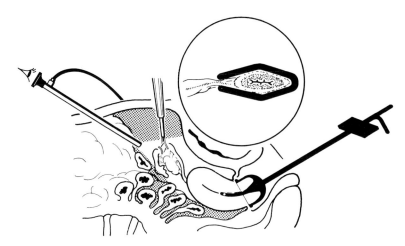

FIG 337.
Spring action in the clip partially releases pressure on tubal lumen, allowing passage of spermatozoa and fertilized egg.

the tube may be partially or totally squeezed beyond the reach of the plastic jaws, as was illustrated for the coagulation technique in Figures 329 and 330. Figure 340 shows the correct application and Figure 341 the incorrect application of the tubal clip. The tube may be prevented from escaping when the clip is closed by keeping the tube under tension with atraumatic grasping tongs introduced through a third puncture, as shown in Plate 317.

Proper clip application (e.g., Bleier clip) is shown in Plates 317–319. The tube is kept under tension with atraumatic grasping tongs (Plate 317) before the plastic clip is applied, with the jaws of the applicator reaching across the tube and anchoring the clip into the mesosalpinx (Plate 318).

It is inherent in this method that well-placed clips (Plate 319) also clamp part of the arteriovenous vascular system, shown in Figure 114. This leads to a disturbance of ovarian metabolism, because it interferes with the nutritional system (see

chapter 12.5.4.), i.e., the incretory and excretory system, of the ovary.

Most of the time, however, clips are applied by the ''single-entry technique,'' i.e., the clips are applied without holding the tube under tension (see Plate 317); this may lead to a misapplication, as shown in Figure 341.

This problem is clearly illustrated in Plate 320. A Bleier clip, which had been applied pelviscopically 2 years earlier, was obviously in an ideal position (Fig 342). The tubal specimen (see Plate 321), which was obtained during a total abdominal hysterectomy for carcinoma of the cervix (stage 1A), shows, however, that the clip had included only the subperitoneal muscularis, comparable to that shown in Figures 329 and 330 for the endocoagulation technique.

When the Bleier clip was closed, the muscularis containing the tubal lumen was squeezed out of the clip, therefore failing to obstruct it.

In addition to the risk that the tubal lumen

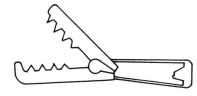

FIG 338.
The Hulka clip, made of plastic jaws and a gold-plated stainless steel spring.

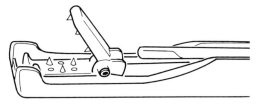

FIG 339.
Applicator for the Hulka clip.

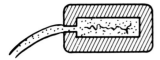

FIG 340.
Tubal clip correctly applied.

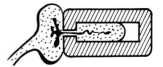

FIG 341.
Tubal clip incorrectly applied.

may escape, (i.e., the failure rate), a foreign body reaction at the implantation site should not be disregarded. From the experiences in the field of orthopedics as well as dentistry, it is well known that implantation of any type of organic or inorganic material may lead, after months or years, to foreign body reactions of varying degrees. All ring and clip methods were introduced into gynecology without prior investigations in this regard, although it was known from the outset that these foreign body implants would not only have to remain for years but for decades!

Most clips are overgrown in a few weeks or months by a layer of peritoneum (Plates 320, 322). In our experiments on rabbits, we clearly observed foreign body reactions after only a few days. The Bleier clip is completely encapsulated after 8 weeks. These tissue reactions are possible because every elastic synthetic material absorbs water and therefore becomes a substrate for biologic reactions. If such plastic clips slip off the tubes after days, weeks, months, or years, they may be found as migrating bodies in every area of the abdominal cavity.

Many manufacturers offer applicators for clips that can be introduced by the "single-entry technique." This makes them well suited for pelviscopic sterilization under local anesthesia or volonelgesia.

Originally, it was hoped that the tubes would

recanalize spontaneously after removal of the clips. These expectations have not materialized. Since clips must principally reach deep into the mesosalpinx in order to be anchored securely, they partially ligate automatically the vascular and nervous supply to the ovary, as shown in Figure 114. The poststerilization syndrome, described in chapter 14.2.15., may therefore be more common after application of long clips (Bhatt, 1981).

14.2.15.2.2. TUBAL STERILIZATION BY SILICONE RING APPLICATION

The fact that silicone rings have a high elasticity and can be stretched considerably stimulated Yoon to replace the suture ligature technique with the application of rings. The application mechanism is shown in the following original photographs. The narrow segment of the tube is grasped with the atraumatic grasping tongs of the ring applicator (Plate 323) and the ring is then released onto the loop of tube (Plate 324) from the lower end of the applicator to which it had been mounted in a stretched condition. As the ring regains its original shape (Plate 325), it constricts and ligates both tubal lumina.

The main advantage of Yoon's Falope-Ring is its technically relatively simple and bloodless mode of application. Some of the reactions that may occur in the constricted tubal tissues are dia-

FIG 342.
A Bleier clip correctly applied.

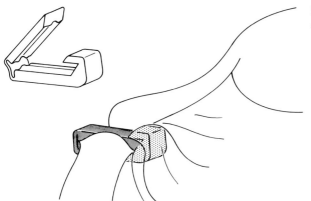

gramed in Figure 343. *A* shows an ideal position of the ring. The vessels are not completely interrupted; the constricted tubal loop is suffering from the effects of this hypoxemic condition and, after a few years, sometimes shows a suspicious histology: the ligated segment of the tube becomes necrotic *(B)* and sloughs off. The ring may also separate from the tube, i.e., it may migrate throughout the abdominal cavity. As shown in *C*, spontaneous recanalization may occur proximal or parallel to the dislodged ring.

With the ring method of tubal ligation, at least 2–3 cm of tube is sacrificed. The loss of this much of the tube may reduce the success rate after a possible microsurgical tubal reanastomosis.

The silicone ring method can be summarized as follows. It is a bloodless, very simple method of creating a barrier against the ascending spermatozoa. However, this method carries certain risks that have not yet been completely investigated and therefore must be accepted by the patient. The ring application may lead to an increased incidence of poststerilization syndrome.

14.2.16. Comments and Conclusions Regarding Endoscopic Tubal Sterilization

The müllerian duct, originally derived from a fold of celomic epithelium in the 3rd to 4th weeks of fetal development, is transformed into a duct in the 7th to 11th weeks of fetal development. From the originally solid strand of tissue developed the tubal lumen, the uterine cavity, and the vaginal barrel. This genetically preprogrammed biologic propensity to form ductal structures seems to remain active in this reproductive organ throughout life. At least Philipp and Semm (1980) could not detect any mitoses in 1,000 electron microscopic sections of fallopian tubes. However, in fallopian tubes that have been traumatized by high-frequency current or by mechanical measures (such as ligation for sterilization purposes), mitoses were always found in varying numbers (see Fig 331). Considering that mitosis lasts for only 10–20 minutes, this must be due to a reactivation of an inherent regenerative potential. The sudden reappearance of so many mitoses must be interpreted as a response to an artificial proliferative stimulus.

This may also be the explanation for the occurrence of pregnancies after surgical sterilizations that have left the tubes so severely damaged that a pregnancy had been deemed impossible. In this case, biologic control mechanisms are able to correct, for the preservation of the species, artificially induced anatomical and functional alterations of the process of reproduction, which are unknown in other organs.

On the basis of this fact, we have to conclude that all operative efforts to establish a barrier between spermatozoa and egg can only be an attempt to reduce the rate of reproduction without being able to completely abolish it. Therefore, every operative measure to cause sterility, including total hysterectomy—Schreiner (1974) describes at least 15 extrauterine pregnancies after hysterectomy—is not a sterilization in the true sense of the word; it is only a reduction of fertility, and the effectiveness varies from method to method. A true sterilization with 100% success is only possible by castration, i.e., the removal of the gonads [and in addition, considering the current option of in vitro fertilization, the uterus as well.—*Ed.*].

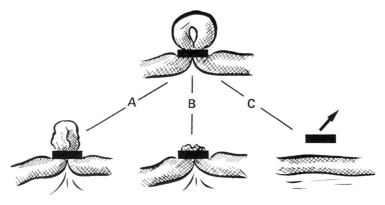

FIG 343.
After application of Yoon's Falope-Ring, the constricted tubal tissue may react in different ways. See text.

14.2.16.1. Comments and Conclusions Regarding Endoscopic Tubal Sterilization by Pelviscopy

Pelviscopic sterilization has been an important improvement in the methods by which sterilization can be accomplished. The physical stress and risks to the patient are small. If modern knowledge and surgical experience are applied, pelviscopic tubal sterilization is a safe method that can even be performed under ambulatory conditions. It is certainly superior to past procedures by laparotomy.

As far as reversibility is concerned, there is no difference between endoscopic methods and techniques performed by laparotomy. An easy, reversible operative method of sterilization has not yet been developed.

In regard to available options for endoscopic sterilization, one must decide between the utilization of destructive heat to accomplish hemostasis with subsequent bloodless transection of the tube or a purely mechanical method, such as a clip or a ring.

If destructive heat is utilized, the general risk from the operative procedure should not be increased by the specific risk inherent in the high-frequency current method (see chapter 12.5.1. ff.).

The modern endocoagulation method not only replaces the technique utilizing high-frequency current, but is far superior to it. The pregnancy rate is less than 0.2% and approaches 0 if the tubes have been transected and the ostia are separated far apart. For a review of all operative methods for the sterilization of women, with rates of pregnancies and complications, refer to Hirsch (1976) and Riedel, Conrad, and Semm (1985). In this statistical overview of the German experience, the endocoagulation technique resulted in a pregnancy rate of only 0.11%, which is the lowest for all sterilization techniques used in Germany.

14.2.16.2. Comments and Conclusions Regarding Endoscopic Tubal Sterilization by Hysteroscopy

The method of transvaginal, i.e., transuterine tubal sterilization by hysteroscopy was discussed in detail in the *Atlas of Gynecologic Laparoscopy and Hysteroscopy*. In the meantime, the methods of high-frequency current and endocoagulation have been augmented by the implantation of liquid or solid splints through the uterine cavity into the tubes.

In summary, it can be stated that, in spite of

several decades of further experimentation since Mikulicz/Radecki's work was published in 1927, the transuterine option of closing the intramural tubal ostium has not yet reached the stage of clinical acceptance. If destructive heat is used with the intention of closing the tubal ostium, a postoperative pregnancy rate of 10%–20% must be expected. If solid splints are implanted into the tubes or first injected in a liquid state and then allowed to polymerize, the difficulties in implanting these devices or their expulsion rate is so high that one cannot yet consider this a safe operative contraceptive method.

14.2.16.3. Counseling of Patients Before Operative Sterilization

Legally, tubal sterilization is a procedure of far-reaching consequences for the patient. It should be performed only after the physician has counseled and educated the patient in detail and has obtained her consent. A written consent must be obtained from the patient; one from the husband may also be desirable. Although only the patient is responsible for her actions and, legally, one does not have to obtain her husband's consent, it must be understood that the physician, by performing the operative procedure, changes the legal situation established by the marriage or the "business contract." If the marriage partner has not consented, legal action may be taken against the physician for his involvement in changing inheritance and property rights. Therefore, the physician is well advised to request the husband's signature in an effort to forestall the possibility that he may demand recourse in the future.

The patient's signature on a preprinted consent form for sterilization in many cases is no real legal protection if, later on, the patient can convince the jury that she had not been adequately informed and would not have consented under such circumstances. The physician who intends to perform the sterilization is therefore well advised to have the patient state again in 4–6 lines in her own handwriting that she has received and understood the printed information, and have this witnessed by a notary public, as is customary for a last will and testament. This form of legal protection by the physician performing sterilization operations may appear complicated and cumbersome; however, it is certainly justified if one considers recent judgments against physicians in cases related to this matter. The patient must be informed at length, both orally and in print, that in every case—even

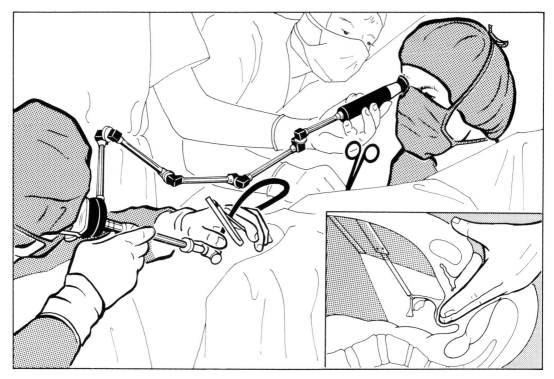

FIG 344.
Creation of a neovagina.

with most meticulous, correct operative techniques—another pregnancy is possible.

As 100 years of experience have shown, the establishment of a barrier between ascending spermatozoa and the ovary reduces the fertility rate to 0.2%–5%, depending on the method; in other words, 100% sterility can be accomplished only by castration, i.e., the removal of the gonads (Semm, 1976). At the same time, the patient should also be informed that, depending on the method applied, other pathologic conditions in the abdomen can be corrected in conjunction with the sterilization operation, for example, symptoms caused by endometriosis.

14.3. PELVISCOPIC MONITORING OF AN OPERATION TO CONSTRUCT A NEOVAGINA

For the construction of an artificial vagina, for example, in the case of Rokitansky-Küster-Mayer-Hauser syndrome, a combined operative procedure is a definite advantage.

The procedure begins with a diagnostic pelviscopy to evaluate the anatomy of the internal genitalia (Plate 326) and to perform a gonadal biopsy. Subsequently the vaginal operation is begun under constant pelviscopic control. This is done partially by the assistant, partially by the surgeon himself, using an articulated or flexible teaching attachment (Fig 344).

The technique with which we have had the

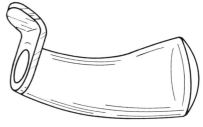

FIG 345.
The Plexiglas prosthesis for a neovagina.

best experience is the dilatation of a vaginal barrel. After the hymen has been opened with an incision in the shape of an H or a star, the noncanalized "vaginal tissue" is dilated with Hegar dilators (Plate 327). Advancement of the dilators can be observed through the articulated or flexible teaching attachment (Plate 328). This dilatation is continued, if possible, up to Hegar No. 20 or No. 30 before the Plexiglas prosthesis (Fig 345) is introduced under pelviscopic control (Plate 330). This has first been covered by a sock made of lyophilized dura (Plate 329) is transformed in 3–6 weeks into a well-peritonealized, spacious vagina. This combined method permits the best utilization of the space available without the risk of perforation. The patient is spared the laparotomy, which was previously required.

15 _____ General Endoscopic Abdominal Surgery

In general surgery, laparoscopy is still practically unknown. The surgeon prefers to open the abdomen with a scalpel. To obtain the best cosmetic result, however, the general surgeon attempts to keep this abdominal incision as small as possible. These efforts can best be appreciated in surgical scars from an appendectomy.

The operative technique for endoscopic adhesiolysis and resection of the omentum (see chapter 14.2.2.1.), which was developed for gynecologic applications over the past four decades, has matured to such perfection that it can now be adopted for general surgical applications. The technique of endoscopic appendectomy, which presently is beyond the realm of the usual gynecologic operations, will certainly provoke considerable discussion. One of the first points of discussion will be that suspicion of appendicitis used to be an indication for a laparotomy. Regardless of whether or not the suspicion was confirmed, the appendix was then routinely removed. How long this general surgical routine can be maintained in the future, when the suspicion of appendicitis can be evaluated by a procedure that is less aggressive than a laparotomy—namely, by the physically less stressful endoscopy—will have to be decided by ongoing discussion.

Certainly surgeons will have to consider further under what circumstances the appendix should or might be removed for prophylactic reasons if the diagnostic endoscopic evaluation fails to confirm the suspicion of appendicitis. Therefore, the fol-lowing discussion should serve as an appraisal of modern endoscopic methods. In particular, it suggests how techniques that have already been developed, such as endoscopic intra-abdominal sutures and tying of knots, could expand the spectrum of general surgery. Examples are postoperative omental and intestinal adhesiolysis without risk of recurrence.

15.1. OMENTAL ADHESIOLYSIS AND RESECTION

Previously, omental adhesiolysis during a pelviscopic procedure was performed only if adhesions prevented inspection of the pelvic organs or if adhesiolysis was technically necessary to achieve tubal sterilization.

As techniques and the safety of adhesiolysis in the area of the omentum improved, the indications for operative pelviscopy were gradually expanded at the University Women's Hospital in Kiel. Patients who did not require specific gynecologic operative procedures but mainly a general surgical intervention were included, such as those with complaints due to postoperative adhesions. This approach was so successful that, from 1978 on, operative pelviscopy was utilized in patients who did not have a specific gynecologic indication for surgery but a suspected surgical condition.

Patient preparation and operative techniques for extensive omental adhesiolysis and resection are described in chapters 14.2.2.1. to 14.2.2.4. and illustrated in Plates 19, 20, and 32. The same techniques apply to general abdominal surgery.

15.2. INTESTINAL ADHESIOLYSIS AND INTESTINAL SUTURE

As the safety of endoscopic intra-abdominal ligating and dissecting techniques in the abdomen with massive adhesions improved, the operative spectrum was expanded to lysis of postoperative adhesions between bowels and both the parietal peritoneum and the visceral peritoneum.

For lysis of adhesions between loops of bowel and the parietal peritoneum, particularly in an area corresponding to the peritoneal suture at the end of a laparotomy, low-power magnification of the endoscopic image with a loupe (see chapter 12.2.4.) is very helpful. Under such conditions, scissor dissection in the line of cleavage can be carried out more exactly than during a laparotomy. Bowel to be dissected can be kept under light tension with atraumatic grasping tongs (Plate 331) introduced through a secondary incision so that the cleavage line (see Fig 20) is demonstrated even better.

To separate bowel from the surface of ovaries (Plate 332), it is advisable to dissect more in the tunica albuginea so that ovarian tissue—usually tissue from the surface of an ovarian cyst—remains on the bowel surface. This is also the usual routine during a laparotomy. The serosal defect is closed with an endosuture and external slipknots (Plate 333) to prevent postoperative complications. Remember the maxim: *In endoscopic abdominal surgery, apply the same techniques as in a laparotomy* (see chapter 14).

The end result of the operation illustrated in Plates 332 and 333 is shown in Plate 334. Postoperative adhesions between a loop of small bowel and the left ovary had caused incapacitating pain. The site of adhesion is clearly demonstrated as traction is placed on the bowel with atraumatic grasping tongs (Plate 335). If necessary, visualization of adhesions may be aided by low-power magnification with a loupe. The dissection is carried out in the area of the tunica albuginea of the ovary, which is clearly visible on the surface of the freed bowel (Plate 336).

Bloodless adhesiolysis techniques are used in the case of intestinal-ovarian adhesions shown in Plate 337: After an endoligature has been applied and tied (see Plate 337) the adherent loop of bowel

is dissected off the ovary (Plate 338) with preservation of the peritoneal cover (Plate 339).

If the sigmoid colon is adherent to the left ovary and the uterine fundus (Plate 340) it is first dissected off the ovary (Plate 341). Then an endoligature is introduced through the suture applicator (Plate 342) and guided around the band of adhesions with 5-mm and 3-mm needleholders (Plate 343). After ligation, the adhesion is transected bloodlessly (Plate 344), and then the denuded surface on the myometrium is endocoagulated, as described in chapter 14.2.10. ff.

If serosal defects remain on the separated loop of bowel, they are repaired either with an endosuture and an externally tied slipknot or with an internal surgical knot (see chapters 12.6.2. or 12.6.3.).

The end result of the adhesiolysis illustrated in Plates 340–344 is shown in Plate 345.

If postoperative adhesions involve epiploic appendices of loops of bowel or omental bridges, as seen in Plate 346 (about 5 years after a total abdominal hysterectomy in a 43-year-old patient with symptoms of partial intestinal obstruction), they will have to be ligated. As is also customary during a laparotomy, they are doubly ligated according to the technique described in chapter 12.6.2. and then transected without bleeding. At first, the highly vascular bridge of adhesions between a loop of jejunum and the sigmoid colon is clearly demonstrated between two atraumatic grasping tongs, as shown in Plate 346. This internal herniation of about 6–8 cm in diameter, which resulted from a total abdominal hysterectomy, was responsible for the partial intestinal obstruction with cramp-like pain. After introduction of an endoligature, the 5-mm needleholder accepts the suture material and guides it around the adhesion (Plate 347). After it has been returned to the 3-mm needleholder (Plate 348) the suture is retracted and a slipknot is tied externally and then reintroduced to close the ligature. The long end of the first ligature is cut (Plate 349) and then a second ligature is applied (Plate 350). The doubly ligated strand of adhesions is kept under tension (Plate 351) and transected (Plate 352). If necessary, the two tissue stumps (Plate 353) can each be secured with an endoloop.

The 43-year-old patient whose case was just illustrated left the hospital 4 days postoperatively and was completely free of symptoms.

A 67-year-old patient with a past history of a right salpingectomy because of tubal pregnancy and simultaneous appendectomy complained of chronic mid and lower abdominal pain. Before the ovarian cyst (Plate 354) was removed, the adhesions between the cecum and the right uterine horn were lysed. An endosuture was placed around the intestinal adhesion (Plate 355), which was then ligated and dissected. The broad peritoneal defect was closed with a few endoloops after the peritoneum had been grasped and reapproximated with the spikes in the biopsy forceps (Plate 356). If this maneuver should fail because of too much tension, the peritoneum is reapproximated with endosutures. The anatomical appearance after intestinal adhesiolysis on the right side and salpingo-oophorectomy on the left side and subsequent irrigation of the pelvis is shown in Plate 357.

We also extended our endoscopic intervention to symptoms caused by postoperative adhesions from operations on the gallbladder and to cases of previous hepatitis with perihepatic adhesions. Endoscopic correction is particularly indicated for postcholecystectomy adhesions. These adhesions, usually between omentum and parietal peritoneum and caused by postoperative drains, are easily ligated and severed without blood loss. To do this, the endoscope is first introduced in the usual manner through the umbilicus to determine the location and extent of the adhesions. Depending on the endoscopic surgical manipulations necessary, the puncture sites for the second and third 5-mm trocars are then selected. Usually, these sites are in the mid-abdominal region (see chapter 15.3.2.).

Most commonly adhesions are found postoperatively after appendectomy (Plate 358). In such cases, the lower pole of the cecum is attached to the peritoneal wound. This can usually be corrected without difficulty. However, only the hook scissors should be used to cut such adhesions. Since the underlying cecum is frequently adherent with a broad base to the parietal peritoneum immediately adjacent to the omental region, it is kept under tension (see Fig 172, steps 1–3) before the grasped tissue is cut, to be absolutely certain that bowel is not injured. In this region, any hemostatic measure using destructive heat, even with the carefully placed crocodile forceps, can only be justified if it is absolutely certain that coagulation does not occur too close to bowel. Squirting hemorrhages in the area are not dangerous and can always be ligated with an endoloop. One should always remember the basic rule: *Prophylactic hemostasis is less time-consuming than the control of hemorrhage!* Even in the area of an appendix scar, it is worthwhile to first apply an endoligature and tie the slipknot externally.

If large areas of the omentum have to be dissected off the parietal peritoneum, it will be necessary to coagulate the large wound area to prevent adhesions. Coagulation should be done with the myoma enucleator, by moving it as one would a steam iron across the bloody tissue (i.e., peritoneal defects). Another recommendation for postoperative adhesion prophylaxis is the instillation into the abdominal cavity of high doses of cortisone—500 mg in 100–200 ml of physiologic saline solution. We have successfully used this routine for 12 years, and we continue the high-dose cortisone regimen for adhesion prophylaxis with oral doses of cortisone for another 3 days postoperatively. For dosages, refer to chapter 17.2.

15.3. ENDOSCOPIC APPENDECTOMY

In the past, few intra-abdominal endoscopic operations were performed because the hemorrhages that sometimes occur during such procedures could not be controlled. Now that classic methods of hemostasis by suture and ligature have been introduced into endoscopic abdominal surgery, it is possible to perform other procedures that expand endoscopy beyond simple adhesiolysis. For the microsurgeon who is skilled in operating under the microscope, the classic appendectomy technique (MacBurney and Sprengel) with inversion of the stump by purse string suture and additional Z-suture does not pose any particular technical difficulties (Grewe and Krämer, 1977).

At present, it may appear presumptuous to perform an endoscopic appendectomy because of the counterargument: Why do it endoscopically with four punctures when the same can be done by a laparotomy with a single small gridiron incision and a small set of instruments.

The arguments for an endoscopic appendectomy, viz., (1) minimal physical stress to the patient, comparable to that of tubal sterilization, (2) the procedure is almost microsurgical (i.e., exact dissection and resection of the appendix are possible), and (3) the absence of postoperative adhesions, have not yet been accepted.

However, if during a pelviscopy one detects that the vermiform appendix is adherent to the adnexal area, this may be an indication to remove the appendix during the same operation. In an evaluation for sterility, for instance, one might find that the vermiform appendix has become adherent to the ovary subsequent to an inflammation (Plate

359) or subsequent to sterilization by Madlener's technique (1919; Plate 360); the adhesions, without doubt, resulted from chronic inflammation in the adnexal area. The advantages of endoscopic appendectomy in this setting are far-reaching:

- The hospitalization time is not prolonged by the endoscopic appendectomy.
- Because of the almost microsurgical technique of removing the appendix, to date we have not observed any postoperative adhesions.
- After 1 week at most, the patient is completely free of discomfort (i.e., able to work).

It should again be stated, in this manual of specific operations, that there are no particular difficulties for a surgeon skilled in microsurgery to remove the appendix endoscopically. It remains to be seen whether or not this technical possibility will become a clinical reality in the future.

15.3.1. Indications, Requirements, and Selection of Patients for Endoscopic Appendectomy

To date, the decision to perform an endoscopic appendectomy has not been necessitated by an acute indication from the field of general surgery but is based on pelviscopic findings, usually in connection with the evaluation of sterility. In the search for a cause for sterility, the appendix may be one such disturbing factor or the cause of the symptoms of which the patient had complained. In the past it was necessary to prepare the patient for a classic appendectomy to be performed at another time to correct the pathologic findings. Today, this procedure can be performed immediately after the diagnostic pelviscopy.

For reasons mentioned above, the following *catalog of indications* is proposed.

- A. Therapeutic appendectomy:
  Sterility patients with adhesions between the appendix and adnexa after a previous laparotomy
  "Long" appendix hanging into the pelvis
  Appendix with extragenital endometriosis
  Subacute and/or chronic appendicitis
  Appendicitis suspected
  Appendicitis discovered incidentally to a pelviscopy or laparoscopy for other indications
- B. Prophylactic appendectomy:
  Appendix with "family disposition"
  Chronic complaints of pain in the right

adnexal area in the absence of pelviscopic findings or anatomical evidence

Requirements for endoscopic appendectomy are:

1. Skills to perform an appendectomy by laparotomy.
2. Appropriate level of training of the endoscopic surgeon, particularly in regard to microsurgical techniques.
3. Ability to transform monocular endoscopic observations into stereoscopic mental images and dexterity in endoscopic suturing and intra-abdominal tying techniques.
4. Appendix located such that it is accessible to the techniques described below.
5. A signed consent form after the patient has been appropriately counseled and prepared for this procedure (see also chapter 3).

15.3.2. Technique of Orthograde Appendectomy

The technique of endoscopic appendectomy follows the same operative steps as the classic procedure, for example, that of MacBurney and Sprengel. Natural catgut and synthetic suture material (Ethicon PDS sutures, which are absorbed slowly over a 7-month period) are tied partially externally and partially intra-abdominally, allowing exact surgical techniques to be used without the risk of postoperative complications. The possibility of performing the operative steps described in the following section under low-power magnification with a loupe permits the surgeon for the first time to remove the vermiform appendix extremely accurately and meticulously.

Due to the almost microsurgical correction of serosal defects, postoperative adhesions are almost completely preventable. The peritoneal suture which, in a laparotomy, is usually directly adjacent to the cecal wound is not present.

Therefore, even from theoretical considerations, there is no possibility for postoperative adhesions to form. This has been confirmed by practical observations which have been documented photographically at the time of numerous repeat pelviscopies.

The trocar for the endoscope is introduced in the lower margin of the umbilicus using the usual Z-puncture technique as in a regular pelviscopy (Fig 346, *1*). The second puncture for the 5-mm

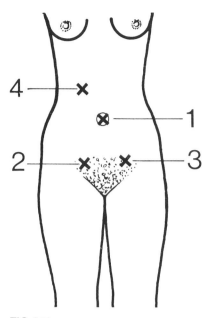

FIG 346.
Puncture sites for orthograde appendectomy.

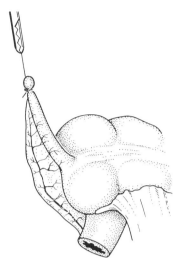

FIG 347.
Endoloop applied to the tip of the appendix for safe manipulation.

trocar sleeve is made in the right suprapubic area (Fig 346, 2). An 11-mm trocar sleeve is introduced in the left suprapubic area (Fig 346, 3) for the extraction of the appendix later on, and a fourth puncture for a 5-mm trocar sleeve is made in the right upper abdomen approximately one handbreadth below the costal margin (Fig 346, 4). In most cases, the appendectomy is preceded by a classic diagnostic pelviscopy with the umbilical puncture for the endoscope and two suprapubic punctures for 5-mm tocar sleeves. If the decision is made to perform an appendectomy, the trocar sleeve in the left pubic area is dilated from 5 mm to 11 mm diameter according to the technique described in chapter 12.8.8., and an additional 5-mm trocar sleeve is placed in the right upper abdomen.

First, the appendix extractor with an atraumatic grasping forceps is introduced through the 11-mm trocar sleeve in the left pubic area. The appendix is elevated from the pelvic cavity (Plate 361), then the tip of the appendix is grasped for the application of an endoloop which was introduced through the right trocar sleeve (Fig 347 and Plate 362). After this guide suture has been trimmed to about 4 cm (Plate 363), the appendix is kept under tension with a needleholder introduced through the appendix extractor. The appendix can be moved with this guide suture without the risk of accidental trauma. If the appendix were

grasped with a grasping instrument that could slip off, there would be the risk of accidentally opening the lumen of the appendix.

After sharp dissection of lateral adhesions (Plate 364), the appendiceal artery is identified by applying tension to the mesenteriolum with an atraumatic forceps. An endosuture (see also chapter 12.6.3.) is introduced through the 5-mm trocar sleeve on the right upper abdomen (see Fig 346); then the needle is advanced through the base of the mesenteriolum (Plate 365 and Fig 348) at an avascular point so that the artery can then be ligated after an external slipknot has been tied (Plate 366). Viewing this procedure under low-power magnification with a loupe allows the surgeon to ligate the appendiceal vessels quite accurately. The slipknot is pushed into the abdomen under endoscopic view. Use of an atraumatic grasping forceps may help avoid curling of the suture or the simultaneous ligature of an epiploic appendix, etc. After the mesenteriolum has been securely ligated, firm traction on the guide suture will keep the appendix under tension so that the mesenteriolum can be unfolded with an atraumatic grasping forceps and the appendix can be skeletonized (Fig 349) with hook scissors to the level of the tinea libera (Plate 367).

If the vascular tree is ligated properly, this can be done almost without loss of blood. The resected fatty tissue can be left alone, or, if it should get in the way, it can be cut off and removed through the 5-mm trocar sleeve.

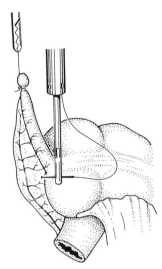

FIG 348.
Needle is advanced through base of mesenteriolum; artery is ligated.

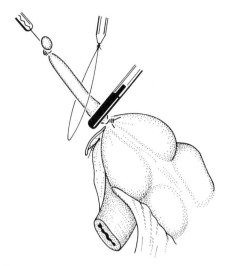

FIG 350.
The appendix is crushed to displace any fecal matter.

After the guide suture has been released, an endoloop is placed around the appendix (Plate 368) and tied directly at the base of the appendix at the level of the tinea libera (Fig 350). The crocodile forceps (see chapter 12.8.9.) crushes the appendix just distally to this ligature (Plate 369) to displace any fecal matter (see Fig 350). After the crocodile forceps has been heated for 20–30 seconds at 90° C—which will almost sterilize the intended site of

transection—the appendix is released again and a second endoloop (see Fig 350) is placed around it (Plate 370) and tied distally to the crocodile forceps (Fig 351). After the crocodile forceps has been removed (see Fig 351) the guide suture is kept under tension and the appendix is sharply transected (Fig 352) between the two ligatures (Plate 371). Shortly before, the appendix extractor was advanced forward and the appendix was pulled halfway into the extractor tube. Then the amputated appendix disappears completely in the extrac-

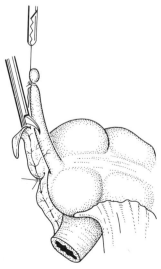

FIG 349.
Appendix is skeletonized to level of the tinea libera.

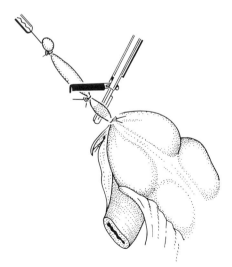

FIG 351.
A second endoloop is placed and tied.

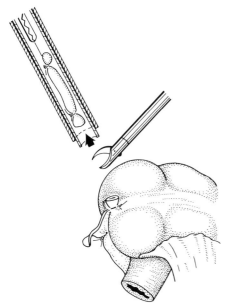

FIG 352.
Appendix is transected between the two ligatures and pulled into the extractor tube.

tor tube (see Fig 352). Any contact between the ligated stump and other tissues is avoided. The appendix is removed from the abdomen completely inside the appendix extractor (see chapters 12.8.11. and 15.4.) without contaminating anything. For reasons of sterility, the scissors used for the transection and the extractor tube are not used for the remainder of the operation.

An applicator with iodine (Fig 353) is intro-

duced into the abdomen through a new appendix extractor sleeve and, for safety's sake, the remaining appendiceal stump is again treated with iodine (Plate 372). The suture (PDS 4–0) with needle for the purse string ligature are introduced through the trocar sleeve in the right upper abdomen (see Fig 346, *4*) and the 5-mm needleholder is introduced through the right suprapubic trocar sleeve (see Fig 346, *2*). The suture is put in the cecal wall in the classic purse string manner (Plate 373), surrounding the appendiceal stump (Fig 354), and a surgeon's knot is tied internally (Fig 355), as previously shown (see chapter 12.6.3. and Fig 146). The plastic push-rod (Plate 374) left over from the endosuture previously used for ligating the mesenteriolum is introduced through the appendix extractor to invaginate the appendiceal stump (Fig 356). The purse string suture is closed by pulling on both ends of the tied PDS suture. Two more surgical knots will secure this suture.

The conical tip of a plastic push-rod of the endosuture or endoloop is suited best for the invagination. When the purse string suture is tied, the conical configuration of the plastic push-rod allows it to escape automatically from the loop; this facilitates the invagination.

To secure the purse string suture, a Z-suture of PDS material is placed in the same manner (Fig 357) and tied. The stitches for the Z-figure (Plate 375) can be placed much better under close observation through the endoscope than is possible under macroscopic conditions when the appendix is removed through a small abdominal incision. This Z-suture is again secured with two more surgical knots (Plate 376).

If any serosal defects remain after this manip-

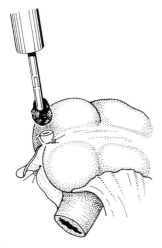

FIG 353.
Appendiceal stump is treated with iodine.

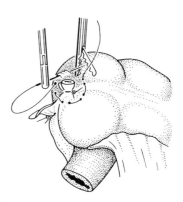

FIG 354.
Purse string suture placed around the appendiceal stump.

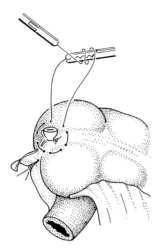

FIG 355.
Surgeon's knot tied internally.

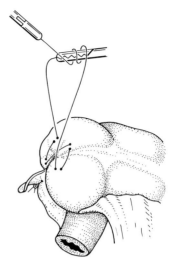

FIG 357.
Z-suture of PDS secures the purse string suture.

ulation, as is sometimes the case in the area of the lateral parietal peritoneum, or if there is excessive mesenteric fatty tissue, the wound is closed either by endosuture and externally tied slipknots, or the defect is carefully secured with another endoloop (Fig 358). This will prevent any possibility of adhesion formation in the future. Then the operative field is thoroughly irrigated using the Aquapurator and physiologic saline solution warmed to 37° C (see chapter 12.4.ff.).

The suture area is again inspected for complete hemostasis (Plate 377). The liver, gallbladder, and the pelvic cavity (uterus, tubes, ovaries) are reviewed, and the operation is terminated by

removing the trocar sleeves under direct vision with the endoscope. After deflation of the gas and removal of the trocar sleeve for the endoscope, the four puncture wounds are closed with skin clips (see chapter 12.8.13. and Figs 196–199).

15.3.3. Technique of Retrograde Appendectomy

The possibility of evaluating the anatomical status of the appendix under low-power magnification also permits clean dissection of the appendix from retrocecal adhesions. This procedure is often difficult under macroscopic conditions through a small abdominal incision, but the true anatomical relationships are easily revealed when the abdomen is

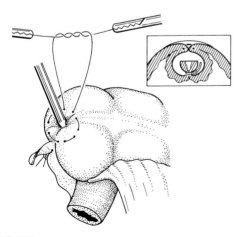

FIG 356.
Appendiceal stump invaginated; purse string suture closed.

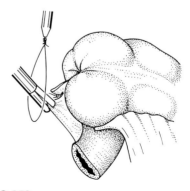

FIG 358.
Serosal defect secured with another endoloop.

insufflated and allows the surgeon a clear overview through the endoscope.

In contrast to the dissection of a retrograde, inverted appendix through a gridiron incision, endoscopic dissection of such an appendix poses no surgical problem. After the peritoneum is incised, the appendix can usually be extracted very easily and its end can be tagged with an endoloop (see Fig 347). The remainder of the procedure is identical with the technique illustrated in Figures 348–358.

When such a condition is encountered for the first time, one should always remember that the patient has been informed of the possibility of a laparotomy and prepared for it. If there is any indication that the procedure may not succeed, the operation can be continued by laparotomy at any time.

In this context, the work of de Kok should be recalled. As early as 1977 de Kok had recommended a combination of laparoscopy and transabdominal appendectomy to improve both access to the appendix as well as the surgical technique. It is assumed that the appendix can be dissected more easily from a confusing situation through a small gridiron incision if its anatomical relationships have first been carefully evaluated.

Today, in the era of intra-abdominal endoscopic suturing and tying, the transabdominal gridiron incision is no longer necessary. The appendix may be operated on under more ideal visual conditions than a minilaparotomy can offer.

The broad-based serosal defects that result from dissection of the appendix from a retrocecal position can be better closed with endosuture under endoscopic conditions. To save time, it is recommended that the surgeon close such serosal defects with individual endosutures and tie the slipknots externally, because more time is needed for tying endosutures internally. Whereas retractors are always necessary for a laparotomy, none are used with endoscopy; consequently, reapproximation of peritoneal wound edges does not cause any problems.

15.4. INSTRUMENTS FOR ENDOSCOPIC APPENDECTOMY

Although the instruments for endoscopic operations were detailed in chapter 12.8., those necessary for an appendectomy should again be re-

viewed, because it is absolutely essential that all of them be available to perform an endoscopic appendectomy.

An appendectomy can be accomplished with a 7-mm endoscope. However, for the beginner, it is essential that a good 10.5-mm endoscope is used, for instance a Hopkins endoscope with a two- to four-power loupe attached (see Fig 51 and chapter 12.2.4.). Additional requirements are electronic monitoring of the pneumoperitoneum (refer to chapter 12.3. ff.) and an endocoagulation apparatus (refer to chapter 12.5.6.1.).

Whether or not sterilization with the crocodile forceps is absolutely necessary will have to be determined by practical application. In any case, a compression device must be available to remove feces from the segment of the appendix that remains between the two ligatures.

An *instrument set for appendectomy* (Fig 359) must be selected from the set of instruments identified in chapter 12.8.ff.

1. Atraumatic grasping tongs
2. 5-mm and 11-mm trocars and sleeves with trumpet valves
3. Crocodile forceps
4. Endoloops
5. Endosutures
6. Hook scissors
7. Double-toothed biopsy forceps
8. Appendix extractors
9. Ethicon PDS (polydioxanon-4) suture (reabsorption time, 6–7 months) for purse string suture and Z-suture
10. 3-mm and 5-mm needleholders
11. Suture applicators

In conclusion, it should be mentioned that the technique described for endoscopic removal of the appendix follows the classic technique, with skeletonizing, invagination, purse string and Z-sutures, and a combination of external and internal knot tying; it allows the highest technical perfection of an appendectomy incorporating the best safety factors. On the other hand, an appendectomy without Z-suture has been accepted in general surgery, and techniques without invagination, i.e., purse string suture, are being discussed. Even the appendectomy using simple clamping, such as a tantalum clip (Weck clip), has been reported in the literature.

There is no doubt that such techniques would reduce the endoscopic appendectomy to a simple

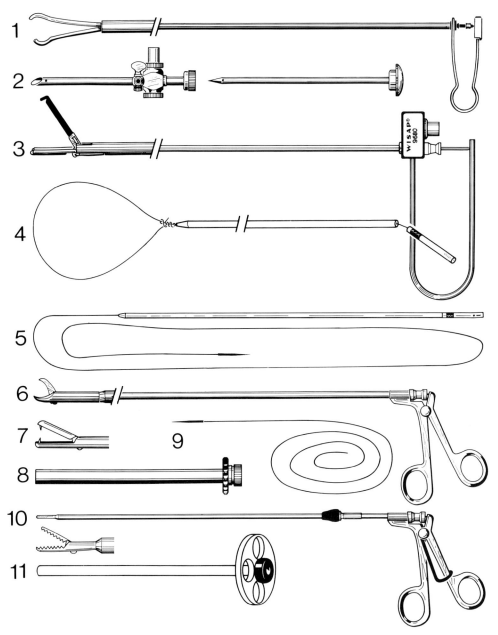

FIG 359.
Instrument set for appendectomy. See text.

endoscopic surgical procedure. The simple application of an endoloop that includes both the appendix and the mesenteriolum would correspond to the technique of performing an appendectomy by ligature only, but without further inversion of the stump, which is being discussed in general surgery. However, it is not the prerogative of a gynecologist to recommend new appendectomy techniques solely because they would simplify the endoscopic procedure.

It was my goal to develop the presently most respected and technically most perfect technique of appendiceal amputation into a routine endoscopic procedure, although this procedure is the most difficult one to be performed with the endoscope. Colleagues in classic general surgery, after gathering sufficient experience, may determine whether or not a simplification of the appendectomy technique is possible without trauma to the abdomen, i.e., the gridiron incision.

15.5. BIOPSY OF PERITONEAL METASTASES

If metastases of a malignant tumor of the abdominal cavity are present or suspected (e.g., ovarian, gastric, or intestinal carcinoma), pelviscopy is indicated. To confirm the diagnosis histologically, a tissue specimen for microscopic evaluation is obtained with biopsy forceps from a suspicious area (Plate 378).

It is of particular value to obtain this biopsy specimen at the time of a routine second-look pelviscopy to monitor the therapeutic response after 6 months of cytostatic chemotherapy. Histology often shows regression of metastases (Plate 379), so-called ghost cells, and is important to determine whether chemotherapy should be continued or whether operative measures are indicated.

15.6. LIVER BIOPSY

Liver biopsy is performed in internal medicine either blindly (blind biopsy) or by laparoscopy. In-dications for liver biopsy have been extensively discussed. During an operative laparoscopy, it is no problem to biopsy specific areas of the liver—under direct vision—for further evaluation of liver disease. Guided by the endoscope introduced in the umbilical area, a Menghini needle is used to obtain a cylinder of tissue from a specific area of the liver (Plate 380). Hemostasis is accomplished in approximately 20 seconds with the point coagulator (Plates 381 and 382).

15.7. LYSIS OF PERIHEPATIC ADHESIONS

Adhesions between liver and the diaphragmatic peritoneum (Plate 383), often quite extensive, develop after hepatitis, either postoperatively or due to other etiology [or after pelvic inflammatory processes due to gonorrhea, chlamydia, etc.—*Ed.*]. These strings of connective tissue are usually avascular and can simply be cut with scissors. If a strand is very thick and vascular, it is first coagulated with crocodile forceps (Plate 384) before it is severed with hook scissors (Plate 385).

This operation is often done in addition to other procedures in the abdomen and relieves the patient of nonspecific mid or upper abdominal or even lower abdominal pain that may have been present for years.

16

Transition From Endoscopy to Laparotomy in the Same Operation

As was discussed in detail in chapters 3 and 5, all patients who undergo endoscopic operative abdominal procedures have been prepared for a laparotomy. One can never predict whether the diagnosis, which is based on palpation, ultrasound, or history, will in fact correspond to the visual findings, that is, whether the presumed diagnosis can be confirmed endoscopically, or if the necessary operative procedure can actually be performed endoscopically. Whether or not transition to a laparotomy is necessary will therefore depend on a variety of indications and conditions.

16.1. TRANSITION FROM ENDOSCOPY TO LAPAROTOMY IN THE SAME OPERATION: AS A PLANNED PROCEDURE

In many cases it is very likely, on the basis of the preoperative findings on palpation or x-ray, ultrasound, or other examinations, that the endoscopic evaluation will be followed by a laparotomy. This, for instance, will be the case if an ovarian carcinoma is suspected, if the differential diagnosis is between myomatous uterus and an ovarian tumor and the latter is confirmed, and so forth. In such cases, the diagnostic procedure is done first to confirm the diagnosis and indication for laparotomy. The endoscopic preoperative diagnostic evaluation can also serve to determine whether the gynecologic operation should be performed by the transabdominal or vaginal route. The abdominal scan

will orient the vaginal surgeon and allow him to ascertain that no adhesions are present which would increase the risk of the vaginal operation. If such adhesions are present, they may be dissected by a more or less extensive adhesiolysis (see chapter 14.2.2.1. and Plates 17–40 and 341–358). Then the vaginal operation can be performed without complications. It should be mentioned again that preliminary ligation and transection of the infundibulopelvic ligaments prior to a vaginal hysterectomy with salpingo-oophorectomy may be very helpful (see chapter 14.2.8.1.).

16.2. TRANSITION FROM ENDOSCOPY TO LAPAROTOMY IN THE SAME OPERATION: AS AN OPTION PREVIOUSLY CONSIDERED

In many cases it may appear likely from preliminary evaluations that the procedure can be accomplished by endoscopy. However, it may become clear during the primary inspection or secondarily after the endoscopic surgical manipulation has begun, that the procedure, according to usual and customary classic surgical routines, must be continued by laparotomy. Since the patient has been informed about and consented to a laparotomy and has been physically prepared in the operating room, everything is ready for a laparotomy, and such borderline situations can be managed easily.

It is not in the patient's best interest to minimize surgical intervention by performing the operation with the endoscope if, for technical reasons, the endoscopic procedure would increase the risk. Technical reasons include:

• Inadequate visibility
• The organ cannot be identified with 100% certainty
• Lack or failure of technical prerequisites (e.g., light source, OP-PNEU Electronic, instruments, etc.)

The wide spectrum of endoscopic operations that can already be performed without complications and with a low risk should not be discredited by overzealous surgeons who try to utilize endoscopy in extreme cases; this often leads to negative results. Whereas in the 1960s an abdomen after a previous laparotomy was considered a contraindication to diagnostic laparoscopy, the technical requirements available today make it possible to expand the former, restricted catalog of operations.

The number of pathologic conditions that are presently amenable to endoscopic intra-abdominal surgery is large, and procedures should be confined to those that can be performed under good technical control. In contrast to diagnostic laparoscopy, the transition from endoscopic abdominal surgery to a laparotomy is no major catastrophe but rather the logical response of a prudent surgeon to a specific diagnosis or situation.

16.3. TRANSITION FROM ENDOSCOPY TO LAPAROTOMY IN THE SAME OPERATION: AS "EMERGENCY LAPAROTOMY"

During an endoscopic procedure as well as during a laparotomy, an emergency situation can arise completely unexpectedly—usually precipitated by a major hemorrhage. The possibilities of a sudden drop in blood pressure, cardiac arrest, and so forth were discussed in chapter 10 and chapter 14.1.3. ff. It should again be emphasized that primary injuries to blood vessels which are caused by instruments rarely bleed acutely and freely into the abdominal cavity. Blood from the injured vessels infiltrates the retroperitoneal space (see Figs 247 and 248), so that the surgeon will frequently misjudge the volume of blood loss. This also applies to the situation in which, for instance, the tip of the trocar has injured one of the large retroperitoneal abdominal blood vessels and the rapidly growing retroperitoneal hematoma is initially obscured by bowel (see chapter 14.1.3.5.).

As a ground rule, one must resort to classic surgical techniques whenever complications occur either from massive hemorrhages or from confusing anatomical situations in the intestinal tract. No time must be wasted in the transition from a diagnostic or operative endoscopy to a laparotomy!

The abdomen is opened *without* any further loss of time (no additional disinfection, scrubbing of hands, etc.) through a longitudinal incision in the linea alba (never through a Pfannenstiel transverse incision). The set of vascular clamps (see chapter 12.8.12.) must be ready for use.

First the mainstem vessels are generously clamped with special vascular clamps—not the usual clamps from the set of gynecologic surgical instruments. A desperately life-threatening condition can be prevented by proceeding quickly and deliberately. Thanks to modern medical techniques, even a cardiac arrest is reversible, provided that the patient has not completely exsanguinated. The reader is again referred to the case described in chapter 12.8.12., e.g., the patent omphalomesenteric duct.

After the hemorrhage has been controlled with clamps, a vascular surgeon can be consulted and the vessels can be repaired calmly and without haste.

In all cases of death due to exsanguination which I have had to evaluate as an expert consultant, the life-threatening complication developed secondarily, for one of the following reasons:

1. The misdiagnosis of "anesthesia incident" was made without any effort to search for another reason, such as hemorrhage.
2. Considerable time was wasted between the onset of the complication and the laparotomy.
3. The abdominal cavity was opened through a transverse rather than a longitudinal incision.
4. Excessive preparation of the operative team (scrubbing, etc.).
5. Failure to observe the patient postoperatively for 24 hours in the intensive care unit.

Such emergency situations that arise during the endoscopic procedure do so most frequently after acute hemorrhage and must be managed by immediate laparotomy.

Unrecognized intestinal and ureteral injuries, however, which constitute the second most common complications, become an indication for "emergency laparotomy" only after a few days. Since they are directly related to the endoscopic surgical intervention, they should also be discussed here.

Even during a laparotomy, accidental injury to a loop of bowel cannot always be prevented. As an example, injuries to the rectal ampulla during an operation for retrocervical endometriosis should be mentioned.

As a rule, after endoscopic surgical abdominal procedures, the patient should be free of discomfort within 48 hours. If any abdominal complaints, leukocytosis, fever, or possibly a drop in hemoglobin and hematocrit should be present at that time, it is very likely that the endoscopic procedure was not a full success and a laparotomy will be necessary. If there is any doubt, a repeat pelviscopy is absolutely necessary to evaluate whether or not further conservatism and observation can be justified.

Since the patient has previously been advised of such a possibility, one should never hesitate too long before resorting to such procedure. In our series of 10,000 laparoscopies, our annual laparotomy rate fluctuates between 2% and 3%.

If a perforated bowel is not repaired within 48 hours and peritonitis has developed, it usually cannot be controlled and may lead to the patient's death.

Many postoperative worries and concerns, particularly after extensive postoperative adhesiolysis, can be avoided by appropriate preoperative diagnostic measures, as demonstrated in the following example.

A 43-year-old patient who had had four previous laparotomies underwent extensive pelviscopic lysis of adhesions between the omentum and the intestinal tract. Two days postoperatively a partial intestinal obstruction developed with leukocytosis and fever, precipitated by an acute cholelithiasis and a gallbladder filled with stones. Cholelithiasis had not been diagnosed preoperatively and the stones had not been noticed on the obstructive series of radiographs because they were obscured by distended loops of bowel. If we had done an emergency laparotomy to search for a bowel perforation, it probably would not have been detrimental to the patient but also would not have cured her. The repeat pelviscopy performed on the third postoperative day helped to determine the course of further therapy.

We have learned from this case to evaluate carefully the liver and gallbladder before every endoscopic operative procedure for the indication of "postoperative adhesiolysis," so as not to misinterpret the etiology of postoperative abdominal symptoms in a patient with an underlying cholelithiasis.

Finally, this may indicate that a laparotomy is not always the solution of a problem, but that an exact indication must be present.

However, one should principally follow the classic rule in surgery, to perform a laparotomy once too often rather than not often enough. The recent introduction of endoscopic intra-abdominal procedures has not changed this rule.

If postoperative bleeding is suspected, a repeat pelviscopy should be performed without delay. After blood has been aspirated, the source of the hemorrhage usually can be recognized and controlled by one of the endoligature methods described in chapter 12.6. If this is technically not possible, a laparotomy through a longitudinal midline incision should be done without delay. This must be the primary incision if the hemorrhage has progressed too far; any delay by performing an exploratory pelviscopy first would be irresponsible.

17 _____ Postoperative Care After Endoscopic Abdominal Surgery

Miniaturizing the operative procedure in regard to the physical stress to the patient should not lead to the impression that the intra-abdominal operative measures are also miniaturized. The defects that occur in the peritoneum are the same as those that occur after a laparotomy. This also applies to omental adhesiolysis or resection. The elimination of most of the postoperative complaints which are usually caused by incisional pain in the abdominal wall should not distract from the fact that extensive healing processes take place intra-abdominally. How huge a biologic effort the organism has to make will occasionally become evident when a repeat pelviscopy has to be performed to rule out hemorrhage, etc. (refer also to chapter 16.3.).

> EXAMPLE.—Four days after a cesarean section, a 31-year-old patient developed a paralytic ileus that had to be investigated by diagnostic pelviscopy. After extensive adhesiolysis in the area of the intestinal tract, which was relatively easily accomplished because the adhesions between loops of bowel were only moderately developed, copious quantities of vernix caseosa were found to be diffusely dispersed as high as the diaphragm. An intestinal lesion could be ruled out. The entire peritoneum showed an inflammatory reaction caused by the vernix caseosa.

Although the patient may not seem to experience any discomfort, intra-abdominal healing processes take place, indicating that a patient who has just undergone an endoscopic operation will require essentially the same postoperative care as is necessary after a laparotomy.

17.1 POSTOPERATIVE CARE AFTER DIAGNOSTIC LAPAROSCOPY

In principle, a diagnostic laparoscopy may be performed under local anesthesia, as has been shown in internal medicine. However, if a diagnostic laparoscopic evaluation is done in the midabdomen and the pelvis, possibly to determine whether or not a subsequent endoscopic abdominal operative intervention is indicated, a second and third puncture are necessary to allow extensive manipulation between bowels, omentum, uterus, adnexa, and so forth, so that the exact diagnosis can be made visually. Since the peritoneum is always very sensitive, even diagnostic laparoscopy in gynecology and general surgery requires intubation anesthesia.

Only small, limited operative procedures such as tubal sterilization (see chapter 14.2.15. ff.) can be performed under local anesthesia, provided that it is highly unlikely that further corrective operative measures in the abdomen will be required.

[The above statements may apply if only local anesthetic agents are used. However, as discussed

228

more extensively in chapters 10.1.1. and 10.1.2., if the local anesthetic is augmented by vocal and neuroleptanalgesia, that is, if "volonelgesia" is utilized instead of plain local anesthesia, even more extensive operations such as extensive adhesiolysis, including partial omentectomy, ovarian and parovarian cystectomy, and removal of lost IUD's may be performed. The experience of thousands of operations under "volonelgesia"—some of them requiring several hours—has taught us that the abdominal viscera are not very sensitive to pain stimuli, provided they are handled gently and slowly but deliberately. The use of local or topical anesthetics on the more sensitive organs in the pelvis (ovaries, tubes, uterosacral ligaments) may be helpful.

If the diagnostic endoscopic evaluation is done to determine the source of chronic abdominal or pelvic pain, this may require the patient's active collaboration in identifying the painful area during surgery; it is optimally done under "volonelgesia" with general anesthesia standby to permit the immediate transition to more extensive operative endoscopic measures or a laparotomy (refer also to chapters 10.2.1. and 10.2.2. and chapters 16.–16.3.).—*Ed.*]

The postoperative care after purely diagnostic laparoscopic procedures for the purposes discussed in this book (see chapter 2) is, therefore, primarily determined by those measures required for the patient's complete recovery from the anesthetic procedure.

The purely physical stress to the patient from one to three puncture sites is usually within tolerable limits for pain and discomfort. As far as incisional care is concerned (see chapter 12.8.13.), no further special care is necessary.

As far as the patient's general condition after abdominal endoscopic operations and postanesthetic care are concerned, no additional nursing care is required. After recovery from anesthetic medications, the patient may be discharged from the hospital, either on the day of the operation or 1–2 days later, depending on the doctor/patient relationship.

17.2. POSTOPERATIVE CARE AFTER ENDOSCOPIC OPERATIONS FOR GENERAL GYNECOLOGIC INDICATIONS

The postoperative care depends on the extent of the gynecologic operative intervention and the duration

of anesthesia required for it. If the physical stress from the procedure is relatively small, such as for an ovarian biopsy (see chapter 14.2.5.) or a tubal sterilization (see chapter 14.2.15. ff.), ambulatory operative techniques have been well accepted in many places. The patient is advised not to eat or drink for at least 8 hours prior to his or her appointment in the surgical facility, is operated on endoscopically, and is discharged from medical care after the effects of anesthetic agents have worn off. This is possible because the physical stress related to pain in two or three trocar puncture sites is tolerable. Occasionally, inadequate absorption of gases (see chapter 12.3.1.) may cause more intense subphrenic pain (Riedel and Semm, 1981) and may require prolonged hospitalization (see Fig 360).

[We encourage early ambulation, even let the patient walk with assistance from the operating table to the recovery room with reclining chairs; this stimulates and accelerates the metabolism of analgesic drugs, absorption of gases, and so on. Whereas patients as well as their physicians and nurses used to have the tendency to allow the patient to "sleep off" the drug effects—that is, the patient was kept in the same position for several hours—early stimulation and ambulation are, at least in part, responsible for the prevention of adhesions after endoscopic operations.—*Ed.*]

All other gynecologic operations, as mentioned in chapter 14.2. ff., may require a postoperative observation of at least 24 hours, if not longer. There are two reasons:

1. Endoscopic operating techniques with cutting instruments, particularly scissors, create the same type of surgical wounds on intra-abdominal organs as a laparotomy would do. Although these wounds heal more rapidly because intestinal and vascular paralysis do not develop, they may still require the same period of rest and inactivity to heal.

2. Endoscopic surgery is still a new operative procedure and more extensive experiences are still lacking. Overzealous attempts to minimize the postoperative phase in favor of ambulatory operative techniques (outpatient surgery) may, in one respect, be detrimental to the method and, in a different respect, may be construed as a basis for law suits if complications should occur.

If lysis of multiple adhesions was necessary, that is, if large peritoneal wounds were produced,

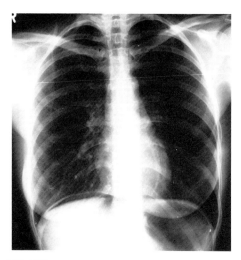

FIG 360.
Subphrenic collection of CO_2 gas postoperatively.

some authorities recommend continuing the intra-operative intra-abdominal treatment with high doses of cortisone (see chapter 14.2.2.1. ff.) by giving decreasing oral doses of cortisone during the following 3 days. Although, as emphasized before, this treatment is purely empirical and not based on any published experimental evidence, we have had good success with the following oral dosage of hydrocortisone preparations:

1. First postoperative day: 50 mg × 4 (i.e., 50 mg q6h)
2. Second postoperative day: 50 mg × 3 (i.e., 50 mg q8h)
3. Third postoperative day: 50 mg × 2 (i.e., 50 mg q12h)

Since, with the exception of intestinal operations, patients after endoscopic operations resume oral food intake on the day of surgery, oral cortisone therapy is no problem.

If the operations were of a purely gynecologic nature (no intestinal adhesiolysis or even appendectomy was performed), the patients may resume oral food intake as soon as anesthetic effects have completely subsided. This will promote intestinal peristalsis and reduce the risk of postoperative adhesion formation. However, since anesthetic effects may persist for some time, the diet should not be too heavy.

After more extensive gynecologic operations, such as salpingo-oophorectomy (see chapter 14.2.7. ff.), myomectomy (see chapter 14.2.10.1.

ff.), or endoscopic termination of an extrauterine pregnancy (see chapter 14.2.11. ff.)—in other words, operations in which the risk of postoperative bleeding is comparable to that after a laparotomy—the patient will remain under close observation for 24 hours, as she would after a laparotomy. One should not be deceived by the absence of postoperative discomfort due to the absence of an abdominal incision and the painful symptoms related to it and, therefore, disregard such strict postoperative supervision. One should share the patient's satisfaction who, in contrast to a patient after a laparotomy, is doing well physically on the evening of the day of surgery, but one should also be aware of the extent of the intra-abdominal procedure and its related risk of postoperative hemorrhage.

Patients who are doing well physically may not want to be disturbed by nurses for monitoring of vital signs and the like, but one should insist on close observation.

Most of the discomfort after intra-abdominal endoscopy with operative intervention is caused by the subphrenic collection of CO_2 gas, which is similar to the discomfort experienced after the use of nitrous oxide gas or oxygen insufflation. In 5%–10% of operations, discomfort may persist for hours or days postoperatively (Riedel and Semm, 1981), although the patient should theoretically be able to absorb 50–100 ml of CO_2 gas per hour. In a few patients, we were able to observe subphrenic collections of CO_2 gas up to 1.5 L in volume (Fig 360) for several days. Some of these patients will complain of unbearable subphrenic pain. Analyses of this gas confirmed without doubt that it was CO_2 gas; this finding refuted the contention that the persistent collection of gas was nitrogen.

A biologic or physical explanation for the prolonged presence in the subphrenic space of an absorbable gas has not yet been found.

For such patients who often complain of severe pain, treatment with effective analgesic drugs is indicated. In our experience, the intensity and duration of pain are not directly proportional to the duration or extent of a procedure.

As already mentioned, the essential advantage of endoscopic abdominal surgery is not a shorter hospitalization time, which, due to peritoneal healing processes, may not differ much from that after a laparotomy. The critical point for the evaluation and appreciation of endoscopic abdominal surgery is the time when patients resume their normal activity. In contrast to laparotomy, resumption of normal activity after endoscopic abdominal surgery usually coincides with the patient's discharge from the hospital.

The fact that in Germany, patients are still granted sick leave for several days is based on long-standing custom rather than need. We can read in the 1980 annual report of the AAGL that the postoperative recovery period after tubal sterilization in the United States was reduced to an average of 2–4 hours.

[In the editor's experience, patients who undergo a laparoscopic tubal sterilization by Hulka clip application under "volonelgesia" usually want to leave the outpatient facility after 20–60 minutes. Refer also to comments above and in chapter 10.1.2. in which it is noted that early ambulation increases the patient's metabolism and promotes faster recovery.—*Ed.*]

17.3. POSTOPERATIVE CARE AFTER AN ENDOSCOPIC OPERATION FOR THE INDICATION: "STERILITY"

Even after the operative correction of tubal pathology by conventional gynecologic abdominal operative techniques, special therapeutic measures are indicated. We distinguish between general postoperative care and the care required when endometriosis is present.

17.3.1. General Postoperative Care

Our 12-year statistics (Fig 361) indicate that the preliminary diagnostic pelviscopy for the evaluation of tubal factors was followed in 80% of cases by operative pelviscopy.

On the one hand, lysis of adhesions was necessary after previous operations; on the other hand, existing tubal pathology could be corrected in the same operation by fimbrioplasty or salpingostomy (see chapter 14.2.4. ff.), coagulation of endometriotic implants, and so on. Since there is always the risk after such procedures that the tubes may recoagulate, our postoperative regimen after operative pelviscopy includes a 5-day course of hydropertubation (Fig 362). A universal pertubation apparatus (see chapter 12.4.2.) is used to instill 20 ml of our hydropertubation solution (Figs 363, 364). The solution to be instilled is prepared freshly from a stock solution that is prepared under sterile conditions, stored in the refrigerator, and shaken before use. It can be stored for approximately 1 week.

For each instillation, 20 ml is removed from the stock solution and 5 ml of it is used to dissolve 5 mg of α-chymotrypsin powder (see Fig 363, step II). This is again mixed with the 15 ml of the stock solution and used as instillation solution. For chromosalpingostomy, 1 ml of methylene blue solution (5%) is also added to the 20 ml of solution to be instilled. This way we combine the visual effect of the blue dye solution, which is necessary for the diagnosis, with a therapeutic one. At the same time, we prevent the problem that diagnostic tubal

12-Year Pelviscopy Statistics 1971–1982 (n = 8,943)

	DIAGNOSTIC PELVISCOPIES	OPERATIVE PELVISCOPIES	TOTAL
1970/71*	192	211	403
1972	173	194	367
1973	196	282	478
1974	247	469	716
1975	236	511	747
1976	168	432	600
1977	241	703	944
1978	315	627	942
1979	362	684	1046
1980	262	706	968
1981	249	611	860
1982	188	684	872
Totals	2829 (31.6%)	6114 (68.4%)	8943 (100%)

*November 1970 to December 1971 (introduction of pelviscopy in Kiel: Nov. 1, 1970).

FIG 361.

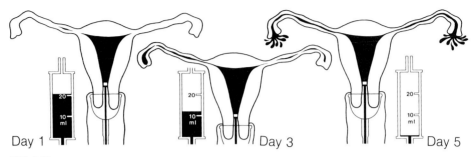

Day 1   Day 3   Day 5

FIG 362.
Hydropertubation therapy after operative pelviscopy.

FIG 363.

Ingredients of Hydropertubation Solution (According to Fikentscher and Semm)

I.		
Hydrocortisone acetate		0.1 gm
Streptomycin sulfate		4.0 gm
Procaine hydrochloride		0.4 gm
Distilled water to		100.0 ml

II. +5 mg α-Chymotrase to each 20 ml of hydropertubation solution I immediately before instillation.

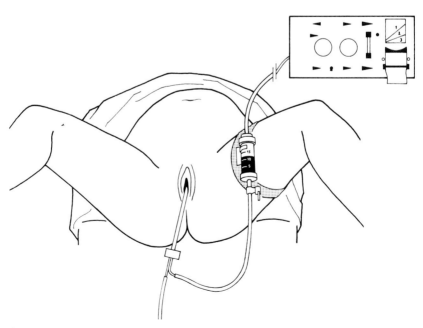

FIG 364.
Postoperative hydropertubation.

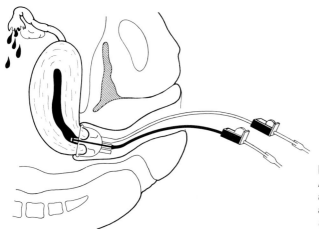

FIG 365.
After instillation of solution, the instillation and suction tubes are clamped and the adapter is left attached to the cervix for 6–8 hours to prevent reflux.

pertubation during pelviscopy with methylene blue solution and physiologic saline solution may initiate an ascending infection.

For postoperative hydropertubation, the patient is positioned on the gynecologic table in the usual manner (see Fig 24) and, depending on the degree of tubal patency (see Fig 270), the solution is instilled at a pressure not exceeding 200 mm Hg. Instillation takes between 30 and 300 seconds.

After the solution has been instilled, the instillation tubes are clamped with roller-type clamps (Fig 365) and the adapter is left attached to the uterine cervix for 6–8 hours to prevent reflux of the instillation solution. During this time the patient remains in bed.

Before the vacuum tube is clamped, the negative pressure is reduced to 0.1 atmosphere (Fig 366) so that no hematoma will develop in the uterine cervix from prolonged exposure to a negative pressure.

For two decades we have repeated these irrigations on a daily basis for 5 days after operative procedures on the tubes. This prolonged hydropertubation has been used in more than 12,000 instillation cases without complications, except for occasional nausea and a moderate number of allergies. The patient is discharged after the fifth prolonged hydropertubation in the evening of the fifth postoperative day.

For the painless instillation of the solution

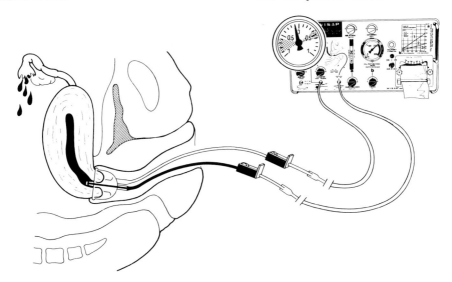

FIG 366.
Negative pressure is reduced to 0.1 atm to prevent the development of a hematoma.

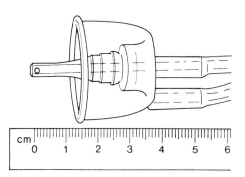

FIG 367.
Cervical adapter.

which remains in the tubes for 6–8 hours, the following *instruments* were developed by WISAP:

A cervical adapter (Fikentscher and Semm, 1959; Fig 367) made of crystal-clear synthetic material is used for atraumatic occlusion of the cervix for gas insufflation, hysterosalpingography, and particularly hydropertubation. A negative pressure is produced by the universal pertubation apparatus (see Fig 92) or manually by a hand pump, as shown in Figure 368; the cervical adapter with its flexible tubes is sucked onto the cervix and then the hydropertubation solution is slowly instilled with controlled pressure monitored by the universal pertubation apparatus. The injection time and the injection pressure indicate at the same time the degree of tubal patency or its improvement.

The duckbill speculum (Semm; Fig 369) is used for the painless application of the cervical adapter. This speculum, which consists of three parts, has a hinge at the level of the vulva so that opening of the speculum is not painful, which usually is the case if the hinges are outside the vulva. This speculum makes it possible to place the cervical adapters, sizes A and B, on the cervix without causing pain.

To introduce the cervical adapter (Fig 370), it is grasped with the adapter forceps and introduced through the duckbill speculum to be attached to the uterine cervix. The roller-type clamps on the tubes prevent reflux of pertubation fluid and, at the same time, maintain the vacuum to keep the cervical adapter attached to the cervix.

In cases of secondary sterility, the cervix is frequently disfigured by previous childbirth (e.g., Emmet's laceration). Since in such cases the cervical adapter may not remain attached to the cervix, a double-balloon catheter (Fig 371) (Fikentscher and Semm, 1955) is atraumatically introduced into the cervical canal and fixed in its position with tenaculum forceps.

The double-balloon catheter is also suited for cases of traumatic or congenital malformations when suction of the cervical adapter to the cervix is technically impossible.

The postoperative care after follicle puncture (see chapter 14.2.14.) depends in part on the extent of the operative procedure, in part on the time schedule, i.e., on the results of in vitro fertilization with possible reimplantation of the fertilized egg in the two- to eight-cell stage.

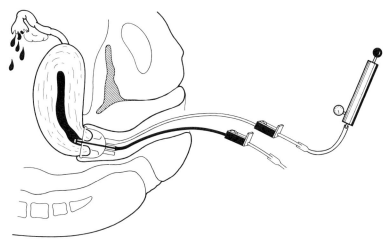

FIG 368.
Negative pressure may be produced manually, by a hand pump, or by the universal pertubation apparatus.

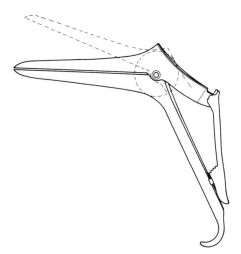

FIG 369.
Duckbill speculum used to apply the cervical adapter.

17.3.2. Postoperative Care According to the "Three-Phase Therapy" for Endometriosis and Sterility

The cause of endometriosis and the mode of its recurrence are not yet completely understood. Five theories of the development of endometriosis which are presently recognized are shown in Figure 372.

In the past, operations for pelvic endometriosis were not very successful in reestablishing fertility. Sterility operations by laparotomy in the presence of endometriosis frequently led to the development of particularly dense postoperative adhesions (see Plate 100), usually resulting in permanent sterility. The possibility of the successful pelviscopic treatment of endometriosis up to Acosta stage III, AFS stages I to IV, or EEC stages I to IV (EEC = Endoscopic Endometriosis Classification) (see chapter 14.2.4.4. and Charts 1 and 2 on pages 159 and 160) for the first time of-

fers completely new options for the treatment of sterility caused by endometriosis. As shown in Figure 373, during the first diagnostic or therapeutic procedure, treatment is primarily directed toward the eradication of endometriotic implants in the abdominal and pelvic cavity. Visible implants are coagulated (see Plates 42, 44, 62, and 64), larger ones are scraped off with biopsy forceps (see Plate 41), invisible implants are diagnosed by the thermocolor test, which is therapeutic at the same time (see Plates 61–64, 76, 386, and 387), and chocolate cysts are excised (see chapter 14.2.6.2.). If endometriosis is extensive, treatment is limited to fimbrioplasty of stenosed tubes.

Finally, another classic example of how endometriotic implants can be "overlooked" is demonstrated in Plates 386 and 387. When pelviscopy was performed on cycle day 7 in a 28-year-old patient with primary sterility, no endometriotic implants were found (see Plate 76). Fifteen milliliters of sanguineous fluid were aspirated from the cul-de-sac. The blood was thought to represent retrograde menstruation, and bilateral blunt dilatation of the tubal ampullae was performed. Since the patient failed to conceive, although all other parameters appeared to be normal, another pelviscopy was performed 11 months later. The appearance at that time (Plate 386) was identical to the appearance 11 months earlier (see Plate 76): blood in the cul-de-sac, no evidence of active endometriotic implants. Only after the thermocolor test was done did extensive implants become apparent (Plate 387). This is a classic example, and one that may also explain why statistical data seem to indicate such widely diverse incidence rates for endometriosis.

Under no circumstances should blocked tubes in the presence of EEC III be opened by salpingostomy. Tubes opened in this manner (see chapter 14.2.4.3.) will immediately reagglutinate during the healing phase. Even after thorough coagulation

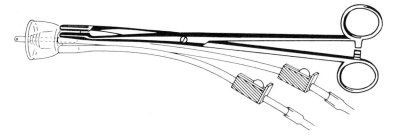

FIG 370.
Cervical adapter is grasped with the special adapter forceps and introduced through the duckbill speculum.

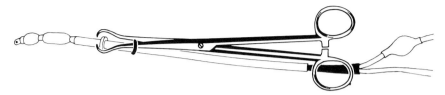

FIG 371.
A double-balloon catheter may be used if the cervix has been disfigured by childbirth.

of endometriotic implants, a few implants will remain. Despite immediate hormonal therapy, these implants will bleed once more, leading to recurrent tubal blockage.

Treatment is restricted to postoperative hydropertubation (see chapters 12.4.2. and 17.3.) and a 4- to 6-month course of hormonal therapy of the endometriosis. This is particularly important when intramural obstruction is present and if adenomyosis or adenoma of the tubal cornu is suspected. Figure 374 shows the mechanism of action of hormonal therapy when progestational agents and antigonadotropins are used.

After completion of the progestational or antigonadotropin therapy, which is followed by withdrawal bleeding, one waits for at least one normal menstrual period. Immediately after that, a second-look pelviscopy is performed between cycle days 4 and 8, at the latest, so that at least 5 days are left

for prolonged hydropertubation (see chapters 12.4.2. and 17.3) before the secretory phase begins. During this second-look pelviscopy, all procedures performed during the first operative pelviscopy (see Fig 373) are checked and then the tubal ampullae are reconstructed either by fimbrioplasty (i.e., blunt dilatation in the presence of phimosis or ampullary stenosis) or by stomatoplasty, as described in chapter 14.2.4.2. to 14.2.4.4.

The operative measures that are possible today as part of the "three-phase therapy" of endometriosis are again outlined in an overall catalog shown in Figure 375.

Finally, it should be reemphasized that operative correction of tubal pathology in the presence of endometriosis, i.e., a "pool of menstrual blood," as shown in Plates 63 and 76, will not be very successful, because the tubal ampullae will reagglutinate rapidly. Since operative pelviscopy

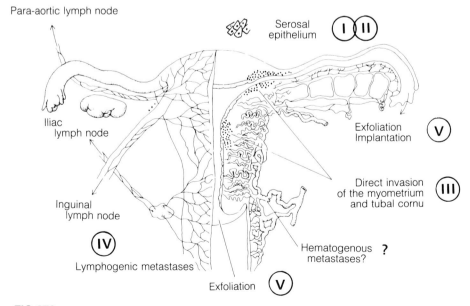

FIG 372.
Pathogenesis of endometriosis: five theories.

1. Operative → eradication of implants only
2. Hormonal.
3. Operative → correction of tubal pathology

FIG 373.
Three-phase therapy of sterility caused by pelvic endometriosis.

can be repeated, the operative steps can be divided into three phases and therefore may be performed much more effectively than would be technically possible by laparotomy. Only if endometriosis is restricted to EEC I and II is it advisable to perform fimbrioplasty and/or salpingostomy in the first sitting. There is a high probability that conception will occur in the subsequent cycles.

Thanks to the three-phase therapy, we observed a pregnancy rate of 48% among 572 women with endometriosis or sterility due to tubal factors.

17.4. POSTOPERATIVE CARE AFTER GENERAL SURGICAL ENDOSCOPIC ABDOMINAL OPERATIONS

Postoperative care after general surgical endoscopic procedures in general follows classic surgical routines. However, we distinguish between operative procedures that directly involve bowels and those performed on the omentum, etc.

17.4.1. General Postoperative Care

Postoperative care after general surgical endoscopic procedures which were not performed for purely gynecologic indications, as described in chapter 15, is principally not much different from postoperative care discussed in chapter 14.

However, particular caution is required when, during intestinal adhesiolysis, lesions occur in the serosa that is attached to the muscularis of the bowel, or if the bowel lumen is opened. According to conventional surgical practice, the defect is closed by endosuture and either external or internal tying of slipknots (see chapter 12.6.2 and 12.6.3.). During the healing phase, the same rules are followed as in general bowel surgery: parenteral fluids are given for 48 hours, as after a laparotomy, to allow sufficient time for the intestinal wound to heal. In this context, the importance of a careful preoperative bowel preparation should be mentioned again, consisting, if necessary, of several days of an "astronaut" diet (see chapter 15.2.) to avoid any postoperative risk. Since bowel was dissected under almost microsurgical conditions (see chapter 12.2.4.) and subsequently su-

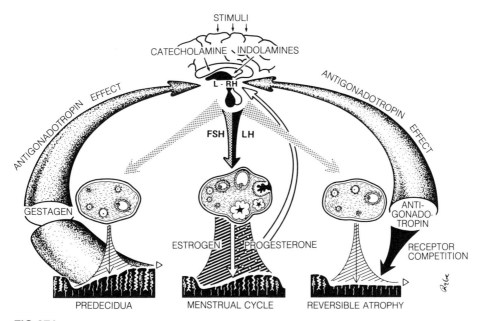

FIG 374.
Hypothalamic-pituitary-gonadal-endometrial axis of endometriosis therapy.

1. Diagnostic and/or operative pelviscopy
    + Chromosalpingoscopy + series of hydropertubations
    - Adhesiolysis
    - Ovariolysis
    - Salpingolysis
    - Fimbrioplasty
    - Resection or enucleation of ovarian cysts, etc.
    - Endocoagulation of endometrial implants
    - Treatment of entire pelvic cavity

2. 3- to 9-month course of endocrine therapy with progestational
   agents or antigonadotropins

3. Repeat operative pelviscopy
    + Chromosalpingoscopy + series of hydropertubations
    - Adhesiolysis
    - Ovariolysis
    - Salpingolysis
    - Fimbrioplasty
    - Salpingostomy or
    - End-to-end anastomosis or tubal implantation by
      laparotomy

FIG 375.
Operative measures possible as part of "three-phase therapy" of endometriosis.

tured and since bowel peristalsis continues postoperatively, wound healing should be complete in 2–3 days.

17.4.2. Postoperative Care After Endoscopic Appendectomy or Intestinal Suture

The endoscopic appendectomy, described in chapter 15.3. ff., corresponds to the classic approach by laparotomy. However, the steps of the operation, beginning with the ligature of the appendiceal artery and skeletonizing of the appendix, up to placement of the purse string suture and Z-suture, are carried out under low-power magnification almost equal to a loupe. Regarding trauma to the bowel, sutures can be placed much more gently than would be possible during a normal laparotomy. As shown in Plates 373–377, the adaptation of the serosa by the purse string suture and the Z-suture is extremely accurate, so that adhesions are extremely unlikely to develop during the postoperative course.

However, since this is a "new operative procedure," it is certainly advisable to completely adhere to the postoperative therapy for the conventional appendectomy by laparotomy. Although there is no pain from a laparotomy and the patient does not offer any complaints, one should avoid any inappropriate action. It takes at least 3–4 days for the open wound produced in the cecum to heal and build up sufficient resistance to the stress of peristalsis, or dilatation, which is stimulated by the resumption of oral food intake. It would be detrimental to the method to miniaturize the procedure and, at the same time, reduce the hospitalization time.

The main advantage of this method is not the reduction of hospitalization time but the fact that the patient will be free of complaints when she leaves the hospital, i.e., she will be able to return to work.

18

Recovery and Restoration to Working Capacity After Endoscopic Abdominal Surgery

In regard to preoperative and postoperative hospitalization for endoscopic abdominal procedures, the widespread experience with ambulatory sterilization may serve as a guideline. Sometimes it is performed under general anesthesia, sometimes under local anesthesia. Whether or not this mode of ambulatory surgery complies with medical standards deserves further discussion.

The decision as to how long a patient should or must be hospitalized after an endoscopic abdominal procedure depends on the pathophysiology of wound healing. The dominant factor used to be incisional pain from the laparotomy, which determined how long a patient had to remain in bed. This abdominal trauma is not present in a patient after an endoscopic operation. However, the organs operated on have been traumatized to an extent comparable to that during a laparotomy. The impact of the physical stress has just been reversed. There is no longer such a stark contrast between the endoscopic procedure on the diseased organ (e.g., ampulla) and the trauma to the abdominal wall. A striking example: a large incisional trauma is incurred with a transverse Pfannenstiel incision or even a longitudinal incision to open the abdominal wall for a relatively small procedure such as a blunt dilatation of the tubal ampullae to correct ampullary stenosis or phimosis.

Perhaps another comparison should be made with a condition encountered in internal medicine. A pneumonia heals pathophysiologically (i.e., histologically) in four phases. Even the use of antibiotics does not change this sequence. Antibiotics only produce a rapid decline in bacterial toxins, which makes the patient feel better, so that subjectively the pneumonia seems to be cured within 8 days.

The recovery period after an endoscopic abdominal operation therefore depends on (1) the recovery from the stress of general anesthesia, and (2) the healing process of defects in the peritoneum, etc.

It can probably be assumed that due to the lesser trauma from the endoscopic procedure, the healing times would be at the lower limit of the usual healing times observed after a laparotomy; however, they are essentially the same as those after a laparotomy.

According to the physical stress, the patient's recuperation to full working capacity depends in part on the pathophysiology of her illness and in part on the time required purely for wound healing. Even after major procedures, such as the endoscopic conservative correction of a tubal pregnancy, the patient should be free of discomfort after 6 postoperative days, at the most. Hence, the recovery period corresponds to that after dilatation and curettage for induced or spontaneous abortion.

[Although I basically agree with most of the essential facts and policies which Semm presents in this book, I strongly disagree with some of the statements made in this section. Based on my own experience and that of many gynecologic surgeons in the United States, I want to take this opportunity to highlight some of the differences in gynecologic practice on opposite sides of the Atlantic Ocean. Pathophysiology of disease and the healing process after surgical trauma must be assumed to be the same on all continents. However, there are definite differences in attitude in regard to the practice of medicine in Germany and in the United States. As repeatedly stated by Semm, the introduction of laparoscopy has had a tremendous impact on the practice of gynecology in both countries but, due to larger size and larger numbers, probably much more so in the United States. In the past, gynecologic surgery was practiced mainly in hospitals. By tradition, hospitals and the personnel working in hospitals are preoccupied with illness and the treatment of illness and, only as a consequence, restitution to health.

During the past 10 to 15 years, emphasis in the United States has shifted to wellness, the maintenance of health and the prevention of illness. This has had a tremendous impact on the attitude of both "providers"—physicians and medical personnel—as well as "consumers"—both patients who want to be relieved of illness and healthy men and women who contract with the physician for a "service" such as a sterilization operation, facelift, etc. They are well before the operation, they expect no complications from the operation, and they desire to return to their usual lifestyle and work without delay.

Semm is correct: We have done a huge biologic experiment in the United States; hundreds of thousands of laparoscopic tubal sterilizations per year with only a brief hospitalization or only a few hours' stay in an ambulatory surgical facility. The result: Healthy women tolerate the "physical stress" of this procedure extremely well! Some of my own patients have returned to their usual office work or similar duties only a few hours after the procedure. Others played tennis or golf. Some went shopping, dining, or dancing; others preferred bed rest for a while. For the past 15 years I have not recommended any restrictions in their activities except that they refrain from sexual activities until they are back home.

By custom and constitutional right, the German citizen still expects to be hospitalized and excused from work until his or her recovery is complete in every respect. In such an environment, Semm's hospital is progressive. The average hospitalization time of his patients is shorter by several days when compared to the average hospitalization time in other German hospitals. On the other hand, his "patients" are hospitalized considerably longer than our "consumers."

I am convinced that attitude has a tremendous impact on postoperative recovery. If physicians as well as patients and consumers think "wellness," the postoperative recovery time can be reduced on both sides of the Atlantic. This applies not only to laparoscopic/pelviscopic procedures, but even to procedures requiring a laparotomy. In the past we used to give corticosteroids during and after operations to reverse previous tubal sterilizations, and we assumed that these steroids "made" patients euphoric. I abandoned this practice several years ago but continue to observe the same euphoria. These women have a strong desire; after the operation they are one step closer to the fulfillment of their desire and are anxious to return to their normal activities, so much so that it often requires considerable persuasive efforts to keep them in the hospital beyond the second or third postoperative day.

With a reasonable attitude on the part of the physicians a well as the "consumers"—including their families, friends, and co-workers—I cannot think of a valid reason why the pathophysiology of wound healing should be more physiologic in a strange environment, a hospital, than in a familiar environment, the individual's home.—*Ed.*]

19 _____ Repeated Endoscopic Abdominal Procedures

At the beginning of the 1940s, Palmer performed celioscopy exclusively under local anesthesia. However, since no patient would consent to the same procedure a second time after only a few years, he completely converted to general anesthesia. The patient should retain a pleasant memory of this procedure.

On the international scene, Palmer's example was followed with few exceptions (e.g., pelviscopic tubal sterilization), so that today, operative pelviscopy or endoscopic abdominal surgery is usually performed under endotracheal inhalation anesthesia.

From a purely mechanical-technical point of view, it could be shown that the procedure can be performed through an umbilical incision as often as necessary. However, it is a prerequisite that the Z-puncture technique (see Fig 240) be used, in which the umbilical fascial plate remains intact, and that the conical trocar be introduced 2–3 cm lateral to the umbilicus through the soft muscle layer (see Plate 10). In more than 10,000 pelviscopic operations, particularly in our sterility practice, the three-phase therapy for pelvic endometriosis, and during in vitro fertilization, we have gathered considerable experience, so that we can recommend repeated pelviscopies by the Z-puncture technique as a routine procedure.

If repeated endoscopic operative procedures are necessary, as they often are in the sterility practice, for cosmetic reasons one can always utilize the same puncture scars in the suprapubic region without altering wound healing. If, for instance, a transverse Pfannenstiel scar or a large appendectomy scar is present, the trocars may be introduced in the scar areas, if that is feasible in the particular operation. However, one must take care that only the skin incision is made in the scar; the Z-track itself is not made through the underlying scar tissue. It is extremely difficult to perforate such tough scar tissue with the conical trocar.

Perforating very vascular scar tissue with a sharp-edged pyramidal trocar, however, may easily result in intracutaneous or intra-abdominal hemorrhages. As mentioned before, this type of trocar should not be used for most cases of endoscopic abdominal surgery.

20 _____ Documentation of Endoscopic Abdominal Surgery

The documentation of endoscopic operations is particularly important. For legal reasons it is done in written form. In addition, photographic documentation has achieved a particularly high value in endoscopy.

20.1. WRITTEN DOCUMENTATION OF THE ENDOSCOPIC OPERATION (= OPERATIVE REPORT)

At the end of the endoscopic abdominal operation, an operative report is prepared just as in general surgery. Better than a purely verbal description is a report augmented by some graphic documentation. To ensure that all technical facts pertaining to the procedure are included, we have designed a "Pelviscopic Operative Report" (Fig 376). It contains all data and sketches of the operation which are needed for documentation and, in addition, it serves as a guideline for the surgeon when he prepares his detailed report.

20.2. PHOTOGRAPHIC, CINEMATOGRAPHIC, AND VIDEOTAPE DOCUMENTATION OF THE ENDOSCOPIC ABDOMINAL SURGERY

Practical surgical knowledge is acquired by assisting in an operation. Learning about individual op-

erative steps occurs at the same time. In general abdominal surgery, the widely opened abdomen is the ideal opportunity for this.

By contrast, the endoscopic diagnostician and surgeon used to do his work all by himself. His work is made even harder because in endoscopic surgery he cannot rely upon his usual binocular (i.e., stereoscopic or three-dimensional) vision, which is so important for an operation. He must determine the size and shape of organs with monocular vision only. Hence, until 1965, the endoscopic surgeon had to acquire his training and skills only by performing laparotomies and by studying books on endoscopy. Since 1965, flexible fiberglass teaching attachments or Wittmoser's articulated optical attachment have been available for a second observer. Depending on the optical quality of these attachments, simultaneous observation is possible and, hence, the opportunity for a second surgeon to assist in modern endoscopic abdominal surgery (see Figs 22, 23, and 377). However, this optical system has the following drawbacks: (1) the available light has to be split by a prism into two optical systems, which reduces the light available to the surgeon by 50%–90%, and (2) the optical field is reduced considerably by splitting the optical beam.

These optical systems for the benefit of a second observer, which are also referred to as "teaching attachments" (see Fig 22), substantially reduce the field of view, the light intensity, and hence the surgeon's vision in general. This, indeed, restricts

DEPARTMENT OF GYNECOLOGY, CENTER FOR OPERATIVE MEDICINE I
OF THE CHRISTIAN ALBRECHTS UNIVERSITY AND MICHAELIS MIDWIFERY SCHOOL, KIEL
Director: Professor Dr. K. Semm

PELVISCOPY REPORT

Ward: _____   Date: _____

Patient: _____ Birth date: _____

Surgeon: _____ Assistant: _____

Anesthesiologist: _____ Instrument nurse: _____

Indication: _____

Dictated by:_____
7/11 mm trocar
Adhesions
5 mm trocar

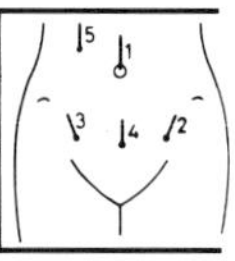

History:

Examination under Anesthesia:

Sounding depth . . . . cm, **application of small/large intrauterine cannula**   (Surgeon . . . .)
Pneumoperitoneum with . . .liters CO_2 gas   Intra-abd. pressure . . mm Hg   Total vol. used . . liters CO_2 gas Endosc. trocar 7 / 11 mm Rt./Lt.
Trocar punctures   ①   ②   ③   ④   ⑤   **Aspiration test:** Pos. / Neg.   **Sounding test:** Adhesions / Neg.   Documentation: Yes / No
Laparoscopic findings:
Pelviscopy:

Chromosalpingoscopy: . . . .ml hydrosolution at . . . . mm Hg pressure in. . . . .min. with/without distention CO_2 pertubation: Patency Grade I - II - III

Lt. Tube: Intramural - Peripheral - Ampullary Stenosis -   **Rt. Tube:** Intramural - Peripheral - Ampullary Stenosis -

Histology:	Yes No
Cytology:	Yes No
Bacteriology	Yes No

Obstruction Free/Restricted - Patency - Peritubular/   Obstruction - Free/Restricted Patency - Peritubular/
Ovarian Adhesions - Endometriosis   Ovarian Adhesions - Endometriosis
Operative prognosis: good / guarded / poor   **Operative prognosis:** good / guarded / poor
Diagnosis:

Laparoscopy: Diagnostic - Operative
Pelviscopy: Diagnostic - Operative

Therapeutic Recommendation:

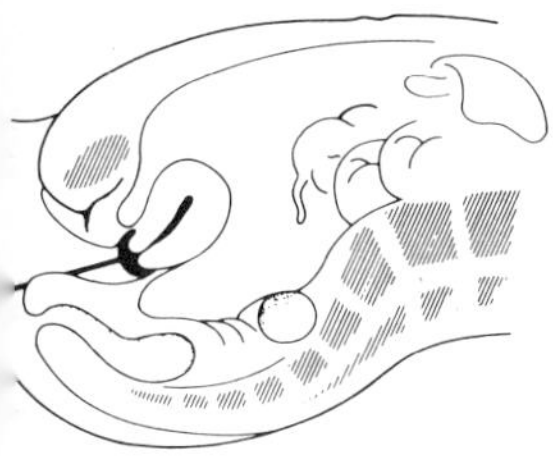

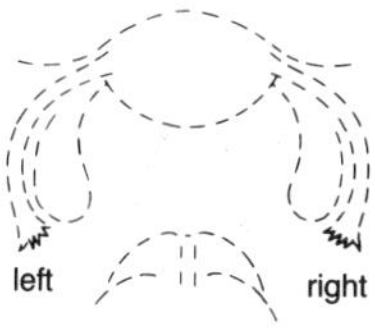

left   right

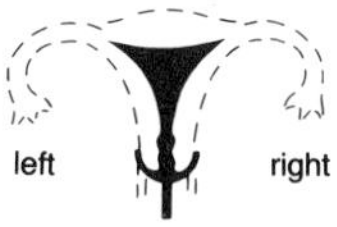

left   right

left   right

• Biopsy   △ Endometrial implant
x Coagulation   ⫰ Adhesions
⟶ Transection   ∞ Endosuture/Ligature

Endoscopic Endometriosis Classification: _____
EEC   I   II   III   IV   Surgeon's signature

FIG 376.
Pelviscopic operative report.

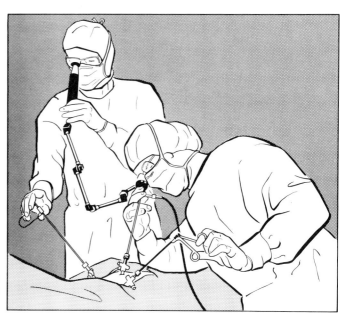

FIG 377.
An articulated optical attachment allows an assistant to view and assist in endoscopic operations.

the surgeon's activity considerably, yet it offers the only opportunity for the assistant or student to share the operative image live.

The individual who tries to learn endoscopic abdominal surgery is well advised to practice first on the Pelvi-Trainer (see chapter 22) and then to utilize the full light capacity of the endoscope when he performs his first procedures, if necessary, even by attaching a loupe for magnification (see chapter 12.2.4.). However, the same magnification can be achieved by attaching a camera with the appropriate telephoto lens with zoom options between 70 and 140 mm (see Figs 52 and

53). A reflex camera armed with such a lens (Fig 378) magnifies the image of the endoscopic eyepiece approximately 2–4 times. Although this affects the panoramic view, it will provide, at the same time, low-power magnification for inspection and an opportunity to document the findings.

In the past, one had to be satisfied that in endoscopic photography a substantial part of the photographic slide remained black (Fig 379) and only in the middle remained a round disc with the image of the internal organs, which were usually underexposed. Today, after many years of development, the frame-filling color slide has become a reality.

FIG 378.
A reflex camera with a telephoto zoom lens magnifies the image of the endoscopic eyepiece and can be used to document findings.

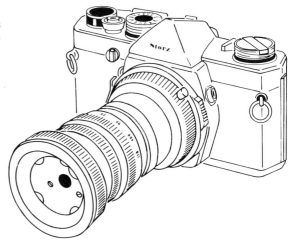

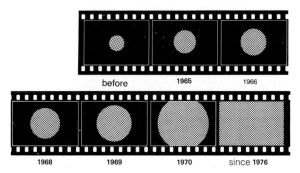

FIG 379.
Gradual historical enlargement of endoscopic image on film. Today frame-filling color slides are a reality.

Semm in 1976 succeeded in producing frame-filling panoramic photographs of pelvic organs (uterus and both adnexa photographed at the same time) by multiple exposures to two successive flashes $\frac{1}{100}$ of a second apart. Until now, the tube-shaped electronic flash has been used, but attempts to concentrate its light output have been fraught with great technical difficulties. Its replacement by the so-called spherical flash (see Fig 39) made it possible to concentrate the light output of the electronic flash to such an extent that even with extension tubes of 110–140 mm (see Figs 52 and 53), format-filling, well-illuminated 24 × 36-mm color slides can be produced with 27 DIN (400 ASA) film.

Today, the light source described in chapter 12.1.3. in combination with an endoscope with integrated fiber light bundles (see chapter 12.2.5. and Fig 40) has eliminated all the problems in pro-ducing endoscopic abdominal panoramic photographs. Modern cameras (e.g., Olympus OM-2S) terminate the flash energy to prevent overexposure. However, underexposure cannot yet be prevented automatically. Such cameras offer the tremendous advantage that photographs that offer close-up details can be made without problems and without overexposure if used with the flash generator shown in Figure 41 and monitored by a through-the-lens computerized flash system. If the sound signal that has been cleverly integrated in the Storz light source is not heard after the exposure, it will be underexposed. The shot can then be repeated with a shorter focal length (= less magnification), or the light source (i.e., the spherical flash) can be checked as to whether or not sufficient light energy is produced. Figure 380 shows my simple test instrument, which we utilize before every series of photographs. This is highly recommended, because

FIG 380.
Semm's instrument for checking illumination capacity of light sources for endoscopic photography.

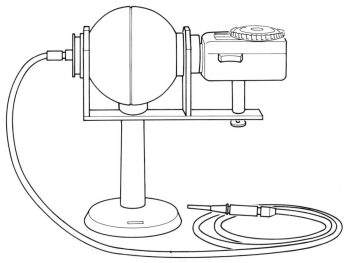

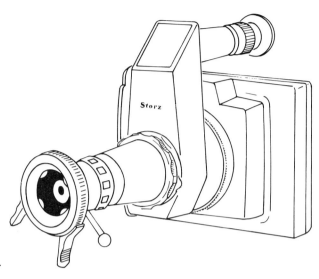

FIG 381.
Polaroid Camera for instant photographs.

the flash tubes available today show a rapid decline in their emission of light energy.

In addition to the format-filling slides, cameras for instant photographs (e.g., Polaroid system) are available (Fig 381). Although the quality of those photographs is not comparable to the quality of slides, they may be of particular value when instant photographs are needed for documentation in the patient's chart.

A similar purpose may be served by 16-mm slides made with an Olympus miniature camera, which requires less light for exposure. If they are used in scientific presentations and publications, their graininess due to higher magnification becomes a disturbing problem.

As mentioned before, the physical problem in producing an endophotograph is the amount of light reflected by the optical system of only 2–3

mm diameter. Whereas the front lens of a camera for normal 24 × 36-mm photographs has a diameter of 20–60 mm, the optical system of an endoscope of 11 mm diameter measures only 2 to maximally 3 mm in diameter and additionally has a length of 300 mm (length of the endoscope) plus 150 mm (telephoto lens). To obtain a disc-shaped image, all the light transmitted into the abdominal cavity is reflected through the optical system (Fig 382) and exposes the film. To expose the entire format, it is necessary that several times the quantity of light required for a disc-shaped image be transmitted into the abdominal cavity, because the format-filling rectangular image is only a segment of the large, fully exposed circular image (Fig 383). Only a portion of the light transmitted is

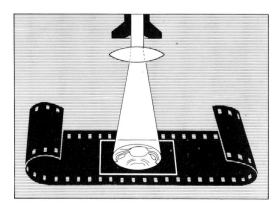

FIG 382.
Disc-shaped image made with normal amount of light.

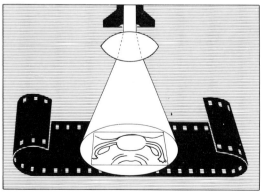

FIG 383.
To expose the entire format of 35-mm film, much more light is needed. The photographic image is then only a portion of the larger, true image.

used for the exposure of the photographic slide. The remainder of the transmitted light is not used for photographic purposes.

The most essential item for good photography in endoscopy is not the camera—in principle, any camera body can be used for endoscopic photography—but the light source. The amount of light transmitted into the body cavity must be great enough that the light reflected through the optical system of the endoscope and the telelens of the camera can expose a format-filling image on the color film. The intra-abdominal flash developed in the 1960s by the Wolf company was ideally suited. However, for the patient's safety (risk of explosion of the flash tube), the light output cannot be increased any further. Unfortunately, it is of no importance today. The internal light source produced color photographs of very high contrast.

The highest value of endoscopic cinematographic documentation is primarily in the area of teaching films. At a time when gynecologic laparoscopy had not yet achieved any significance, during the years 1966–1970, it was mainly teaching films that demonstrated the high clinical diagnostic value of this method to a broad audience (see chapter 2). With the development of high-pressure gas discharge lamps in the middle of the 1960s it became technically possible to produce format-filling, well-exposed endoscopic motion pictures. This was possible at a time when the endoscopic photograph could impart only little information and when in endoscopic textbooks the endoscopic image could not be adequately appreciated, as only retouched color photographs were presented.

In summary, it should be emphasized that there is no other operative field in medicine in which photography and cinematography played the same essential role to introduce the method into clinical practice, as has been the case for laparoscopy and pelviscopy.

The photographic films (Kodak and Fuji) which are available today are the 27-M-DIN color reversal film (400 ASA) and the 22–27 DIN (160–400 ASA) 16-mm color film.

The cinematographic documentation of operative steps during endoscopic surgery will always require a most experienced surgeon who is also experienced in cinematography, because the image produced in the movie cameras available so far is very small and is a poor substitute for direct vision during microsurgical manipulations. Splitting the light beam, as through an articulated optical attachment, is technically not possible because this method absorbs too much light for the exposure of movie film. Therefore, the production of good endoscopic teaching films will remain in the hands of a few highly specialized teams.

In contrast, electromagnetic imaging (Fig 384) offers a welcome improvement to make diagnostic and operative steps available to a broad audience. However, one must accept that the image on the television screen is of considerably lower quality than a 16-mm motion picture. This applies both to image resolution and to the color spectrum.

We must distinguish between two different systems of color video cameras:

1. This is a so-called *single-tube video camera,* which electronically splits the image transmitted to the color television tube into component colors according to empirical values. However, since endoscopic images are mainly in the red scale, to the exclusion of other colors, these images are frequently unsatisfactory.

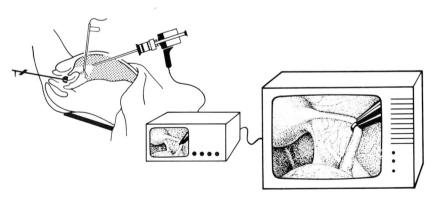

FIG 384.
Electromagnetic imaging with lightweight video camera.

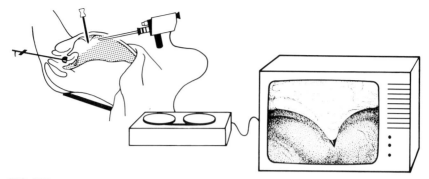

FIG 385.
Simultaneous videorecording equipment.

2. The *triple-tube color television camera:* In this system, the transmitted light is split by a prism into the three primary colors, red, blue, and yellow, which are processed by three television tubes and only then reassembled into an image on the television screen or monitor. The color images of the abdominal cavity produced with such methods correspond to a high degree to the real color spectrum inside the abdomen.

The difference between the two camera systems for practical application is not only the price but also their weight. While the color video camera presented under 1 can be built very light and coupled directly to every endoscope (see Fig 384), the heavy professional cameras mentioned under 2 always require the transmission of the image through, for instance, an articulated optical attachment. A flexible fiberglass attachment, furthermore, produces a honeycombed dissolution of the image, which is typical for fiber light optical systems.

If one is willing to forego the brilliance of the image, however, the television technique is an excellent improvement that allows the transmission of diagnostic findings and operative steps. The option for simultaneous videorecording (Fig 385) preserves the image at the same time and makes it available for teaching and study purposes at any time.

There is no doubt that the transmission and videorecording of the television image imposes a considerable burden on the diagnostician and surgeon because he

   a. can observe the image only on the television screen if the camera is directly attached to the endoscope, which considerably diminishes the available information;

   b. can hardly operate endoscopically because of the complete absence of stereoscopic perception;

   c. due to the transmission of the image through an articulated optical attachment to the camera, depending on the camera, the surgeon will lose 50%–90% of the transmitted light which would otherwise be available for his own observation purposes. Furthermore, the visual field is restricted and handling of the endoscope is more difficult.

   d. must use high-intensity light sources, which are an additional burden to himself and his personnel and are quite expensive.

The last 20 years have brought considerable progress in the documentation of endoscopic findings. The revolution in photographic and cinematographic imaging is already in the transition from Daguerre's silver reduction on film to the magnetic image. Ten year ago I used a tractor-trailer parked in the courtyard of the hospital for videorecording, from which cables as thick as a thumb were run to the operating room, terminating in equipment weighing hundreds of pounds. Today, the whole system, including that for transmission to the auditorium, is installed on an instrument table and weighs only several kilograms. We also have color films available with 1,000 ASA sensitivity. Tomorrow we will have a magnetic disc (CD, Cupple Device) of 4 × 4 cm on which approximately 100 images can be stored, which can immediately be viewed on the television screen without prior development. This technique will relieve us of many of the problems in endoscopic photography, because its sensitivity can be controlled by microprocessors instead of requiring photochemical processing.

21 _____ Assessment of the Operative Risk in Endoscopic Abdominal Surgery

The endoscopic operative risk can be viewed from several perspectives. The greatest drawback to endoscopic operative techniques is the monocular view of the operative field. However, this can essentially be compensated for by the use of two operative instruments. The possibility of inspecting organs to be operated on from a certain distance and under low-power magnification up to $6\times$ certainly lowers any risk due to optical misinterpretations if compared to a laparotomy, which is usually performed without magnification with a loupe or microscope.

A prerequisite for endoscopic operations is complete familiarity with and skill in the same procedure under laparotomy conditions. The common practice that a surgeon not yet skilled in abdominal surgery would perform operative endoscopic procedures such as tubal sterilization was limited to the development phase: on the one hand, laparoscopy was introduced worldwide within only a few years; on the other hand, the development from purely diagnostic measures to operative ones was usually accomplished by self-training. It should be stated categorically that even a skilled diagnostic laparoscopist cannot, from one day to the next, perform salpingo-oophorectomies or appendectomies. He must have extensively assisted such procedures—as is also customary for total ab-

dominal hysterectomy and similar procedures—before he can perform them on his own.

For endoscopic surgery in the abdomen, the following levels of training should be established.

1. Complete skills in corresponding operative techniques on the same organ by laparotomy
2. Excellent training in diagnostic pelviscopy or laparoscopy
3. Sufficient experience as an assistant or opportunity for observation of a skilled endoscopic abdominal surgeon
4. The availability of all instruments and equipment in sufficient number—as has also been customary for decades for laparotomy

The risk of endoscopic misjudgment during cutting or blunt dissection of adhesions can lead to intestinal injuries or to the transection of a ureter. However, such mishap cannot be ascribed solely to the method, for it is a risk inherent in all abdominal surgery. The only difference is whether perforation of the urinary bladder or transection of the ureter or incidental incision into bowel by laparotomy can immediately be corrected during the same procedure by laparotomy. If such injuries occur during pelviscopy, the transition to a laparotomy is necessary. It is essential and absolutely necessary that such lesions be recognized immediately. The same is also true, however, for laparotomy.

Since hemostasis by coagulation—also endo-coagulation—should largely be avoided in areas outside the pelvic cavity, late perforations after co-agulation necrosis of bowel should be a rare com-plication.

In summary, the same operative risks present in any laparotomy are also present in endoscopic abdominal surgery. Some of them can be corrected endoscopically, others require immediate laparot-omy. Since the patient is always prepared for a laparotomy, such procedure poses no real risk to the patient.

The fate of the endoscopic surgeon is identical to that of the conventional abdominal surgeon:

It is not the sudden incident that affects the success of the operation, but the meticulous control of every step of the operation and the determined actions to keep everything under control.

Endoscopic abdominal surgery is a substantial technical enhancement of gynecologic surgery and general surgery. For the patient it has resulted in a considerable reduction in physical stress, because in many cases it makes a large abdominal incision unnecessary.

22 _____ Pelvi-Trainer

The Pelvi-Trainer is a training device for operative pelviscopy that allows surgeons both to teach and to practice all endoscopic procedures, including the new techniques of endoloop ligation and endosuture techniques.

Surgical skills are usually acquired in 3 steps:

1. Theoretical study of printed operative manuals and teaching films,
2. Intensive observation of coordinated, skilled operative teams, and
3. Actively assisting in surgery with the operative field exposed.

Since the abdominal wall is not opened in operative pelviscopy, opportunities for close observation of the operative procedure and active assistance in it are extremely limited. The assistant's active participation in suturing and tying of knots is almost impossible from his position during the endoscopic surgery. These critical handicaps in the teaching and practice of endoscopic surgery have been overcome by the development of a mechanical teaching aid, the Pelvi-Trainer.

22.1. DESCRIPTION OF THE PELVI-TRAINER

The Pelvi-Trainer consists of a stainless steel tray in which a placenta or surgical specimens can be placed. A claw forceps is mounted at the theoretical anatomical site of the vagina for the fixation of surgical specimens. Above the tray is a clear plastic panel with two rubber plates which are preperforated at the theoretical suprapubic, umbilical, and paraumbilical sites for the introduction of trocars of 5 to 11 mm diameter. For cleaning purposes, these rubber plates are easily exchangeable.

A steel bar is mounted on the right side of the model for the attachment of the flexible support arm for the endoscope. A small fluorescent light source is mounted at the cranial end or the left side of the model so that an expensive cold light source is not needed for practice purposes. Below the transparent "abdominal wall" three metal rods are mounted and four skin clips are suspended from bead chains. When placenta and amniotic membranes are attached to these devices, they simulate extensive adhesions (Fig 386).

22.2. PELVI-TRAINER PRACTICE: THREE STEPS

1. The operating instruments, 30 cm long, are introduced through the appropriate sites and the surgeon carries out the operation under binocular vision through the transparent "abdominal wall" (Fig 387, 1). The trainee learns to appreciate new anatomical relationships not previously noticed when the abdominal wall was laid wide open during laparoscopy.

2. Next, the trainee tries to repeat the same manipulations with the aid of the pelviscope. This is held in place by the flexible support arm and directed toward the structures to be operated on. This leaves the surgeon's hands free to operate with the surgical instruments. The surgeon may sit on a stool and rest his shoulder against a supporting device which can be attached to the Pelvi-Trainer. If the surgeon has any difficulties with orientation or manipulation of instruments, "cheating" is possible: the appropriate corrections can usually be made by observing the instruments through the transparent "abdominal wall" with both eyes (Fig 387, 2).

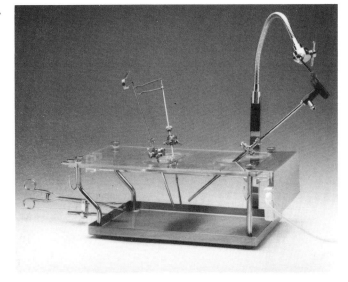

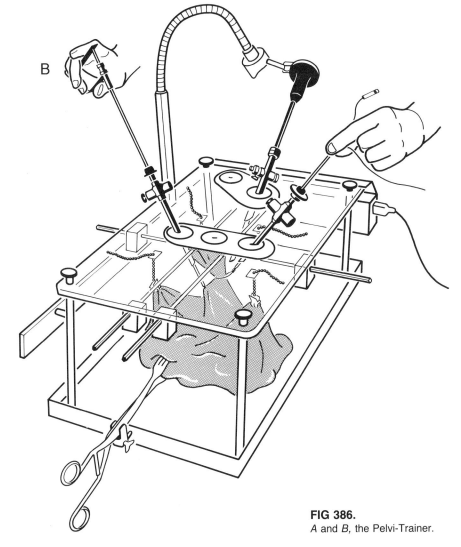

FIG 386.
A and *B,* the Pelvi-Trainer.

252

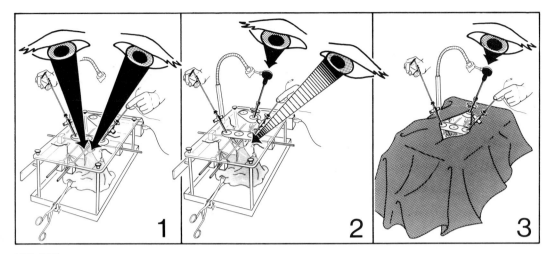

FIG 387.
Steps in learning to perform pelviscopic operations with the aid of the Pelvi-Trainer. See text.

If, after a few hours of training with the endoscope it is no longer necessary to "cheat" in this binocular fashion, the surgeon may advance to the third step of the training program.

3. After the operative specimen has been affixed to the Pelvi-Trainer, the model is covered with a split surgical drape before the endoscope and the ancillary operative instruments are introduced in the same manner as in vivo. Then the surgical procedures are performed under monocular pelviscopic vision in a sitting or semirecumbent position (Fig 387, *3*).

22.3. RECOMMENDED TRAINING PROGRAM

Practice Session 1

A placenta is placed into the Pelvi-Trainer with the maternal parts in the tray and the fetal membranes exposed so that the trainee can practice on the amniotic membranes and umbilical cord how to grasp, take biopsies, and work with scissors and knives, in the following order:

1. with both eyes,
2. through the endoscope with occasional "cheating", and
3. only through the endoscope after the Pelvi-Trainer has been covered.

Practice Session 2

The placenta is introduced into the model and the amniotic membrane and umbilical cord are sus-

pended below the "abdominal wall" in such a manner as to simulate longitudinal and transverse adhesions. The trainee repeats exercise 1 and then learns to perform "bloody" and "bloodless" adhesiolysis by applying endoloops, endoligatures, and endosutures.

Practice Session 3

A placenta is placed into the Pelvi-Trainer, segments of the amniotic membranes are excised, and the "wounds" are closed with endosutures.

Practice Session 4

A fresh operative specimen consisting of uterus, tubes, and ovaries is mounted in the Pelvi-Trainer by grasping the cervix with the claw forceps and suspending the tubes by the chained clips. Ovarian biopsy, tubal sterilization, etc. can be practiced.

Practice Session 5

On an operative specimen similar to that used in exercise 4, the trainee focuses on the tubal ampulla and practices dilatation, sounding, salpingostomy, oophorectomy, salpingo-oophorectomy, etc.

Practice Session 6

Pathologic operative specimens are introduced and the trainee practices incising the tunica albuginea, dissecting ovarian cysts, and excising pedunculated and subserous and intramural myomas, followed by wound closure with endosutures.

Practice Session 7

On a placenta with a relatively thin umbilical cord, appendectomy techniques can be practiced.

Summary

An intensive training program with a Pelvi-Trainer allows a gynecologic surgeon familiar with the pelvic anatomy and skilled in conventional abdominal-pelvic surgery to acquire the skills necessary for endoscopic surgery. The trainee will develop a certain sense for the spatial relationships when working under monocular endoscopic conditions and will acquire the skills to work with endoscopic instruments, particularly endoloops, needles, and sutures. It is no longer necessary to learn and practice new endoscopic techniques in vivo in the operating room. Once adequate dexterity has been achieved by practicing on the Pelvi-Trainer, these new endoscopic techniques can be transferred to the hospital operating room.

23 ——————————— Color Atlas

384 COLOR PHOTOGRAPHS
2 RADIOGRAPHS
1 BLACK AND WHITE
PHOTOGRAPH

Intraoperative findings and surgical procedures that have been described in the preceding chapters have been documented by original color photographs. The color prints are accompanied by 377 line drawings in which the same anatomical structures, pathologic conditions, and instruments are represented by symbolic print patterns and a numerical key to facilitate their identification and interpretation. Color photographs are identified, in the preceding text, by Plate and a number that will help the reader locate the individual color prints in this atlas.

The key to the code of print patterns and numerals is located on page 485, which will simplify the study of both color photographs and line drawings. Text and drawings included in the atlas describe and clarify specific procedures. The contents of the descriptive texts which accompany the color photographs are subdivided into separate headings in *italics: History, findings, operation, caution,* and *comment*. In addition, the reader is frequently referred to other photographs and chapters.

12.3.1. Expansion Media to Produce the Pneumoperitoneum (Choice of Gas)

Plate 1.   **Introduction of a trocar**

History: A 41-year-old infertile woman underwent a previous laparotomy at age 37 years to correct sterility.

Findings: This photograph clearly demonstrates the mobility of the peritoneum, particularly if the patient is obese.

Operation: The 5-mm trocar is introduced suprapubically from the left side and dislocates the subfascial peritoneum for about 10 cm without perforating it.

Caution: This picture should always be remembered when the Veress needle or the first trocar for the laparoscope is introduced in the area of the umbilicus.

See also Plates 95, 268, 290.

12.3.1.2. Transvaginal Insufflation of the Pneumoperitoneum Through the Posterior Vaginal Fornix (Insufflation of the Cul-de-Sac of Douglas)

Plate 2.   **Transvaginal gas insufflation to establish the pneumoperitoneum**

History: A 30-year-old patient had had two previous laparotomies.

Operation: The Veress needle has been introduced through the vaginal fornix and is seen adjacent to the right adnexal area.

Caution: It is clearly demonstrated that this puncture site is not without risk because the pelvic and intra-abdominal tissues are in direct contact with one another before gas insufflation (before this photograph was taken).

See also Plate 3.

Plate 3.   **Transvaginal gas insufflation to establish the pneumoperitoneum**

Operation: After the uterus has been elevated from its previous position (shown in Plate 2), it can be seen that the Veress needle, which was introduced through the posterior vaginal fornix, has inadvertently perforated an epiploic appendix of the rectal ampulla.

Plate 4.   **Tubal sterilization by unipolar high-frequency current**

Findings: Shown is a left fallopian tube that has just been cauterized with unipolar high-frequency current. Significant segments of the isthmic portion of the tube and of the adjacent mesosalpinx show a white discoloration. In addition, there are several black areas indicative of carbonization, which occurs when tissues are exposed to temperatures of several hundred degrees Celsius.

Comment: There is no doubt that the entire tubal segment and the mesosalpinx visible in this photograph have been exposed to temperatures above 57° C, i.e., that thermobionecrosis has been initiated.

256

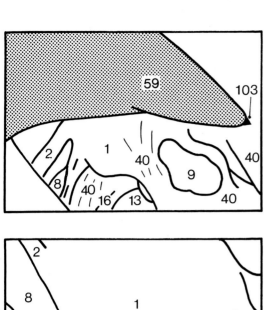

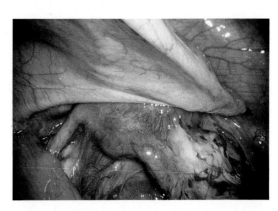

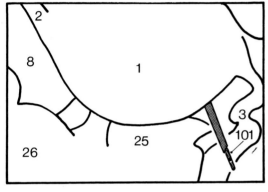

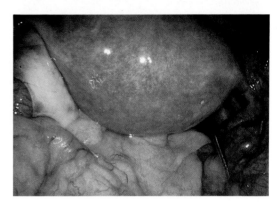

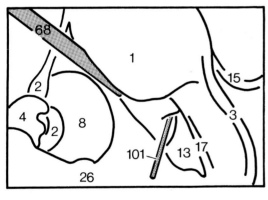

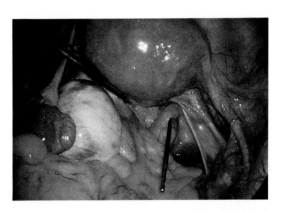

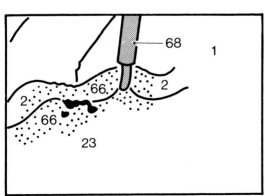

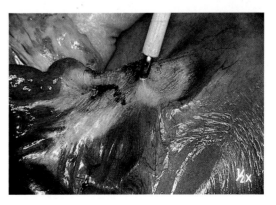

12.5.6.2. Histologic Changes After Heat-Induced Hemostasis

Plate 5.   **Coagulation by high-frequency current**
History: Five days earlier, an area of myometrium was coagulated with unipolar high-frequency current.
Findings: The coagulated area is sloughing off and the wound becomes a crater. Fibrin exudes into the defect and is invaded by histiocytes and fibroblasts which may initiate the formation of adhesions.

Plate 6.   **Hemostasis by endocoagulation at 100° C**
History: Five days earlier this tissue was coagulated by the endocoagulation method.
Findings: Tissues affected by thermonecrosis due to temperatures up to 100° C do not slough off. They are invaded from the periphery by histiocytes and fibroblasts while the process of regeneration occurs from within.
Comment: Peritoneal adhesions to the surface of an organ will not occur if the surface is biologically inactive.

12.6.1. Hemostasis by Loop Ligature

Plate 7.   **Hemostasis by ligation with an endoloop**
History: A 33-year-old patient had primary sterility.
Findings: A vascular adhesion between the right adnexa and an epiploic appendix of the sigmoid colon has already been sharply transected.
Operation: An endoloop has been introduced into the pelvis, and the severed epiploic appendix, which has been grasped with a biopsy forceps, is pulled through the loop.

Plate 8.   **Hemostasis by ligation with an endoloop**
Operation: The loop (shown in Plate 7) has been pulled tight, securely ligating the epiploic appendix. The long end of the catgut suture will be cut with hook scissors.

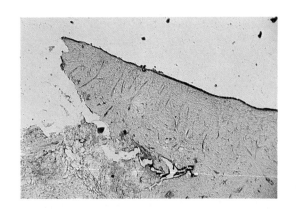

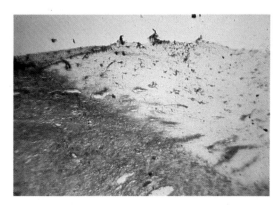

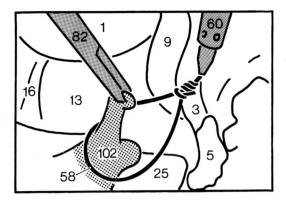

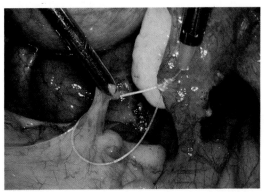

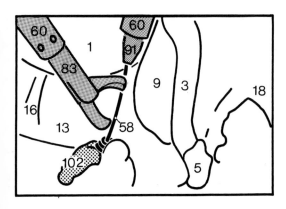

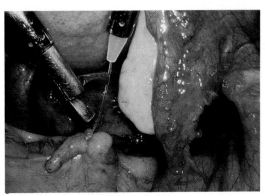

Plate 9.   **Hemostasis by ligation with an endoloop: End result**
Operation: The ligated epiploic appendix, shown in Plates 7 and 8, has been grasped with biopsy forceps and resected distal to the ligature. It will be removed through the trocar sleeve.

12.8.1. Sleeves for Endoscopes and Operative Instruments

Plate 10.   **Postoperative adhesiolysis**
History: Status after laparoscopic sterilization performed via a subumbilical transfascial midline insertion of the trocar for the endoscope.
Findings: A view from the lower abdomen into the upper abdominal cavity reveals postoperative adhesions that had formed after the previous laparoscopy. After the trocar for the laparoscope had been withdrawn, at the end of the previous laparoscopy, it must have left a subumbilical, transfascial midline defect in which a segment of the greater omentum was caught.
Operation: The secondary puncture was dilated from 5 mm to 7 mm diameter to accommodate a second endoscope. It is clearly evident that the first trocar for the laparoscope had been introduced in the paraumbilical area according to the Z-puncture technique.
Caution: If periumbilical omental adhesions must be lysed, inspection through a suprapubic endoscope is always necessary.

12.8.8. Instruments for Dilatation

Plate 11.   **Trocar sleeve dilatation**
Operation: Trocar sleeve dilatation of a puncture site of 5 mm or 7 mm diameter to accommodate the larger trocar sleeve of 11 mm diameter.
Caution: This dilatation technique (see also Plate 218) is completely safe if these precautions are observed: the guide rod is used with great caution to palpate the right pelvic wall; then it is retracted sufficiently so that it will merely serve as a guide for the threaded dilatation cannula, but will not cause an accidental injury to the opposite side of the pelvic wall, such as a hole in the peritoneum of the bladder dome.
See also Plates 12 and 218.

Plate 12.   **Trocar sleeve dilatation: Risk**
Operation: During the dilatation from a 7 mm trocar sleeve to a trocar of 11 mm diameter, the guide rod, demonstrated well in Plate 11, was not sufficiently retracted, causing this accidental injury.
Findings: Perforation in the peritoneum of the bladder dome.

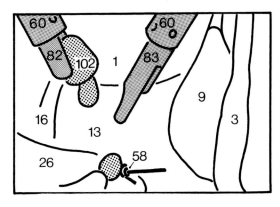

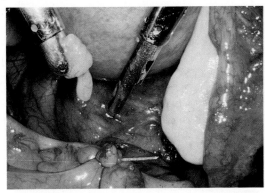

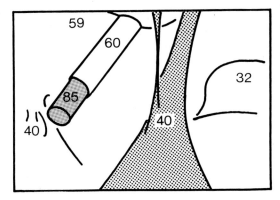

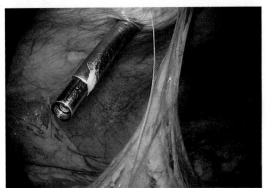

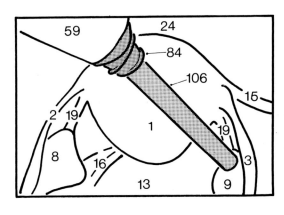

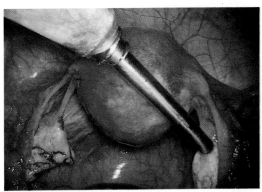

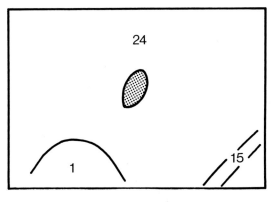

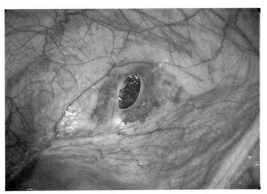

14.1.5. Second and Third Punctures To Establish a Diagnosis as an Indication for the Operative Phase

Plate 13.   **Transabdominal hemostasis**

History: A 28-year-old woman had had two previous laparotomies, an appendectomy at age 16 years and an ectopic tubal pregnancy at 27 years.

Operation: The suprapubic puncture was made on the right side in the area of the appendectomy scar. The cone-shaped trocar impaled the lateral umbilical artery.

Caution: If a sharp, triangular pyramidal trocar had been used, this artery would have been cut immediately. The conical trocar merely impales the vessel.

Comment: Since endocoagulation failed to accomplish hemostasis, transabdominal suture was necessary.

See also Plates 14 and 15.

Plate 14.   **Transabdominal hemostasis**

Operation: The conical trocar has been withdrawn and, under optical control with the laparoscope, the large abdominal needle is introduced through the entire thickness of the abdominal wall and the needle tip is guided around the bleeding vessel.

See also chapter 12.8.7.

Plate 15.   **Transabdominal hemostasis: End result**

Operation: The large abdominal needle, which had been introduced through the entire thickness of the abdominal wall, has already penetrated the abdominal wall in reverse direction from the peritoneum to the external skin. There it is grasped with a needleholder and the suture is tied under strong traction.

Comment: Bleeding usually stops immediately. Only in rare cases will a double ligature be necessary. Note the topography of this artery; it originates caudally.

14.2.2.2. Adhesiolysis Without Prior Hemostasis (Bloody Adhesiolysis)

Plate 16.   **Bleeding with adhesiolysis and attempt to achieve intra-abdominal hemostasis in the greater omentum by endocoagulation**

Operation: The crocodile forceps grasps a wide band of adhesions between the omentum and appendectomy scar.

Caution: Before coagulation, one must be quite certain that the intestinal tract is at least 1 cm from the crocodile forceps. Although heat dissipates from the crocodile forceps into the surrounding tissues only by convection (in contrast to high-frequency currents), this margin of safety must be observed, because tissues tend to shrink considerably during the coagulation process. The intestinal tract may then very rapidly approach the coagulation instrument.

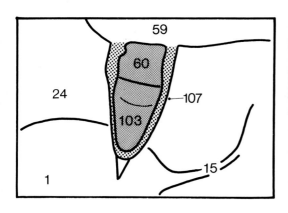

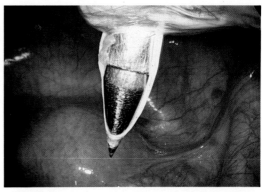

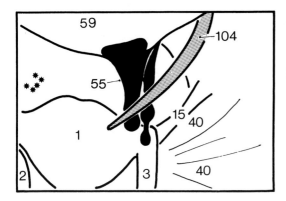

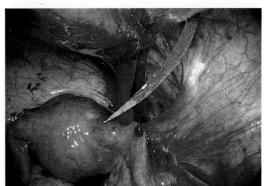

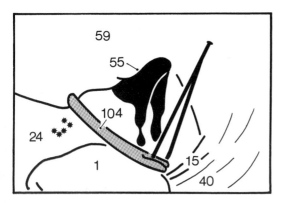

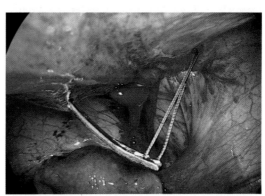

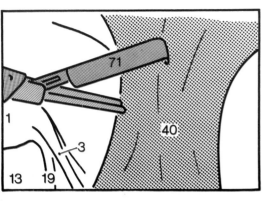

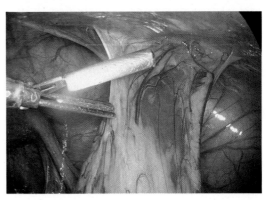

Plate 17. **Bleeding with adhesiolysis**

Operation: The large band of fatty tissue shown in Plate 16 is wrapped around the crocodile forceps as around a haircurler to increase the area in which the lumina of blood vessels are obliterated.

Comment: Fatty tissue is not well suited for endocoagulation because it contains only small amounts of protein, which must be coagulated to obliterate blood vessels and effect hemostasis.

Plate 18. **Bleeding with adhesiolysis**

Operation: After endocoagulation for 20–40 seconds (see Plates 16 and 17), the adhesive band is severed step by step with hook scissors.

Comment: If hemorrhage occurs during this procedure, hemostasis is accomplished with the aid of an endoloop, according to the technique shown in Plates 19 and 20.

Plate 19. **Lysis of adhesions without prior hemostasis**

History: A 29-year-old woman with secondary infertility had a broad-based omental adhesion (see Plate 20) to the left ovary, discovered 18 years after laparotomy for a perforated appendix.

Operation: The adhesion was sharply dissected off without prior coagulation. An endoloop and an atraumatic grasping forceps (if necessary, a biopsy forceps may be used) have been introduced through a second and third puncture. The forceps is advanced through the catgut loop until the bleeding omental pedicle can be grasped and pulled through the catgut loop. *See also* Plate 20.

Plate 20. **Lysis of adhesions without prior hemostasis**

Operation: The bleeding omental pedicle, which had been dissected off the ovary (see Plate 19), has been pulled through the catgut loop. The external end of this catgut loop is pulled while the surgeon simultaneously pushes on the plastic tube, thus advancing the pretied knot until the base of this pedicle is ligated. The protruding omental segment is cut off and removed through the trocar sleeve. *See also* Plate 9.

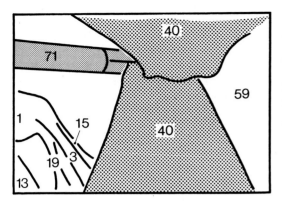

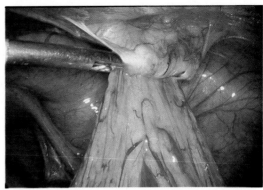

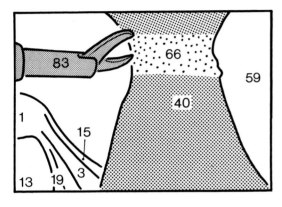

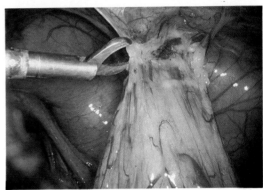

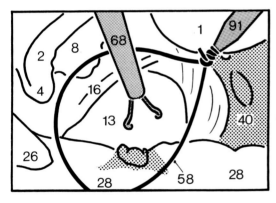

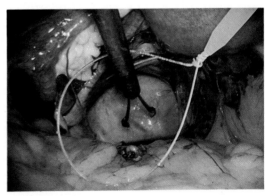

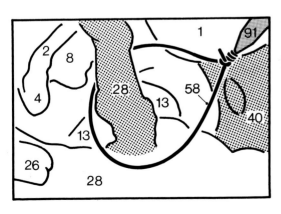

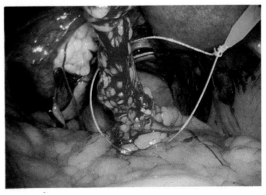

Plate 21. **Lysis of adhesions without prior hemostasis**

History: A 35-year-old patient had undergone an appendectomy at age 29, and ovarian wedge resections for Stein-Leventhal syndrome with simultaneous Baldy-Webster uterine suspension at age 33.

Findings: Both ovaries have grown together and onto the posterior wall of the uterus. An epiploic appendix of the sigmoid colon is also adherent to this convolution.

Operation: This fatty tissue is kept under tension with atraumatic grasping forceps to clearly demonstrate the cleavage line on the ovarian surface. It is sharply dissected off the ovary.

See also Plates 22, 71, and 72 for the continuation of this operation.

Plate 22. **Lysis of adhesions without prior hemostasis**

Operation: The epiploic appendix of the sigmoid colon has been sharply dissected off the ovary without prior coagulation, as shown in Plate 21. It is now pulled with atraumatic forceps through a catgut loop that has been introduced through a third puncture site. The pedicle will be ligated at its base and the protruding segment will be resected, as previously shown in Plate 9.

See also Plates 71 and 72.

14.2.2.3. Adhesiolysis After Prophylactic Hemostasis (Bloodless Adhesiolysis)

Plate 23. **Lysis of vascular adhesions after hemostasis**

History: The patient had had two previous laparotomies: an appendectomy at age 15 and a cesarean section at age 24.

Findings: The greater omentum is adherent to a wide area of the scar in the anterior abdominal wall.

Operation: To prevent excessive loss of blood, an endoligature is introduced with a needle-holder of 3 mm diameter through an applicator sleeve. A 5-mm-diameter needleholder has been placed behind the adhesions and has just received the end of the suture, which has been introduced through the sleeve on the right.

Caution: Although adhesiolysis without prior hemostasis is possible, it is not advisable. Such adhesions are often very vascular and bleed briskly after sharp dissection. The blood loss may be quite substantial before the bleeding vessels can be identified and ligated.

Plate 24. **Lysis of vascular adhesions after hemostasis**

Operation: The 5-mm needleholder has guided the suture (see Plate 23) around the broad adhesion and returned it back to the 3-mm needleholder, after approximately 60 cm of the endosuture was introduced into the peritoneal cavity. Its free end will then be pulled out through the trocar sleeve.

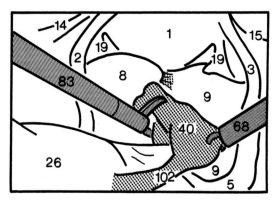 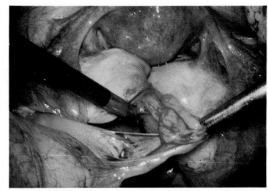

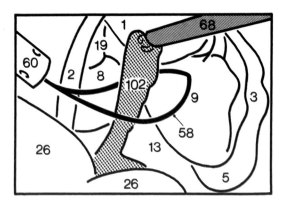 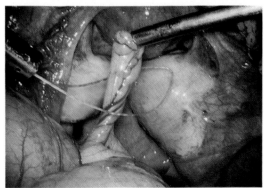

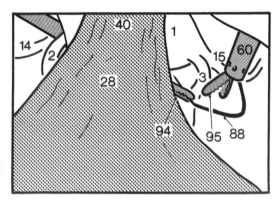 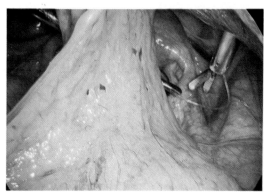

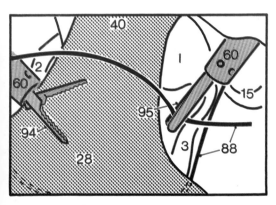 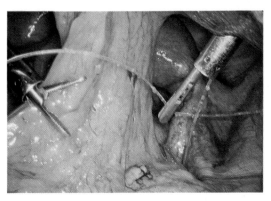

267

Plate 25. **Lysis of vascular adhesions after hemostasis: End result**
Operation: An external slipknot has been tied and pushed down with the plastic applicator cannula, ligating the broad base of the omental adhesion. It is shown being dissected off the anterior abdominal wall without any significant bleeding.
Comment: Should there be any bleeding from collateral blood vessels in the abdominal wall, hemostasis can usually be achieved by endocoagulation with the crocodile forceps without risk to vital structures. If necessary, another endoloop can be applied. If the pedicle of tissue in the endoligature is very large, one or two additional catgut loops should be applied, as is usual in a laparotomy.

Plate 26. **Lysis of vascular adhesions after hemostasis**
History: After a previous total abdominal hysterectomy with bilateral salpingo-oophorectomy, the patient complained of symptoms suggestive of partial intestinal obstruction.
Findings: The omentum is broadly adherent to the ileocecal area of the ascending colon.
Operation: A segment of the adhesion is isolated with atraumatic grasping forceps and the site for the ligature is chosen.

Plate 27. **Lysis of vascular adhesions after hemostasis**
Operation: An endosuture (after its needle has been cut off) has been introduced with a 3-mm needleholder through a second trocar sleeve. The segment of omental adhesions (shown in Plate 26) has been elevated with a 5-mm needleholder, which was introduced through a third trocar sleeve on the left side. The 5-mm needleholder is opened to receive the free end of the endosuture.

Plate 28. **Lysis of vascular adhesions after hemostasis**
Operation: The endosuture (shown in Plate 27) has been pulled through the bridge formed by the omental adhesions with the 5-mm needleholder, which is just disappearing into the left trocar sleeve. The 3-mm needleholder is prepared to regrasp the free end of the endosuture. After approximately 60 cm of suture material has been fed into the peritoneal cavity, the free end of the suture is withdrawn through the trocar sleeve and the slipknot is tied externally.

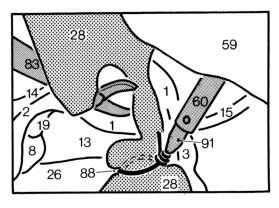

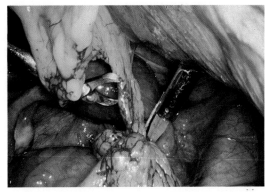

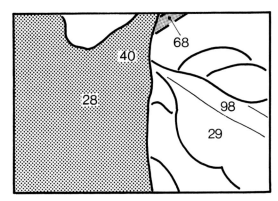

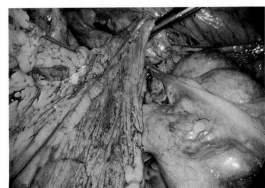

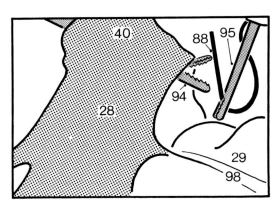

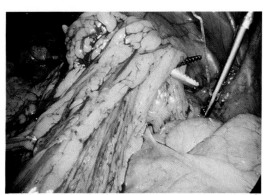

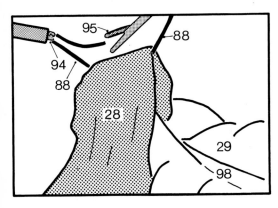

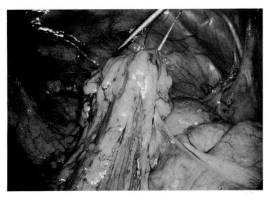

Plate 29. **Lysis of vascular adhesions after hemostasis**

Operation: The externally tied slipknot has been pushed with its plastic applicator tube into the peritoneal cavity, and the omental bridge has been ligated. The first ligature is cut with hook scissors.

Caution: The surgeon must ascertain that the ligature has been applied only to the omentum and that it does not include a loop of small intestines, etc., which may have been inadvertently pulled into the ligature.

Plate 30. **Lysis of vascular adhesions after hemostasis**

Operation: After the first ligature has been applied (see Plates 27–29), another endosuture is introduced with the aid of the 3-mm needleholder so that a second ligature can be applied. The omental bridge is again elevated with a 5-mm needleholder, which is ready to grasp the end of the endosuture.

Plate 31. **Lysis of vascular adhesions after hemostasis**

Operation: After the second endoligature has been applied with the plastic tube to the omental bridge, traction is applied to the omental adhesion with the aid of the plastic tube and the long end of the suture, which has not yet been cut. Hook scissors are used to cut the omental tissue between the two ligatures.

Comment: If necessary, both omental pedicles may be resecured by applying additional endoloops.

14.2.2.5. Pelviscopic Adhesiolysis in Preparation for a Laparotomy Either During the Same Operation or at Another Time

Plate 32. **Lysis of vascular adhesions after hemostasis**

History: A 42-year-old woman, para 3, had a history of right salpingo-oophorectomy and recent conization of the cervix. Microscopic examination revealed a microcarcinoma that was not completely surrounded by a margin of healthy tissue. A vaginal hysterectomy was considered for this multiparous patient.

Findings: Pelvic examination revealed findings suggestive of adhesions in the area of the previous salpingo-oophorectomy. This diagnosis was confirmed by pelvic laparoscopy.

Operation: Broad-based omental adhesions to the uterine fundus were endoligated and dissected without bleeding. With knowledge of the anatomical situation, the surgeon could then remove the uterus vaginally without difficulties.

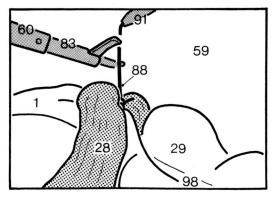

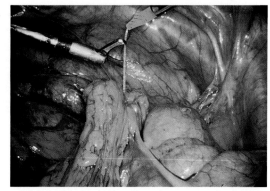

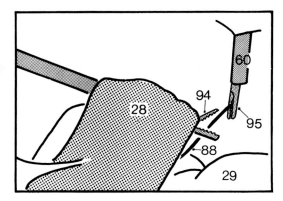

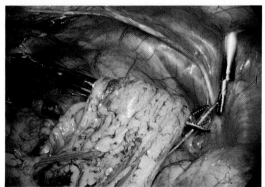

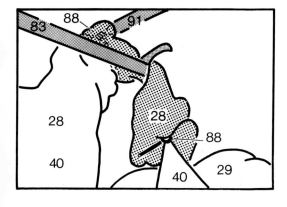

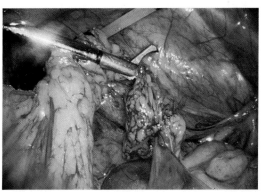

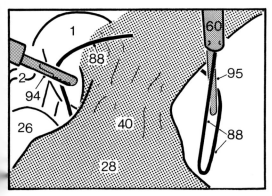

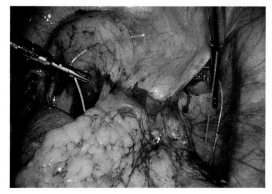

Plate 33. **Lysis of adhesions without prior hemostasis**
History: The patient had undergone two previous laparotomies for correction of sterility.
Findings: Diagnostic pelvic laparoscopy reveals extensive adhesions.
Operation: At the end of the present diagnostic laparoscopy, extensive endoscopic adhesiolysis is performed.
Comment: Correction of the bilateral intramural tubal occlusions is planned for a later laparotomy under microsurgical conditions, focusing only on reimplantation of the tubes.
See also Plates 34–36.

Plate 34. **Lysis of adhesions without prior hemostasis**
History: A 31-year-old patient with primary sterility had pelvic peritonitis at age 30 years.
Findings: Hysterosalpingography revealed bilateral intramural tubal occlusion. Extensive bilateral adhesions are seen at diagnostic pelvic laparoscopy and corrected by adhesiolysis without prior hemostasis.
See also Plate 35.

Plate 35. **Lysis of adhesions without prior hemostasis**
Operation: The adhesions shown in Plate 34 are held under tension with an atraumatic grasping forceps so that they may be separated from the pelvic structures with hook scissors. Bleeding omental pedicles are ligated with Roeder's endoloop. After completion of the adhesiolysis without prior hemostasis, the abdominal and pelvic cavities are repeatedly irrigated with saline solution. Finally, 500 mg of cortisone dissolved in 100–200 ml of saline solution is instilled into the pelvis (see chapters 14.2.2.1. ff. and 17.2.). It is hoped that the pelvis will be free of adhesions when the patient returns for a laparotomy and microsurgical correction several months later.

Plate 36. **Lysis of adhesions without prior hemostasis: Follow-up findings**
Findings: Eleven months later, the patient whose previous condition was shown in Plates 34 and 35 is undergoing a laparotomy with microsurgical correction of the tubal obstruction. No adhesions are noted between the intestinal and genital tracts.
Operation: Both tubes can be mobilized and reimplanted.

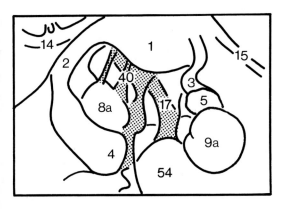

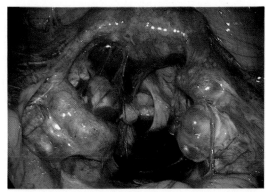

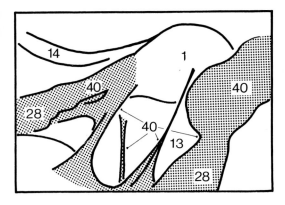

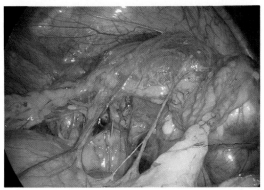

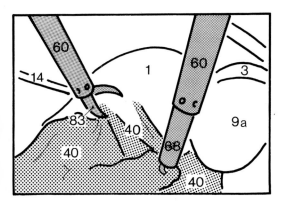

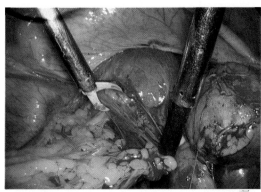

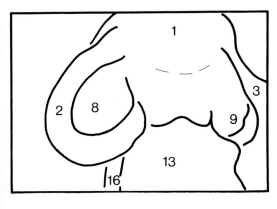

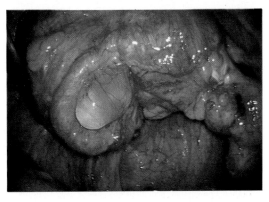

273

Plate 37. **Adhesiolysis with and without prior hemostasis**
History: A 32-year-old patient with secondary infertility was seen 5 years after a right salpingectomy was performed for tubal ectopic pregnancy.
Findings: Extensive peritoneal and omental adhesions.
Operation: Some of the broad-based omental adhesions will be dissected off the anterior abdominal wall after hemostatic coagulation; others will first be dissected sharply and then the pedicles will be ligated with endoloops.
See also Plates 38–40.

Plate 38. **Adhesiolysis with and without prior hemostasis**
Findings: The broad-based omental adhesions to the anterior abdominal wall, which had previously prevented the view and access into the pelvic cavity, have been lysed. Pelvic congestion is visible in the left adnexal area.
Operation: A broad-based adhesion of a segment of omentum to the right side of the uterine corpus at the site of the previous salpingectomy will be coagulated with the crocodile forceps.
See also Plates 37, 39, and 40.

Plate 39. **Adhesiolysis with and without prior hemostasis: End result**
Findings: The coagulated omental adhesion has been dissected off the uterine surface with hook scissors. It is clearly evident that the ovarian blood vessels have been severely damaged by the previous salpingectomy.
See also Plates 37, 38, 40, and 301–314.

Plate 40. **Adhesiolysis with and without prior hemostasis: Follow-up**
History: Appearance 7 months after laparoscopic adhesiolysis.
Findings: No adhesions are visible. The intramural segment of the left tube is obstructed by a small adenoma.
Operation: Laparotomy with Pfannenstiel* incision with microsurgical intramural implantation of the left tube will be performed immediately after this diagnostic laparoscopy.
See also Plates 37–39.

---

*H.-J. Pfannenstiel, Chairman of Obstetrics and Gynecology at the University of Kiel from 1907 until his death in 1909.

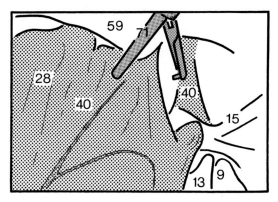
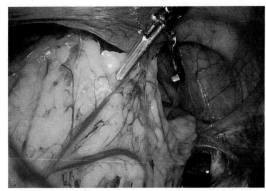

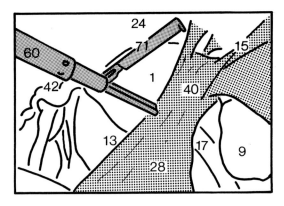
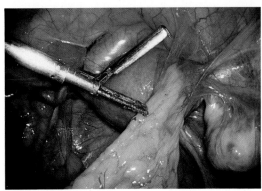

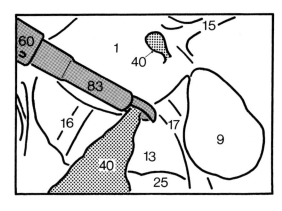
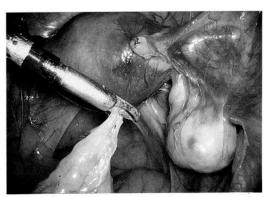

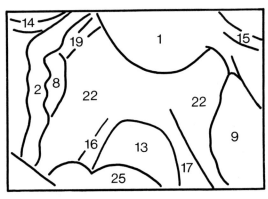
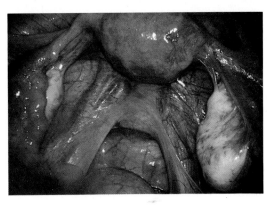

14.2.3.1. Excision of Endometriotic Implants

Plate 41. **Superficial abrasion and biopsy of endometriotic implants**
History: A 29-year-old woman was seen with primary infertility.
Findings: Widespread endometriotic implants in the dome of the bladder (Endoscopic Endometriosis Classification, EEC II).
Operation: Abrasion of the endometriotic implants with a biopsy forceps. Some larger areas are denuded of peritoneum.
See also Plate 42.

Plate 42. **Superficial abrasion and biopsy of endometriotic implants**
Operation: The raw surfaces caused by abrasion and superficial biopsy of endometriotic implants are coagulated with a point coagulator in a sweeping motion, as in ironing.
See also Plate 41.

Plate 43. **Excision of endometriotic implants**
Findings: Widespread retrocervical endometriosis (EEC III) in which the rectal ampulla is pulled anteriorly and attached to the cervix and posterior uterine wall.
Operation: Under careful observation of the rectal ampulla, the peritoneal adhesions are dissected bluntly with the aid of atraumatic forceps.
Caution: If it should become necessary to use scissors, the dissection should be done layer by layer under low-power magnification.
See also Plate 44.

Plate 44. **Excision of endometriotic implants**
Operation: After the rectal ampulla has been separated from the posterior wall of the uterus and the cervix, the retrocervical endometriotic implants (EEC III) shown in Plate 43 are removed with biopsy forceps and then their "basalis" is coagulated with a point coagulator. Finally, the peritoneal defect will be closed with interrupted catgut sutures.
See also Plates 53–57.

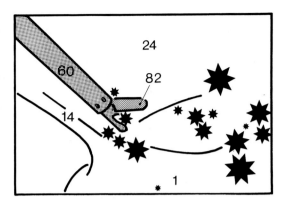

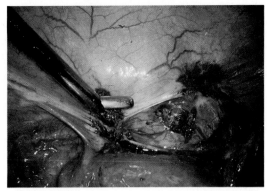

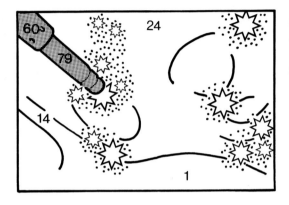

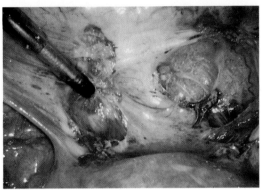

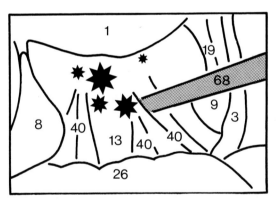

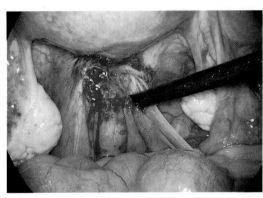

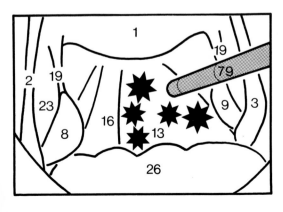

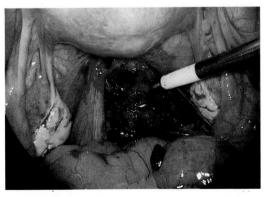

Plate 45. **Intestinal endometriosis**

Findings: A 27-year-old patient was seen with primary infertility. Illustration shows the typical appearance of intestinal endometriosis (EEC IV) on the sigmoid colon.

Caution: These implants penetrate to the muscularis and must not be coagulated.

Plate 46. **Endometriosis of appendix**

Findings: Endometriosis of the appendix (EEC IV). Involvement of the appendix is relatively common; however, it can hardly be recognized during the proliferative phase of the cycle.

Caution: A very meticulous search under low-power magnification may be necessary to detect such implants.

See also Plates 76, 386, and 387.

Plate 47. **Cornual adenoma**

Findings: Endometriosis in the cornual region of the uterus (EEC III) usually presents as a prominent bulge of the cornual region.

Comment: During chromopertubation and chromosalpingoscopy, particularly when the insufflation pressure has risen to 200–300 mm Hg, the cornual area first changes to a white color, then bluish when the dye is filling the tubular endometriotic glands, which penetrate diffusely into the muscular layers.

See also Plate 48.

Plate 48. **Uterine adenomyosis**

Operation: The cornual adenoma (EEC III) and blue discoloration of the uterine fundus are clearly visible, as is the blue discoloration of the uterine veins and lymphatic vessels. In contrast, the isthmic segment of the left tube shows a whitish discoloration. The right tube is patent.

Comment: If adenomyosis is extensive and the blue dye solution for chromopertubation is injected at a pressure of 200–300 mm Hg, it will diffuse into the myometrium. Such pertubation pressure may cause temporary ischemia of the intramural and isthmic portion of the tube.

See also Plate 47.

278

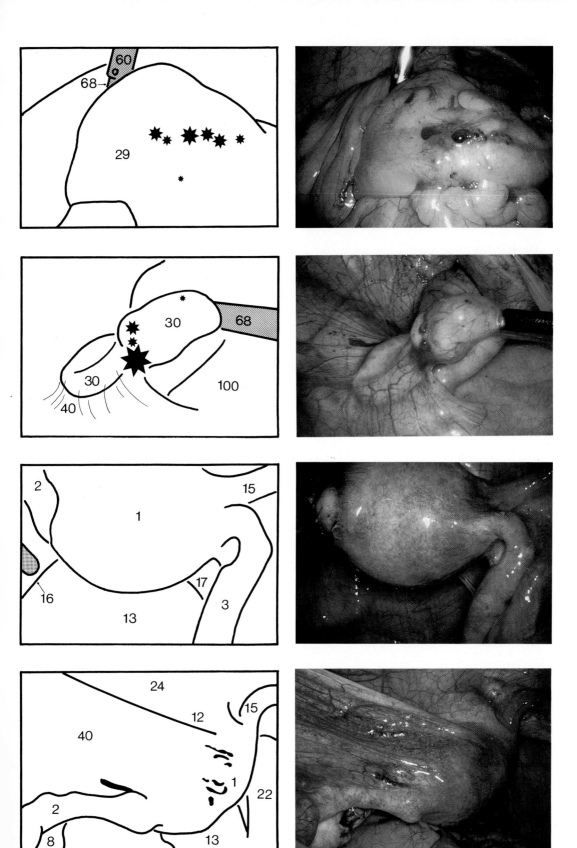

Plate 49. **Salpingitis isthmica nodosa**

Findings: Severe tubal adenomyosis (EEC III) is present in both tubes. Only a small amount of blood is seen in the cul-de-sac, whereas small endometriotic implants are barely visible in the proliferative phase of the cycle.

Operation: Both tubes were patent on ascending chromopertubation-chromosalpingoscopy.

Comment: In spite of tubal patency, the 34-year-old patient failed to conceive for years.

14.2.3.2. Coagulation of Endometriotic Implants

Plate 50. **Removal of retrocervical endometriotic implants**

Findings: Endometriotic implants in the anterior wall of the uterus and the dome of the bladder (EEC II). The endometriotic implants are destroyed by the endocoagulation technique.

Operation: The temperature of the point coagulator is preset at 120° C. Endometriotic implants are coagulated individually or in a sweeping "ironing" motion when widespread implants have to be treated. If deep-seated implants are present, they are coagulated after the peritoneum is opened. The thermocolor test shows a clear distinction between the healthy peritoneum and endometriotic implants (hemosiderin effect) (see Plates 53–57).

See also Plates 61–64, 76, 386, and 387.

Plate 51. **Removal of retrocervical endometriotic implants**

History: A 35-year-old patient had tried to conceive for 5 years and had chronic lower abdominal and pelvic pain, particularly with coitus.

Findings: Retrocervical nodules were palpable on vaginal examination and endometriotic implants were noted between both uterosacral ligaments (EEC II).

Operation: The implants are grasped with a biopsy forceps and opened.

See also Plate 106, showing the patient's status 8 months later.

Plate 52. **Removal of retrocervical endometriotic implants**

Operation: After the peritoneum has been opened widely, the endometriotic implants (EEC II) are resected, and all implants in the pelvis are coagulated with the point coagulator.

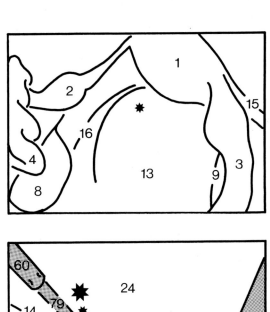
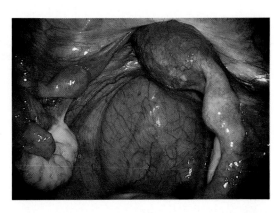

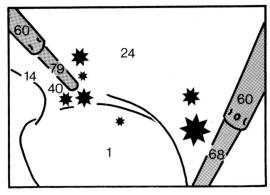
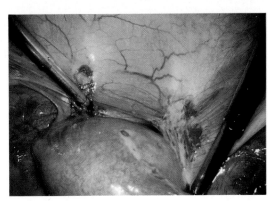

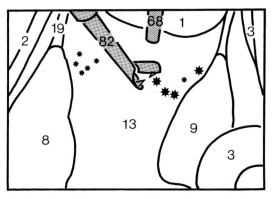
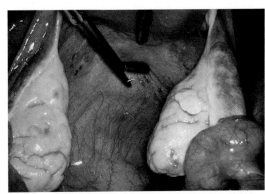

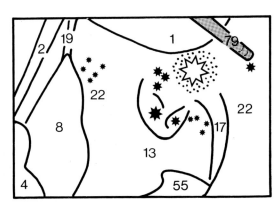
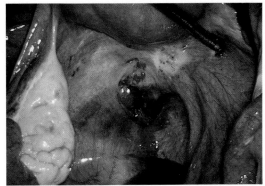

Plate 53. **Removal of retrocervical endometriotic implants**
Operation: The large peritoneal defect remaining after removal of retrocervical endometriotic implants (EEC II) is reapproximated by endosutures; the short, straight needle held
with the 3-mm needleholder has penetrated the right margin of the incision and will be
grasped by the 5-mm needleholder.

Plate 54. **Removal of retrocervical endometriotic implants**
Operation: After external tying of Roeder's slipknot, the knot is pushed into the peritoneal
cavity with the aid of the plastic applicator tube and the wound edges are approximated.

Plate 55. **Removal of retrocervical endometriotic implants**
Operation: After the first suture has been tied, the free end is cut with hook scissors. Since
the retrocervical wound edges were still gaping, a second suture was applied.
See also Plate 56.

Plate 56. **Removal of retrocervical endometriotic implants**
Operation: The second end of the suture has been introduced, and the needle, held in the
3-mm needleholder, has already penetrated the right margin of the wound, which remained
wide open after removal of the deep endometriotic implants and application of the first
suture. The 5-mm needleholder is ready to receive the needle.

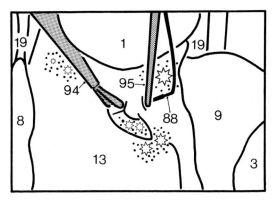
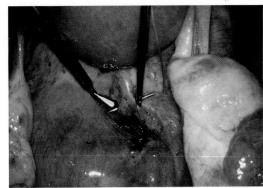

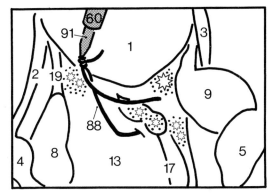
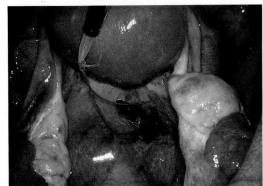

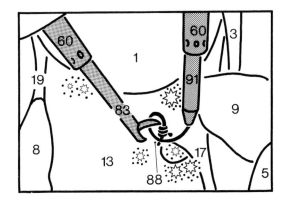
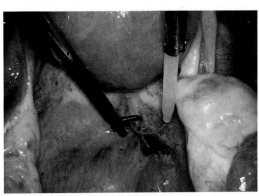

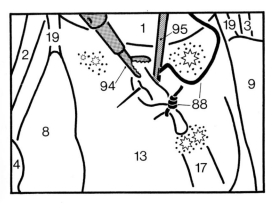
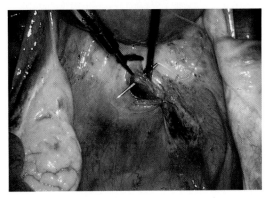

Plate 57. **Removal of retrocervical endometriotic implants: End result**

Operation/Findings: Appearance immediately after removal of deep retrocervical endometriotic nodules with closure of the peritoneal defect by endosutures.

Comment: Brown endometriotic implants within white fields are clearly visible after coagulation of the peritoneum (thermocolor test, hemosiderin effect).

See also Plates 51–56. Plate 106 shows the follow-up appearance 8 months later; conception occurred during the following cycle.

Plate 58. **Ovarian endometriosis**

Findings: Endometriotic implants are frequently found on the surface of the ovaries (EEC II).

Operation: These implants are easily coagulated with a point coagulator, which transmits heat to the surface of the ovary only by conduction, indicating heat-induced bionecrosis.

Caution: Coagulation with high-frequency current will heat up the entire ovary, causing serious damage. One or two atraumatic forceps should always be used to dislocate the ovary and to demonstrate endometriotic implants. About 20% of endometriotic implants occur behind the ovary and can be demonstrated only after appropriate elevation of the ovary.

See also Plate 60.

Plate 59. **Ovarian endometriosis**

Findings: Endometriosis penetrates deeply into the ovary (EEC III).

Operation: This biopsy forceps has spoon-shaped jaws at least 1.5 cm long. The teeth, just inside the distal lips, penetrate and hold the ovarian tissue, which can then be punched out by advancing the trocar sleeve.

See also chapter 14.2.5.

Plate 60. **Retro-ovarian endometriotic implants**

History: A 29-year-old patient was seen with primary sterility.

Findings: No evidence of endometriosis was detected through the infraumbilical laparoscope until an attempt was made to elevate the left ovary. It was found to be adherent to the broad ligament.

Operation: With the aid of two biopsy forceps, the ovary was freed from the adhesions and extensive endometriotic implants were noted.

Comment: Since 20% of endometriotic implants are located behind the ovaries (EEC II), a diagnosis is not possible from the umbilical perspective without adequate mobilization of the ovaries with ancillary instruments introduced through the second and third puncture sites.

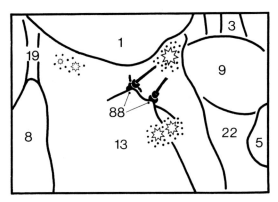

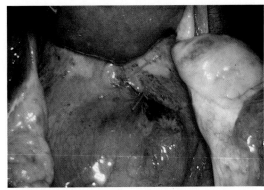

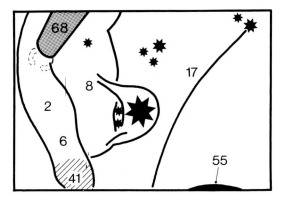

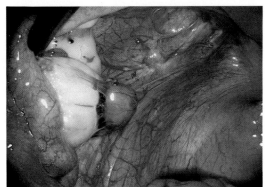

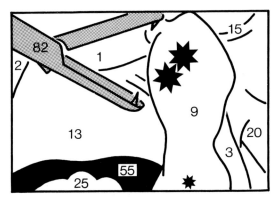

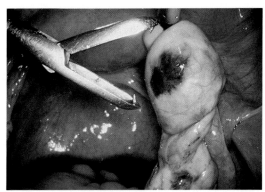

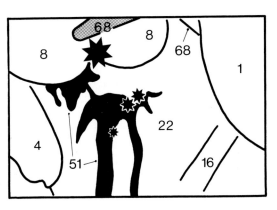

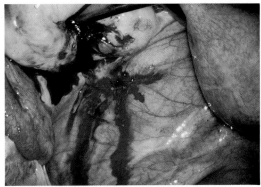

Plate 61.   **Thermocolor test for identification of endometriosis**
History: A 26-year-old patient was seen with primary infertility. Plate was made on the seventh day of her menstrual cycle.
Findings: Faint endometriotic implants in the dome of the bladder (EEC II) can be detected only with low-power magnification.
See also Plate 149.

Plate 62.   **Thermocolor test for identification of endometriosis**
Operation: Endocoagulation at 100° C changes the color of the peritoneum from pink to white. The endometriotic implant changes to a brown color (hemosiderin effect) and can be clearly distinguished from the surrounding white peritoneum.
Comment: A discoloration of the peritoneum due to endometriosis was barely distinguishable from the surrounding peritoneum during the proliferative phase of the cycle. Low-power magnification (Plate 61) raised the level of suspicion of endometriotic implants in the dome of the bladder. In such doubtful cases, the thermocolor test is very helpful.
See also Plates 63 and 64.

Plate 63.   **Thermocolor test for identification of endometriosis**
History: A 28-year-old patient with secondary infertility who had failed to conceive for 6 years was examined on cycle day 7.
Findings: Twenty-five milliliters of old menstrual blood was noted in the cul-de-sac and aspirated (EEC II). No source for this blood, such as endometriotic implants, could be detected on superficial inspection with the laparoscope.
Since fresh menstrual blood in the cul-de-sac usually originates from endometriotic implants, the thermocolor test was indicated.
See also Plate 64.

Plate 64.   **Thermocolor test for identification of endometriosis: End result**
Findings: After thermal coagulation, endometriotic implants show a brown discoloration (the hemosiderin effect). They show up clearly against the surrounding white peritoneum.
Comment: Endometriotic implants in the pelvis, and particularly in the area of the uterosacral ligaments, were suspected only from careful inspection of all pelvic organs with low-power laparoscopic magnification. The suspicion could be confirmed by the thermocolor test when the peritoneum was coagulated at 100° C.

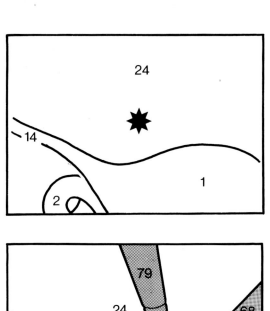

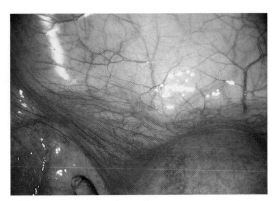

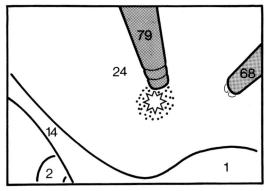

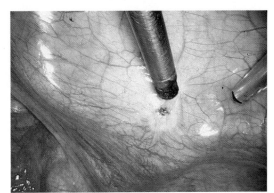

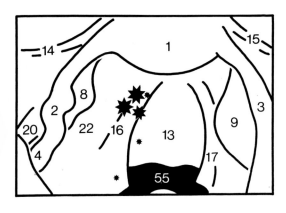

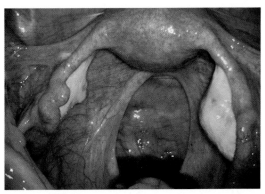

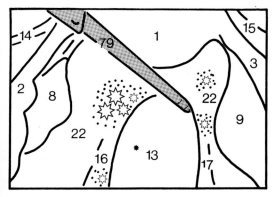

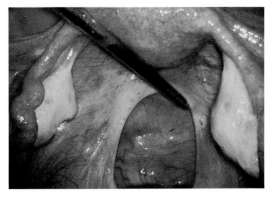

14.2.4.1. Endoscopic Salpingo-ovariolysis

Plate 65. **Salpingo-ovariolysis**

History: A 28-year-old patient was seen with primary infertility resulting from previous pelvic peritonitis.

Findings: Extensive velamentous adhesions between the posterior wall of the uterus and the rectal ampulla are noted, many of them extending to other loops of bowel. Marked pelvic congestion is also present, particularly of the venous plexus in the left broad ligament, where some vessels are 5–7 mm in diameter.

Operation: With careful observation of the rectal ampulla, the adhesions are coagulated with the crocodile forceps. Atraumatic forceps applied to the fringe of epiploic appendices keeps the rectal ampulla under tension so that the sheets of adhesions can be pulled as far away from the intestinal wall as possible.

Plate 66. **Salpingo-ovariolysis**

Findings: The vascular sheets of adhesions, which have resulted from previous pelvic inflammatory diseases, have already been coagulated (see Plate 65).

Operation: The adhesions are kept under considerable tension with atraumatic forceps and cut with hook scissors without causing any bleeding. The pool of blood in the cul-de-sac strongly suggests the presence of superficial endometriosis (EEC II).

Plate 67. **Salpingo-ovariolysis**

History: A 31-year-old patient had primary infertility for 5 years.

Findings: Very vascular adhesions between the left tube and the sigmoid colon indicate an inflammatory etiology.

Operation: The tube is grasped with atraumatic grasping tongs and the sheets of adhesions are kept under tension. They can first be coagulated with the crocodile forceps without risk to adjacent bowel; then they can be dissected without bleeding.

Plate 68. **Salpingo-ovariolysis**

Findings: The tube has been separated from bowel, as shown in Plate 67.

Operation: The tubal ampulla is grasped with atraumatic forceps, and dense adhesions are seen between the ampulla and the left ovary. Because of manipulation and tension on the dilated tubal ampulla (i.e., a sactosalpinx), traces of blue dye solution escape as the crocodile forceps is used to coagulate layers of adhesions.

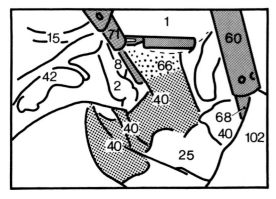

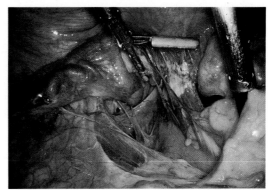

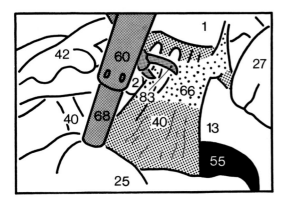

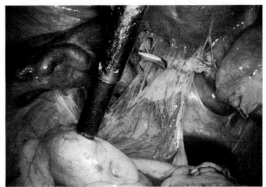

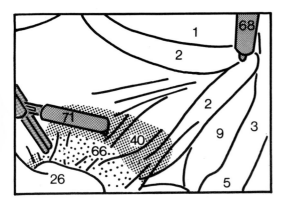

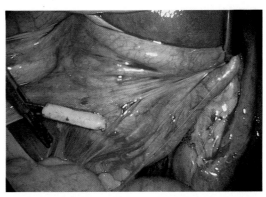

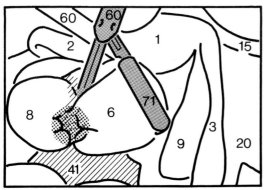

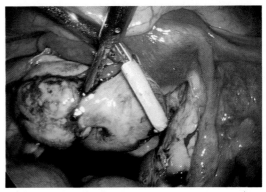

Plate 69.   **Salpingo-ovariolysis**
Operation: After the tubo-ovarian adhesions have been carefully coagulated, the tubal ampulla can be sharply dissected off the ovary without causing any bleeding. Methylene blue solution has been instilled into the uterus under continuous pressure, controlled by an appropriate injection pump (see chapter 12.4.2.), and is now flowing from the fimbrial end of the tube, which is beginning to expand. The layers of adhesions are again brought into view by keeping the tubal ampulla under tension with atraumatic grasping forceps. In some cases, a special instrument designed for the enucleation of myomas (for endocoagulation and cutting) may be utilized.

Plate 70.   **Salpingo-ovariolysis**
Operation: After the tubal ampulla has been dissected off the ovary, one can begin with the eversion of the fimbria and dilatation of the tubal ampulla.
See also Plates 75, 80, 86, and 91–93.

Plate 71.   **Salpingo-ovariolysis**
Findings: This plate illustrates the continuation of the procedure shown in plates 21 and 22. The tubal ampulla is attached to the ovary by some of its fimbria.
Operation: The atraumatic grasping forceps is used to keep the adhesions under tension. Since some of the fimbria are very vascular, the bridge of adhesions is coagulated for 20 seconds with the crocodile forceps at a temperature of 100° C before it can be severed.
Comment: Occasionally it is less traumatic to the tissues if the adhesions are coagulated and dissected with the myoma enucleator.

Plate 72.   **Salpingo-ovariolysis**
Findings: The bridge of adhesions has been coagulated (see Plate 71).
Operation: The tubal ampulla is kept under tension with the atraumatic grasping forceps so that the adhesions can be cut with hook scissors at the level of the tunica albuginea without causing any bleeding.

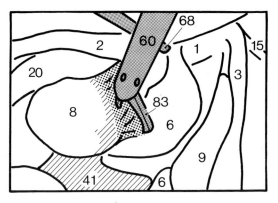
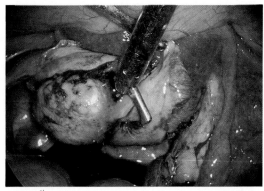

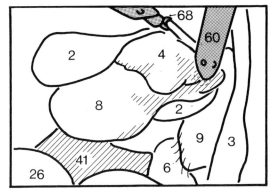
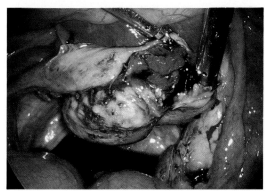

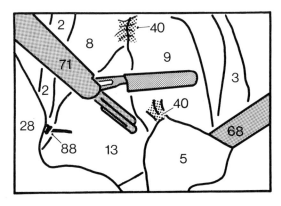
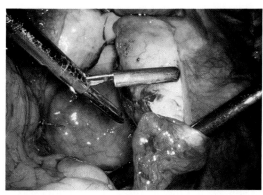

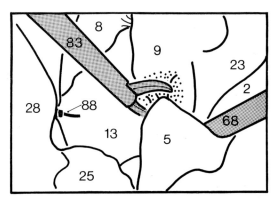
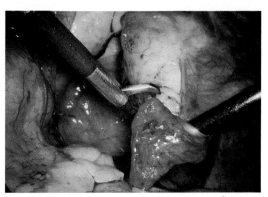

14.2.4.2. Endoscopic Fimbrioplasty

Plate 73.   **Blunt fimbriolysis**

History: A 33-year-old patient was seen with primary infertility.

Findings: Salpingitis isthmica nodosa distorts the right tube, which is quite distended after instillation of methylene blue solution under 200 mm Hg pressure. The left tube is clearly obstructed by an intramural nodule of endometriosis.

Operation: Atraumatic grasping tongs and atraumatic grasping forceps are used to demonstrate the course of the tube. Only traces of the blue solution are trickling from the fimbrial end (see p. 231–232 for the contents of the methylene blue solution).

Plate 74.   **Blunt fimbriolysis**

Operation: The atraumatic grasping tongs and the atraumatic grasping forceps are used to distend the tubal ampulla. However, due to an ampullary stenosis or phimosis, the blue solution does not yet escape freely, corresponding to a patency grade I (according to Fikentscher and Semm).

See also Plate 75 for continuation of procedure.

Plate 75.   **Blunt fimbriolysis: End result**

Operation: The atraumatic grasping forceps is used to bring the tubal ostium into the same axial position in which the atraumatic grasping tongs will be introduced. The closed tongs will then be advanced 2–3 cm into the right tubal ampulla. The tongs will then be opened and withdrawn in the opened position, as demonstrated in Plate 80. The methylene blue solution now flows freely and without distention of the infundibular portion of the tubal ampulla. This is a clear indication that the stenosis or phimosis has been eliminated.

See also Plate 74.

Plate 76.   **Endometriosis of the genital tract and phimosis of the tubal ampulla**

History: A 28-year-old patient was seen with primary infertility.

Findings: Blood is pooled in the cul-de-sac.

Comment: A pool of blood in the cul-de-sac is typical for superficial endometriosis of the genital tract and indicates recent bleeding from endometriotic implants. Up to 50 ml of menstrual blood can often be aspirated from the cul-de-sac. Whenever there is a large pool of blood in the cul-de-sac it is an almost certain sign of superficial endometriosis of the genital tract. One must search for it carefully under low-power magnification (see Plates 386 and 387). Other differential diagnostic possibilities must be excluded, such as fresh bleeding caused by insufflation of the pneumoperitoneum or the introduction of the trocar for the laparoscope. A collection of blood in the cul-de-sac is often interpreted as retrograde menstruation. In the case illustrated, no endometriotic implants were diagnosed or coagulated. However, 11 months later, when another laparoscopy was performed, the previously missed diagnosis of endometriosis was made by the thermocolor test.

See also Plates 386 and 387, which show the findings on repeat laparoscopy.

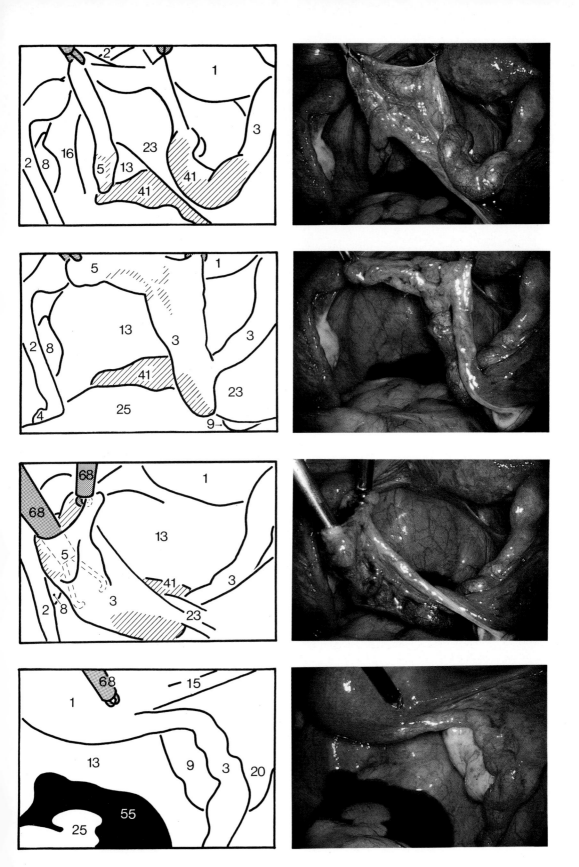

Plate 77. **Endometriosis of the genital tract and phimosis of the tubal ampulla**

Findings: Although the ampullary segments of the tubes appear to be perfectly normal in Plates 71, 72, 74, and 79, these tubes are closed, or at least severely obstructed in the preampullary region. The blue dye solution is injected at a pressure of 250 mm Hg which, as shown here, will cause considerable distention of the tubes before traces of the dye solution begin to trickle from the fimbrial ends.

Comment: Hysterosalpingography would have indicated the wrong diagnosis: bilateral tubal patency. Only pelviscopy permits an accurate diagnosis of the site and degree of the stenosis, which can then be corrected at the same time.

See also Plates 73–75 and 80.

Plate 78. **Blunt dilatation of the tubal ampulla**

History: A 28-year-old patient was seen with primary sterility; she had undergone an appendectomy at age 16.

Findings: Superficial endometriosis of the genital tract, stage EEC I.

Operation: The methylene blue solution, instilled for chromopertubation with a pressure of 200 mm Hg, causes considerable distention of the right tube, but only traces escape through the ampullary portion. The right ovary is demonstrated with an atraumatic grasping forceps.

Plate 79. **Blunt dilatation of the tubal ampulla**

Operation: One begins to correct the obstruction by stretching the ampullary portion of the right tube between two atraumatic grasping forceps until the blue dye solution can escape. It had been contained behind the obstruction at a pressure of 200 mm Hg. Since the complete expansion of the ampulla cannot be accomplished by merely stretching the fimbria . . .

Plate 80. **Blunt dilatation of the tubal ampulla: End result**

Operation: . . . atraumatic grasping tongs are introduced in a closed position, as clearly shown in this Plate, then the instrument is opened and retracted in an open position. The spring-like mechanism of the atraumatic grasping tongs prevents laceration of the stenosed tubal walls. Occasionally it will be necessary to repeat the introduction of the closed forceps and retraction of the opened forceps several times before the preampullary stenosis can be completely eliminated.

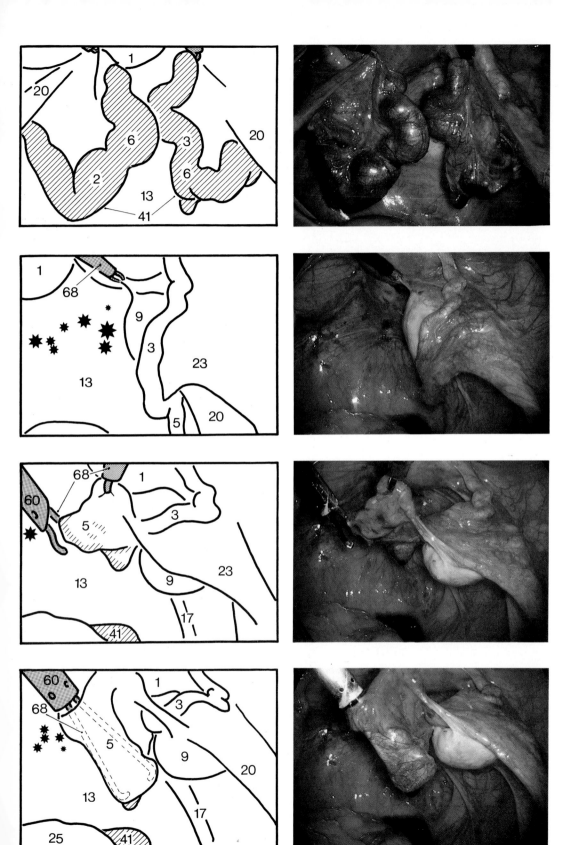

Plate 81. **Salpingoplasty by blunt dilatation**
History: A 29-year-old patient with secondary infertility had undergone four previous lapa-rotomies for appendectomy at age 14, suspected ectopic pregnancy at age 24, adhesiolysis at age 25, and right salpingectomy for ectopic tubal pregnancy at age 26.
Findings: Hysterosalpingography confirms the status after right salpingectomy and a hy-drosalpinx/sactosalpinx on the left side.

Plate 82. **Salpingoplasty by blunt dilatation**
Operation: The sactosalpinx of the left tube, which was diagnosed from the hysterosalpin-gographic appearance in Plate 81, is demonstrated with the aid of an atraumatic suction cannula attached to the ampullary segment. When dye solution is injected through a uterine cannula with a pressure monitor set at 250 mm Hg, ascending chromosalpingoscopy reveals distention of the left fallopian tube to a level of approximately 1 cm before the ampulla.

Plate 83. **Salpingoplasty by blunt dilatation: End result**
Operation: The sactosalpinx, shown in Plates 81 and 82, has been opened by blunt dilata-tion with two atraumatic grasping forceps. Atraumatic grasping forceps is repeatedly intro-duced into the tubal ampulla to a level of 2–3 cm (see Plates 75 and 80) until agglutination of the fimbriae has been completely eliminated. As is seen in this Plate, the methylene blue solution drips freely from the fimbriae, corresponding to a patency grade I (according to Fikentscher and Semm).

14.2.4.3. Endoscopic Salpingostomy

14.2.4.3.1. DISTAL SALPINGOSTOMY
Plate 84. **Salpingoplasty/salpingostomy**
History: A 25-year-old patient with primary sterility was seen 5 years after laparotomy was performed for appendicitis with perforation.
Findings: Extensive adhesions in the middle and lower peritoneal cavity prevent a view into the pelvis.
Operation: The omental adhesions are kept under tension with atraumatic grasping forceps so that adhesiolysis can be accomplished with hook scissors, mostly at the level of avascular cleavage lines on the parietal peritoneum.

296

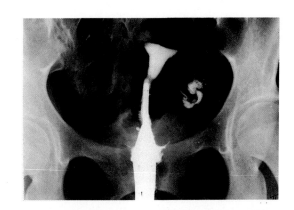

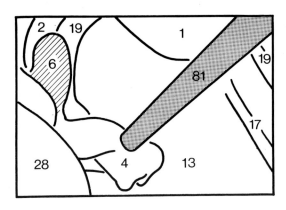

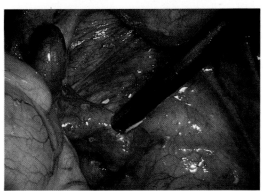

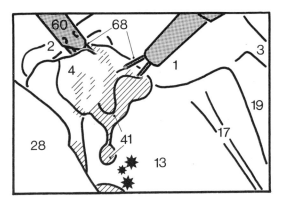

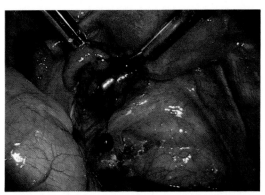

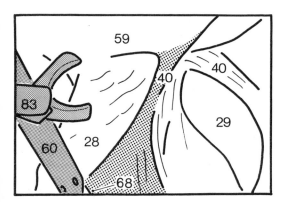

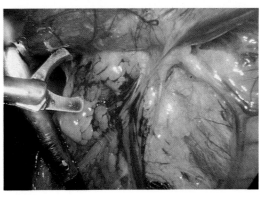

Plate 85.   **Salpingoplasty/salpingostomy with suture**
Findings: After chromopertubation, monitored at 300 mm Hg, the entire length of the left tubal ampulla and its scarred fimbrial end are visible. The right tube presents as sactosalpinx.
Operation: The ampulla is elevated with atraumatic grasping forceps and a navel-like dimple of the fimbriae can be recognized. Methylene blue hydropertubation solution (for ingredients, see chapter 17.3.) emerges from a pinhead-sized area, through which the fimbriae can be clearly recognized with low-power magnification of a loupe attached to the ocular end of the endoscope.

Plate 86.   **Salpingoplasty/salpingostomy with suture**
Findings: After the inverted, fibrosed fimbriae have been dilated and teased apart with two atraumatic grasping forceps, as shown in Plates 74, 79, and 83, constricting scars have been eliminated almost without blood loss.
Operation: After repeated introduction of the right atraumatic grasping forceps into the tube, as shown in Plates 75 and 80, the endosalpinx is grasped approximately 2 cm inside the ostium and everted. An excellent cuff can be made on the ampullary portion of the tube. The gas flow monitor shows a pressure of 150 mm Hg at a flow rate of 120 ml/min, which corresponds to a tubal patency grade I, according to Fikentscher and Semm.

Plate 87.   **Salpingoplasty/salpingostomy with suture: End result**
Operation: The everted fimbriae of the left tube, shown in Plates 85 and 86, will be secured by endosutures. This ensures that the success of this operation will not be reversed, during the next few hours, by another collapse and retraction of the fimbriae. A combined gas-fluid pertubation shows the emergence of a foamy blue dye solution corresponding to a grade I tubal patency. This concludes the operation on this tube.
Comment: In this case, the endosuture was accomplished by external tying of the slipknot. However, the endosuture technique with Ethicon PDS 4–0 suture and internal tying of the knot would have been preferable. This suture material will be absorbed after 5–7 months.

Plate 88.   **Salpingostomy with suture**
Findings: The right tube, which was shown in an overview in Plate 85, is considerably distended by the blue dye solution injected at a pressure of 300 mm Hg (sactosalpinx). The fimbrial end is completely sealed by scar tissue; however, the old ostium can be clearly recognized by a dimpled scar.

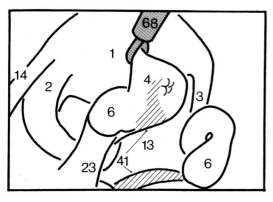
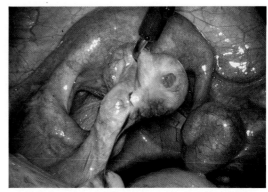

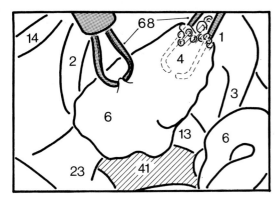
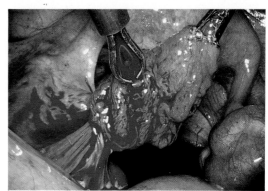

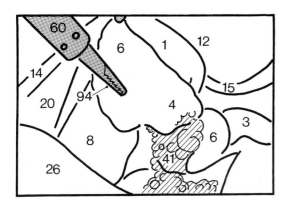
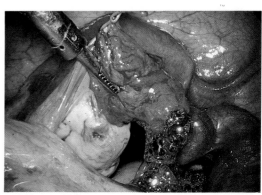

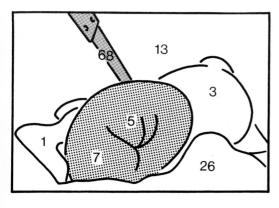
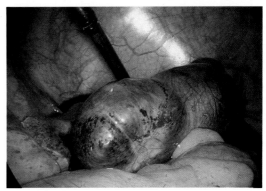

Plate 89.   **Salpingostomy with suture**

Operation: Hemostasis in this ''umbilical area'' of the ampullary portion of the right tube is accomplished by coagulating a strip approximately 2 cm long and 4 mm in diameter with a point coagulator, set at 100° C, before the tubal ampulla is opened widely with scissors in the area of the old tubal ostium.

See also Plate 90.

Plate 90.   **Salpingostomy with suture**

Operation: The chromopertubation solution is instilled at a monitored pressure of 250 mm Hg to fully distend the ampullary portion of the tube. The distended tube is elevated with atraumatic grasping forceps and the scarred, retracted ostium can be opened widely with scissors without causing any bleeding. The blue dye solution will emerge immediately.

Plate 91.   **Salpingostomy with suture**

Operation: The sactosalpinx of the right tube, shown in Plates 88–90, has been split open. The ampullary portion will be everted widely with the aid of a 3-mm needleholder (right) and atraumatic grasping tongs (left). The dilated ampulla is clearly seen.

Comment: Inspection under low-power magnification reveals that the normal fimbrial architecture has been lost and that the ampullary portion is lined with only a smooth, flat epithelium. This will decrease the potential to conceive through this tube to almost 0%.

Plate 92.   **Salpingostomy with suture**

Operation: The salpingostomy, shown in Plates 88–91, is terminated by attaching the everted tubal ampulla to the serosa of the tube by using endosutures and external tying of the knots. The free end of the second endosalpinx suture will be cut with hook scissors.

Comment: Endosutures are used to maintain the everted status of the tubal ampulla, as has already been shown in Plate 87, after salpingoplasty/salpingostomy by blunt dilatation, just as is customarily done when infertility surgery is performed through a laparotomy incision. It is preferable to secure the everted fimbria with Ethicon PDS 4–0 to 6–0 endosutures and to tie the knots internally, but this technique had not been developed by Semm at the time the photographs were taken.

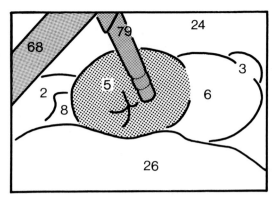

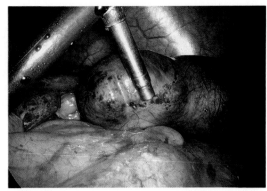

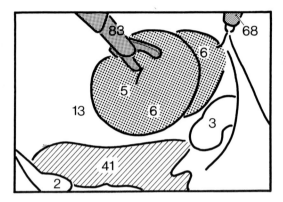

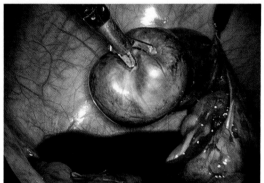

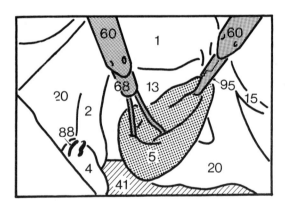

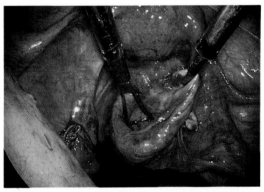

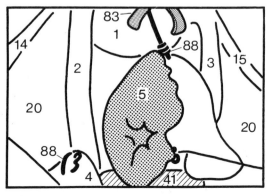

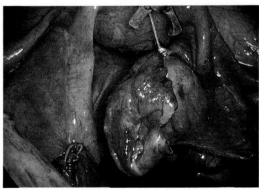

Plate 93. **Salpingostomy with suture: End result**
Findings: End result after extensive adhesiolysis in the mid and lower abdomen and salpin-goplasty/salpingotomy of a sactosalpinx of the left and right tube, in which the ampullary portions of both tubes were incised with scissors and the everted ampullary portions of the tubes were fixed to the tubal surface with endosutures.
Operation: The methylene blue chromosalpingoscopy solution emerges freely from both sides, corresponding to a tubal patency grade I.
See also Plates 84–92.

Plate 94. **Salpingostomy and extensive adhesiolysis on the left side**
History: A 26-year-old patient was seen with primary infertility 15 years after an appendec-tomy was performed.
Findings: The hysterosalpingogram reveals a huge sactosalpinx on the left side and only minimal filling of the right tube, with ampullary obstruction.

Plate 95. **Salpingostomy and extensive adhesiolysis on the left side**
Findings: Massive peritoneal adhesions prevent inspection of the pelvic organs with the pelviscope.
Operation: Introduction of the secondary trocar under visual control clearly demonstrates mobility of the parietal peritoneum. In this case, it was pushed ahead of the conical trocar into the peritoneal cavity a distance of about 10 cm before it was perforated by the trocar.
Caution: Transpose this photograph to the primary puncture with the Veress needle in the subumbilical area, particularly if the puncture is not made perpendicular to the peritoneum but in a more tangential direction! Consider the possibility of intestinal or vascular injuries!
See also Plate 1.

Plate 96. **Salpingostomy and extensive adhesiolysis on the left side**
Operation: Adhesions extending particularly toward the area of the appendectomy scar on the right side, and which are far removed from the intestines, are first coagulated with the crocodile forceps before they are cut with scissors. The omental pedicles are then secured with Roeder's endoloops.

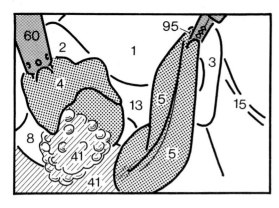
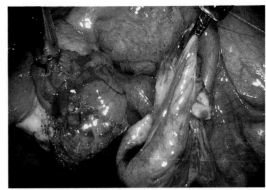

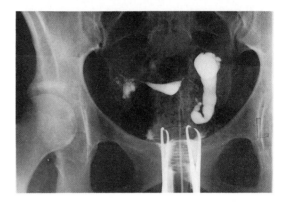

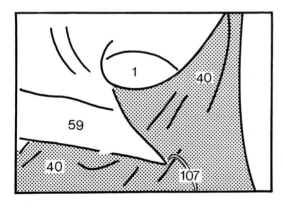
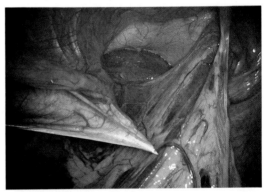

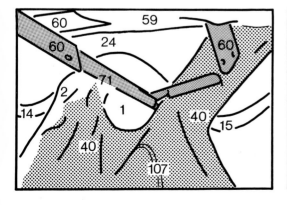
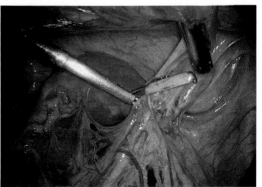

Plate 97. **Salpingostomy and extensive adhesiolysis on the left side**

Operation: All intra-abdominal adhesions (shown in Plates 95 and 96) have been dissected and the sacculated left tube (shown in Plate 94) has been distended at constant, monitored pressures of 250 mm Hg. With the assistance of atraumatic grasping forceps, the ampulla is held in a suitable position for inspection and operation so that the dimpled scar is clearly visible and can be coagulated with a point coagulator.

Plate 98. **Salpingostomy and extensive adhesiolysis on the left side**

Operation: After adequate coagulation with the point coagulator, the ampulla of the left tube is fixed with atraumatic grasping forceps. The tube is distended with chromopertubation solution, kept under constantly monitored pressure of 250 mm Hg, and opened widely with hook scissors. This is followed by eversion and fixation of the ampullary portion according to the endosuture technique illustrated in Plates 86 and 87 or Plate 91, respectively, using at least two atraumatic grasping tongs or grasping forceps and needleholder. PDS 4–0 to 6–0 sutures are used and the knots are tied externally or, preferably, internally.

Plate 99. **Salpingostomy and extensive adhesiolysis on the left side: End result**

Operation: After careful, bloodless eversion of the ampullary portion of the left tube, the free margins of the ampulla are secured by two to three endosutures to the corresponding adjacent sites of tubal serosa.

Comment: The sutures will maintain the operative result, i.e., patency of the everted fimbrial end, which was closed earlier. Inspection under low-power magnification reveals that in this case, too, the normal fimbrial architecture no longer exists, as a consequence of previous inflammatory changes in the sactosalpinx. A cuboidal tubal epithelium without cilia has replaced the fimbrial epithelium. This will considerably decrease the patient's potential for conception.

Plate 100. **Abdominal adhesions after previous operation to correct sterility**

History: A 29-year-old patient was seen after three previous laparotomies, performed for an appendectomy at age 18, for renal surgery at age 24, and for an anterior suspension of the uterus at age 28. The immediate postoperative course after microsurgical bilateral salpingostomy and anterior suspension of the uterus was febrile.

Findings: An overview reveals extensive adhesions in both adnexal areas.

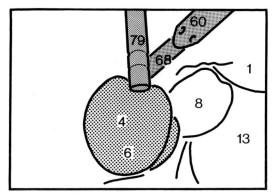
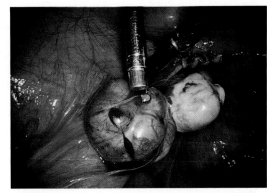

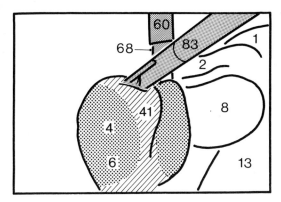
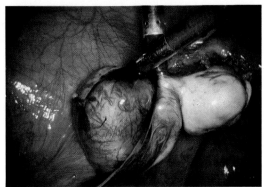

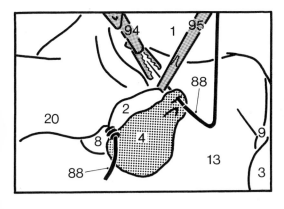
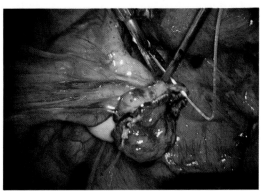

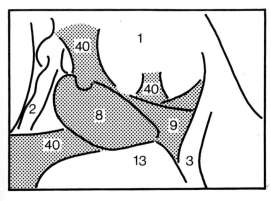
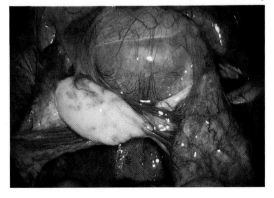

Plate 101. **Bilateral stomatoplasty**

Operation: Ascending chromopertubation at a pressure of 250 mm Hg distends both fallopian tubes. The right tube has been grasped with an atraumatic grasping forceps. After adhesiolysis of an omental pedicle, a small area of hemorrhage has been coagulated and there is minimal bleeding from both ovaries after ovariolysis and salpingolysis. The right tubal cornu shows some blue discoloration, compatible with adenomyosis (EEC II). After extensive ovariolysis and salpingolysis, salpingostomies were performed at the free end of both tubes. Since adenomyosis or interstitial salpingosis with stenosis was present intraoperatively, chromopertubation revealed only grade III tubal patency.

Comment: Surgery was followed by treatment with Danazol for 6 months. Thereafter the patient was readmitted for follow-up pelviscopy and laparotomy with microsurgical tubal reimplantation.

See also Plate 102, which shows the appearance on follow-up 11 months later.

Plate 102. **Bilateral stomatoplasty: Follow-up status of Plate 101**

History: Eleven months earlier, extensive ovariolysis, salpingolysis, salpingostomy, and omental adhesiolysis had been performed, followed by a 6-month course of Danazol treatment.

Findings: Internal pelvic organs are completely free of adhesions, and ascending chromopertubation reveals normal patency for dye solution in both tubes (tubal patency for CO_2 gas: grade I).

Comment: The antigonadotropin therapy apparently eliminated the adenomyosis in the tubal cornu (see Plate 101); therefore, this favorable result of the previous pelviscopic stomatoplasty made another surgical procedure unnecessary.

14.2.4.3.2. ISTHMIC SALPINGOSTOMY

Plate 103. **Isthmic neosalpingostomy on the right side**

History: A 35-year-old patient had undergone two previous laparotomies, including left salpingectomy, in an effort to correct secondary sterility.

Findings: On the right side, only a tubal stump is visible.

Operation: Since the patient requested that a "last attempt" be made, it was decided to perform a neosalpingostomy in the midsegment of the tube. The closed tubal stump had to be coagulated initially with the crocodile forceps for about 10 seconds at 100° C before the terminal segment could be resected without blood loss.

Plate 104. **Isthmic neosalpingostomy on the right side**

Operation: After careful coagulation of approximately 3 mm of tubal tissue, the closed terminal tubal segment was cut off with hook scissors, without blood loss. The chromopertubation solution, which had filled the uterine cavity and the right tube under a pressure of 250 mm Hg, immediately squirted from the patent tubal stump, mixed with gas bubbles. This terminates the operative procedure.

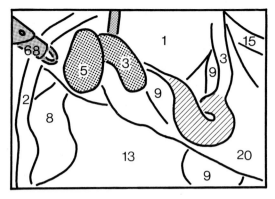
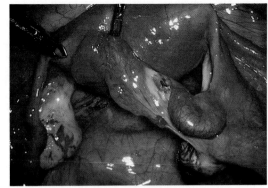

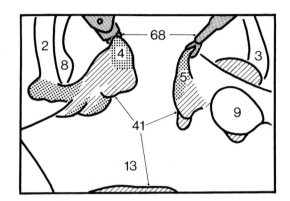
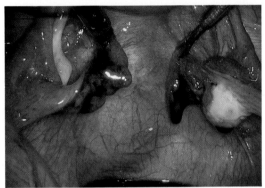

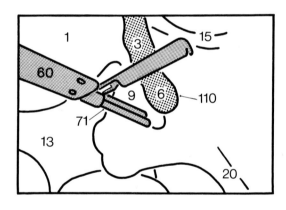
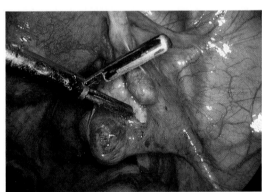

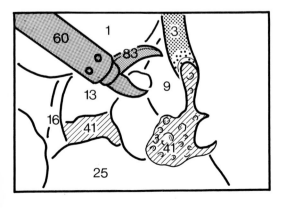
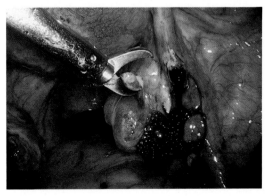

Plate 105. **Isthmic neosalpingostomy on the right side: End result**

Findings: The tubal fistula, which was created in Plates 103 and 104, is demonstrated again under four-power magnification. One can quickly recognize the coagulated zone of about 1–2 mm in depth with hemostasis in its blood vessels. The tubal lumen has a diameter of about 1 mm.

Comment: This patient conceived 7 months after the procedure and was delivered at term of a healthy son.

Caution: This result—although extremely rare—should encourage every gynecologic surgeon to make a last effort, even in such dismal surgical situations. This is particularly true when a laparoscopic procedure can spare the patient the risk of a laparotomy.

14.2.4.4. Endoscopic Tubal Surgery in the Presence of Endometriosis

Plate 106. **Tubal patency in the presence of pelvic endometriosis (see Plates 51–57)**

History: A 35-year-old patient was seen with primary infertility for 5 years. Eight months earlier she underwent excision of deep-seated retrocervical endometriotic implants, and the peritoneal defect was closed with endosutures, as shown in Plates 51–57.

Findings: Both tubes are patent; however, typical endometriotic changes are still present: the methylene blue solution, mixed with CO_2 gas bubbles, emerges at a pressure of 200 mm Hg. Due to a preampullary stenosis or phimosis, which is characteristic for endometriosis, the ampullary portions of both tubes are severely distended.

Comment: A phimosis seems to represent a protective mechanism against the foreign body reaction that is always present in the cul-de-sac. It is necessary to remove the menstrual blood. In the present case, bilateral blunt salpingoplasty was performed, with introduction and separation of the prongs of the atraumatic grasping tongs, as shown in Plates 75 and 80. After the dilatation, the chromopertubation solution emerged without distending the ampullary portion of the tube, representing a grade I patency. This was interpreted as proof of removal of the ampullary stenosis. The patient conceived during the following cycle and gave birth to a healthy son.

14.2.5. Pelviscopic Ovarian Biopsy

Plate 107. **Biopsy of an ovary supported by the uterus and pelvic wall**

History: A 51-year-old patient had undergone a cholecystectomy in 1969 and a laparotomy with right salpingo-oophorectomy in 1981.

Findings: The left ovary was enlarged and had a suspicious surface pattern. Therefore, biopsy was indicated.

Operation: Since it is difficult to grasp the ovary, the uterus has to be positioned deep in the cul-de-sac and turned toward the left side, displacing the ovary anteriorly and laterally, where it is sufficiently fixed and can be grasped with a forceps. This maneuver will make unnecessary a third puncture, through which the ovary could also be grasped with an atraumatic forceps and brought into the same position.

Comment: The biopsy forceps with jaws of 15 mm length and two internal spikes is introduced through a secondary suprapubic 5-mm trocar sleeve. The ovarian surface selected for the biopsy is fixed between the two spikes, and the jaws of the biopsy forceps are then closed as much as possible.

Plate 108. **Biopsy of an ovary supported by the uterus and pelvic wall**

Operation: An assistant advances the trocar sleeve into the abdomen and at the same time applies traction on the biopsy forceps. The distal cutting edge of the trocar sleeve will punch out the specimen of ovarian tissue, which is grasped within the biopsy forceps.

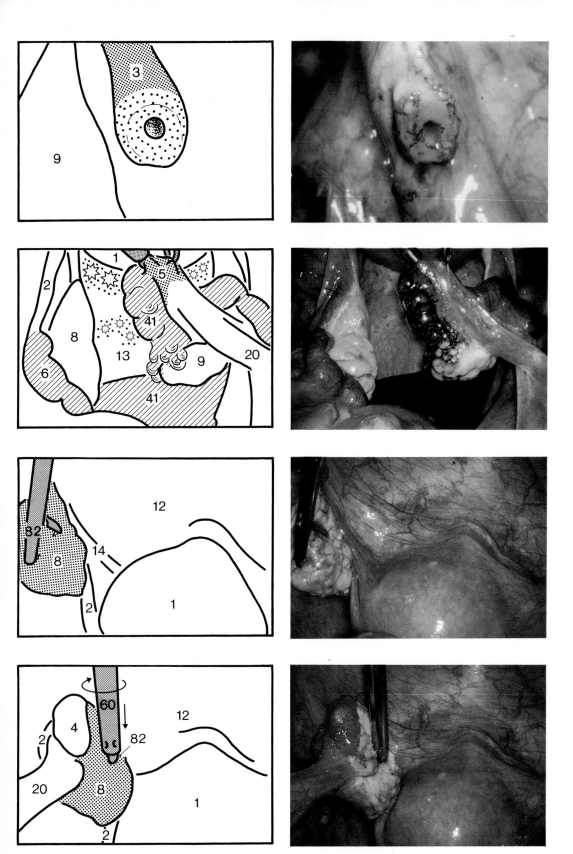

Plate 109.   **Biopsy of an ovary supported by the uterus and pelvic wall: End result**
Operation: The defect left by the biopsy, shown in Plates 107 and 108, is coagulated with the point coagulator for about 20 seconds at 100°–110° C. Only the ovarian tissue that is in direct contact with the heated probe will be coagulated; no other parts of the ovary will be exposed to the heat. This is in contrast to coagulation with high-frequency current, which used to damage larger areas beyond the primary biopsy site.

Plate 110.   **Biopsy of an ovary suspended by its ligaments**
History: A 31-year-old patient was seen 9 years after a laparotomy for Stein-Leventhal syndrome.
Operation: If the biopsy forceps is introduced from the contralateral side to the ovary to be biopsied, it is usually possible to grasp the ovary at any site selected. In this photograph, the spiked jaws of the biopsy forceps have already grasped the ovary at the preselected site. The trocar sleeve is advanced and ready to punch out a cylinder of tissue.

Plate 111.   **Biopsy of an ovary suspended by its ligaments**
Operation: The large defect left by the biopsy, shown in Plate 110, was coagulated with the point coagulator for 20 seconds at 110° C, which achieved complete hemostasis. Adhesions to such coagulated biopsy wounds have never been observed.

14.2.6.1. Puncture of Ovarian Cysts

Plate 112.   **Aspiration of an ovarian cyst**
History: A 32-year-old patient with primary infertility underwent a laparotomy for Stein-Leventhal syndrome at age 22 years.
Findings: There is a smooth right ovarian cyst 8 cm in diameter with adhesions to the posterior wall of the uterus.
Operation: The adhesions are kept under tension with a grasping forceps so that they can be dissected off the posterior wall of the uterus in a relatively avascular plane.
Histology: Cystic endometrioma.
The continuation of this operation is illustrated in Plates 125–128. Plate 225 shows follow-up findings after 12 months.

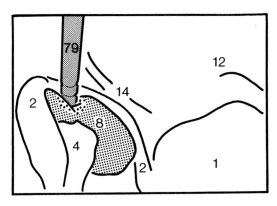

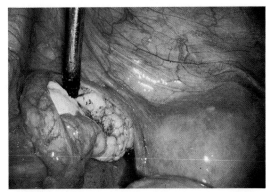

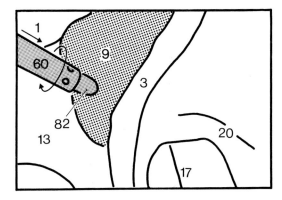

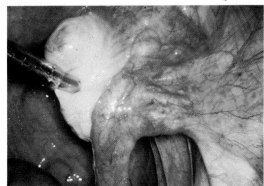

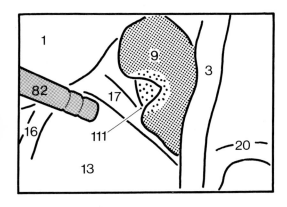

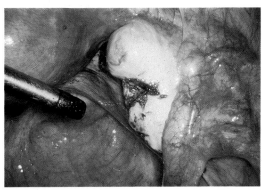

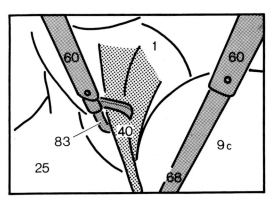

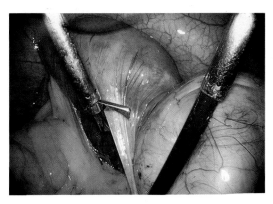

Plate 113. **Aspiration and excision of an ovarian cyst**

History and Findings: In a 32-year-old patient, sonography revealed a left ovarian cyst 8–9 cm in diameter; the cyst was confirmed by diagnostic pelviscopy.

Operation: The left ovarian cyst was first punctured and aspirated with the long aspiration needle which, because of the size of the ovarian cyst, was connected to the Aquapurator aspiration apparatus. A clear yellow serous fluid was obtained. Therefore . . .

Plate 114. **Aspiration and excision of an ovarian cyst**

Operation: . . . the ovarian cyst was incised and laid wide open for careful inspection of its inner surface under low-power magnification. The internal surfaces were smooth and devoid of any papillary or solid structures.

Plate 115. **Aspiration and excision of an ovarian cyst**

Operation: The cyst (shown in Plates 113 and 114), which was evacuated and opened widely, is now removed completely. The cyst wall is grasped with biopsy forceps at the appropriate layer and then curled around the biopsy forceps, just as hair is curled around a curling iron. Should the cyst wall tear during this maneuver, the same procedure may be repeated until all remnants have been removed.

Plate 116. **Aspiration and excision of an ovarian cyst: End result**

Operation: After aspiration and excision of the entire cyst wall (shown in Plates 113–115), the ovarian defect is closed with an endosuture. Here, the 5-mm needleholder has just received the needle after it has penetrated the wound edges with the aid of a 3-mm needle-holder. Next, about 50 cm of suture will be advanced into the abdominal cavity and the needle with its suture will be grasped with the 3-mm needleholder and withdrawn through the applicator sleeve. An external slipknot will be tied and then pushed back into the pelvic cavity to close the ovarian defect.

Histology: Cyst wall with elements of a granulosa-theca cell cyst.

312

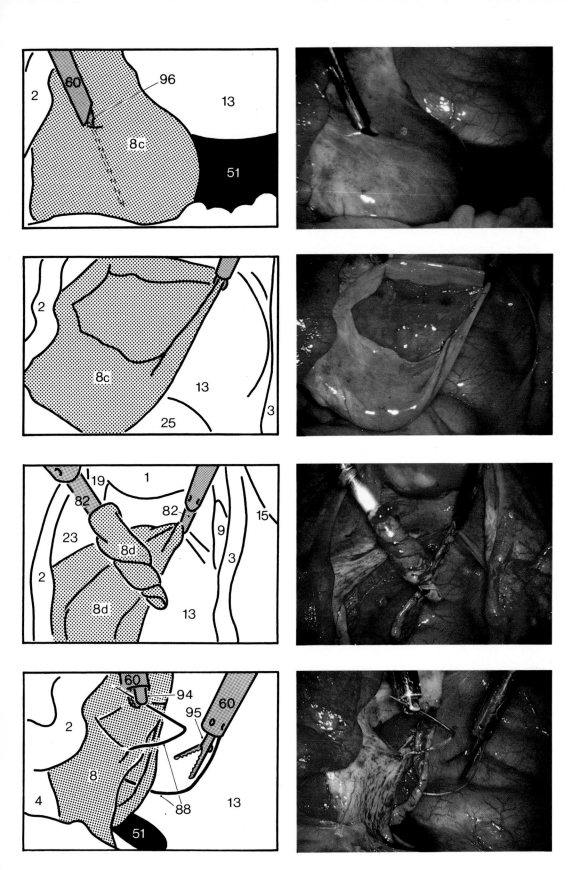

14.2.6.2. Excision of Ovarian Cysts and Ovarian Suture

Plate 117. **Excision of ovarian cyst and suture**

History and Findings: A 20-year-old patient had a left ovarian cyst 6 cm in diameter that was diagnosed on sonography and confirmed by pelviscopy.

Operation: At first the cyst is punctured and aspirated with an aspiration needle connected to the Aquapurator aspiration apparatus. Since the cyst contained sebaceous material, it was not incised and opened, as shown in Plate 114. Only about 5 cm of the tunica albuginea of the left ovary will be incised with hook scissors and the cyst will be dissected.

See also Plate 118.

Plate 118. **Excision of ovarian cyst and suture**

Operation: After sebaceous material was obtained by diagnostic aspiration of the ovarian cyst (shown in Plate 117), the tunica albuginea is incised to a length of 5–7 cm. This can be achieved almost without blood loss.

Plate 119. **Excision of ovarian cyst and suture**

Operation: After the tunica albuginea has been incised sufficiently (shown in Plate 118), it can be retracted with the aid of two biopsy forceps, exposing the entire cyst, until . . .

Plate 120. **Excision of ovarian cyst and suture**

Operation: . . . eventually, the entire unruptured ovarian cyst protrudes from the ovary. With the aid of a large spoon-jawed forceps and the Aquapurator aspiration apparatus and copious amounts of irrigation fluid (1–2 L), the cyst and its contents are extracted through the 11-mm trocar sleeve.

Histology: Cystic teratoma with derivatives of all three germ layers.

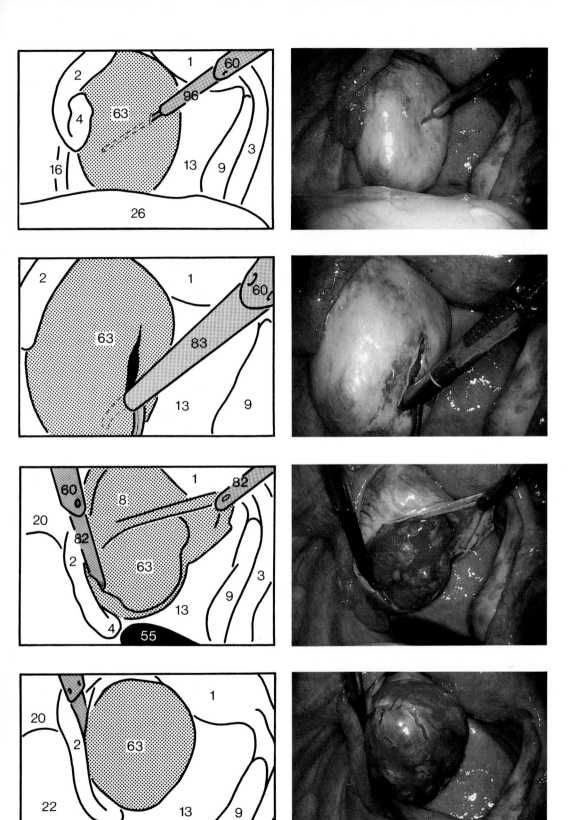

Plate 121.   Excision of ovarian cyst and suture

Operation: After enucleation of the dermoid cyst (shown in Plates 117–120), remnants of the cyst wall are sharply resected, although this can often be accomplished bluntly by traction with two biopsy forceps.

Plate 122.   Excision of ovarian cyst and suture

Operation: After enucleation of the ovarian cyst (shown in Plates 117–120), followed by resection of the cyst wall (shown in Plate 121), the pelvic cavity is thoroughly irrigated to allow a clearer view of the pelvic organs. The ovarian incision can be inspected for satisfactory hemostasis. Thereafter . . .

Plate 123.   Excision of ovarian cyst and suture

Operation: . . . the ovarian incision is closed with an endosuture. The endosuture has been introduced with a 3-mm needleholder into the peritoneal cavity; it has just perforated the right margin of the wound. Here, the needle is being grasped with the 5-mm needleholder, which will return it to the 3-mm needleholder in the appropriate position for the next stitch.

Plate 124.   Excision of ovarian cyst and suture: End result

Findings: The photograph shows the pelvic anatomy after bilateral excision of ovarian cysts (dermoid cysts) in a 20-year-old patient (procedure shown in Plates 117–123). After thorough irrigation, the pelvic peritoneum is smooth and clean. There is complete hemostasis in both ovaries.

Operation: Under pelviscopic view, the instruments are removed from the peritoneal cavity and the CO_2 gas is deflated.

Comment: It was noted that the cyst contained sebaceous material. The cyst was not incised and opened, as illustrated in Plate 14; instead, only about 5 cm of the tunica albuginea of the left ovary was incised with hook scissors. It should be noted that there is only minimal bleeding during endoscopic operations on the ovary.

See also Plate 120 for histologic findings.

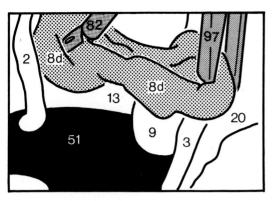

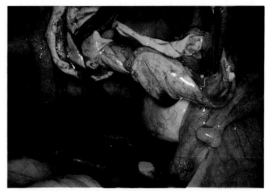

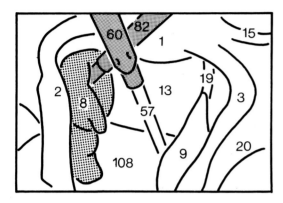

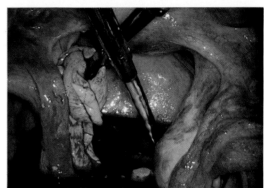

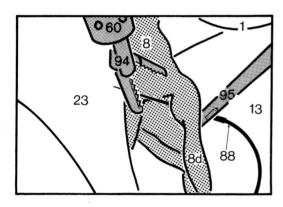

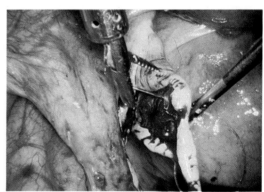

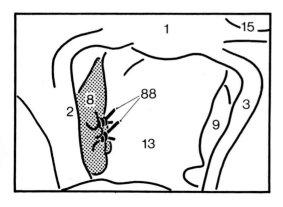

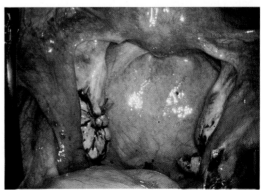

Plate 125. Excision of a chocolate cyst

History and Findings: A 32-year-old patient had a right ovarian cyst 8 cm in diameter (shown in Plate 112).

Operation: After ovariolysis and puncture of the cyst with the aspiration needle, some brown fluid escapes under pressure. Since numerous endometriotic implants were found in the pelvic cavity, it is almost certain that this is a chocolate cyst.

Histology: Endometrial cyst of the right ovary with focal concentrations of siderophages.

Plate 126. Excision of a chocolate cyst

Operation: To prepare this 8-cm-diameter ovarian chocolate cyst for dissection, its contents are aspirated almost completely.

Comment: Occasionally the chocolate material in the cyst is too viscous for aspiration; in that case the cyst must be incised. The chocolate material will drain into the cul-de-sac and can then be aspirated. Sometimes it is helpful to dilute it first with saline solution.

Plate 127. Excision of a chocolate cyst

Operation: Because of the large size of the cyst, major portions of the attenuated, function-less cyst wall must be resected. This is accomplished, step by step, with hook scissors while the deflated cystic sac is held firmly with the large spoon forceps.

Plate 128. Excision of a chocolate cyst

Findings: After the chocolate cyst has been opened widely and its inner wall has been exposed for inspection, only a few foci a few square millimeters in diameter seem to contain tissues typical for endometriosis. Two separate layers can be recognized in this photograph: the tunica albuginea and the actual wall of the chocolate cyst.

Operation: Therefore, it is usually quite easy to grasp the appropriate layer to enucleate the entire chocolate cyst by curling it around a grasping instrument, as shown in Plate 115. Finally, the ovarian wound edges are approximated with a suture, as shown in Plate 123.

Comment: Bleeding from small implants over months, possibly years, has caused the accu-mulation of chocolate material until it reached a diameter of 8 cm. This photograph may also explain why occasionally only minimal coagulation after aspiration of chocolate cysts will prevent recurrences, provided that the procedure has really destroyed the endometriotic implants.

See also Plate 225, which shows follow-up findings 12 months later.

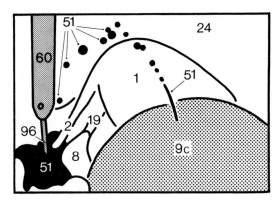
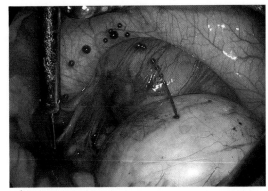

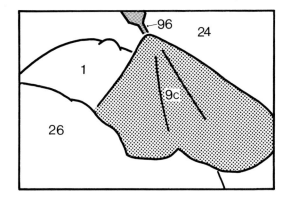
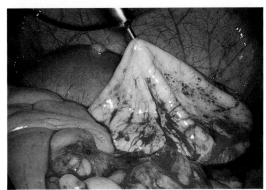

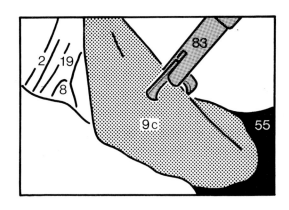
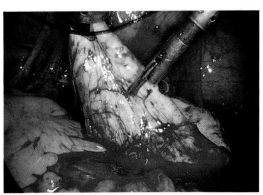

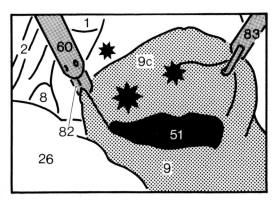
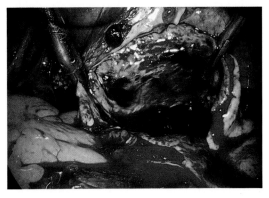

Plate 129. **Excision of a chocolate cyst and treatment of sterility**

History: A 35-year-old patient underwent appendectomy at age 29 and laparotomy with partial ovarian resection and an anterior uterine suspension (Baldy-Webster) because of suspected Stein-Leventhal syndrome at age 33. Because the patient had failed to conceive and had chronic lower abdominal and pelvic pain, diagnostic and possibly operative pelviscopy was scheduled.

Findings: After partial resection of the ovaries, massive postoperative adhesions formed between the two ovaries and between the ovaries and a loop of small bowel, as well as epiploic appendices of the sigmoid colon.

Plate 130. **Excision of a chocolate cyst and treatment of sterility**

Operation: The first step consisted of adhesiolysis of the small intestine (illustrated in Plates 335 and 336). Then the two ovaries were separated from one another with scissors. This dissection, at the same time, included the tunica albuginea over a larger area of the right ovary, exposing the chocolate cyst contained within the ovary.

Plate 131. **Excision of a chocolate cyst and treatment of sterility**

Operation: The entire chocolate cyst could be enucleated according to the technique illustrated in Plates 118–120. The pelvic cavity was thoroughly irrigated before . . .

Plate 132. **Excision of a chocolate cyst and treatment of sterility**

Operation: . . . the defect in the right ovary was closed with an endosuture (shown in Plate 123). The needle, held with the 3-mm needleholder, has just penetrated both wound edges and will be received by the 5-mm needleholder.

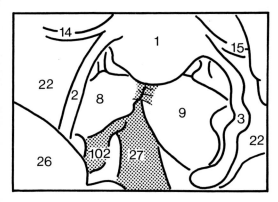
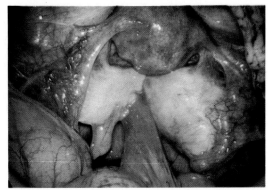
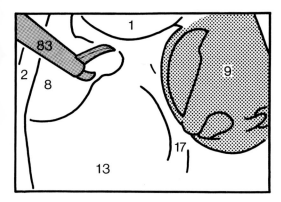
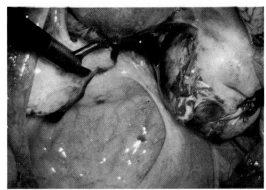
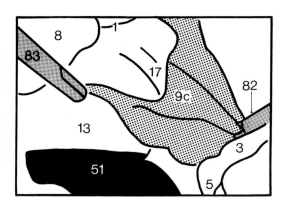
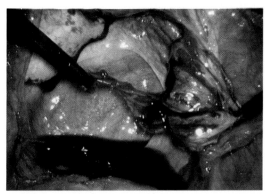
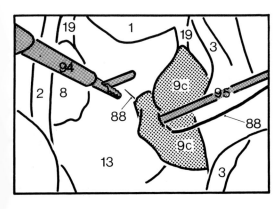
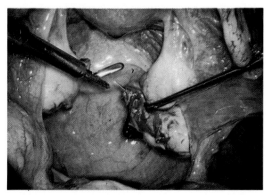

Plate 133. **Excision of a chocolate cyst and treatment of sterility: End result**

Operation: After bilateral salpingoplasty and chromopertubation, the pelvic cavity is thoroughly irrigated with warm normal saline solution at 37° C.

Comment: At the end of the operation, the pelvic organs are completely free of adhesions and both tubes are patent (patency grade I). Because of the smooth surfaces, there is no risk of recurrent adhesions.

See also Plates 335 and 336, illustrating lysis of the adhesions to the intestinal tract. The entire operative procedure is illustrated in Plates 21, 22, 71, 72, 129–133, 335, and 336.

Plate 134. **Enucleation of a dermoid cyst (see also Plates 117–124)**

Findings: The incisor tooth with its alveolar process and a fragment of the jaw were carefully dissected after the entire dermoid cyst had been extracted with claw forceps.

See also Plate 135 and the preoperative x-ray film of the pelvis, Fig 289.

Plate 135. **Enucleation of a dermoid cyst**

Operation: A completely developed incisor tooth with its alveolar process and a fragment of jaw bone has been grasped with claw forceps and extracted from the dermoid cyst, which is shown in Plates 136–142. It was then removed through the 11-mm trocar sleeve.

Comment: This tooth and its bony anlage were detected radiologically earlier on a contrast uropyelogram.

See also Fig 289.

Plate 136. **Enucleation of a dermoid cyst**

History: A 27-year-old patient had a strong desire to have children.

Findings: A dermoid cyst about 9 cm in diameter was noted in the right ovary.

Operation: For diagnostic reasons, the cyst was punctured with an aspiration needle attached to a 10-ml syringe, and an oily sebaceous material with hairs was obtained. Therefore, it was decided to proceed immediately from a diagnostic to an operative pelviscopy.

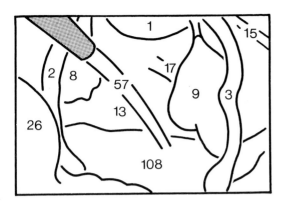

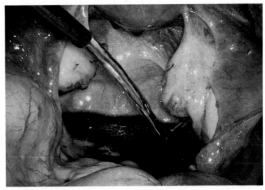

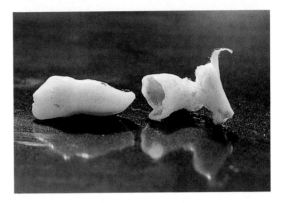

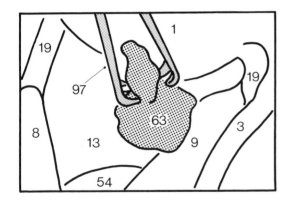

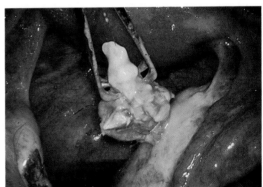

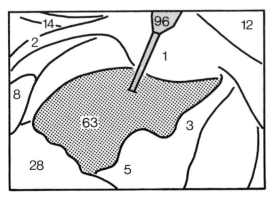

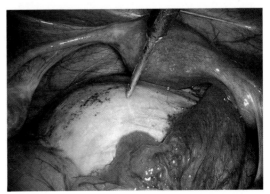

Plate 137. **Enucleation of a dermoid cyst**

Operation: After an 8-cm incision is made through the tunica albuginea, the entire dermoid cyst can be enucleated. This can be accomplished with two biopsy forceps, partially with blunt, partially with sharp dissection. The strands of tissue, which are still visible in this photograph, correspond to the vascular pedicle of the dermoid cyst. They were then severed without blood loss.

Plate 138. **Enucleation of a dermoid cyst**

Operation: After enucleation of the entire dermoid cyst (shown in Plate 137), the empty sac is grasped with two forceps and carefully inspected. Its walls are completely smooth.

Plate 139. **Enucleation of a dermoid cyst**

Operation: The attenuated, functionless cyst wall is then generously resected and the base of the dermoid cyst is peeled off the underlying normal ovarian tissue, using the hair curler technique illustrated in Plate 115. This reduces the ovary to a more manageable size.

Plate 140. **Enucleation of a dermoid cyst**

Operation: The actual dermoid cyst, as well as the tooth and its anlage (shown in Plates 134 and 135), and its accumulation of hair, are scooped up with the large spoon-jawed forceps and removed through the 11-mm trocar sleeve.

Caution: One must pay close attention that no remnants of the dermoid cyst will be spread into the central and upper abdominal regions. This can usually be prevented by avoiding a steep Trendelenburg position. If in doubt, the entire abdominal cavity can be irrigated with the patient placed in the reversed Trendelenburg position.

See also Fig 29.

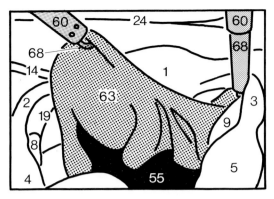
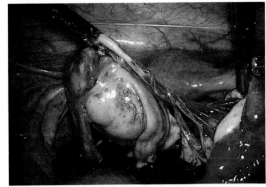

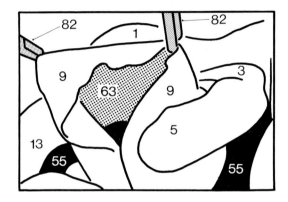
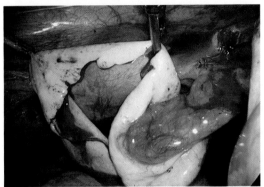

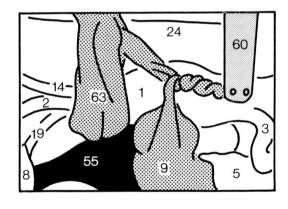
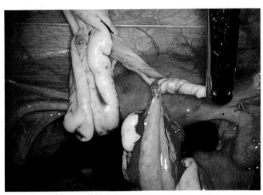

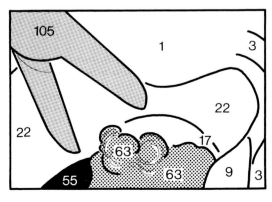
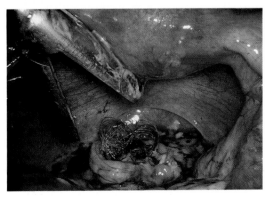

Plate 141. **Enucleation of a dermoid cyst**

Findings: After the cyst, which originally had a diameter of 9–10 cm, was excised from the right ovary and the pelvic cavity was thoroughly cleansed, inspection confirmed complete hemostasis.

Operation: The wound edges in the ovary are grasped with the large claw forceps and are reapproximated with endoloops.

Comment: Complete hemostasis is achieved when irrigation of the pelvic cavity with warm saline solution at 37° C is repeated and the aspirated fluid remains clear.

Plate 142. **Enucleation of a dermoid cyst: End result**

Findings: After enucleation of a dermoid cyst 9–10 cm in diameter and thorough irrigation of the pelvic cavity with 3 L of warm saline solution (illustrated in Plates 135–141), pelviscopic inspection reveals smooth, glistening peritoneal surfaces and an internal genital tract of normal appearance.

Comment: Five days postoperatively, the patient left the hospital without complaints. She has not had any recurrences during a 3-year follow-up period.

Histology: Cystic teratoma with elements of all three germinal layers.

14.2.6.3. Removal of Ovarian Cysts by Oophorectomy or Salpingo-oophorectomy

Plate 143. **Removal of an ovarian cyst by salpingo-oophorectomy**

History: A 51-year-old patient had a small pelvic tumor 3.5–4 cm in diameter that was detected on sonography and confirmed by diagnostic pelviscopy.

Operation: The cyst was first punctured and aspirated through a long aspiration needle attached to a 10-ml syringe. The contents consisted of a clear, serous fluid. After the cyst wall was opened, the inner surfaces of the cyst were inspected under low-power magnification and found to be completely smooth. In consideration of the patient's age, the decision was made to proceed immediately from a diagnostic to an operative pelviscopy with right salpingo-oophorectomy.

See also Plate 151, which shows the appearance at follow-up pelviscopy, 13 months later.

Plate 144. **Removal of an ovarian cyst by salpingo-oophorectomy**

Operation: After aspiration of the cyst contents, the large claw forceps reaches through the endoloop, which had been introduced through the fourth trocar sleeve. The claw forceps will simultaneously grasp both the tube and the ovary, which will then be pulled toward the opposite side of the pelvis so that the mesosalpinx will be put under maximum tension. The atraumatic grasping tongs will be used to position the catgut loop around the adnexal pedicle.

See also Plate 145.

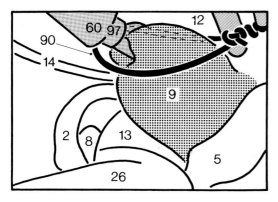

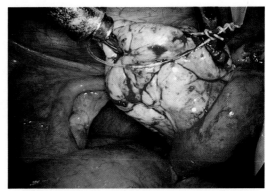

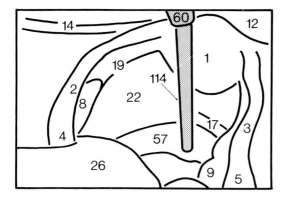

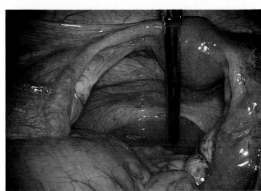

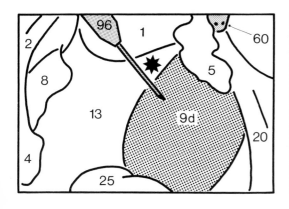

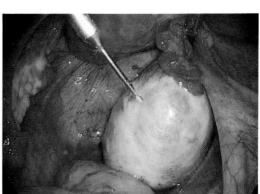

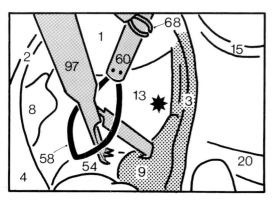

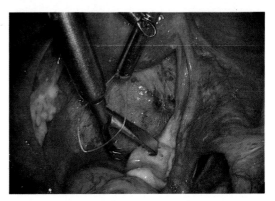

Plate 145. **Removal of an ovarian cyst by salpingo-oophorectomy**
Operation: The large claw forceps has pulled the right adnexa with the empty ovarian cyst through the endoloop, and the atraumatic grasping tongs are placing the looped suture as close to the pelvic wall as possible so that the infundibulopelvic ligament and the utero-ovarian ligament can be ligated far laterally.

Plate 146. **Removal of an ovarian cyst by salpingo-oophorectomy**
Operation: After the maneuver shown in Plates 144 and 145 has been repeated three times, the salpingo-oophorectomy by the triple-loop technique is completed. The free end of the third endoloop has not yet been cut. The atraumatic grasping tongs are still in the same position to which the loop has been advanced.

Plate 147. **Removal of an ovarian cyst by salpingo-oophorectomy**
Operation: Under traction with a biopsy forceps, the tube has just been cut. The large scissors presently resect the ovary from its mesovarium without loss of blood.

Plate 148. **Removal of an ovarian cyst by salpingo-oophorectomy**
Operation: After resection of the adnexa, a small vascular pedicle remains distal to the three ligatures; it is coagulated with the point coagulator to prevent adhesions to this area.
Caution: Do not coagulate too intensely, because this may loosen the catgut sutures! Superficial coagulation is quite sufficient to prevent the deposition of fibrin.
See also Plates 164, 173, and 188.

328

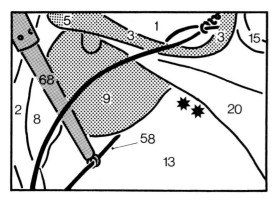
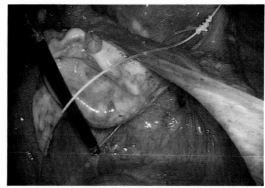

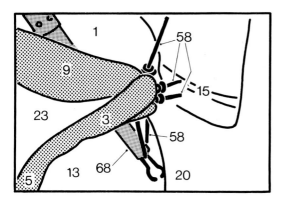
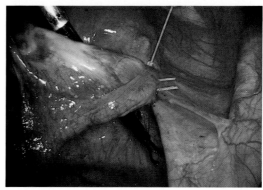

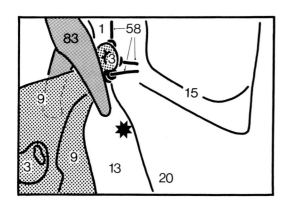
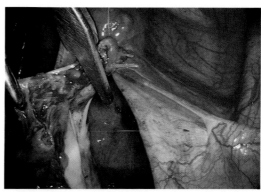

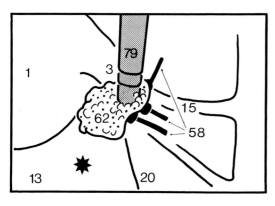
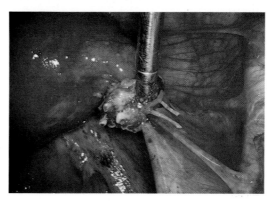

Plate 149. **Removal of an ovarian cyst by salpingo-oophorectomy**
Operation: After the right salpingo-oophorectomy has been completed, endometriotic implants in the cul-de-sac are coagulated. The thermocolor test result is clearly recognized: healthy peritoneum changes to a white color, endometriotic implants appear with a brown discoloration (hemosiderin effect).

Plate 150. **Removal of an ovarian cyst by salpingo-oophorectomy: End result**
Operation: After right salpingo-oophorectomy for an ovarian cyst 3.5–4 cm in diameter (shown in Plates 143–148), the pelvic cavity is irrigated thoroughly with the aid of the Aquapurator apparatus until the entire peritoneum is smooth and clean.
Comment: This step is very important so that the body does not reabsorb debris during the postoperative period; it contributes greatly to the speedy postoperative recovery of the patient.

Plate 151. **Removal of an ovarian cyst by salpingo-oophorectomy: Status at follow-up**
History: At age 51 years, this patient underwent a right salpingo-oophorectomy for an ovarian cyst 3.5–4 cm in diameter (shown in Plates 143–150).
Findings: Thirteen months postoperatively, the remaining tubal stump is 5 mm long. The pelvic cavity is completely free of adhesions. There is hardly any scarring in areas from which the right adnexae were resected. There is about 10 ml of a clear serous fluid in the cul-de-sac.

Plate 152. **Removal of an ovarian cyst by salpingo-oophorectomy**
History: A 69-year-old patient had a left adnexal tumor 6 cm in diameter, detected on physical examination and confirmed by sonography.
Findings: Inspection through the pelviscope revealed a left ovarian cyst 6.5–7 cm in diameter with a smooth surface and a small accessory ovary.
Comment: In view of the patient's age and the completely normal adnexa on the right side, the surgeon decided to perform a left salpingo-oophorectomy.

330

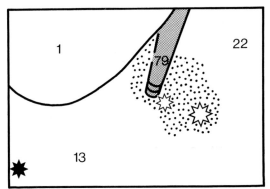

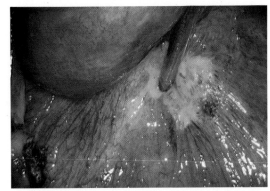

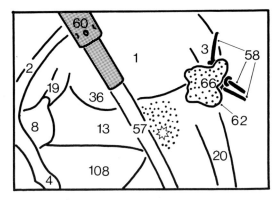

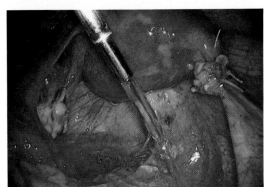

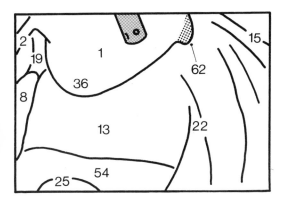

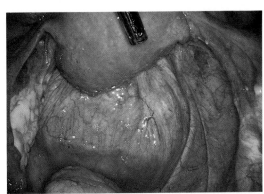

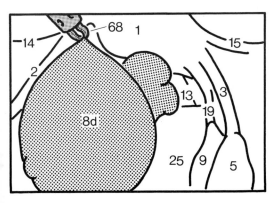

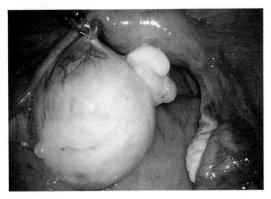

Plate 153. **Removal of an ovarian cyst by salpingo-oophorectomy**

Operation: After puncture, aspiration, and inspection of the inner wall of the ovarian cyst, three operative instruments are introduced through three additional trocar sleeves. The endoloop has been introduced through a 5-mm suprapubic trocar sleeve on the same side from which the adnexa are to be removed: in this case, the left side. Atraumatic grasping tongs have been introduced through the right suprapubic 5-mm trocar sleeve to assist in the placement of the endoloop around the base of the adnexal pedicle. A large claw forceps has been introduced through a suprasymphyseal 11-mm trocar sleeve in the linea alba to grasp the ovary.

Plate 154. **Removal of an ovarian cyst by salpingo-oophorectomy**

Operation: The adnexal pedicle has been ligated by the triple-loop technique (illustrated in Plates 143–150) and the left adnexa have just been resected en bloc with hook scissors distal to the three ligatures around the vascular pedicles. Only 2–3 ml of blood can be recognized in the cul-de-sac, resulting from retrograde drainage of blood from the excised adnexa.

Plate 155. **Removal of an ovarian cyst by salpingo-oophorectomy**

Operation: Because of its size, the small accessory ovary (see Plate 152) must first be separated from the adnexa and removed with the large spoon forceps through the 11-mm trocar sleeve. Because of the elliptical configuration of the orifice of this beveled trocar sleeve, further morcellation of the specimen was not necessary.

Plate 156. **Removal of an ovarian cyst by salpingo-oophorectomy: End stage**

Findings: After excision of the left adnexa with an ovarian cyst 6–7 cm in diameter and irrigation of the pelvis, final inspection reveals a vascular pedicle that has been triple-ligated and endocoagulated; all peritoneal surfaces are smooth and clean.

Comment: The postoperative trauma is limited almost entirely to the healing process in the vascular pedicles. As already demonstrated in Plate 151, healing occurs almost without scar formation.

Caution: During this healing process, which requires about 5 days, the patient should be kept in the hospital for observation.

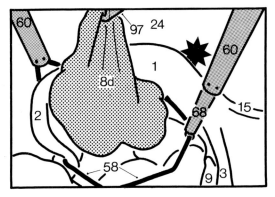
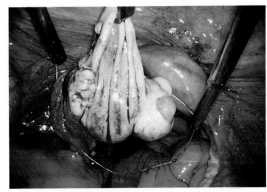

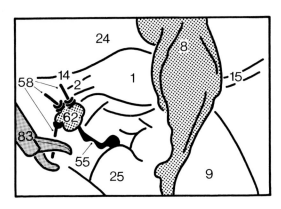
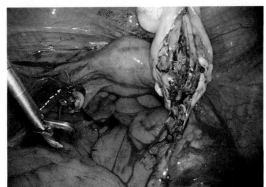

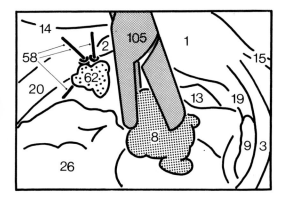
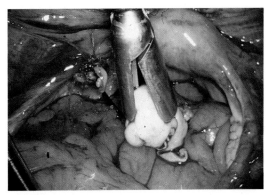

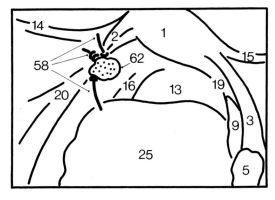
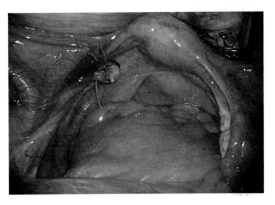

14.2.7. Pelviscopic Oophorectomy

Plate 157. Oophorectomy

History: A 34-year-old patient had had an appendectomy at the age of 18 years. Presently she requires therapy for recurrent breast carcinoma. Since tests for estrogen receptors were positive, castration by bilateral oophorectomy was indicated.

Operation: At this stage of the operation, the right ovary has been removed by the triple-loop technique and has been deposited in the cul-de-sac. In preparation for the left oophorectomy, an endoloop has been introduced through the left suprapubic trocar sleeve. The large claw forceps is reaching through the loop to grasp the ovary. Atraumatic grasping tongs have been introduced through the right suprapubic trocar sleeve to assist in the placement of the loop.

Plate 158. Oophorectomy

Operation: Under strong traction with the claw forceps, which has grasped the left ovary, the endoloop is pushed down onto the mesovarium while, on the opposite side of the mesovarium, the plastic applicator tube pushes the slipknot into the lateralmost position on the mesosalpinx/mesovarium.

Plate 159. Oophorectomy

Operation: As the endoloop is tightened (i.e., as the slipknot is applied), the ovary is pulled vigorously with the large claw forceps toward the center of the pelvis. The atraumatic grasping tongs retract the tube away from the area where the ligature is being applied.

Plate 160. Oophorectomy

Operation: After the first ligature, a second endoloop is applied, again with vigorous traction on the ovary and with the guidance of atraumatic grasping tongs.

Caution: It is important that the second ligature and, finally, the third ligature each be applied closer toward the pelvic wall than the previous one, so that the mesovarian pedicle will be developed as long as possible.

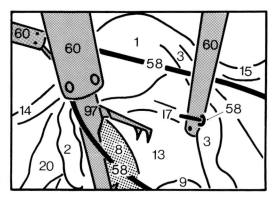
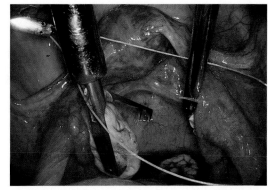
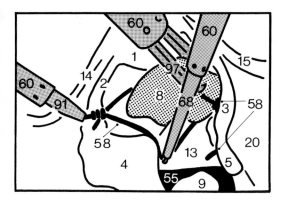
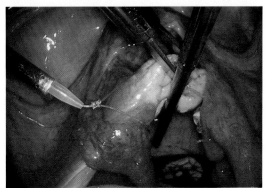
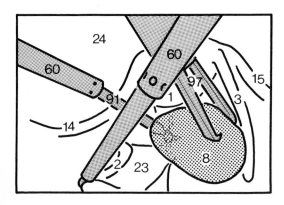
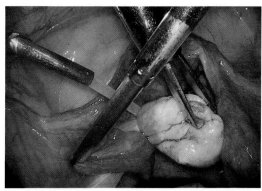
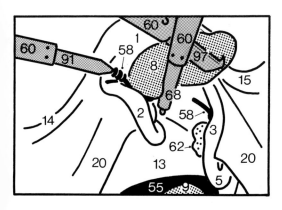
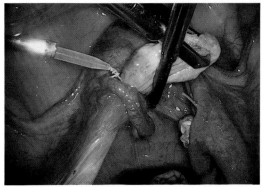

Plate 161. Oophorectomy

Findings: The right ovary, which has already been resected, can be recognized in the cul-de-sac.

Operation: After the second endoloop has been tied, the third ligature will be applied. Again, with maximal traction placed on the ovary by the large claw forceps toward the center of the pelvis, the loop is guided around the pedicle with the aid of atraumatic grasping tongs.

Caution: One must again make sure that the third ligature is applied between the pelvic wall and the first two ligatures so that the pedicle can be developed as long as possible.

Plate 162. Oophorectomy

Operation: After completion of the triple-loop technique, the left mesovarium is transected step by step with hook scissors. Vigorous traction with the claw forceps toward the center of the pelvis puts sufficient tension on the pedicle to facilitate cutting with hook scissors.

Caution: It is important that the scissors always be introduced through the trocar sleeve on the same side from which the ovary will be resected so that the scissors can cut the pedicle at a right angle. This precaution will prevent both the inadvertent cutting of the ligatures as well as cutting into the ligaments.

Plate 163. Oophorectomy

Operation: The ovarian resection was accomplished without any bleeding. Next, the ovaries will be morcellated with the tissue punch, as shown in Plate 165.

Plate 164. Oophorectomy: End result

Findings: After morcellation of both ovaries (as shown in Plate 165) and thorough irrigation of the pelvis with 1 L of saline solution, the entire peritoneum is smooth and clean and the peritoneal cavity is free of blood.

Operation: To prevent adhesions, both pedicles are coagulated superficially with a point coagulator.

Comment: This precautionary measure ensures that the pedicles will be covered with coagulated protein onto which no healthy peritoneum will grow.

See also Chapter 12.5.6.2. and Plates 148, 173, and 188.

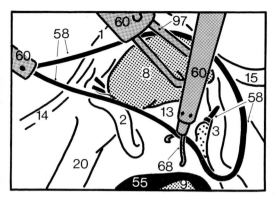
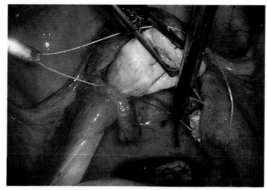

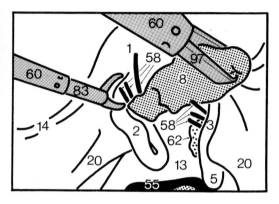
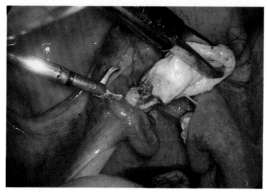

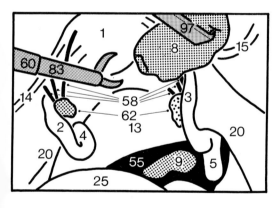
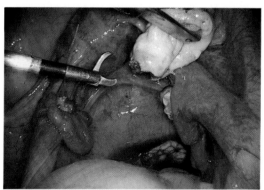

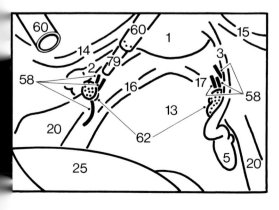
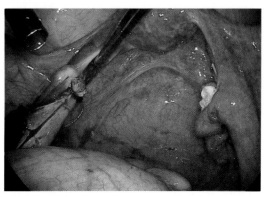

Plate 165. **Oophorectomy, morcellation**

Operation: After resection of the ovaries by the triple-loop technique (see Plates 157–164), the left ovary is grasped with a biopsy forceps and pressed into the cutting orifice of the tissue punch. The tissue fragments of 0.5 to 1 cm^3 in diameter are punched out of the ovary and stored inside the hollow shaft of this instrument. One has to pay attention that, after each bite, the tissue collector returns to its original position; otherwise tissue fragments may be trapped in the cutting orifice and then fall into the abdominal cavity (see also chapter 12.8.5.). Then the pelvic cavity is irrigated with 1–2 L of normal saline solution until the entire peritoneum is smooth and clean. To prevent adhesions, the pedicles will be coagulated as shown in Plates 148, 164, 173, and 188.

Histology: Normal ovarian tissue corresponding to the patient's age.

Plate 166. **Oophorectomy with complications**

Findings: Bleeding from the right ovarian artery after it has retracted from the ligated pedicle.

Operation: An endoloop has been introduced through a suprapubic trocar sleeve on the side that requires the additional ligature. The bleeding or spurting vessel is grasped through the endoloop and the ligature is applied beyond the tip of the grasping forceps.

Comment: As in general surgery, slipping of sutures and ligatures may also occur in endoscopic operations. This is possible with oophorectomy as well as salpingo-oophorectomy if the ligature is not pulled tight enough or if the distance between the ovarian ligament and the infundibulopelvic ligament is so great that too much tension was put on the ligature. In such cases, the pedicle may retract from the three ligatures immediately after the ovary or the adnexa, respectively, had been resected. Hemorrhage may ensue from the ascending branches of the uterine artery, i.e., the ovarian branch of the uterine artery, the tubal artery, etc. (see Plate 100) and from the ovarian artery, i.e., from the infundibulopelvic ligament. In contrast to a laparotomy, however, hemorrhage from these vessels during an endoscopic operation is of lesser magnitude. In such cases it will always be possible to grasp both the caudal as well as the cranial vascular pedicle with a forceps and to ligate the vessels with separate endoloops.

Plate 167. **Oophorectomy with complications**

Operation: The infundibulopelvic ligament, which had retracted from the previous ligature, has been regrasped and religated with the loop shown in Plate 166. The free end of the suture will be cut with hook scissors: if necessary, a second ligature may be applied as an extra precaution.

Plate 168. **Oophorectomy with complications: End result**

Operation: After the three previous ligatures have slipped off the mesosalpinx, the infundibulopelvic ligament has already been religated, as shown in Plate 167. Next, the more caudal vascular pedicle will be ligated according to the same technique as shown in Plates 166–167: introduction of the endoloop on the same side, grasping of the spurting vessel, and ligature.

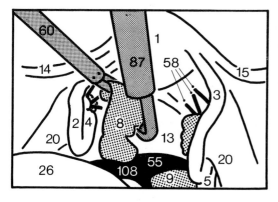
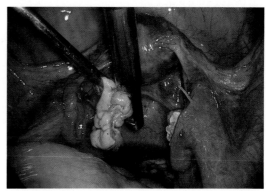
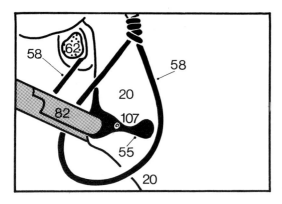
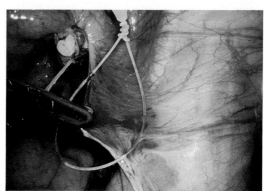
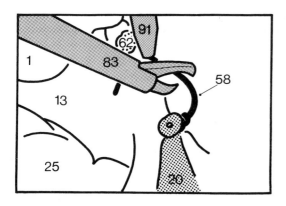
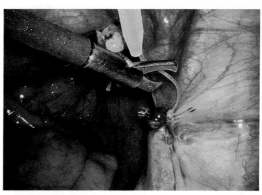
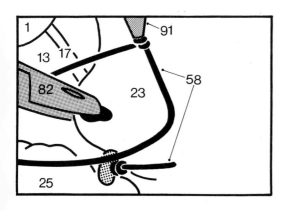
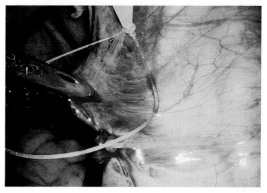

Plate 169. **Oophorectomy after total abdominal hysterectomy**

History: A 53-year-old patient underwent a cholecystectomy at age 34, an appendectomy at age 42, and, at age 49, a total abdominal hysterectomy with right salpingo-oophorectomy and left salpingectomy because of a large myomatous uterus of about 10 cm diameter. In consideration of the patient's age, the left ovary had been spared at that time. When the patient was suffering from a recurrent carcinoma of the breast with positive findings for estrogen receptors, resection of the remaining ovary was indicated.

Findings: An overview of the pelvis reveals the status after total abdominal hysterectomy, right salpingo-oophorectomy, and left salpingectomy. The pelvis was completely free of adhesions.

Plate 170. **Oophorectomy after total abdominal hysterectomy**

Operation: On the side of the planned oophorectomy, the endoloop has been introduced and the ovary has been pulled through the loop by strong traction with the large claw forceps.

Plate 171. **Oophorectomy after total abdominal hysterectomy**

Operation: Under strong traction with the large claw forceps, three endoloops have been applied to the mesovarium. The hook scissors are ready to cut the free end of the third endoloop. The suspensory ligament of the ovary is kept under considerable tension.

Plate 172. **Oophorectomy after total abdominal hysterectomy**

Operation: After the ovarian pedicle has been transected with hook scissors, the ovary is grasped with a biopsy forceps and pushed into the cutting orifice of the tissue punch. With each of the repetitive punching movements, portions of 0.5–1 cm^3 of the ovary are loaded into the hollow shaft of the tissue punch.

Histology: Ovarian tissue without germinal elements.

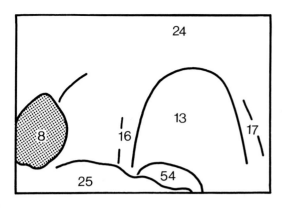

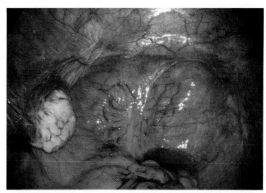

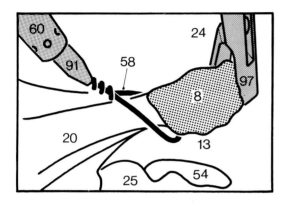

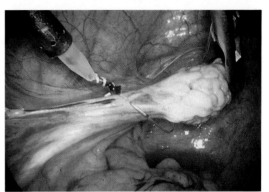

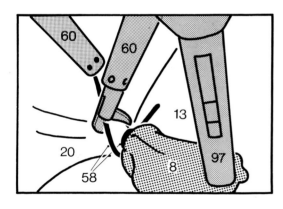

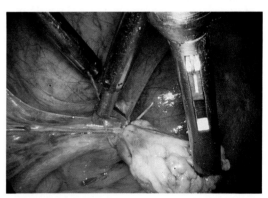

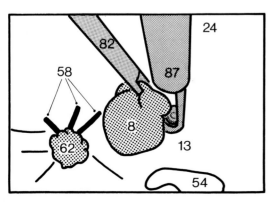

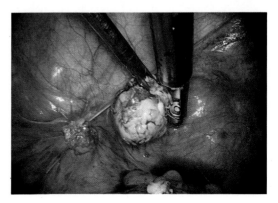

Plate 173.   **Oophorectomy after total abdominal hysterectomy**

Operation: After morcellation and removal of the ovary, as shown in Plate 172, the mesovarian pedicle is superficially coagulated with the point coagulator for 10–20 seconds at 100° C to prevent the formation of adhesions.

See also: chapter 12.5.6.2. and Plates 148, 164, and 188.

Plate 174.   **Oophorectomy after total abdominal hysterectomy: End result**

Operation: At the completion of the left oophorectomy, shown in Plates 169–173, the pelvic cavity is carefully irrigated with 1–2 L of warm saline solution at 37° C until the entire peritoneum is smooth and clean.

Caution: Particular attention should be paid to the careful removal of any ovarian fragments that may have been dropped into the cul-de-sac during the morcellation procedure.

Comment: After oophorectomy or salpingo-oophorectomy, we usually keep our patients in the hospital for 5 days because that much time is required for the healing process of the ligated pedicle.

See also Plate 151 for an overview after salpingo-oophorectomy.

14.2.8.1. Transection of the Infundibulopelvic Ligament

Plate 175.   **Ligation of the infundibulopelvic ligament**

History: This 54-year-old patient was hospitalized with a descensus of the uterus and vagina and scheduled for a vaginal hysterectomy with anterior and posterior colporrhaphy.

Findings: Preoperative pelvic examination revealed an irregular ovarian tumor of about 6.5 cm in diameter which, on ultrasound evaluation, was interpreted as a solid tumor. Since a malignancy had to be suspected, a diagnostic pelviscopy was indicated. It revealed a bizarre, small left ovary of about 1.2 cm diameter from which an ovarian fibroma of 5–6 cm diameter arose. The position of this ovarian tumor high in the pelvis prevented its removal by the vaginal route. Therefore, the decision was made to perform a combined pelviscopic-vaginal salpingo-oophorectomy.

Operation: The infundibulopelvic ligament is put under tension and the needle of the endosuture has just been placed behind the ligament so that it may be ligated after an external slipknot has been tied. Thereafter, a second ligature will be applied more caudally, about 3 cm apart. After bloodless transection . . .

Plate 176.   **Ligation of the infundibulopelvic ligament: End result**

Operation: . . . the pedicle of the infundibulopelvic ligament will be reinforced by another endoloop.

Comment: With transection of the infundibulopelvic ligament and ligation of the ovarian artery and veins before the vaginal operation, the left adnexa was sufficiently mobilized to permit the removal of the ovarian tumor by the vaginal route, intact and without risk.

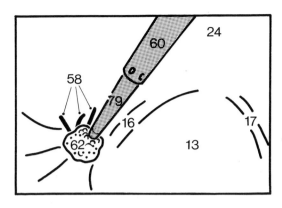
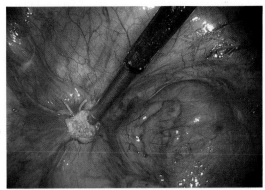
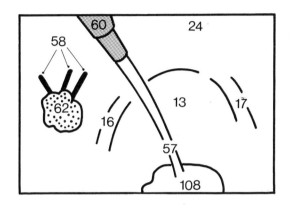
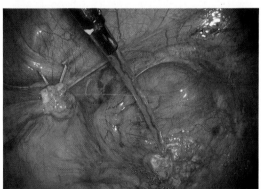
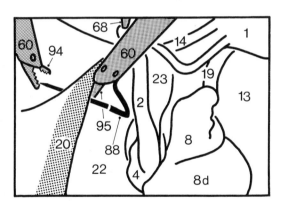
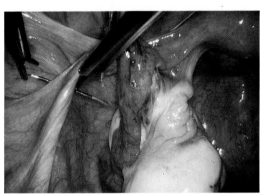
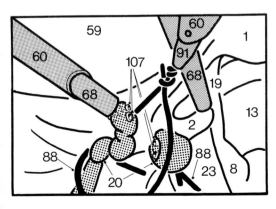
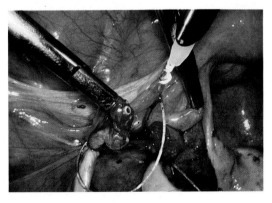

14.2.8.2. Salpingo-oophorectomy

Plate 177.   Salpingo-oophorectomy

History: A 37-year-old patient had a recurrence of a breast carcinoma. Estrogen receptor tests were positive. Hormone withdrawal therapy was indicated and a bilateral salpingo-oophorectomy was scheduled.

Operation: After introduction of the endoloop on the same side on which the salpingo-oophorectomy was to be done (see Plate 157), the ovary and tube are grasped with the claw forceps and pulled as far as possible toward the contralateral side of the pelvis. At the same time, atraumatic grasping tongs, which have been introduced through a third suprapubic trocar sleeve, push the ligature loop as far as possible toward the lateral pelvic wall. This ensures that even the first ligature is applied in the lateralmost position on the mesosalpinx. The right adnexa, which have already been resected, are lying in the cul-de-sac.

Plate 178.   Salpingo-oophorectomy

Operation: The tube and ovary are again grasped with the large claw forceps and vigorously pulled toward the center of the pelvis, and a second ligature is applied.

Caution: One must make sure that each consecutive ligature is applied closer to the pelvic wall than the previous one so that the pedicle will be elongated toward the infundibulopelvic and utero-ovarian ligaments.

Plate 179.   Salpingo-oophorectomy

Operation: After completion of the triple-loop technique, the ovary is kept under strong tension with the large claw forceps and then the adnexal pedicle is transected. For this purpose, the scissors are introduced on the same side on which the adnexal pedicle must be transected. This will allow transection of the pedicle at a right angle, and it prevents the inadvertent cutting of the ligature suture or injury to the broad ligament.

Plate 180.   Salpingo-oophorectomy

Operation: After the left adnexa have been resected, the ovary is grasped with the large claw forceps and the tube is separated from the ovary with hook scissors. In this manner, the fallopian tube may be withdrawn through the elliptical orifice of the 11-mm beveled trocar sleeve, usually without difficulties, in one piece and without prior morcellation.

344

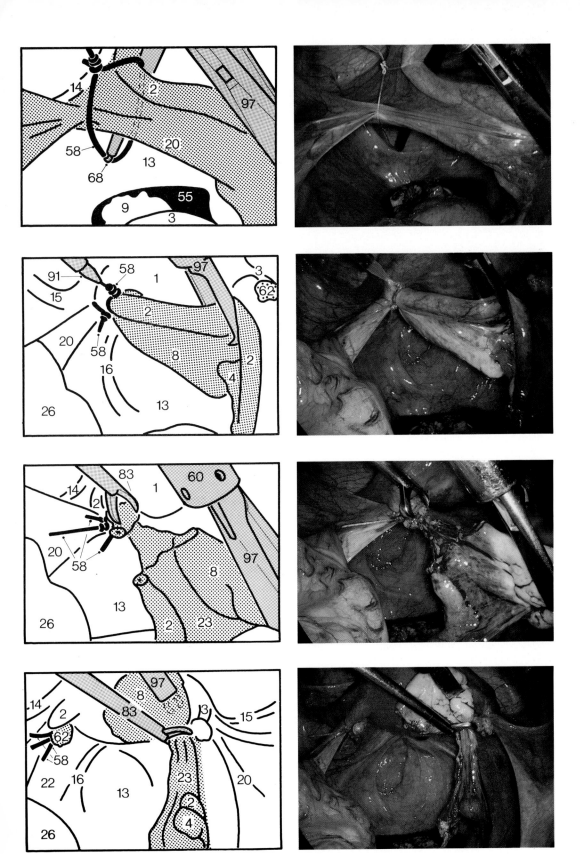

Plate 181. **Salpingo-oophorectomy: End result**

Operation: As shown in Plate 180, the tube has been separated from the ovary and may be withdrawn through the 11-mm trocar sleeve without difficulties; the ovary will have to be morcellated, as shown in Plates 165 and 172. Finally, the pelvis will be thoroughly irrigated with 1–2 L of normal saline solution and the pedicles will be coagulated.

Plate 182. **Salpingo-oophorectomy after previous total hysterectomy**

History: A 41-year-old patient had an appendectomy at age 16 years and a total vaginal hysterectomy for sterilization purposes 6 years before the current presentation.

Findings: There is a right ovarian tumor 3.5–4 cm in diameter and a left ovary of 1.5 × 2.5 cm.

Operation: For diagnostic purposes, the right ovary is punctured with the aspiration needle and the fluid is aspirated into a 10-ml syringe.

See also chapter 12.8.3.

Plate 183. **Salpingo-oophorectomy after previous total hysterectomy**

Operation: The large claw forceps reaches through the endoloop to grasp the right adnexa so that it can be pulled through the endoloop as far toward the center of the pelvis as possible.

Plate 184. **Salpingo-oophorectomy after previous total hysterectomy**

Operation: With vigorous traction on the adnexal structures (tube and ovarian cyst) with the large claw forceps, the infundibulopelvic ligament and remnants of the utero-ovarian ligament are elongated as much as possible. The atraumatic grasping tongs guide the endoloop toward the depth of the cul-de-sac.

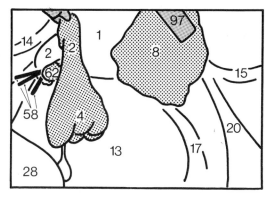
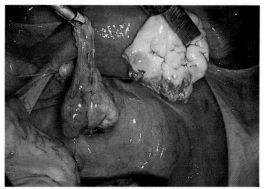

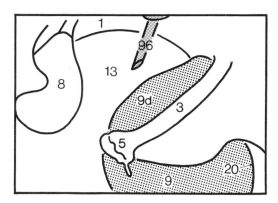
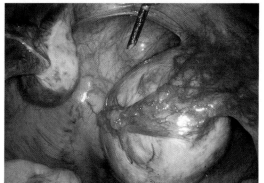

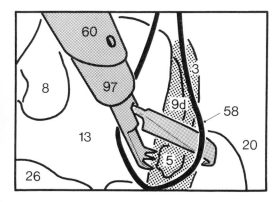
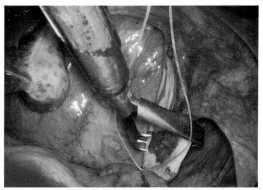

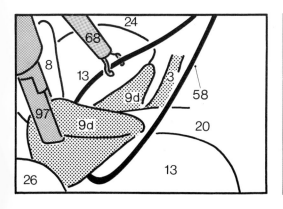
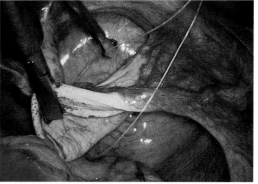

Plate 185. **Salpingo-oophorectomy after previous total hysterectomy**

Operation: While the large claw forceps exerts maximal traction on the adnexa until they touch the left pelvic wall, the atraumatic grasping tongs pull the endoloop toward the right pelvic wall. The plastic suture applicator also pulls the slipknot into the lateralmost position while the loop is slowly tightened.

Plate 186. **Salpingo-oophorectomy after previous total hysterectomy**

Operation: The first loop, which was shown in Plate 185, has been tied and cut; the second loop is being applied.

Caution: It is particularly important that vigorous traction be exerted on the adnexal structures toward the left pelvic wall and that the loop be grasped with the atraumatic grasping tongs (not yet accomplished in this photograph) and pushed deeply into the right mesosalpinx.

Plate 187. **Salpingo-oophorectomy after previous total hysterectomy**

Operation: After completion of the triple-loop technique, the ovary is kept under strong traction with the claw forceps so that the pedicle can be severed at a right angle. There was only a small amount of retrograde bleeding from the resected adnexa. These adnexal structures could be removed in one piece with the large spoon forceps via the elliptical orifice of the 11-mm beveled trocar sleeve.

Plate 188. **Salpingo-oophorectomy after previous total hysterectomy: End result**

Findings: After completion of the right salpingo-oophorectomy, shown in Plates 182–187 (after previous vaginal hysterectomy) and thorough irrigation of the pelvis with 1 L of warm saline solution at 37° C, the pedicle is finally briefly coagulated at 100° C to prevent adhesions.

See also Plates 148, 164, 173, and 213.

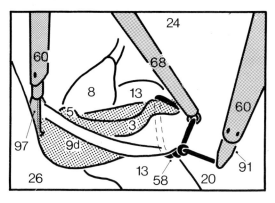

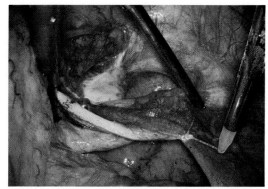

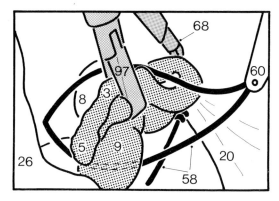

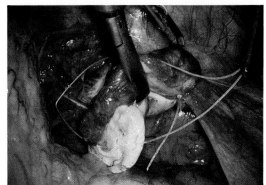

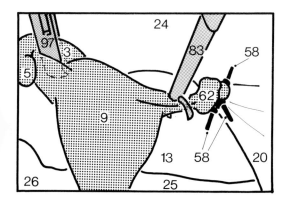

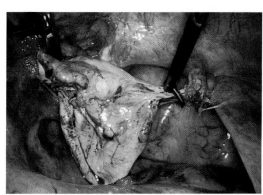

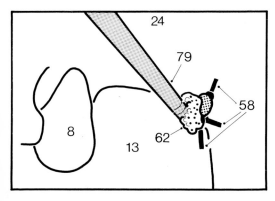

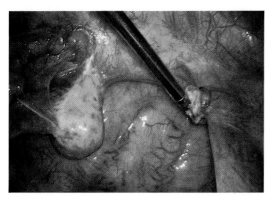

Plate 189. **Salpingo-oophorectomy for ovarian endometriosis**

History: A 46-year-old patient underwent a laparoscopic tubal sterilization operation at the age of 38 years; she is suffering from recurrent ovarian endometriosis.

Findings: Since the endometriosis was restricted to the right ovary and the cul-de-sac, whereas the left adnexa appeared to be perfectly normal, the decision was made to perform a right salpingo-oophorectomy.

Operation: The endoloop is introduced on the same side on which the salpingo-oophorectomy is planned. The large claw forceps is grasping the tube and ovary. It is evident that the loop cannot be closed without trapping the tubal ampulla. Therefore, it is always necessary to utilize the atraumatic grasping tongs for proper application of the loop.

See also Plate 190.

Plate 190. **Salpingo-oophorectomy for ovarian endometriosis**

Operation: The atraumatic grasping tongs are guiding the catgut loop (which was introduced in Plate 189) behind the right ovary and almost to the pelvic wall to ensure that the ligature will be applied at the base of the mesosalpinx.

Plate 191. **Salpingo-oophorectomy for ovarian endometriosis: End result**

Findings: This is the final stage after a right salpingo-oophorectomy for ovarian endometriosis, as shown in Plates 189 and 190. The vascular pedicle has been ligated well; the raw surfaces have already been coagulated with the point coagulator to prevent formation of adhesions.

Plate 192. **Salpingo-oophorectomy**

History: A 47-year-old patient underwent a radical mastectomy with amputation of the right arm at age 45 years; she now has metastatic breast carcinoma with positive estrogen receptors. To eliminate hormonal stimulation, bilateral salpingo-oophorectomy was indicated.

Operation: After introduction of the endoloop on the same side from which the adnexa is to be removed, the large claw forceps is trying to grasp the adnexal structures.

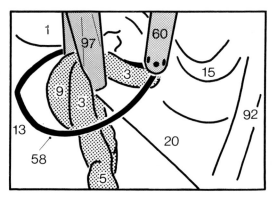
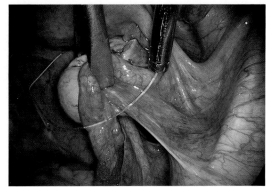

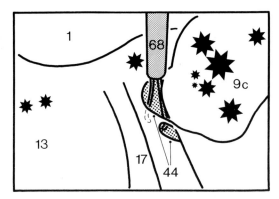
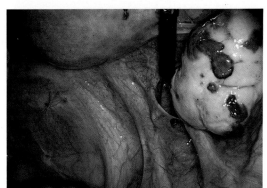

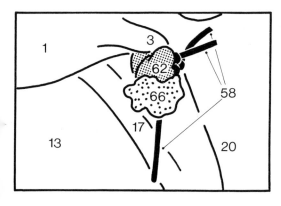
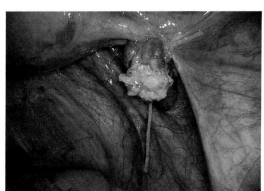

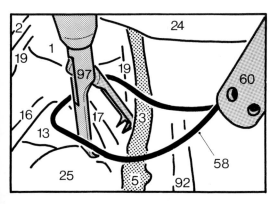
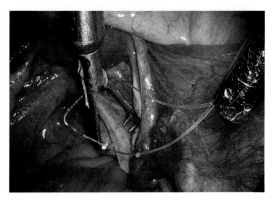

Plate 193.   Salpingo-oophorectomy

Operation: At first it was not possible to simultaneously grasp both tube and ovary with the claw forceps. In such cases, one must be satisfied with elevation of the tube only. The catgut loop is placed behind the ovary with the atraumatic grasping tongs while the slipknot is pulled with the plastic applicator rod firmly against the pelvic wall. If the application of such loop is not optimal, it may at least serve as a traction suture for additional ligatures. *See also* Plate 194.

Plate 194.   Salpingo-oophorectomy

Operation: The first endoloop placed in such a manner around the tube will serve in this particular case only as a traction suture for the additional three ligatures, because some ovarian tissue has been included in the original ligature.

Histology: Ovarian tissue corresponding to the patient's age. No evidence of metastases.

Plate 195.   Salpingo-oophorectomy

History: A 34-year-old patient had recurrent breast cancer after mastectomy at age 31 years.

Findings: The right salpingo-oophorectomy has been completed. The right adnexal structures are lying in the cul-de-sac. It should be noted that the right salpingo-oophorectomy has been accomplished by the triple-loop technique without loss of blood. There are adhesions between the left tubal ampulla and the lateral pelvic wall.

Operation: The left adnexa have been grasped with the large claw forceps and the endoloop will be guided around (i.e., behind) the left adnexa with the atraumatic grasping tongs. The peritoneal adhesions can also be included in the ligature loop because they are so mobile.

Plate 196.   Salpingo-oophorectomy

Operation: After completion of the left salpingo-oophorectomy (shown in Plate 195), the right ovary is grasped with a biopsy forceps and pressed into the jaws of the tissue punch. The ovarian tissue will be morcellated into fragments of 0.5–1 cm^3 size which will be stored in the hollow shaft. The tube can usually be removed in one piece through the 11-mm trocar sleeve, as has already been described in Plate 181.

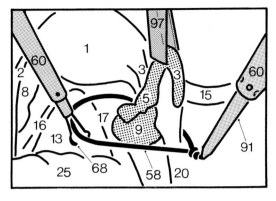
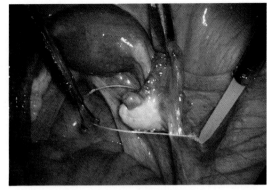
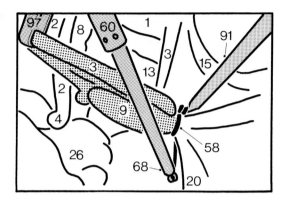
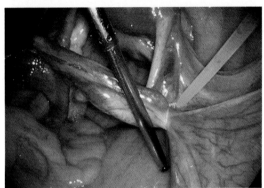
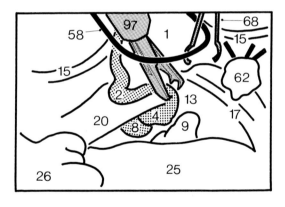
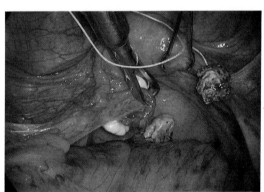
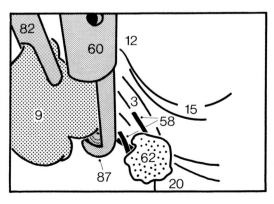
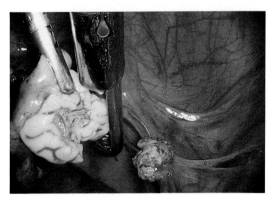

Plate 197.   Salpingo-oophorectomy: End result

Findings: This photograph shows an overview of the pelvis after bilateral salpingo-oopho-rectomy performed with the use of three suprapubic trocar sleeves.

Operation: One 5-mm trocar sleeve has been introduced on each side, left and right, in the hairy suprapubic region, utilizing the Z-technique; an 11-mm trocar sleeve was introduced in the lower linea alba.

Comment: This symmetric introduction of the trocar sleeves allows the surgeon to manipu-late and operate on both adnexa with equal, optimal facility.

14.2.9. Salpingectomy for Hydrosalpinx

Plate 198.   Salpingectomy for hydrosalpinx

History: A 44-year-old patient had an appendectomy at age 18 years and a total hysterec-tomy 6 years before the current presentation.

Findings: A large banana-shaped hydrosalpinx, noted on the left side, can be removed without difficulties by the endoscopic triple-loop technique. The left ovary is slightly en-larged and cystic, but there are no pathologic changes in the right ovary (see Plate 203). The surgeon decided to perform a left salpingo-oophorectomy.

Plate 199.   Salpingectomy for hydrosalpinx

Operation: The endoloop has been introduced on the same side on which the salpingo-oophorectomy is to be done; in this case, on the left side. The large claw forceps reaches through the endoloop to grasp the hydrosalpinx and pull it vigorously toward the center of the pelvis. This maneuver will perforate the tubal wall, allowing the fluid contents to drain out and decreasing the size of the hydrosalpinx to a more manageable size, so that the endoloop can be pushed well behind the tube and ovary with the aid of the atraumatic grasping tongs.

Plate 200.   Salpingectomy for hydrosalpinx

Operation: The first endoloop has been closed. One can clearly see the strong traction that the large claw forceps exerts on the hydrosalpinx. This photograph was taken at the moment the suture was cut.

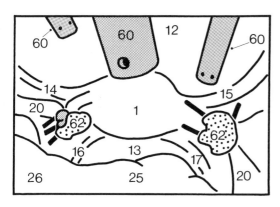

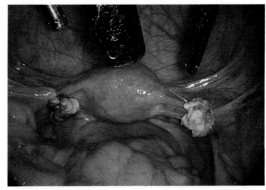

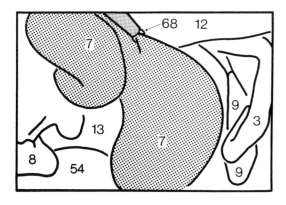

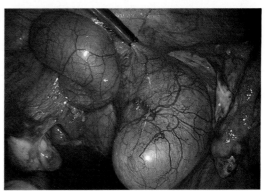

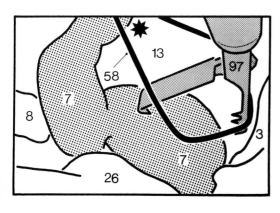

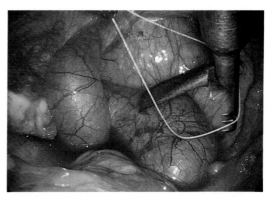

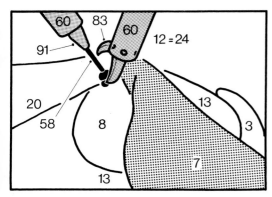

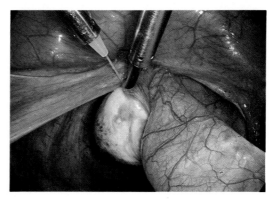

Plate 201. **Salpingectomy for hydrosalpinx**

Operation: After three endoloops have been applied, the tube and ovary are kept under strong traction with the aid of the large claw forceps so that the vascular pedicle can be severed. The scissors are introduced on the side on which the salpingo-oophorectomy is being performed so that cutting can be done at a right angle to the tissue pedicle to prevent the inadvertent cutting of the ligatures or the mesosalpinx.

Plate 202. **Salpingectomy for hydrosalpinx**

Operation: After removal of the hydrosalpinx through the 11-mm trocar sleeve (see Plate 181) and morcellation of ovarian tissues (see Plate 196), the pelvis was thoroughly irrigated until all peritoneal surfaces were smooth and clean. At this moment, the left vascular pedicle is being coagulated with a point coagulator to prevent adhesions from occurring.

Plate 203. **Salpingectomy for hydrosalpinx: End result**

Findings: The final appearance after left salpingo-oophorectomy to remove a hydrosalpinx of about 9–10 cm maximum diameter that had occurred after a previous vaginal hysterectomy. After irrigation of the pelvis with 1 L of normal saline solution, the entire endometrium is smooth and clean.

Comment: The postoperative physical stress to the patient consists only of the healing process in the adnexal pedicle and the four small abdominal wounds resulting from the trocar sleeves.

Plate 204. **Salpingectomy for hydrosalpinx**

History: A 50-year-old patient underwent an appendectomy at age 24 years. Pelvic examination subsequently revealed a right adnexal tumor, which was confirmed by sonography.

Findings: Diagnostic pelviscopy reveals a small cyst of 3–4 cm diameter. In consideration of the patient's age, it was decided to proceed directly from a diagnostic to an operative pelviscopy, i.e., salpingo-oophorectomy.

Operation: After introduction of the endoloop, the hydrosalpinx has been grasped with the large claw forceps. The atraumatic grasping tongs pull the endoloop as far toward the lateral pelvic wall as possible; at the same time an attempt is made to use the plastic applicator rod to also place the slipknot as far laterally as possible.

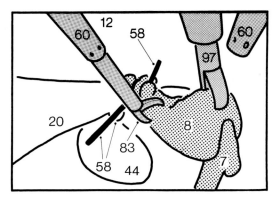

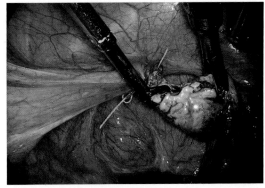

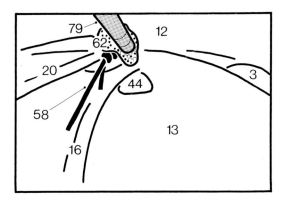

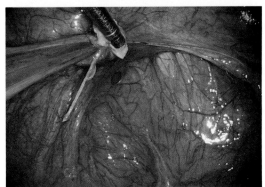

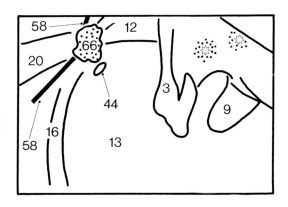

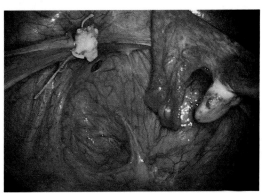

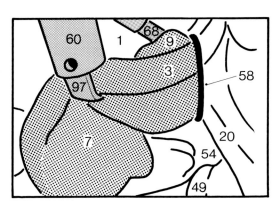

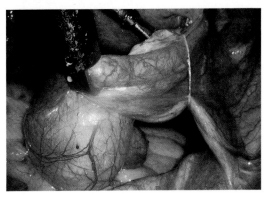

Plate 205. **Salpingectomy for hydrosalpinx**
Operation: With strong traction exerted by the large claw forceps, the ligature has been placed behind the ovary and the hydrosalpinx. The free end of the suture will be cut to about 1 cm length with hook scissors.

Plate 206. **Salpingectomy for hydrosalpinx**
Operation: After triple ligation of the adnexal pedicle by the triple-loop technique, as shown in Plates 204 and 205, the hook scissors are cutting the adnexal structures at a right angle to the vascular pedicle, without causing any active bleeding.

Plate 207. **Salpingectomy for hydrosalpinx: End result**
Operation: The entire right adnexal structures have been grasped with the large claw forceps and can be removed through the 11-mm trocar sleeve. Overhanging ovarian tissue is only incised with hook scissors, so that the entire right adnexa can be pulled in one piece through the 11-mm trocar sleeve.

Plate 208. **Salpingectomy after torsion of the pedicle**
History: A 35-year-old patient had an appendectomy at age 17 years and a vaginal tubal sterilization at age 27 years. Physical examination revealed a subacute abdomen with an elongated pelvic tumor.
Findings: Diagnostic pelviscopy revealed a hematosalpinx with torsion of the stalk, status post tubal sterilization. After careful evaluation, it was decided to proceed with operative pelviscopy, i.e., a salpingectomy.

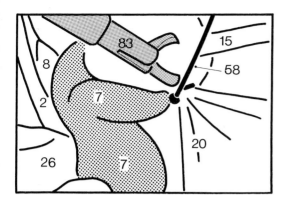

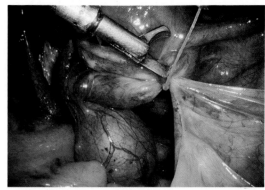

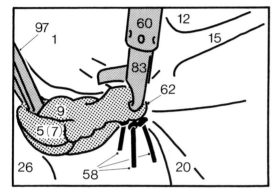

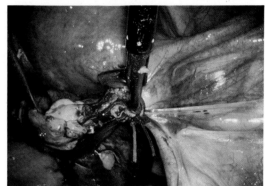

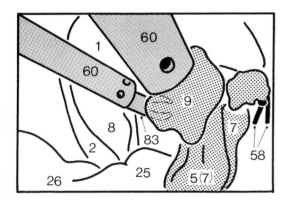

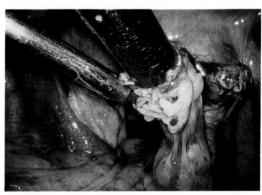

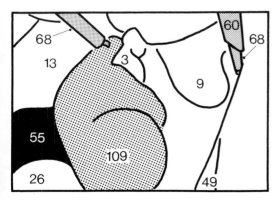

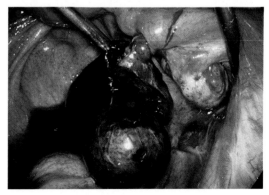

Plate 209. **Salpingectomy after torsion of the pedicle**
Operation: The endoloop has been introduced on the same side on which the salpingectomy is to be performed. The large claw forceps reaches through the loop to grasp the hematosalpinx.

Plate 210. **Salpingectomy after torsion of the pedicle**
Operation: The second endoloop has been placed optimally at the end of the stalk and hook scissors are cutting the suture at 1 cm length. Grasping of the hematosalpinx with the large claw forceps has allowed most of the blood from the hematosalpinx to drain into the cul-de-sac.

Plate 211. **Salpingectomy after torsion of the pedicle**
Operation: The twisted stalk of the hematosalpinx has been ligated three times by the triple-loop technique and resected with scissors, cutting at a right angle to the longitudinal axis of the pedicle. This was accomplished without active bleeding.

Plate 212. **Salpingectomy after torsion of the pedicle**
Operation: The right hematosalpinx that had occurred after torsion of the stalk subsequent to a previous vaginal tubal sterilization operation has been resected as shown in Plates 208–211. Because of the gelatinous consistency of the tubal tissues, it is better to utilize the large spoon forceps instead of the large claw forceps to remove the tube piecemeal through an 11-mm trocar sleeve.

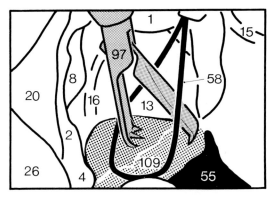
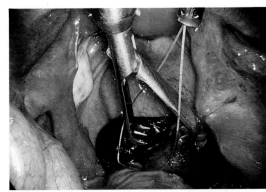

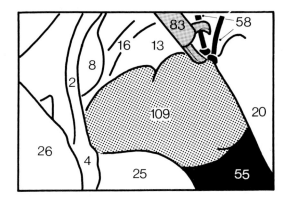
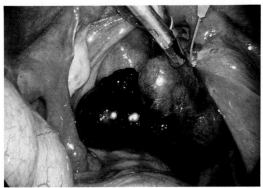

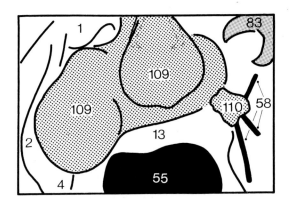
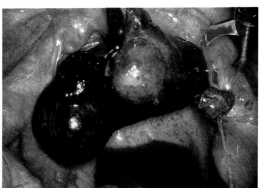

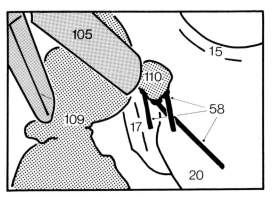
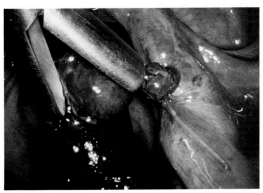

Plate 213. **Salpingectomy after torsion of the pedicle: End result**
Operation: After irrigation of the pelvis with 2 L of warm saline solution at 37° C, the pelvic structures and all peritoneal surfaces are smooth and clean. The tubal pedicle is being coagulated with the point coagulator to prevent the formation of adhesions. The right ovary is covered with membranous adhesions. The left adnexa is unremarkable.

Plate 214. **Salpingectomy for hydrosalpinx**
History: A 33-year-old patient underwent a laparotomy for adhesiolysis and tubal steriliza-tion 6 years earlier and was found to have a cystic pelvic tumor, confirmed by sonography.
Findings: Diagnostic pelviscopy revealed a right hydrosalpinx of 2.5 × 5.5 cm, which may have resulted from the tubal sterilization in the presence of an occlusion of the tubal am-pulla.
Operation: The diagnostic pelviscopy will immediately be followed by operative pelvi-scopy, i.e., total removal of the hydrosalpinx.
See also Plates 215–220.

Plate 215. **Salpingectomy for hydrosalpinx**
Operation: The endoloop has been introduced on the side on which the salpingectomy is to be performed. The hydrosalpinx has been pulled through the loop with atraumatic grasping tongs. In this case, the loop can be placed without the aid of the atraumatic grasping tongs, obviating the need for a fourth abdominal puncture.

Plate 216. **Salpingectomy for hydrosalpinx**
Operation: The second endoloop is placed immediately lateral to the previous one to ligate the firm tubal pedicle.
Comment: This operation was performed without technical difficulties through only two suprapubic 5-mm trocar sleeves.

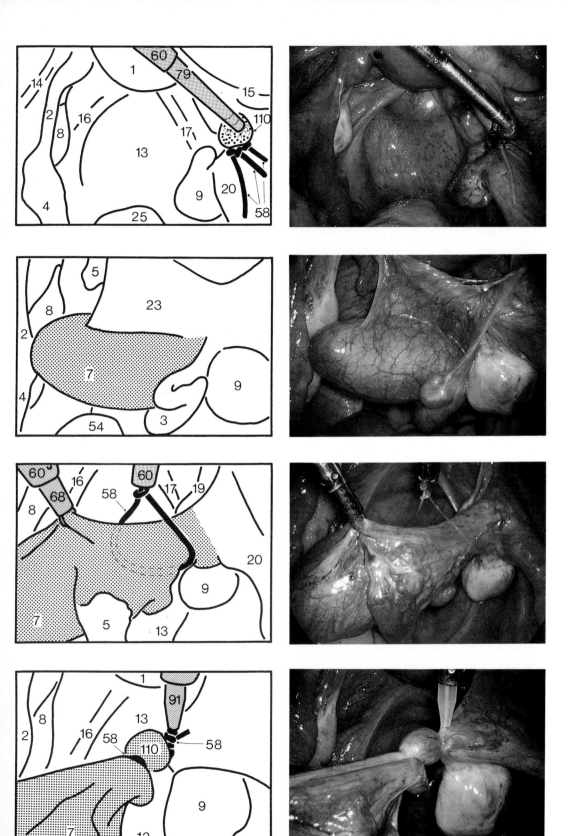

Plate 217. **Salpingectomy for hydrosalpinx**
Operation: After double ligation of the mesosalpinx, the hydrosalpinx is severed with scissors cutting at right angles and without active bleeding. The few milliliters of blood in the cul-de-sac resulted from retrograde drainage from the resected tissues.

Plate 218. **Salpingectomy for hydrosalpinx**
Operation: In preparation for the removal of the hydrosalpinx from the pelvis, a 5-mm trocar sleeve, introduced in the right suprapubic area, will be dilated to 11 mm diameter with the special dilatation set. The threaded 11-mm dilatation trocar is advanced over the guiding rod and is presently perforating the parietal peritoneum.
See also Plate 11.

Plate 219. **Salpingectomy for hydrosalpinx**
Operation: The resected hydrosalpinx is now being grasped with the large claw forceps and retracted in one piece through the 11-mm trocar sleeve. During this maneuver, its contents drain into the pelvis.

Plate 220. **Salpingectomy for hydrosalpinx: End result**
Operation: After complete extraction of the hydrosalpinx, the pelvis is irrigated with approximately 1 L of warm saline solution at 37° C until all peritoneal surfaces are smooth and clean. The right tubal stump, which, after the previous tubal sterilization operation, consists only of a fibrous strand of tissue, will finally be coagulated to prevent the growth of adhesions.

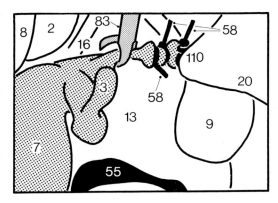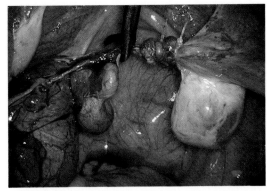

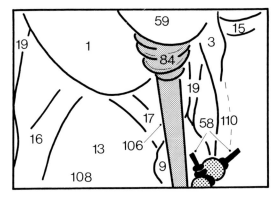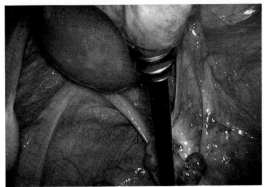

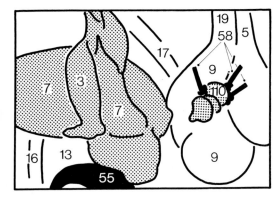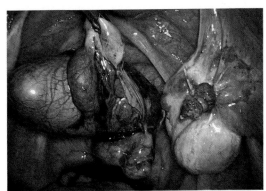

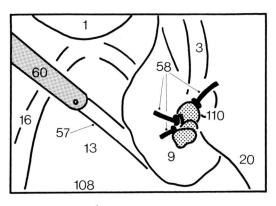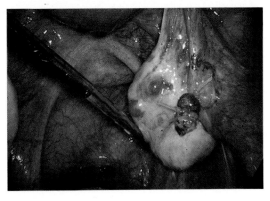

14.2.10. Pelviscopic Operation on the Uterus

Plate 221. **Enucleation of a myoma (pedunculated myoma)**

History and Findings: A 26-year-old infertile patient underwent an appendectomy at age 19 years, a laparotomy to correct sterility at age 20 years, and a second laparotomy with bilateral tubal implantation at 23 years. Fourteen months before the present operation, a follow-up pelviscopy revealed a small pedunculated myoma of 8–10 mm diameter. Both tubes were patent at that time.

Operation: After adequate coagulation of the stalk, either with crocodile forceps or the myoma enucleator (see Plates 233 and 244), the myoma is grasped with the large claw forceps and twisted off its base without causing any bleeding.

Plate 222. **Enucleation of a myoma (pedunculated myoma): End result**

Operation: The myoma, coagulated as shown in Plate 221 and twisted off with the large claw forceps, can now be removed through the 11-mm trocar sleeve.

Comment: The coagulated area about 2 cm in diameter on the surface of the uterine fundus will remain detectable for about 8–12 days (see Plate 6); then fibroblasts and histiocytes will migrate into this area from the periphery until the devitalized tissue has been completely replaced by healthy peritoneum, as documented in Plates 223 and 224.

Plate 223. **Enucleation of a myoma (pedunculated myoma): Follow-up**

History: Twenty-two months earlier the patient underwent a bilateral microsurgical tubal reimplantation to correct intramural tubal obstruction by deep endometriotic implants. Seventeen months later a small pedunculated myoma was enucleated after broad-based coagulation of its stalk, as demonstrated in Plates 221 and 222.

Findings: The uterine fundus is well peritonealized, except for a few vascular irregularities in the peritoneum. There are no adhesions. Superficial endometriosis has occurred, as evidenced by the pool of blood in the cul-de-sac.

Additional follow-up findings after enucleation of the myomas are shown in Plates 224, 237, and 243.

Plate 224. **Enucleation of a myoma: Follow-up**

History: Status 8 months after enucleation of an intramural myoma

Findings: This is a close-up photograph of the coagulation site shown in Plates 225–232. Only fibrosed contours can be recognized in the peritoneum, but no adhesions, which, as a general rule, would almost always be seen after enucleation of a myoma and closure of the uterine incision with sutures under laparotomy conditions.

See also Plates 223, 237 and 243.

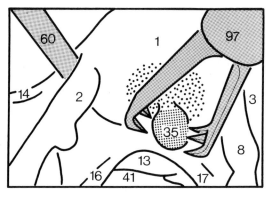

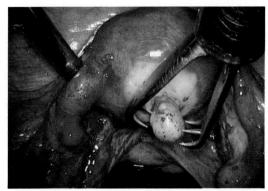

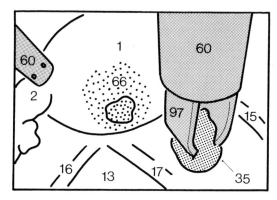

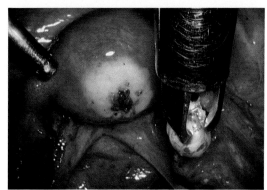

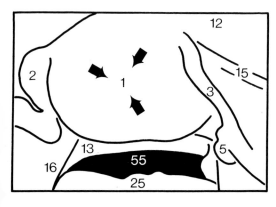

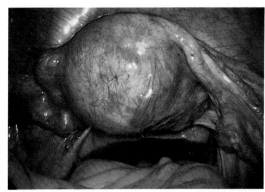

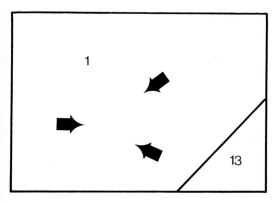

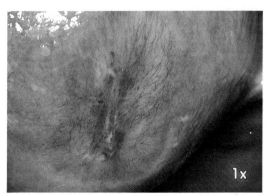

14.2.10.1. Pelviscopic Enucleation of Myomas (Plates 225–228)

Plate 225. **Enucleation of a myoma (intramural myoma) with suture of the uterus: Overview**

History: A 33-year-old patient underwent laparotomy because of Stein-Leventhal syndrome at age 22 years. At age 32 years, 12 months before the current presentation, a chocolate cyst was excised from the right ovary by operative pelviscopy (see Plates 125 and 128). Since the patient failed to conceive, another pelviscopic evaluation was indicated.

Findings: The pelvic organs are free of adhesions. A 4-cm intramural myoma is noted that is probably responsible for the considerable impairment of the tubal patency within the intramural segments of both tubes. Therefore, it was decided to enucleate the myoma.

Histology: Leiomyoma.

See also Plates 226–232.

Plate 226. **Enucleation of a myoma (intramural myoma) with suture of the uterus**

Operation: For hemostatic purposes, a narrow strip of the capsule of the myoma, about 8 cm long and less than 1 cm wide, has been coagulated with the crocodile forceps.

Comment: The myoma enucleator would have been more suitable than the crocodile forceps; however, it was not yet available at that time.

Plate 227. **Enucleation of a myoma (intramural myoma) with suture of the uterus**

Operation: Assisted by atraumatic grasping tongs, a longitudinal incision is made with hook scissors in the coagulated strip of the uterine fundus, splitting both the uterine serosa and the capsule of the myoma. After careful coagulation, this is a practically bloodless procedure.

Plate 228. **Enucleation of myoma (intramural myoma) with suture of the uterus**

Operation: After the capsule of the myoma has been peeled off, the large claw forceps grasps the myoma. The myoma enucleator, heated to 120° C, is used to carefully separate the myoma from its capsule. It may occasionally be necessary to cut some tougher tissue bridges with scissors. However, such tissue connections should always first be coagulated sufficiently to prevent any troublesome hemorrhage.

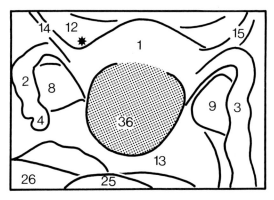
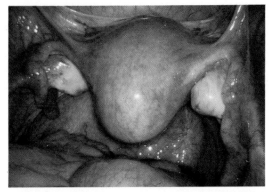

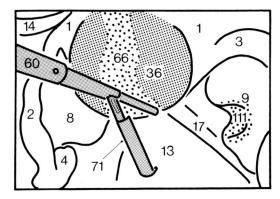
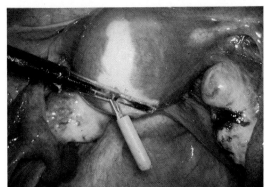

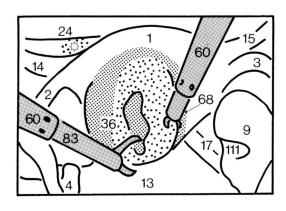
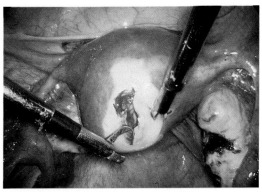

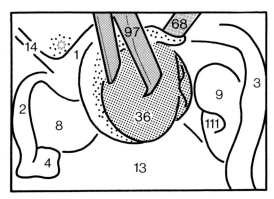
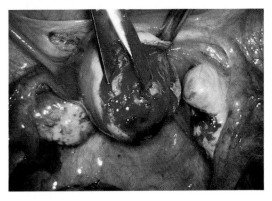

Plate 229. **Enucleation of a myoma (intramural myoma) with suture of the uterus**
Operation: The myoma has been grasped with the large claw forceps and removed from its capsule by rotation and peeling movements with the heated myoma enucleator. If this instrument is not available, an open crocodile forceps may be utilized. Although the adenomyoma was fairly soft, the wound cavity will bleed very little if it has been carefully prepared as described.

Plate 230. **Enucleation of a myoma (intramural myoma) with suture of the uterus**
Operation: The remaining wound cavity is again thoroughly recoagulated with the point coagulator or myoma enucleator until complete hemostasis has been achieved. This can be checked by irrigation of the wound cavity with saline solution. After complete hemostasis has been achieved and the pelvis has been thoroughly cleansed, the wound will be closed. *See also* Plate 231.

Plate 231. **Enucleation of a myoma (intramural myoma) with suture of the uterus**
Operation: After enucleation of the 4-cm-diameter myoma (see Plates 225–230), the large gaping wound remaining must be closed with two endosutures. A 3-mm needleholder has introduced the catgut suture armed with the straight needle into the pelvis and grasped the needle to penetrate the right margin of the wound, which is being steadied by the 5-mm needleholder. Since complete hemostasis has been achieved, and since the healing process after an endoscopic operation seems more favorable than after a laparotomy, a rather crude adaptation of the wound edges is sufficient. The slipknot will be tied externally.

Plate 232. **Enucleation of a myoma (intramural myoma) with suture of the uterus: End result**
Findings: Final appearance of the pelvic organs after enucleation of a subserous 4-cm-diameter adenomyoma, as shown in Plates 225–231. The wound edges have been approximated well by two endosutures.
Comment: Since peristalsis of the intestinal tract is resumed immediately postoperatively and since intestinal and vascular paralysis—which is usually provoked by an open laparotomy—does not develop after a laparoscopy, the wound in the uterus can be expected to heal by primary intention and without adhesions.
See also Plate 224, which shows the smooth uterine surface on follow-up endoscopic evaluation 8 months later; *and see* Plates 236 and 237.

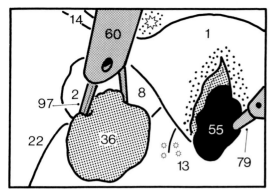
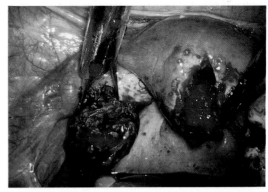

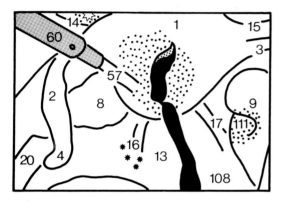
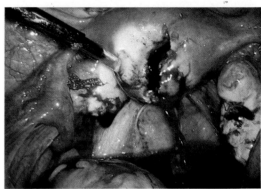

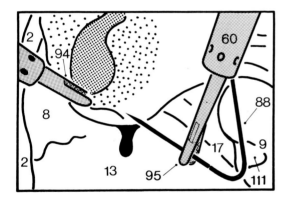
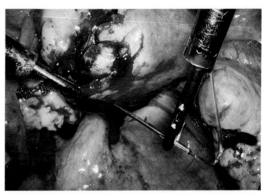

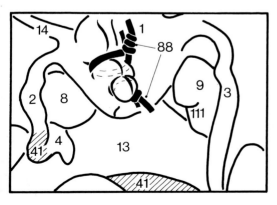
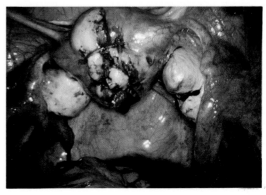

Plate 233. **Enucleation of myoma (pedunculated myoma)**
History: A 45-year-old patient presented with primary sterility.
Findings: A subserous pedunculated myoma about 2 cm in largest diameter arises from the uterine fundus.
Operation: The stalk of the myoma is coagulated with a crocodile forceps; then it can be grasped with a biopsy forceps and twisted off without blood loss.
Caution: Since only the straight jaw of the crocodile forceps is heated, it is recommended that the forceps be applied twice, each time in an opposite direction, whenever a thicker stalk must be coagulated.

Plate 234. **Enucleation of myoma (pedunculated myoma): End result**
Operation: After the pedunculated myoma has been twisted off with the claw forceps, the remaining wound crater is again carefully recoagulated with a point coagulator to denature the tissue proteins in the area of the wound to a depth of at least 1 mm.

Plate 235. **Enucleation of myoma (pedunculated myoma)**
History: A 27-year-old patient presented with sterility.
Findings: A large pedunculated myoma of about 2.5 × 3.5 cm diameter arises from the uterine fundus. A small subserous myoma is noted close to the left tubal cornu. The greater omentum adheres to the anterior parietal peritoneum.
Operation: To improve access to the pelvis, the abdominal adhesions are lysed first. Then the stalk of the myoma is coagulated with crocodile forceps.
Caution: In this case, a coagulation time of at least 2–3 minutes will be necessary to accomplish coagulation of proteins and complete hemostasis throughout the entire diameter of the stalk.
Histology: Leiomyoma, highly vascularized.

Plate 236. **Enucleation of myoma (pedunculated myoma): End result**
Operation: After adequate coagulation of its stalk, the myoma was grasped with the large claw forceps and twisted off its base. If the base of the myoma is broader than anticipated, it may be necessary to cut the base with scissors.
Comment: If the myoma is highly calcified, it cannot be morcellated. Access to the pelvic cavity can then be gained through a posterior colpotomy through which the myoma, which is secured by the claw forceps, can be removed. At the end of the myomectomy a bilateral salpingoplasty was performed.
Caution: A thick, vascular myoma stalk must be cut with great caution, and often it is helpful to recoagulate the tissues with the heated myoma enucleator. One should not hesitate to coagulate even extended areas of the uterus because they usually heal without scar formation, as shown in Plates 223, 224, 237, and 243.
See also Plate 237, which gives an endoscopic overview of the pelvic organs 6 weeks after the present operation.

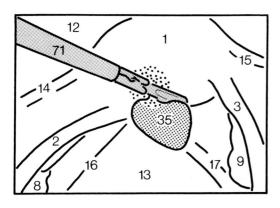

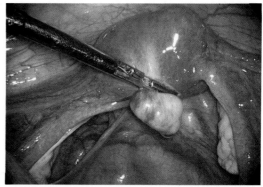

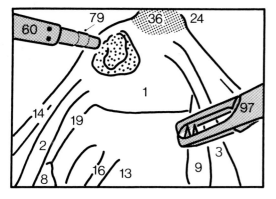

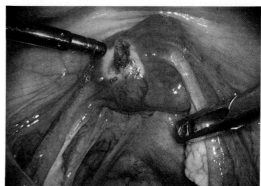

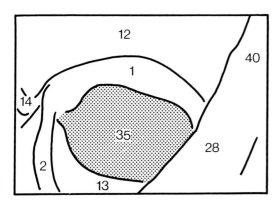

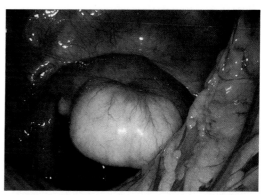

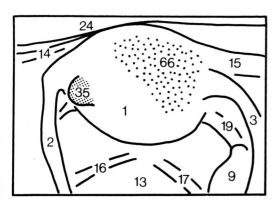

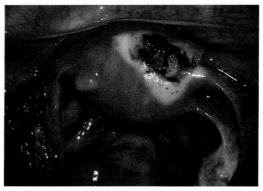

Plate 237. **Enucleation of myoma (pedunculated myoma): Follow-up of Plate 236**
History: Six weeks after enucleation of a myoma and salpingoplasty (see Plates 235 and 236), the patient had to undergo another pelviscopy for suspicion of an ectopic tubal pregnancy.
Findings: A lutein cyst was noted in the right ovary. The uterine fundus was completely epithelialized and there was no evidence of adhesions.
Additional follow-up findings after enucleation of myomas are shown in Plates 223, 224, and 243.

Plate 238. **Enucleation of myoma (cervical adenoma) with suture of the uterus**
History: A 39-year-old patient with uterine adenomyosis was undergoing diagnostic pelviscopy for evaluation of primary sterility. A cervical myoma appeared to have grown rapidly.
Findings: A cervical myoma about 2 × 3 cm in diameter was noted just above the dome of the bladder.
Operation: The myoma capsule has already been coagulated and incised with hook scissors.

Plate 239. **Enucleation of myoma (cervical adenoma) with suture of the uterus**
Operation: The dissection begun in Plate 238 has progressed to the point that the myoma can be grasped with the large claw forceps. The heated myoma enucleator is used to peel it out of the uterine wall. Proceeding in a slow, deliberate, meticulous manner will usually be a bloodless operation.

Plate 240. **Enucleation of myoma (cervical adenoma) with suture of the uterus: End result**
Findings: The supracervical leiomyoma has been completely enucleated and its wound bed has been adequately coagulated.
Operation: After repeated irrigation with normal saline solution, the wound edges are now approximated with an endosuture. The 3-mm needleholder has just advanced the needle through the right and left wound edges and the 5-mm needleholder is pulling the needle through the tissue. The 3-mm needleholder will then grasp the needle and suture to retract it through the trocar sleeve so that the slipknot can be tied externally.
Histology: Leiomyoma with focal hyalinization.

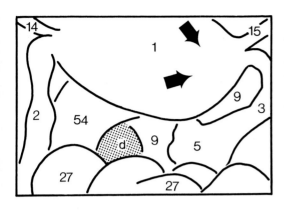
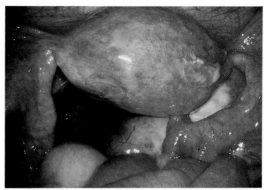

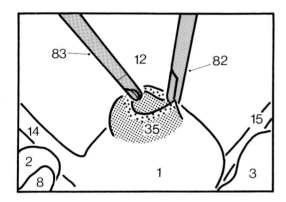
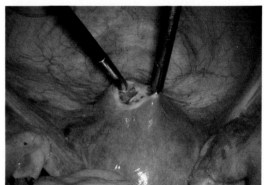

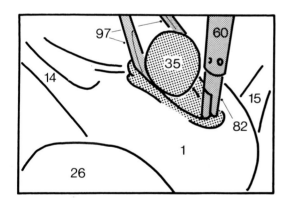
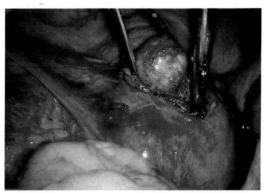

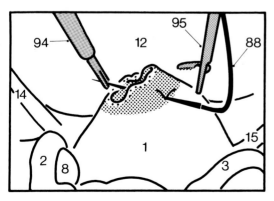
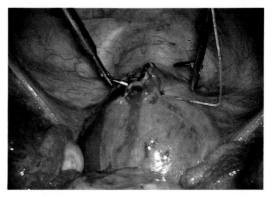

Plate 241. **Extensive omental and intestinal adhesiolysis and enucleation of myoma**

History: A 27-year-old patient with primary sterility had an appendectomy at age 7 years and a partial oophorectomy at age 26 years.

Findings: Extensive pelvic adhesions between the sigmoid colon, the left and right adnexa, and the posterior wall of the uterus have apparently resulted from a postoperative pelvic peritonitis. Hydrosalpinx was also noted on both sides.

Operation: Bilateral salpingostomy was performed, as shown in Plates 88–93 and Plates 97–99. The myoma could be removed in the usual manner, as shown in Plates 233 and 234. Perfect hemostasis was achieved using first the crocodile forceps and then the point coagulator.

See also Plate 243, which shows the appearance on follow-up 5 months later.

Plate 242. **Extensive omental and intestinal adhesiolysis and enucleation of myoma**

Operation: The myoma of 7–10 mm diameter (see Plate 241) has been enucleated after coagulation of its capsule; the uterine defect was recoagulated with the point coagulator. Complete hemostasis has been achieved.

See also Plate 243, which shows the appearance 5 months later.

Plate 243. **Extensive omental and intestinal adhesiolysis and enucleation of myoma: Follow-up**

Findings: On follow-up evaluation 5 months after extensive omental and intestinal adhesiolysis and enucleation of the myoma (see Plates 241 and 242), and bilateral salpingostomy performed according to techniques shown in Plates 88–93 and Plates 97–99, the pelvic organs are completely free of adhesions and both tubes are patent. No adhesions can be recognized in the area from which the myoma has been enucleated, nor is there any scarring in peritoneal surfaces.

See also Plates 223, 224, and 237 for other examples of follow-up findings after enucleation of myomas.

Plate 244. **Enucleation of myomas, ovarian biopsy, and bilateral salpingoplasty**

History: A 36-year-old patient with primary infertility had an appendectomy at age 7 years.

Findings: Pelvic endometriosis, bilateral tubal phimosis, and multiple subserous and pedunculated myomas with diameters between 5 and 25 mm were noted.

Operation: The largest of the pedunculated myomas has been grasped with the large claw forceps to stretch its stalk, which has just been coagulated with the crocodile forceps.

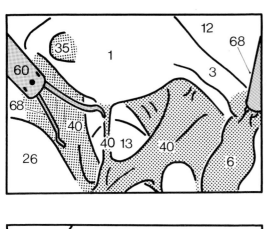
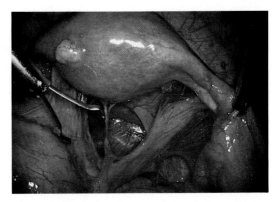
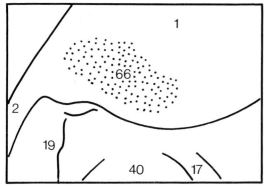
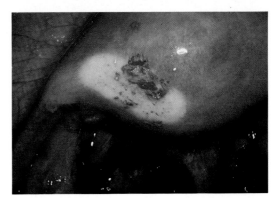
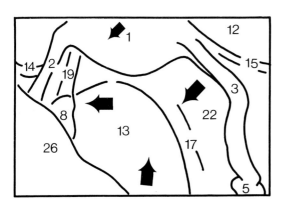
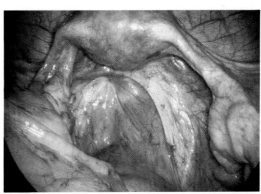
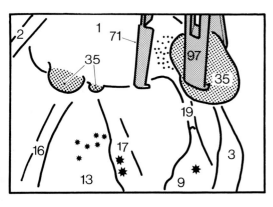
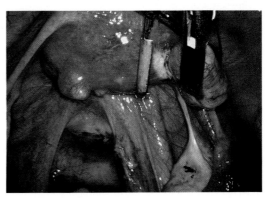

Plate 245. **Enucleation of myomas, ovarian biopsy, and bilateral salpingoplasty**
Operation: The largest myoma has been grasped with the biopsy forceps introduced through the left 5-mm trocar sleeve. The myoma tissue is being pressed into the cutting orifice of the tissue punch for morcellation. This tissue punch has been introduced after one of the 5-mm trocar sleeves has been dilated up to accommodate the 11-mm trocar sleeve.

Plate 246. **Enucleation of myomas, ovarian biopsy, and bilateral salpingoplasty: End result**
Findings: This is an overview of the pelvic organs after enucleation of multiple myomas, right ovarian biopsy, coagulation of endometriotic implants, and bilateral salpingoplasty with ascending chromosalpingoscopy. Endocoagulation at 100° C has resulted in complete hemostasis in all wounds of the uterine fundus and the right ovary. Protruding from the left side of the photograph is the atraumatic grasping forceps, which was used for blunt dilatation of the phimosed ampullary segments of the tubes.

Plate 247. **Enucleation of a myoma from the dome of the bladder**
History: A 29-year-old patient with primary infertility underwent diagnostic pelviscopy for the evaluation of an ovarian tumor.
Findings: A myoma of about 2 × 3 cm diameter is noted adjacent to the bladder dome in the area of the retrosymphyseal peritoneum.
Operation: After the peritoneum has been coagulated and incised, two biopsy forceps are used to retract the peritoneum from the myoma. The myoma can then be grasped with the large claw forceps and bloodlessly twisted off. The peritoneal wound can then be closed without difficulties with two endosutures.
Comment: Endoscopic reevaluation 6 months later showed a peritoneum without scars.
Histology: Leiomyoma.

Plate 248. **Uterine adhesiolysis**
History: After a previous cesarean section, the patient suffered from chronic pelvic and coital discomfort.
Findings: During diagnostic pelviscopy, bands of adhesions were noted in the mid and lower abdominal regions. A solid strand of tissue almost 1 cm in diameter extends from the uterine fundus to the parietal peritoneum in the region of the linea alba.
Operation: This apparently very vascular adhesive band is first carefully coagulated so that
. . .

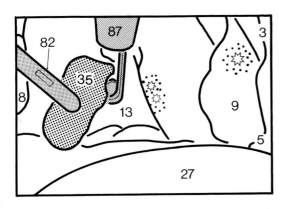

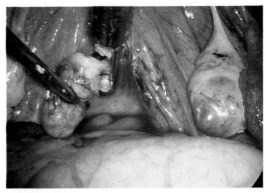

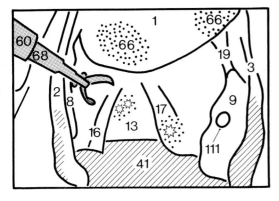

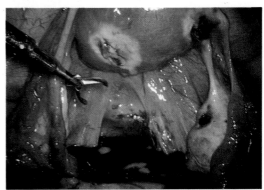

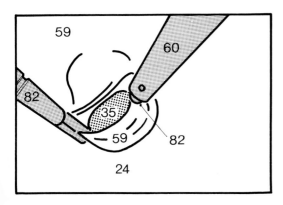

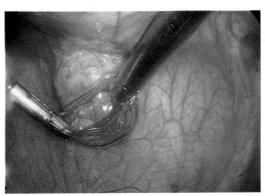

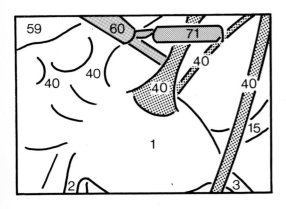

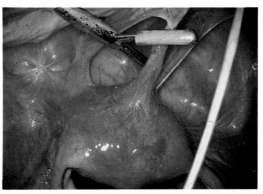

Plate 249. Uterine adhesiolysis: End result

Operation: . . . sharp dissection with hook scissors can be accomplished without bleeding.

Comment: This procedure immediately relieved the patient of her discomfort.

14.2.10.2. Pelviscopic Removal of a "lost IUD"

Plate 250. "Lost IUD" removal with a hysteroscope

History: The patient has been wearing an intrauterine contraceptive device (IUD); however, its tail could no longer be palpated or visualized. Sonographically, the IUD appeared to be in the endometrial cavity.

Findings: On hysteroscopic exploration, the IUD and its tail were found lying in the endometrial cavity. The left tubal ostium is also clearly visible.

Operation: The IUD was removed through the cervical canal.

Comment: In the field of intrauterine contraception, it is presently assumed that the IUD is in its proper position if the synthetic monofilamentous tail protrudes through the cervical canal into the vagina. If the tail can no longer be palpated or visualized, one refers to it as a "lost IUD." Several possibilities and conditions have to be addressed and evaluated: Is the IUD still present in the uterine cavity and effective as a contraceptive? Has the IUD been expelled through the cervical canal and lost through the vagina, unnoticed? Has the IUD partially or totally perforated the uterine wall? Has the IUD transmigrated into the uterine ligaments? Internal genital organs? Pelvic cavity? Or abdominal cavity?

[This IUD probably could have been removed easily in the office by introducing a 3-mm grasping forceps into the uterine cavity, opening it inside, palpating and grasping the IUD, and removing it transcervically. This would have saved the patient the expense and trauma of sonography, x-rays, the hysteroscopic procedure, and local or general anesthesia.—*Ed.*]

See also Plates 251 ff. and 257.

Plate 251. "Lost IUD": Transabdominal removal

History: A 29-year-old patient had an appendectomy at age 12 years. Immediately after the termination of an intrauterine pregnancy in the 10th week of gestation, a Cu-7 IUD was inserted into the uterus. Four months later, the IUD tail could no longer be detected in the external cervical os. Radiologic examination revealed the IUD within the pelvis, and the sonogram seemed to indicate an intrauterine position of the IUD.

Findings: On hysteroscopic examination, however, only the last 2 cm of the IUD tail was still in the uterine cavity.

Operation: The diagnostic hysteroscope was replaced by an operative hysteroscope so that the end of the IUD tail could be grasped and pulled; however, the IUD and its tail could not be mobilized. It was assumed that the IUD had transmigrated through the uterine wall. It was decided to proceed immediately with a diagnostic pelviscopy, which revealed that the short arm of the Cu-7 clearly protruded subperitoneally from the posterior wall of the uterus.

Plate 252. "Lost IUD": Transabdominal removal

Operation: The area of peritoneum and uterine muscle that is still covering the protruding short arm of the plastic IUD is first carefully coagulated to a depth of 2–3 mm with the point coagulator heated to 120° C. To accomplish this, the point coagulator is moved across the uterine surface in the manner of a steam iron.

380

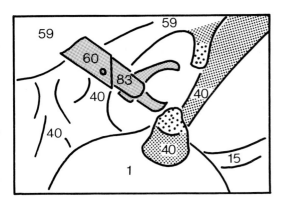

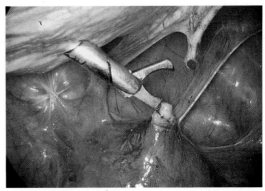

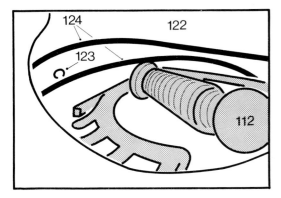

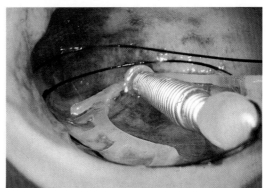

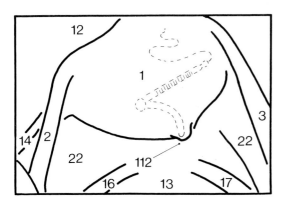

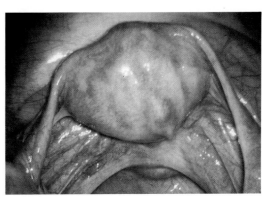

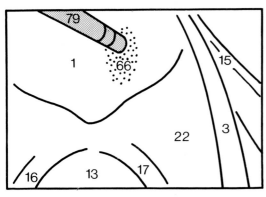

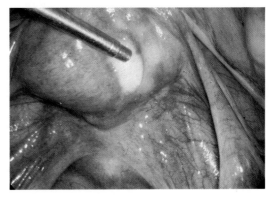

Plate 253. **"Lost IUD": Transabdominal removal**

Findings: Hemostasis of the uterine wall has been achieved by heat coagulation.

Operation: Tissues are carefully teased apart with the atraumatic biopsy tongs until the tip of the short arm of the plastic IUD is exposed sufficiently so that it can be grasped with a biopsy forceps.

Plate 254. **"Lost IUD": Transabdominal removal**

Operation: The free short arm of the Cu-7 IUD, shown in Plates 251–253, was grasped with a biopsy forceps and extracted from the myometrium. Another biopsy forceps was used to stabilize the uterine fundus against the posterior surface of the symphysis.

Plate 255. **"Lost IUD": Transabdominal removal**

Operation: The Cu-7 IUD has been completely extracted, followed by the string, which will also be pulled through the uterine wall into the abdomen with the biopsy forceps. The 5-mm puncture site is then dilated further to accommodate the 11-mm trocar sleeve so that the Cu-7 can be removed with ease.

[If a 3-mm grasping forceps or a 3-mm or 5-mm needleholder had been introduced through the 5-mm trocar sleeve, the IUD probably could have been removed through the 5-mm trocar sleeve without further dilatation to 11 mm. Another alternative, which this editor prefers in most cases, is the use of a 10-mm operating laparoscope with a 6-mm operating channel, introduced through the primary infraumbilical puncture site. IUDs and small tumors or larger fragments of tissue are easily removed through its 11-mm trocar sleeve.— *Ed.*]

Plate 256. **"Lost IUD": Transabdominal removal: End result**

Operation: After the "lost IUD" has been extracted transabdominally, as shown in Plates 251–255, the intramural tract is again carefully recoagulated with the point coagulator.

Comment: Such coagulation is recommended for its sterilizing effect in an effort to prevent transmural contamination with bacteria. Since a short segment of the IUD string has been positioned in the uterine cavity, it is conceivable that bacteria could enter the abdominal cavity.

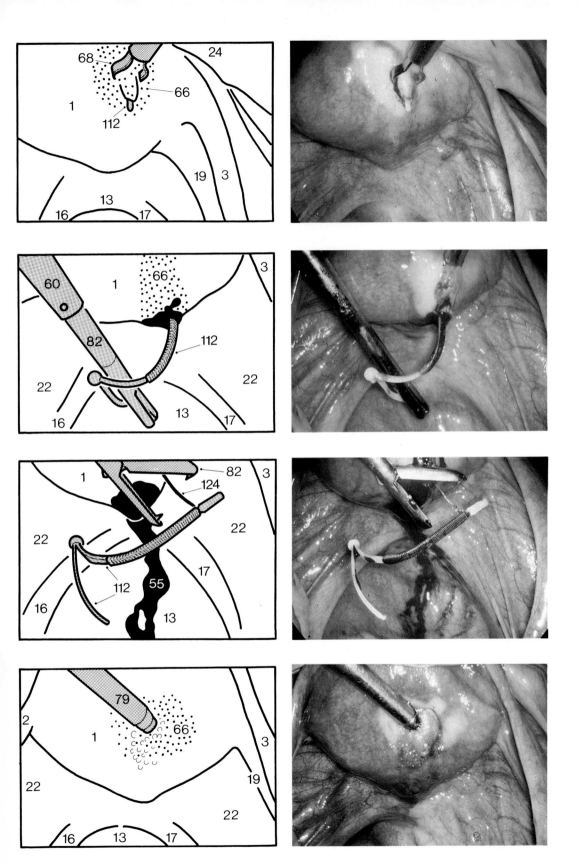

Plate 257. Lost IUD

History: A 26-year-old patient was seen 2 years after the introduction of a Lippes loop into the uterus and 6 months after a vaginal delivery. Preliminary evaluation failed to detect the IUD in the uterine cavity or anywhere in the pelvis.

Findings: The IUD was completely overgrown by the omentum.

Operation: Endoloops were utilized to accomplish a partial omentectomy. The IUD could then be removed without difficulties by the pelviscopic route.

14.2.10.3. Suture of the Uterus After Perforation With a Curette

Plate 258. Suture of the uterus after perforation with a curette

History: A 38-year-old patient was seen whose uterus had been perforated with a large blunt curette during the second recurettage after an abortion at 3 months' gestation.

Findings: Diagnostic pelviscopy was immediately performed under the same anesthesia; the curette was discovered protruding from the uterine fundus. It was also noted that the peritoneum of the bladder dome was adherent to the uterine fundus (= status after cesarean section with curved low transverse incision according to Fuchs).

Plate 259. Suture of the uterine wall after perforation with a curette

Operation: After the curette has been withdrawn through the myometrium under endoscopic vision, the wounds on the surface of the uterine fundus as well as the wound canal will be sufficiently coagulated with the point coagulator. This is done for two reasons: for hemostasis, and for sterilization of the wound canal.

Plate 260. Suture of the uterine wall after perforation with a curette

Operation: After complete hemostasis has been achieved in the area of the uterine corpus, which had been perforated by the curette (see Plate 258), the uterine wound is closed with an endosuture tied with an external slipknot.

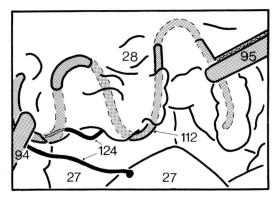

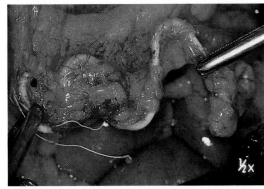

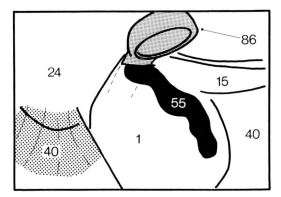

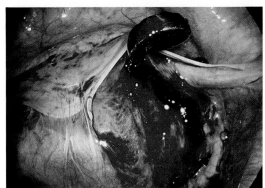

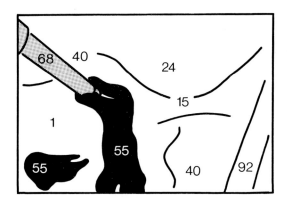

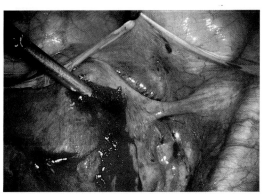

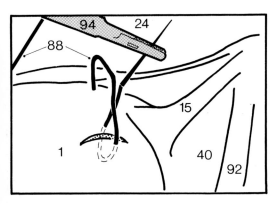

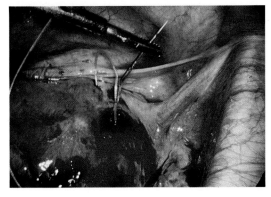

Plate 261.   Suture of the uterine wall after perforation with a curette: End result

Findings: The wound caused by the perforation with a large curette of the uterine wall (see Plate 258) has been closed with one endosuture and an externally tied slipknot. After irrigation, the pelvis is clean.

Comment: The immediate postoperative recovery was uneventful and the patient was discharged from the hospital on the third postoperative day. Follow-up examination after 6 weeks did not reveal any abnormalities. Two months after this pelviscopic operation, a new IUD (multiload) was introduced without any complications.

14.2.11.1.2. ECTOPIC PREGNANCY OF THE TUBE IN THE MIDDLE SEGMENT

Plate 262.   Conservative operation for tubal ectopic pregnancy

History: A 24-year-old patient was seen in the ninth week of gestation. An ectopic tubal pregnancy was diagnosed by ultrasound.

Findings: Pelviscopy confirmed the presence of an ectopic pregnancy in the middle segment of the right tube. There was a considerable amount of blood in the abdomen and the cul-de-sac. The uterus was distorted by a large cervical myoma.

Plate 263.   Conservative operation for tubal ectopic pregnancy

Operation: The Aquapurator apparatus was used to thoroughly irrigate the pelvis to permit a clearer view of the pelvic organs. Then a strip 5 mm wide and 4 cm long was coagulated with the point coagulator on the antimesosalpingeal side of the tube in the area of the ectopic pregnancy.

Comment: This coagulation will require 3–4 minutes to achieve hemostasis throughout all layers of the tubal wall.

Plate 264.   Conservative operation for tubal ectopic pregnancy

Operation: In the area of the coagulated, hemostatic strip, the tube is incised longitudinally with hook scissors. There is no bleeding.

Comment: A radial incision is presently under discussion.

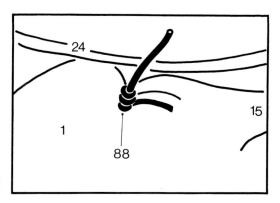

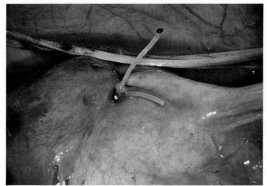

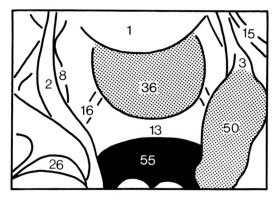

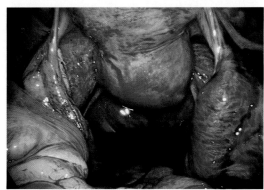

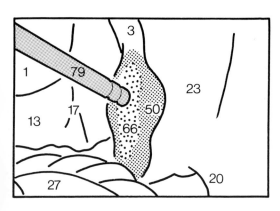

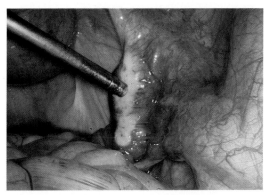

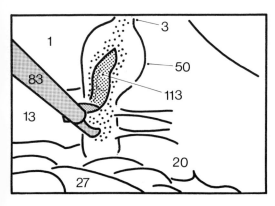

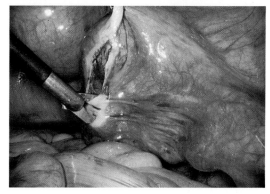

Plate 265. **Conservative operation for tubal ectopic pregnancy**

Operation: After a bloodless longitudinal incision is made into the tube, its wall contracts rapidly, usually expressing all products of conception. Remaining tissues of the tubal pregnancy are removed with a biopsy forceps. Meticulous techniques are very important. The wound cavity and the tube are constantly irrigated through the Aquapurator apparatus, as shown in Plate 273, to maintain an optimum view of the operative field.

Caution: As long as bleeding continues, there are chorionic tissue fragments present, comparable to curettage of an incomplete abortion of an intrauterine pregnancy.

Comment: Occasionally tubal contractions may occur spontaneously and the products of conception may be expelled through the fimbria or through a rupture of the attenuated tubal wall. In older, more advanced pregnancies, the use of the large spoon forceps may be necessary to remove the products of conception from the wound cavity in the tube.

See also Plate 275.

Plate 266. **Conservative operation for tubal ectopic pregnancy: End result**

Operation: After evacuation of the tubal pregnancy, as shown in Plates 263–265, the wound edges from the longitudinal incision into the tube are reapproximated with two endosutures.

Comment: Due to the rapid contraction of the tube after removal of the products of conception, i.e., the restitution of the tube, the wound will shrink until only a small slit remains, even in those cases in which the tube may have been enlarged to 4–5 cm (see Plates 274 and 276). Regardless of the size of the defect, Semm recommends approximating the wound edges by endosutures to prevent the development of tubal fistulas.

[In the experience of the editor and other surgeons, complete hemostasis must be ascertained; however, suture adaptation of the wound edges does not seem to be necessary, as spontaneous closure of the defect seems to be the rule—*Ed.*]

Plate 267. **Conservative operation for tubal ectopic pregnancy**

History: A 37-year-old patient had an appendectomy at age 18 and a pelviscopic operation because of secondary infertility at age 36. At present, physical examination and ultrasound raised the suspicion of a left tubal pregnancy of 8 weeks' gestation.

Findings: The pelvic organs were covered with blood, apparently originating from a beginning rupture of the left tubal pregnancy.

Plate 268. **Conservative operation for tubal ectopic pregnancy**

Operation: First, two 5-mm trocars for ancillary operative instruments are introduced by the Z-puncture technique in the suprapubic region.

Comments: The extreme mobility of the parietal peritoneum is evident in this photograph. Imagine that the same mechanism will apply to the introduction of the Veress needle in the periumbilical area, particularly if the puncture technique is not perpendicular to the skin but in a tangential direction!

See also Plates 1, 95, and 290.

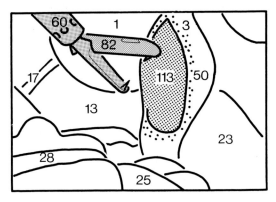
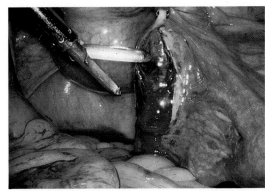

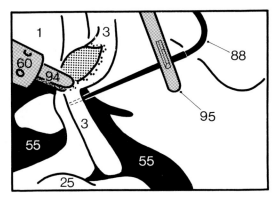
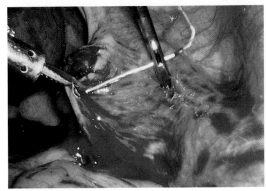

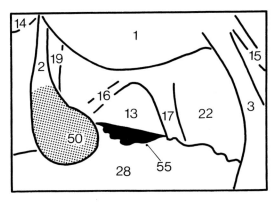
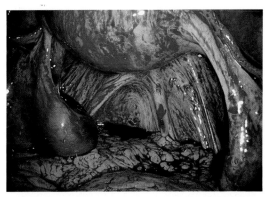

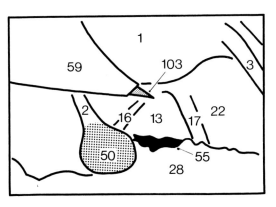
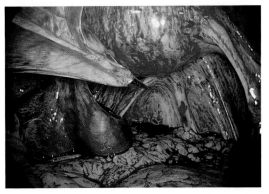

Plate 269. **Conservative operation for tubal ectopic pregnancy**
Operation: The pelvic cavity was first irrigated with 1 L of warm saline solution at 37° C to improve the visibility of the pelvic organs. Then the tubal wall was coagulated and incised in the longitudinal direction exactly over the bulge from the tubal pregnancy, as shown in Plates 263 and 264. Biopsy forceps are used to extract all products of conception in one piece.

Plate 270. **Conservative operation for tubal ectopic pregnancy: End result**
Operation: In this case, the wound edges have been approximated with biopsy forceps and the longitudinal tubal incision will be closed with an endoloop. Since there had been considerable bleeding from the beginning perforation of the tubal wall by the ectopic pregnancy, as shown in Plate 267, the pelvic cavity as well as the mid and upper abdomen were irrigated again to remove as much of the blood as possible.
See also Plates 271 and 272, showing the pelvic organs 17 months later.

Plate 271. **Conservative operation for tubal ectopic pregnancy: Follow-up**
History: Seventeen months earlier the patient underwent pelviscopic operation with the conservative removal of the left tubal pregnancy of 8 weeks' gestation, as shown in Plates 267–270.
Findings: All pelvic organs are completely free of adhesions. There are only minimal peritoneal scars in the area where the tube had been sutured.

Plate 272. **Conservative operation for tubal ectopic pregnancy: Follow-up**
Operation: Chromosalpingoscopy reveals that the left tube is clearly patent for the ascending methylene blue chromopertubation solution. This was followed by gas pertubation, which showed a grade I tubal patency (according to Fikentscher and Semm).

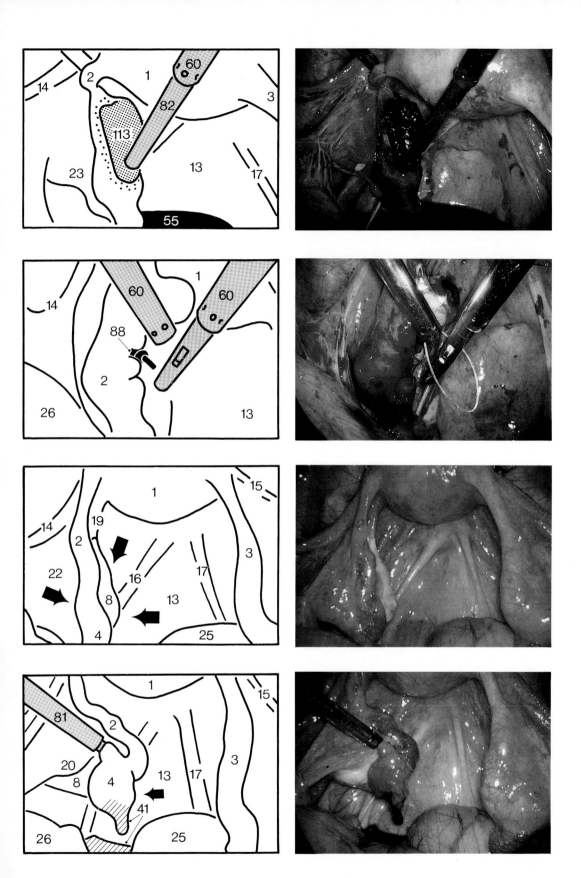

Plate 273. **Conservative operation for tubal ectopic pregnancy**

History: A 33-year-old patient had a tubal pregnancy of 9 weeks' gestation.

Operation: 800 ml of blood was aspirated from the pelvis. Only after the pelvis was adequately irrigated by means of the Aquapurator apparatus was it possible to recognize a ruptured tubal pregnancy in the left tube.

Plate 274. **Conservative operation for tubal ectopic pregnancy**

Operation: The pelvic cavity has been thoroughly irrigated. The atraumatic grasping tongs are used to demonstrate the ruptured ectopic pregnancy in the preampullary portion of the left tube, which is enlarged to about 4–5 cm in diameter.

Plate 275. **Conservative operation for tubal ectopic pregnancy**

Operation: After coagulation and incision, as shown in Plates 264 and 265, fetal and trophoblastic elements—in this photograph, the amniotic sac, which still contains the fetus—are systematically removed with the large spoon forceps.

Plate 276. **Conservative operation for tubal ectopic pregnancy**

Findings: After the egg-sized segment of the tube has been incised and the products of conception, which have partially separated spontaneously, have been removed, contractions have restored the tube almost to its normal size and shape.

Operation: The edge of the incision has been grasped with atraumatic grasping tongs to keep the tube under tension for better exposure of the wound bed. Irrigation with large quantities of saline solution is repeated to permit a good view inside the tubal lumen and to ascertain that the products of conception have been completely removed.

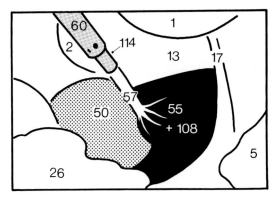
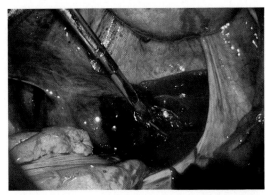

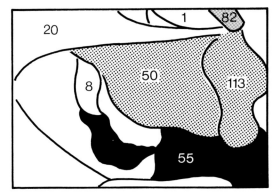
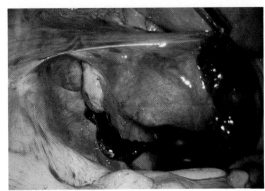

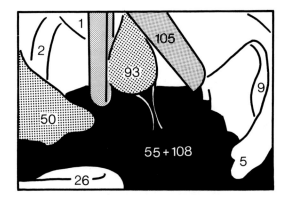
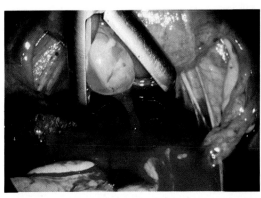

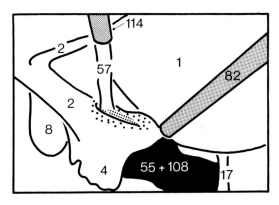
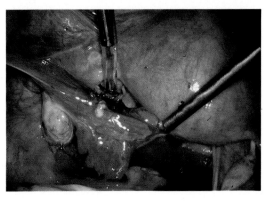

Plate 277. **Conservative operation for ectopic tubal pregnancy: End result**

Findings: After coagulation and incision of the left tube, the products of conception have been removed and the edges of the longitudinal wound will be reapproximated with endo-suture.

Operation: The 5-mm needleholder is just accepting the needle, which had been pushed through the wound edges by the 3-mm needleholder. A slipknot will be tied externally.

14.2.11.2. Salpingectomy for Tubal Pregnancy

Plate 278. **Radical operation for ectopic tubal pregnancy**

History: A 40-year-old patient had an appendectomy at age 34 years. In the current presentation, an ectopic tubal pregnancy was diagnosed in the ninth week of gestation.

Findings: The pelvis is flooded by 810 ml of fresh and old clotted blood.

Operation: To facilitate aspiration of the blood, it is diluted with copious amounts of physiologic saline solutions. An atraumatic grasping forceps is used to keep the uterus and epiploic appendices away from the orifice of the suction cannula.

Plate 279. **Radical operation for ectopic tubal pregnancy**

Findings: After thorough irrigation of the pelvis and aspiration of the blood, the uterus and the left tube, which is distorted by an egg-sized ectopic pregnancy of 9 weeks' gestation, can be inspected.

Comments: Since the patient had indicated that she had completed her family, and in consideration of her age, she had given preoperative consent for a salpingectomy.

Plate 280. **Radical operation for ectopic tubal pregnancy**

Operation: Three endoloops have been applied behind the products of conception according to the triple-loop technique for salpingectomy, as previously illustrated in Plates 208–220. For optimal application of the ligatures, the tube containing the pregnancy is kept under traction with the large spoon forceps.

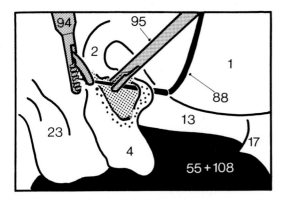

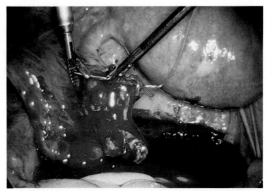

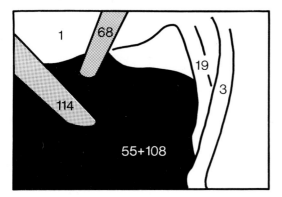

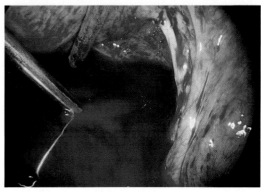

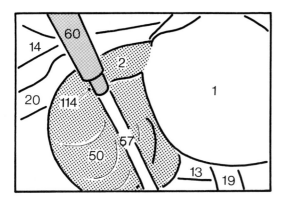

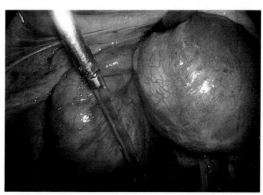

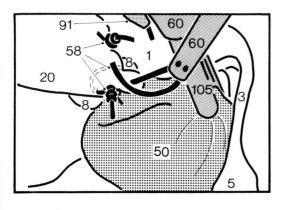

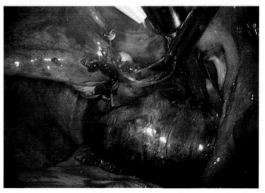

Plate 281. Salpingectomy for ectopic tubal pregnancy

Findings: After triple-ligature, the tube containing the products of conception has been re-sected and incised. The anatomical arrangement of tissues in an ectopic tubal pregnancy can be clearly recognized in this photograph. The external layer consists of the tubal wall; inside of it, there are trophoblastic and chorionic tissue elements and the transparent amniotic sac with yellow contents.

Operation: In preparation for the removal of the products of conception through the 11-mm trocar sleeve, the amniotic sac will first be separated and extracted.

Plate 282. Salpingectomy for ectopic tubal pregnancy

Operation: The amniotic sac, shown in Plate 281, has been incised and the fetus has been aspirated with the irrigation-aspiration cannula of the Aquapurator; the umbilical cord is still attached inside the amniotic sac. The fetus will then be grasped with the large spoon forceps and removed in one piece through the 11-mm trocar sleeve. Trophoblastic tissues and the resected tube will be extracted in the same manner.

Plate 283. Salpingectomy for ectopic tubal pregnancy: End result

Findings: After thorough irrigation of the entire pelvic and abdominal cavity up to the diaphragm (see Figs 28 and 29), all peritoneal surfaces are smooth and clean. Next to the left ovary, the tubal stump can be recognized; it has already been coagulated with the point coagulator to prevent adhesions.

Plate 284. Salpingectomy for ectopic tubal pregnancy: Pathologic specimen

History: A 41-year-old patient had a radical operation for an ectopic tubal pregnancy in the fourth week after conception.

Findings: The tube was resected by the triple-loop technique: It contains the products of conception and two hydatid cysts of Morgagni. The whole specimen was removed through the 11-mm trocar sleeve.

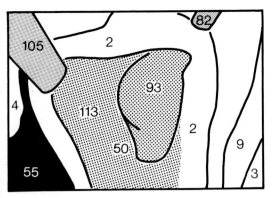

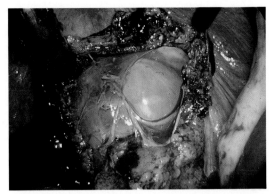

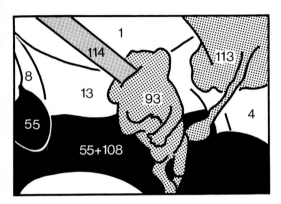

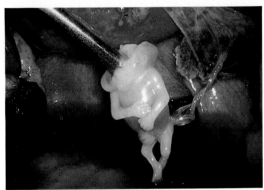

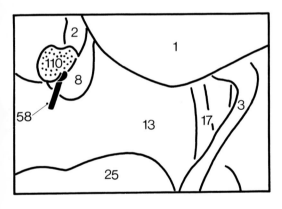

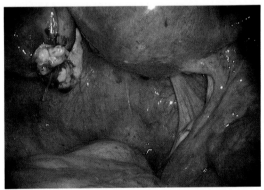

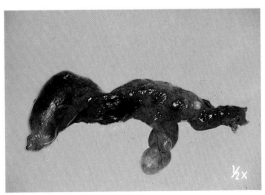

½x

397

14.2.12. Excision of Hydatid Cysts of Morgagni

Plate 285. **Excision of hydatid cysts of Morgagni**

Operation: The stalk of the hydatid cyst will be coagulated with the crocodile forceps.

Comment: Hydatid cysts of Morgagni are derivatives of the Wolffian ducts and have some potential for malignant transformation. They should always be removed at the end of any diagnostic pelviscopic evaluation.

Caution: Since the stalk is vascularized by an artery, which always bleeds briskly when cut, it is obligatory to coagulate the stalk of the hydatid cyst. If the hydatid cysts are resected without coagulation, the bleeding artery will retract into the area of the tubal ampulla, where it is difficult to reidentify it.

Plate 286. **Excision of hydatid cysts of Morgagni: End result**

Operation: The vascularized stalk of the hydatid cyst has been coagulated according to the instructions for Plate 285 and is kept under tension with a biopsy forceps or grasping tongs. It can be severed with hook scissors in the area of the tubal ampulla without causing any bleeding.

Plate 287. **Excision of hydatid cysts of Morgagni**

History: A 30-year-old patient with sterility had several adnexal cysts.

Findings: A left ovarian cyst of about 4 cm in diameter (see Plates 290–293) is seen in the cul-de-sac. A hydatic cyst about 2×3.5 cm in diameter is attached to the right adnexa by multiple stalks and adhesions.

Operation: The stalks of the hydatid cyst are kept under tension with atraumatic grasping tongs and coagulated with the crocodile forceps close to the tubal ampulla.

Plate 288. **Excision of hydatid cysts of Morgagni: End result**

Operation: With tension applied to its stalks, the hydatid cyst is resected with hook scissors, intact and without blood loss.

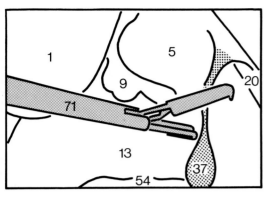

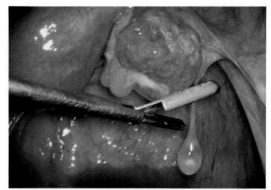

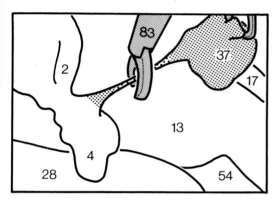

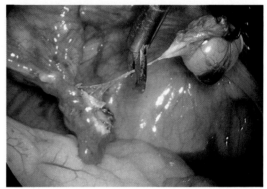

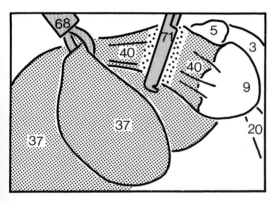

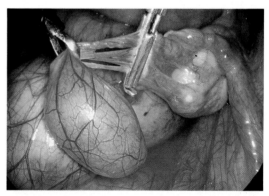

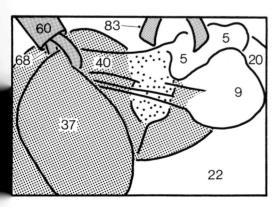

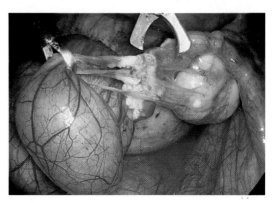

Plate 289. **Excision of inflammatory serosal cysts**

Findings: Serosal cysts frequently develop after pelvic inflammatory disease. They are avascular and readily stained with methylene blue solution, which may be used as a diagnostic test.

Operation: The stalks of serosal cysts are kept under tension with atraumatic biopsy tongs. Since the cysts are avascular, the stalks can be cut without prior coagulation.

14.2.13. Pelviscopic Excision of Parovarian Cysts

Plate 290. **Excision of a parovarian cyst**

History: A 30-year-old patient with infertility had several pelvic cysts.

Findings: This right parovarian cyst of about 4 cm in diameter was completely encased in peritoneum.

Operation: A second 5-mm trocar is introduced in the left suprapubic area.

See also Plates 287 and 288.

Plate 291. **Excision of a parovarian cyst**

Operation: The atraumatic grasping tongs are used to stabilize the parovarian cyst so that a 6–8-cm-long strip of the vascularized peritoneum can be coagulated with the point coagulator. It will then be incised with hook scissors and bloodlessly stripped off the cystic tumor, as previously demonstrated with ovarian cysts, such as in Plates 118–120.

Plate 292. **Excision of a parovarian cyst**

Operation: The parovarian cyst has been peeled out of its retroperitoneal position and its stalk will be ligated with three endoloops (triple-loop technique). It can then be excised without bleeding.

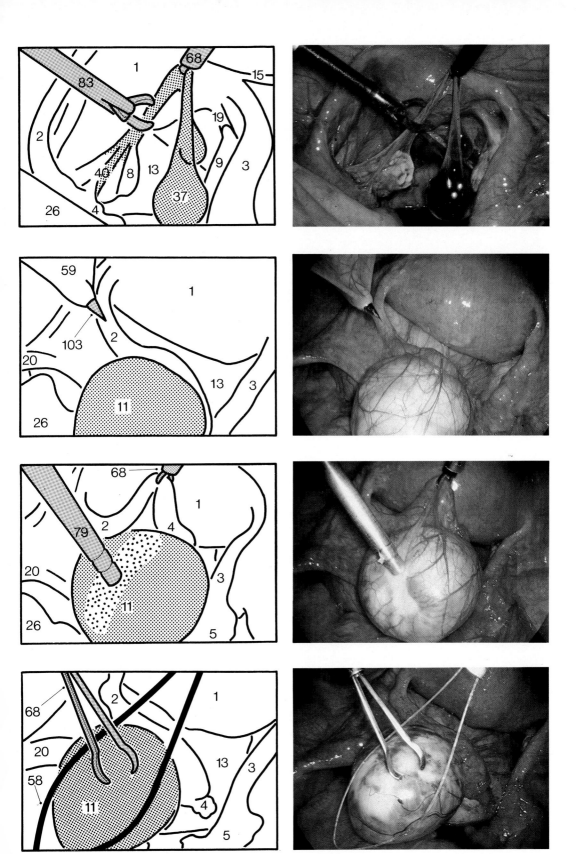

Plate 293. **Excision of a parovarian cyst: End result**

Operation: After the parovarian cyst of about 4 cm diameter, shown in Plate 290, has been dissected from its retroperitoneal position and its stalk has been ligated with three endo-loops, the cyst is grasped with the large spoon forceps. With strong traction applied, the entire cystic structure has been resected with hook scissors cutting at a right angle. The cyst sac can now be removed without difficulties through the 11-mm trocar sleeve. The remaining vascular stalk will be coagulated with the point coagulator to prevent adhesions.

14.2.14. Aspiration of Oocytes for In Vitro Fertilization

Plate 294. **Puncture of follicles for aspiration of oocytes**

History and Findings: The presence of mature follicles was diagnosed by hormonal analysis and ultrasound.

Operation: The ovary is manipulated with an atraumatic suction cannula or grasping tongs attached to the utero-ovarian ligament until the mature follicle is in the proper position for puncture with the aspiration needle. The follicle should not be punctured at its most convex point but more tangentially to prevent the follicular fluid from squirting out when the puncture is made. This risk is also minimized by using the Aquapurator, which produces a negative pressure of -3 to -5 mm Hg in the aspiration needle.

Plate 295. **Puncture of follicles for aspiration of oocytes**

Operation: The follicle, shown in Plate 294, has been completely evacuated and the aspiration needle has been withdrawn from the ovary without significant bleeding. If no ovum is found, the follicle will be filled up again with approximately 5 ml of the appropriate culture medium, which will then be reaspirated.

Plate 296. **Puncture of follicles for aspiration of oocytes**

History: A 25-year-old patient with primary sterility previously underwent bilateral salpingectomy for tubal tuberculosis.

Findings: There are several mature follicles after clomiphene hyperstimulation.

Operation: The aspiration needle is approaching the ovary for the tangential puncture.

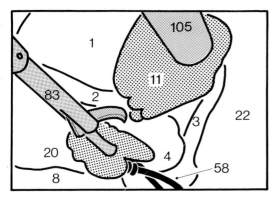
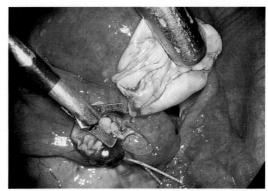

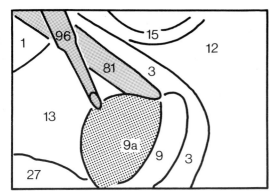
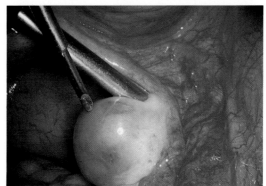

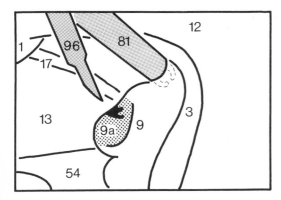
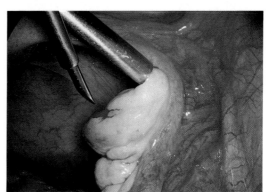

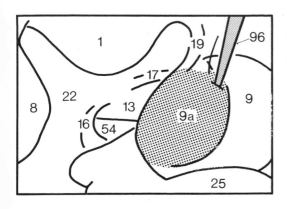
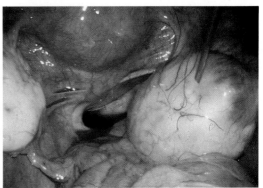

Plate 297. **Puncture of follicles for aspiration of oocytes**
Findings: The follicle, shown in Plate 296, has been completely evacuated without bleeding and its cavity has collapsed.

Plate 298. **Puncture of follicles for aspiration of oocytes**
History: A 34-year-old patient underwent bilateral salpingectomy for bilateral tubal pregnancies.
Findings: Several follicles have matured after hyperstimulation with clomiphene.
Operation: The aspiration needle is penetrating the caudal follicle in a tangential direction.

Plate 299. **Puncture of follicles for aspiration of oocytes**
Operation: The follicle, shown in Plate 298, has collapsed after aspiration. Another mature follicle is present in the cranial pole of the ovary which, on a sonogram, had a diameter of 2.4 cm.

Plate 300. **Spontaneous rupture of an ovarian follicle**
History and Findings: A few seconds before this photograph was taken, the mature follicle, i.e., the thecal layer of the follicle, of this 25-year-old patient had ruptured spontaneously. The ovum is visible in the emerging follicular fluid. Next to it is another, almost mature follicle.

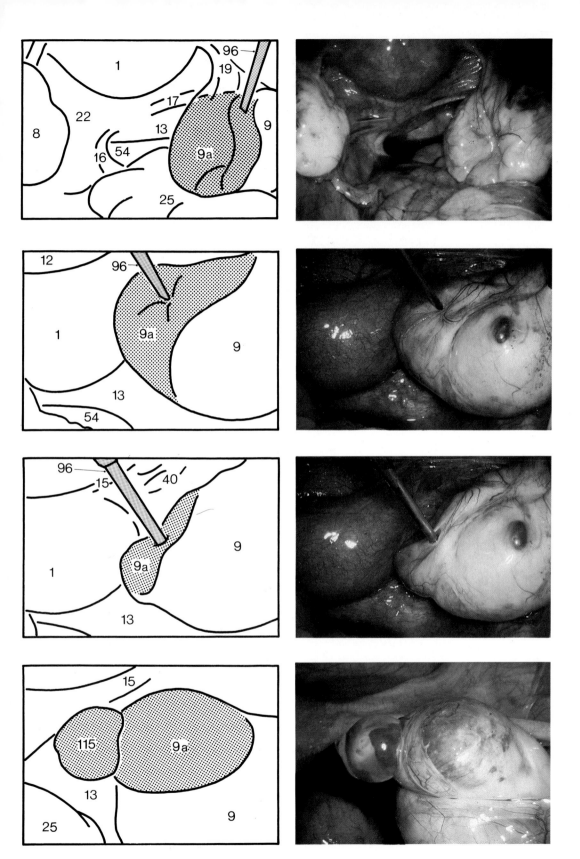

14.2.15.1.1. TUBAL STERILIZATION BY UNIPOLAR HIGH-FREQUENCY COAGULATION

Plate 301. **Postoperative condition after high-frequency sterilization**

History: A 34-year-old patient underwent an appendectomy at the age of 19 years and a tubal sterilization by unipolar high-frequency coagulation for medical indication about 4 years prior to the present admission.

Findings: A tubal segment approximately 6 cm long has been transformed into a thin strand of fibrous tissue and the adjacent vascular plexus (see Fig 114) has vanished. Larger blood vessels can no longer be recognized in the mesovarium adjacent to the uterus, indicating that the nervous and vascular supply of the ovary was severely altered by the sterilization operation (semicastration effect).

Plate 302. **Postoperative condition after high-frequency sterilization**

History: Four years earlier, the 36-year-old patient had a tubal sterilization operation by unipolar high-frequency cauterization for medical indications.

Findings: Two thirds of the tubal length adjacent to the uterus has been transformed into a strand of fibrous scar tissue. The entire vascular system in the mesosalpinx (see Fig 114) was "cooked" at that time, resulting in destruction of the arterial and nervous supply of the ovary and, consequently, a severe impairment of its secretory functions (semicastration effect).

Plate 303. **Postoperative condition after high-frequency sterilization**

History: A 42-year-old patient had an appendectomy at the age of 17 years and a tubal sterilization by unipolar high-frequency cauterization 6 years before the current admission.

Findings: The right tube has been completely destroyed and only a fibrous strand is left above the ovary. In regard to the vascular and nervous supply of the ovary, the comments about Plate 302 apply here, too.

Plate 304. **Postoperative condition after high-frequency sterilization**

History: Five years before the current admission, a 37-year-old patient had a tubal sterilization by unipolar high-frequency cauterization for medical indications.

Findings: The tube has been damaged so severely that only a small fimbrial segment remains. Most of the tube has been transformed into a fibrous strand. The entire vascular system for the tube and ovary, as shown in Figure 114, has been destroyed. The comments for Plate 302 apply here as well.

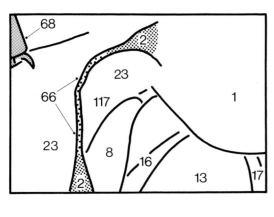

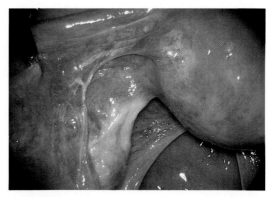

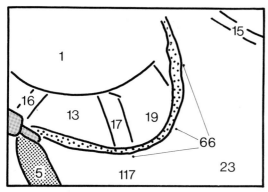

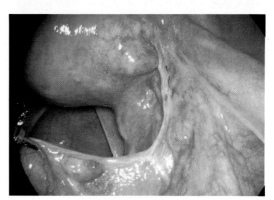

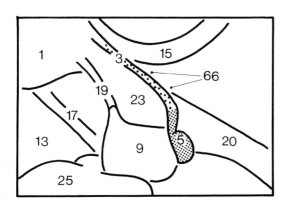

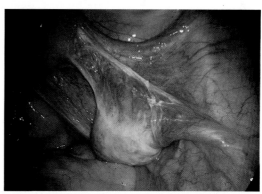

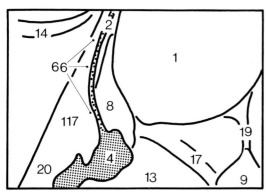

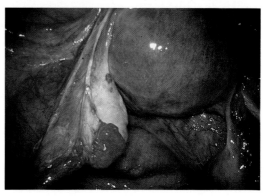

Plate 305. Intraoperative changes during tubal sterilization by high-frequency coagulation

History: The patient is in the early postpartum period.

Findings: Adjacent to the puerperal uterus, the tube was coagulated with atraumatic grasping tongs and unipolar high-frequency current for 20 seconds in each of two sites. One can clearly see the severely coagulated areas of white discoloration separated by carbonized, black tissues, which are produced by sparking when temperatures exceed 400° C.

Comment: There is clear evidence in Plates 301–304 that tissues that show a white discoloration are not the only structures affected by the heat, but that extended zones adjacent to the site of cauterization will also be heated above 57° C, which is the temperature at which proteins are denatured.

14.2.15.1.2. TUBAL STERILIZATION BY BIPOLAR HIGH-FREQUENCY COAGULATION

Plate 306. Tubal sterilization by bipolar high-frequency coagulation

Operation: The left fallopian tube has been grasped with a grasping forceps for bipolar tubal sterilization (in this case, designed by Hirsch) and sterilized by high-frequency coagulation. It is quite obvious that the coagulation of the tube extends beyond the grasping forceps.

Comment: This extended thermal effect corresponds to the pathways that the high-frequency current follows through the electrolytic contents of the tissues of the fallopian tubes and the mesosalpinx. In addition, as already mentioned, extended areas are heated above the 57° C temperature limit. Although not immediately visible, thermal necrosis will also occur in these zones whenever the temperature at which thermolabile enzymes are denatured is exceeded. In the present case, the surgeon felt that the use of high-frequency current for the sterilization precluded simultaneous treatment of the extensive pelvic endometriosis, because high-frequency current should not be applied to any pelvic organs other than the tubes.

[Such restriction will not necessarily be shared by numerous skilled surgeons who have successfully and safely utilized both high-frequency current and laser at low-intensity ranges for many years.—*Ed.*]

14.2.15.1.3. INTERVAL TUBAL STERILIZATION BY COAGULATION (ON THE NONPUERPERAL UTERUS)

Plate 307. Tubal sterilization by endocoagulation

History: A 39-year-old patient underwent a cesarean section at age 34 years. Presently she has a medical indication for a tubal sterilization operation.

Operation: The right tube is grasped and coagulated with the crocodile forceps for the second time. It should be noted that it is in contact only with the muscular wall of the tube (see Figs 113–117 and Figs 326–330). Since there is no contact with the mesosalpinx, the vascular plexus for the tube and ovary, as shown in Figure 114 ff., remains intact.

Plate 308. Tubal sterilization by endocoagulation

Operation: After the muscular wall of the right tube has been coagulated in two sites of 4 mm each, about 2–3 cm distal to the surface of the uterus, the crocodile forceps is removed and the coagulated area of the tube is severed with hook scissors.

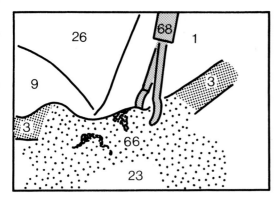

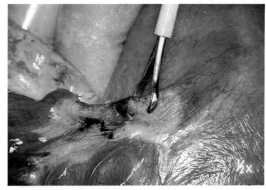

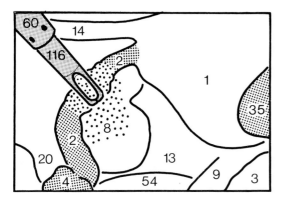

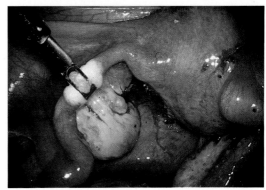

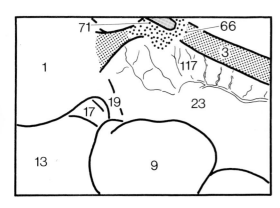

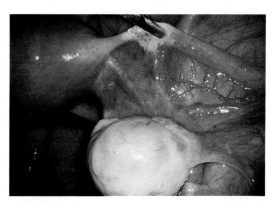

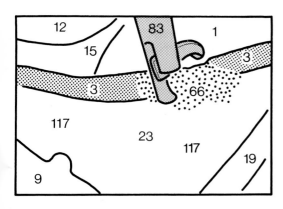

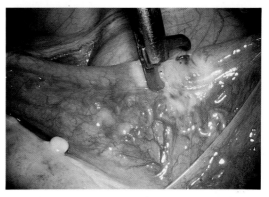

Plate 309. **Tubal sterilization by endocoagulation: End result**
Operation: The coagulation shown in Plates 307 and 308 produced complete hemostasis. All layers of the tube have just been cut with hook scissors (see Figs 117, 326, and 328).
Caution: It is obligatory to confirm with low-power magnification that all layers of the tube have been transected and that the lumen is visible.
See also Plates 312–314, depicting the conditions of the tubes at endoscopic follow-up in comparable cases.

Plate 310. **Pregnancy after tubal sterilization by unipolar high-frequency coagulation: Follow-up**
History: A 36-year-old patient underwent a tubal sterilization 18 months before this examination, which revealed the uterus to be enlarged to 11 weeks' size.
Findings: Half of the left tube has been transformed into a filiform strand of fibrous scar tissue. The right tube has apparently not been sufficiently coagulated by the high-frequency current and has recanalized, although this cannot be detected by endoscopic inspection.
See also chapter 14.2.15.1.1

Plate 311. **Pregnancy after tubal sterilization by unipolar high-frequency coagulation: Follow-up**
History: A 36-year-old patient underwent a left salpingectomy for tubal pregnancy at age 25 years, and two cesarean sections at ages 28 and 29 years. The right tube had been sterilized with high-frequency current; however, her uterus is presently enlarged to 11 weeks' gestational size.
Findings: The left tube is surgically absent and the isthmic portion of the right tube appears to consist only of a solid strand of scar tissue. However, it must have recanalized, permitting spermatozoa to ascend to the ampullary portion as well as the fertilized egg to descend into the uterus.

Plate 312. **Postoperative condition after tubal sterilization by endocoagulation: Follow-up**
History: A 34-year-old patient had an appendectomy at age 13 years and a nephrectomy at age 17 years. Thirty-seven days prior to the present evaluation, on the 19th day of her menstrual cycle, she underwent tubal sterilization by the endocoagulation technique with a crocodile forceps. Her uterus is now enlarged to 8 weeks' gestational size.
Findings: Small foci of necrotic tissue can be clearly recognized on both tubal stumps. Whereas the vascular plexus in the mesosalpinx is well preserved, the whitish discolored tubal stumps adjacent to the site of transection will soon epithelialize, as shown in Plates 6, 313, and 314.

410

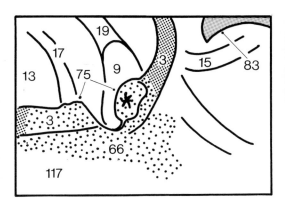
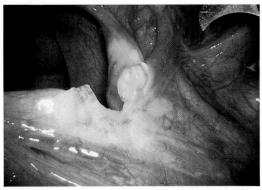

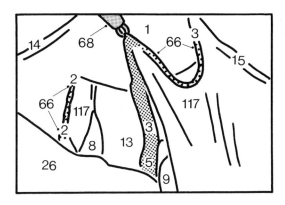
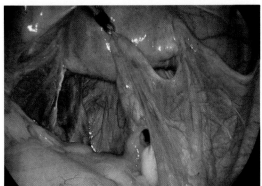

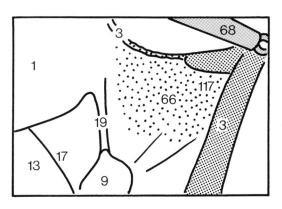
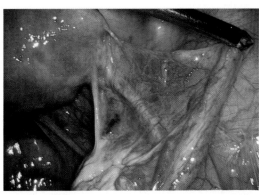

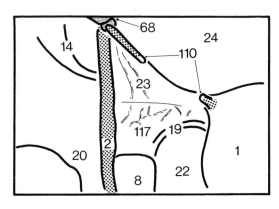
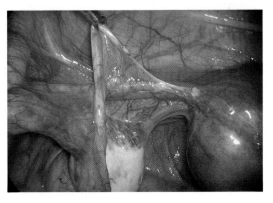

Plate 313. **Postoperative condition after tubal sterilization by endocoagulation: Follow-up**

History: Three years before the current presentation, the 46-year-old patient underwent tubal sterilization by the endocoagulation technique and transection of the tubes with hook scissors.

Findings: The well-peritonealized tubal stumps can be clearly recognized. The mesosalpinx adjacent to the tube is completely normal.

Plate 314. **Postoperative condition after tubal sterilization by endocoagulation: Follow-up**

History: Three years ago, the 37-year-old patient underwent a tubal sterilization by the endocoagulation technique with crocodile forceps, followed by transection of the tubes.

Findings: The transected tubal stumps are peritonealized without scar formation and the adjacent mesosalpinx has a normal blood supply. There is a stigma in the left ovary resulting from a very recent spontaneous ovulation. Pelvic organs in such excellent condition as shown in this photograph and in Plate 313 would be ideal for a microsurgical end-to-end anastomosis of the tubes, if this became necessary. It may be possible in the future to accomplish this by pelviscopy: resection of the closed tubal stumps according to the technique described in Plates 103–105, followed by reapproximation of the reopened ends of the tubal segments with 6-0 PDS sutures.

14.2.15.2. Tubal Sterilization by Ligation

Plate 315. **Tubal sterilization by ligation by Pomeroy's technique**

History: The 36-year-old patient needed a tubal sterilization for medical indications.

Operation: A tubal sterilization according to Pomeroy's technique can be performed without difficulties with the endoloop. After the ligature loop has been introduced into the pelvis and a tube has been pulled through the loop with atraumatic biopsy tongs, the slipknot is tied and the loop closed. The loop has been applied to the tube approximately 2 cm from the surface of the corpus uteri, and then it can . . .

Plate 316. **Tubal sterilization by ligation by Pomeroy's technique: Final condition**

Operation: . . . be transected with hook scissors and without bleeding. In this endoscopic adaptation of Madlener's technique of tubal sterilization, the tubes are not crushed first before a 3-cm segment is sacrificed. Since a catgut ligature is used here instead of silk in Madlener's technique, [this is actually Pomeroy's technique—*Ed.*] the probability of recanalization is very low. However, sufficient clinical experience with this endoscopic adaptation of Pomeroy's technique of tubal sterilization has not yet been gathered.

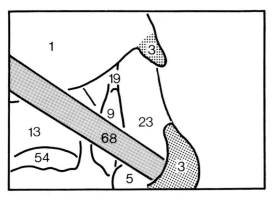

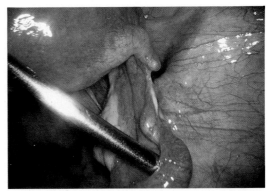

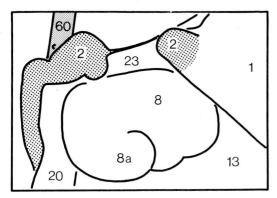

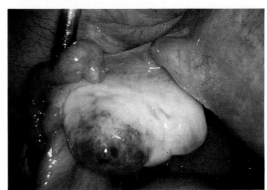

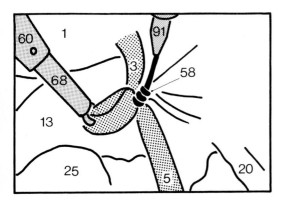

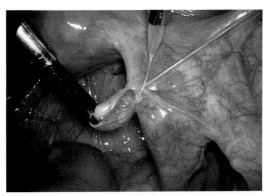

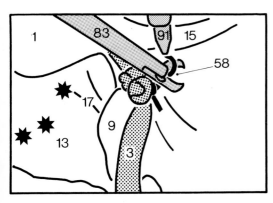

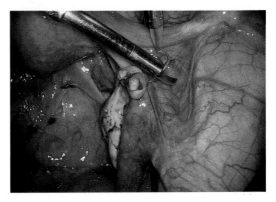

14.2.15.2.1. TUBAL STERILIZATION BY CLIP APPLICATION

Plate 317. Tubal sterilization by Bleier clip application

History: The 32-year-old patient has a medical indication for tubal sterilization.

Operation: For optimal application of the Bleier clip, the tube must be kept under tension with atraumatic grasping tongs. This fixation of the tubes will facilitate application of the clip so that it will grasp the entire tubal diameter. It will also prevent the tubal muscularis from contracting and escaping from the clip before it has been securely closed.

See also Plates 320 and 321.

Plate 318. Tubal sterilization by Bleier clip application

Operation: With firm tension applied to the right tube, the Bleier clip was pushed across the muscular wall of the tube and anchored to the mesosalpinx, as clearly shown in Plate 319, when the grasping jaws of the clip applicator instrument were closed.

Plate 319. Tubal sterilization by Bleier clip application: Final condition

Operation: With firm tension applied to the tube with atraumatic biopsy tongs, a Bleier clip was applied with a special applicator instrument of 11 mm diameter. The clip compresses the entire diameter of the isthmic portion of the tube and is securely anchored to the meso-salpinx. This clip also occludes the tubal artery, an important contributor to the ovarian blood supply.

See also Figure 114.

Plate 320. Tubal sterilization by Bleier clip application: Postoperative follow-up

History: Two years earlier, this 32-year-old patient had a tubal sterilization by Bleier clip application. Because of a carcinoma of the cervix uteri, Stage Ia, she will need a hysterectomy and bilateral oophorectomy.

Findings: The Bleier clip appears to be properly applied to the right tube and is partially overgrown by peritoneum (see also Plate 322).

Operation: A hysterectomy with bilateral salpingo-oophorectomy will be performed to obtain a tubal specimen with the Bleier clip attached.

[This photograph raises the suspicion that the clip may have been applied to a more distal, wider segment of the tubal ampulla instead of the narrower, isthmic tubal segment, as is usually recommended. Incomplete occlusion could result in an increased risk of poststerilization pregnancy.—*Ed.*]

See also Plate 321.

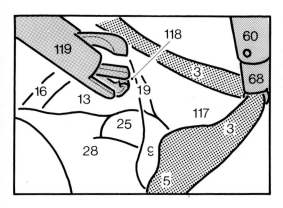
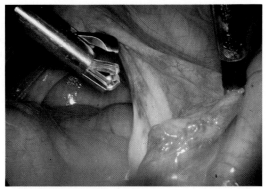

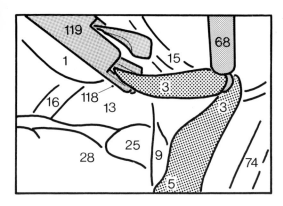
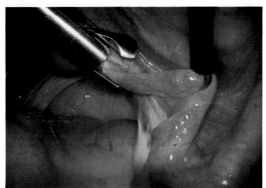

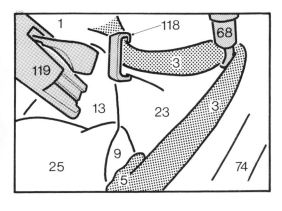
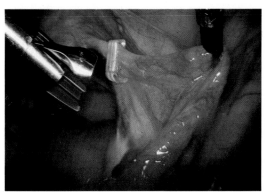

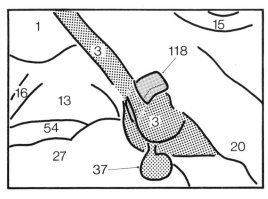
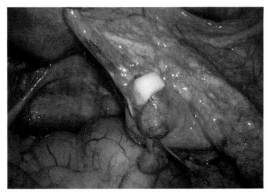

Plate 321. **Tubal sterilization by Bleier clip application (postoperative histology)**

Findings: This histologic specimen shows that the Bleier clip, which seemed to occlude the tube in Plate 320, had grasped only part of the muscular wall of the right tube. The actual tubal lumen must have escaped before the clip was closed.

Comment: Such inadequate application is possible if the tube is not grasped with atraumatic grasping tongs (see Plates 317 and 318). However, such precautionary measures are not taken routinely. The histologic picture presented here could explain the high failure rate of the Bleier clip method.

[Due to a different design of the Hulka clip, which has longer jaws armed with short spikes inside, the tube is less likely to retract when the clip is closed.—*Ed.*]

See also explanations of Figures 340–342, regarding clips, and Figures 329 and 330, pertaining to the tubal transection technique after coagulation.

Plate 322. **Tubal sterilization by plastic clips: Foreign body reaction (operative specimen)**

History: A 32-year-old patient needed a salpingectomy 14 months after the application of Bleier clips.

Findings: Due to a foreign body reaction the clip was completely overgrown by peritoneum. It is assumed that some bleeding started after the application of the clip, which had to be stopped with nonabsorbable suture.

14.2.15.2.2. TUBAL STERILIZATION BY SILICONE RING APPLICATION

Plate 323. **Tubal sterilization by silicone rubber ring**

History: The 38-year-old patient has a medical indication for tubal sterilization.

Operation: The grasping tongs of the 11-mm ring applicator instrument are grasping the right tube about 2–3 cm from the surface of the uterine fundus.

Plate 324. **Tubal sterilization by silicone rubber ring**

Operation: The grasping tongs of the 11-mm ring applicator instrument have grasped the tube and pulled a segment approximately 1 cm long into the hollow shaft of the ring applicator. The outer sleeve of the applicator instrument will then be advanced to release the ring, applying it to the loop of the tube.

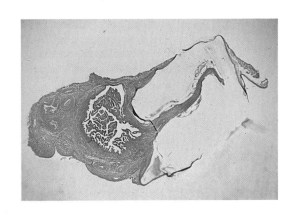

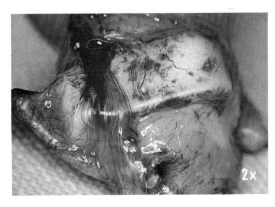

2x

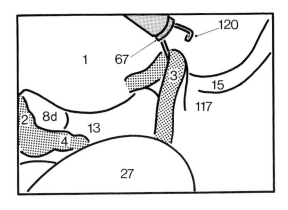

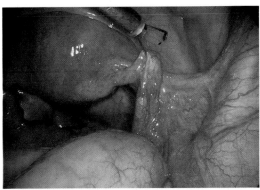

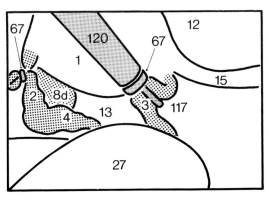

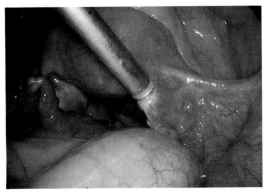

Plate 325. Tubal sterilization by silicone rubber ring: End result

Operation: The grasping tongs of the ring applicator instrument are just releasing the loop of the tube. It is quite obvious that the tubal loop, which has been constricted by the Silastic rubber ring, has become anemic.

14.3. PELVISCOPIC MONITORING OF AN OPERATION TO CONSTRUCT A NEOVAGINA

Plate 326. Construction of a neovagina

History: The patient has Rokitansky-Küster-Mayer-Hauser syndrome.

Findings: In this pelviscopic overview of the internal genitalia, it can be seen that the uterus has been replaced by a genital ridge and bilateral uterine buds adjacent to the adnexa of almost normal appearance.

Operation: During the operation to construct a neovagina, an assistant will constantly observe the internal genital organs and make appropriate recommendations to the vaginal surgeon. In more difficult situations during the operation, the vaginal surgeon will utilize the flexible optical extension, i.e., teaching attachment (see Figs 23 and 344), to monitor his own progress with every phase of his dilating maneuvers, as shown in Plates 328 and 330.

Plate 327. Construction of a neovagina

Operation: After the hymen has been incised in a star pattern or H pattern, a vaginal barrel will be dilated with Hegar dilators, starting with Hegar No. 4 up to about Hegar No. 30. Each time, the Hegar dilators will be advanced under endoscopic control, as shown in Plate 328.

Plate 328. Construction of a neovagina

Operation: The surgeon uses the flexible optical extension on the pelviscope and advances the Hegar dilators, under endoscopic control, in the direction of the ''vagina'' to be constructed. He monitors his surgical procedure transabdominally—without laparotomy—to prevent perforation of the genital ridge.

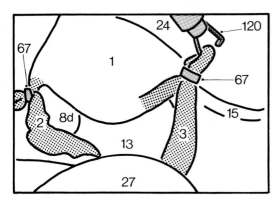

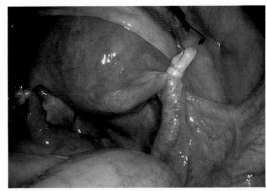

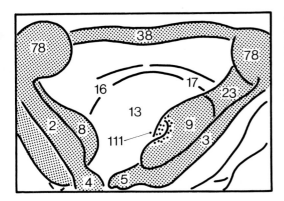

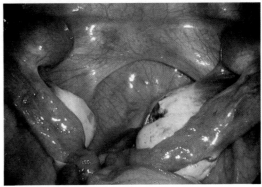

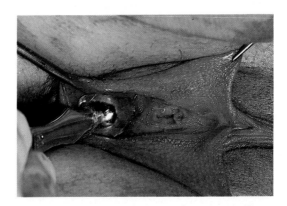

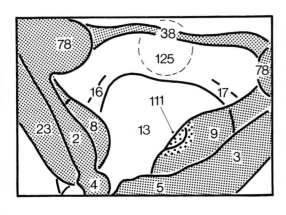

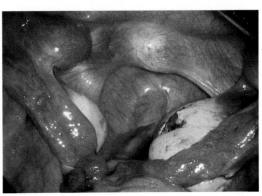

Plate 329. Construction of a neovagina

Operation: A plastic vaginal prosthesis that has been individually selected to comply with the maximal diameter of the "vagina" will be covered with a membrane of lyophilized dura.

Comment: A vagina constructed in this fashion will usually be homogeneously epithelialized after 3–6 weeks and ready for its natural purpose. Obviously, it will have to be dilated continuously for at least 1 year, either actively by coitus or passively by wearing an appropriate stent, because the surrounding tissues have a tendency to shrink.

Plate 330. Construction of a neovagina: End result

Findings: This is the end result after the construction of a neovagina in a patient with vaginal and uterine aplasia. Under pelviscopic control, the small cavity that was present in the vaginal region was sounded and maximally dilated. This photograph shows the pelviscopic view of the vaginal prosthesis, covered with a dura membrane, which has been introduced into the neovagina without perforation of the genital ridge, i.e., the peritoneum.

15.2. INTESTINAL ADHESIOLYSIS AND INTESTINAL SUTURE

Plate 331. Lysis of intestinal adhesions

History: A 42-year-old patient had had three previous laparotomies: for an excision of a right ovarian cyst at the age of 24 years, for an appendectomy at 25 years, and for an adhesiolysis at 36 years. She was suffering from chronic pelvic and lower abdominal pain, sometimes even with symptoms of partial intestinal obstruction.

Findings: Several loops of small bowel were adherent to the parietal peritoneum in the area of the previous peritoneal suture.

Operation: The line of cleavage between the intestinal serosa and the parietal peritoneum is exposed by placing tension on the bowel with the atraumatic grasping tongs. A loupe is attached to the eyepiece of the laparoscope and, under low-power magnification, adhesions are dissected, millimeter by millimeter, with hook scissors (5 mm diameter) or microscissors.

Caution: One must be certain that the adhesions are always cut along or in the abdominal wall and not within the intestinal serosa.

Plate 332. Sharp intestinal adhesiolysis without prior hemostasis

History: A 29-year-old patient with secondary infertility had a perforated appendix at the age of 10 years.

Findings: There is a broad-based adhesion between the descending colon and the right ovary.

Operation: The ovary is grasped and elevated with an atraumatic grasping forceps so that the base of the adhesions between the bowel serosa and the ovary is clearly demonstrated. The intestinal serosa is dissected off with hook scissors; dissection may be facilitated by the use of a low-power loupe attached to the eyepiece of the laparoscope. The incision should be made at the level of the tunica albuginea, which does not bleed, rather than at the level of the vascular bowel serosa.

See also Plate 336.

420

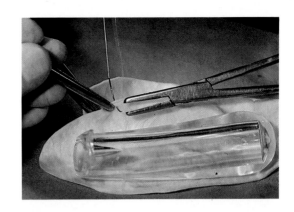

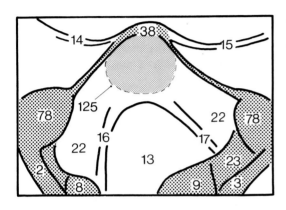

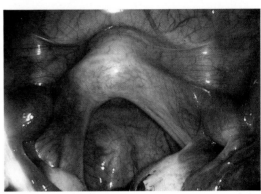

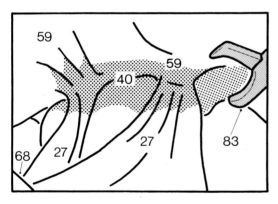

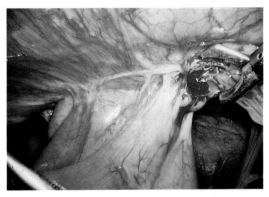

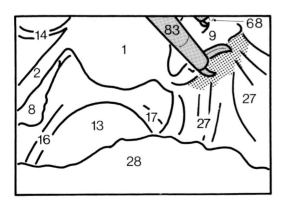

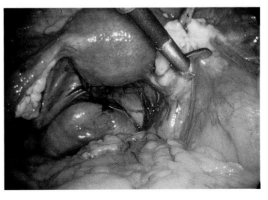

Plate 333. **Sharp intestinal adhesiolysis without prior hemostasis**
Operation: After the ileocecal area and the cecum have been dissected off the right ovary, the defect in the bowel serosa is closed with an endosuture. Here, the needle of the endosuture, guided by the 3-mm needleholder, has just perforated the serosal wound edges and will be received by a 5-mm needleholder. The slipknot will be tied externally and then advanced to reapproximate the gaping serosal edges, as shown in Plate 334.

Plate 334. **Sharp intestinal adhesiolysis without prior hemostasis: End result**
Findings: Lysis of the cecum from the right ovary, as shown in Plates 332 and 333, has been completed, and the serosal defect has been repaired with two endosutures. In addition, a myoma has been enucleated from the anterior wall of the uterine fundus (technique illustrated in Plates 221–246).
Operation: The pelvic cavity is irrigated with copious amounts of warm saline solution until the entire peritoneum is smooth and clean.

Plate 335. **Sharp intestinal adhesiolysis without prior hemostasis (see also Plates 21 and 22)**
History: The 35-year-old patient had an appendectomy at age 29 years and a laparotomy with ovarian wedge resection for Stein-Leventhal syndrome with simultaneous Baldy-Webster uterine suspension at age 33 years.
Findings: Both ovaries are attached to one another by postoperative adhesions; a loop of small bowel and an epiploic appendix are also included in the extensive adhesions.
Operation: Strong traction is applied to the loop of small bowel with atraumatic grasping tongs and the line of cleavage on the left ovary is exposed. The hook scissors are cutting closer to the tunica albuginea than to the intestinal surface so that, . . .

Plate 336. **Sharp intestinal adhesiolysis without prior hemostasis**
Operation: . . . as shown in Plate 335, small fragments of tunica albuginea will remain attached to the serosa of the dissected loop of small bowel. This technique helps prevent more serious defects in the bowel serosa. The epiploic appendices were dissected according to the technique of sharp adhesiolysis without prior hemostasis, shown in Plates 19–22.
See also Plates 129–133, which show the continuation of the operation (ovariolysis and excision of a chocolate cyst). The end result of the entire operation is shown in Plate 133.

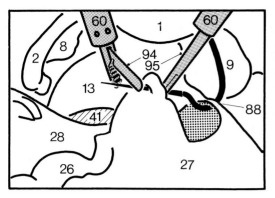
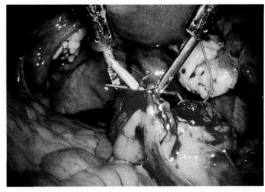
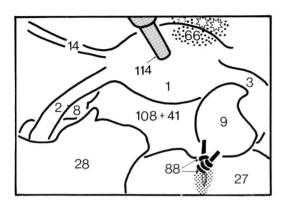
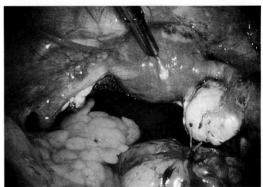
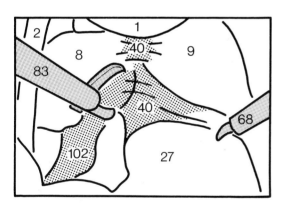
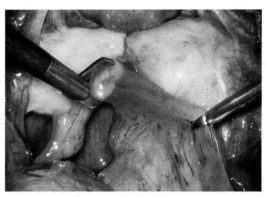
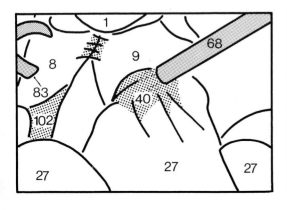
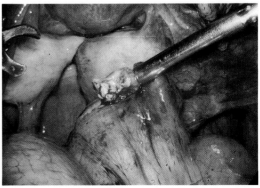

Plate 337. **Adhesiolysis of bowel after hemostasis**

History: A 34-year-old patient with primary infertility underwent laparotomy at age 30 for correction of the sterility.

Findings: A loop of small bowel adheres to the right adnexa by a vascular bridge of tissue.

Operation: In cases like this, the adhesion will be ligated before it is cut. The suture material for the ligature has already been introduced with a 3-mm needleholder through the right trocar sleeve into the abdominal cavity and its free end has been grasped with the 5-mm needleholder and placed behind the strand of adhesions. After about 60 cm of the suture material has been advanced into the abdominal cavity, the end of the suture will be regrasped with the 3-mm needleholder and retracted through the trocar sleeve, and a slipknot will be tied externally.

Plate 338. **Adhesiolysis of bowel after hemostasis**

Operation: After the slipknot has been tied externally, it will be pushed down with the plastic tube until the strand of adhesions is securely ligated. The suture will then be cut with hook scissors.

Plate 339. **Adhesiolysis of bowel after hemostasis: End result**

Operation: After the adhesion between the loop of small bowel and the right ovary has been ligated, as shown in Plates 337 and 338, the adhesion is kept under tension with atraumatic grasping tongs and cut with hook scissors. The loop of small bowel will immediately retract into the upper abdomen.

Plate 340. **Sharp lysis of omental and bowel adhesions with and without hemostatic ligature**

History: About 4 years before the current presentation, the 35-year-old patient underwent a laparotomy for correction of primary sterility but failed to conceive.

Findings: Diagnostic pelviscopy reveals very extensive peritoneal adhesions, which will be corrected by operative pelviscopy.

Operation: The sigmoid colon, which is attached by massive adhesions to the left adnexa and to the posterior wall of the uterus, is grasped with atraumatic grasping tongs so that the adhesions to the left ovary are clearly exposed and can be cut with hook scissors, step by step and without prior hemostasis.

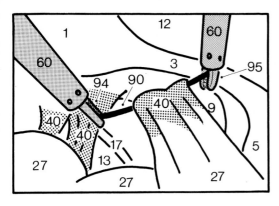

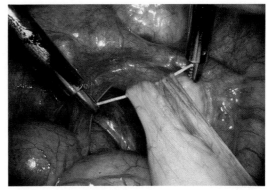

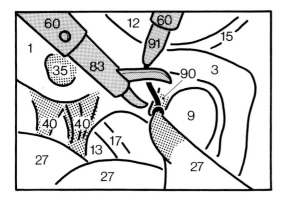

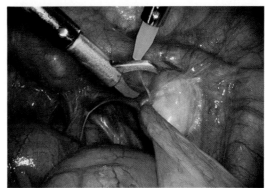

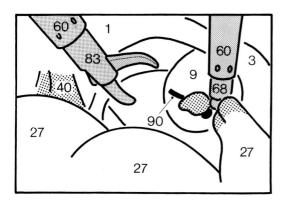

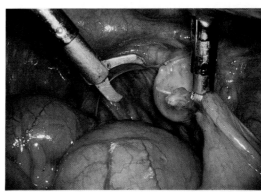

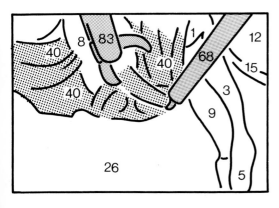

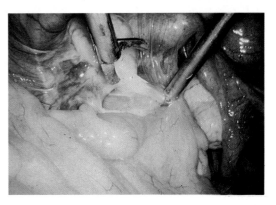

Plate 341. **Sharp lysis of omental and bowel adhesions with and without hemostatic ligature**
Operation: After the sigmoid colon has been separated from the left ovary, with minimal bleeding, the broad adhesion between the sigmoid colon and the posterior wall of the uterus will be dissected. Two atraumatic grasping forceps are used to explore the exact anatomical relationship of the organs in the pelvis.

Plate 342. **Sharp lysis of omental and bowel adhesions with and without hemostatic ligature**
Operation: Since the preliminary exploration of the pelvis has shown that the adhesions in the sigmoid colon and the uterine fundus are suited for the application of a ligature, an endosuture has been introduced with the 3-mm needleholder through the applicator sleeve. The 5-mm needleholder on the left side will be passed underneath the strand of adhesions.

Plate 343. **Sharp lysis of omental and bowel adhesions with and without hemostatic ligature**
Operation: Meanwhile, the 5-mm needleholder has received the end of the suture from the jaws of the 3-mm needleholder, as shown in Plate 342, and pulled underneath the bridge of adhesions. About 60 cm of the suture material has already been pushed into the abdominal cavity, and the 5-mm needleholder is just returning the end of the suture to the 3-mm needleholder, which will retract it through the applicator so that the slipknot can be tied externally.

Plate 344. **Sharp lysis of omental and bowel adhesions with and without hemostatic ligature**
Operation: The ligature of the broad, vascular bridge of adhesions, shown in Plates 342 and 343, is completed with application of the slipknot; however, the long end of the suture has not yet been cut, so that it can be used for traction. The hook scissors are placed to dissect the bridge of adhesions off the posterior uterine wall without causing any bleeding.

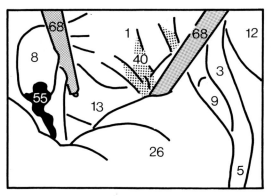

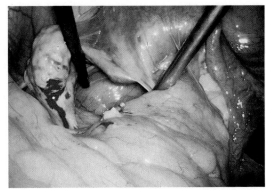

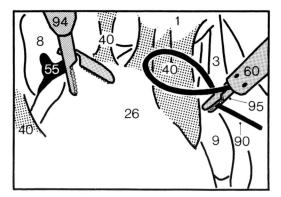

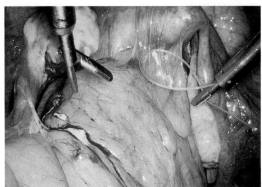

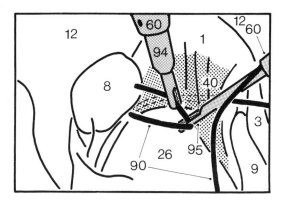

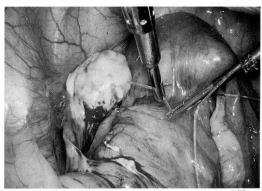

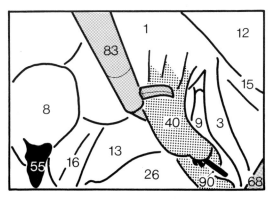

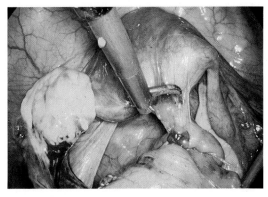

Plate 345. **Sharp lysis of omental and bowel adhesions with and without hemostatic ligature: End result**

Operation: A small bleeder in the uterine fundus has been coagulated with the point coagulator and the pelvis has been irrigated. All operative fields are dry and clean after sharp lysis of omental and bowel adhesions with and without hemostasis, as shown in Plates 342–344.

Plate 346. **Lysis of bowel adhesions after hemostasis**

History: A 43-year-old patient underwent laparotomy with myomectomy at age 31 years, a cesarean section at age 34, and a total abdominal hysterectomy at age 38. Since that time, she has suffered from lower abdominal and pelvic pain with signs of partial bowel obstruction. Adhesions were suspected and a diagnostic laparoscopy was recommended.

Findings: Bridge-like adhesions between small bowel and the sigmoid colon were confirmed.

Operation: A pocket in which loops of bowel probably have been caught periodically is demonstrated with two atraumatic grasping forceps.

Plate 347. **Lysis of bowel adhesions after hemostasis**

Operation: After the endoligature suture has been introduced with the 3-mm needleholder, the 5-mm needleholder is passed behind the bridge of adhesions, shown in Plate 346, and grasps the end of the catgut ligature.

See also Plates 7, 8, and 16–40.

Plate 348. **Lysis of bowel adhesions after hemostasis**

Operation: After the ligature has been passed behind the tissue bridge with the 5-mm needleholder and another 50–60 cm of suture material has been introduced into the abdomen, the end of the catgut ligature will again be grasped by the 3-mm needleholder and withdrawn through the applicator sleeve so that the slipknot can be tied externally.

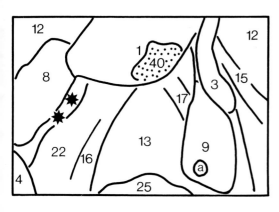
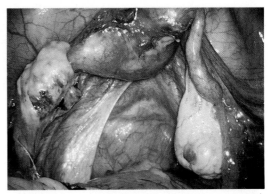
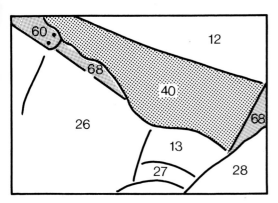
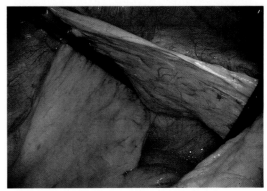
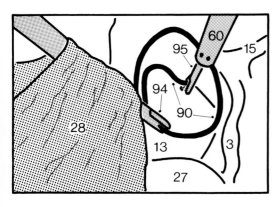
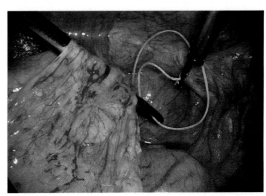
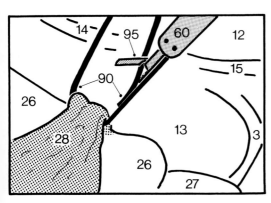
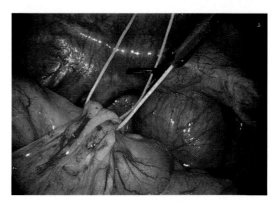

Plate 349. **Lysis of bowel adhesions after hemostasis**

Operation: After the slipknot has been tied externally, it is pushed down on the long end of the suture material with the plastic applicator sleeve and the first ligature is applied. The long end is then cut off with scissors.

Plate 350. **Lysis of bowel adhesions after hemostasis**

Operation: The extremely vascular bridge of adhesions must, according to common general surgical principles, be ligated twice before it can be dissected. Here the 5-mm needleholder has been passed behind the bridge of adhesions and is grasping the end of a catgut ligature, which has been introduced with the 3-mm needleholder.

Plate 351. **Lysis of bowel adhesions after hemostasis**

Operation: The bridge of adhesions, which is 15 mm or more in diameter, has been doubly ligated with two endoligatures. It is again demonstrated between two atraumatic grasping tongs before . . .

Plate 352. **Lysis of bowel adhesions after hemostasis**

Operation: . . . it is stabilized in an optimum position under strong tension between two atraumatic grasping tongs so that it can be transected with hook scissors.

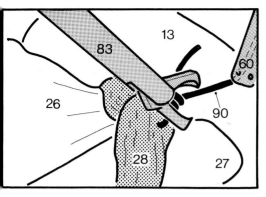
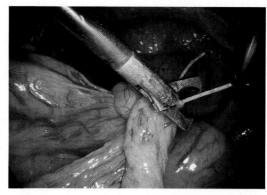

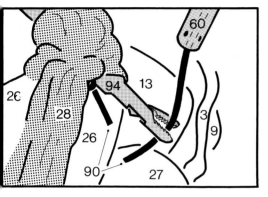
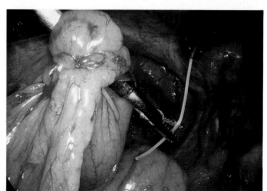

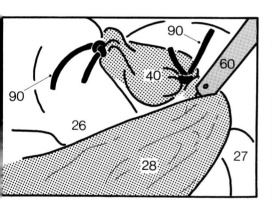
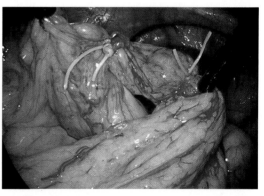

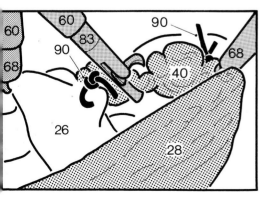
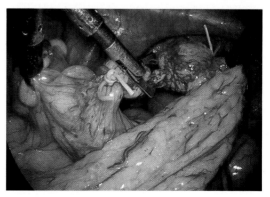

Plate 353. **Lysis of bowel adhesions after hemostasis: End result**

History: After a total abdominal hysterectomy and bilateral salpingo-oophorectomy, the patient was chronically suffering from symptoms caused by peritoneal adhesions with intermittent partial intestinal obstruction.

Findings: This is an overview after broad intestinal adhesions (shown in Plate 346) have been ligated and transected, as shown in Plates 347–352.

Operation: For safety's sake, both tissue pedicles will each be religated with an additional endoloop.

Comment: Two days later, the patient was discharged from the hospital completely relieved of symptoms and without risk of recurrence.

Plate 354. **Lysis of bowel adhesions after hemostasis with peritoneal suture**

History: A 67-year-old patient underwent an appendectomy at age 37 years and a tubal sterilization by laparotomy at age 39. Since that time, she has been suffering from lower abdominal and pelvic discomfort when sitting. A left ovarian cyst of 3.5–4 cm diameter was diagnosed by ultrasound.

Findings: The left ovarian cyst is confirmed and there are dense adhesions between the cecum and the site of the previous tubal ligation performed 28 years earlier.

Operation: The decision was made to proceed with the operative pelviscopy, consisting of ligation and dissection of the adhesions and excision of the left adnexa.

Plate 355. **Lysis of bowel adhesions after hemostasis with peritoneal suture**

Operation: The adhesions shown in Plate 354, were explored and an endosuture was placed. The 5-mm needleholder has pulled the needle through the puncture site and is transferring the endosuture to the 3-mm needleholder. After another 50 or 60 cm of the suture material is fed into the abdomen, the suture and needle will be withdrawn through the applicator so that a slipknot can be tied externally. After this ligation, the adhesive band will be separated from the right round ligament and the area of the right broad ligament. However, tension on the tissues caused a wide dehiscence of the peritoneum.
See also Plate 356.

Plate 356. **Lysis of bowel adhesions after hemostasis with peritoneal suture**

Operation: The gaping peritoneal defect in the area of the right broad ligament, which had occurred after dissection of the ascending colon, will be closed with an endoloop, which has already been introduced into the pelvis. The two spikes inside the jaws of the biopsy forceps will be used to reapproximate and fix the widely separated edges of the peritoneum until the endoloop has been securely applied.

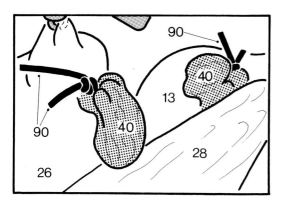

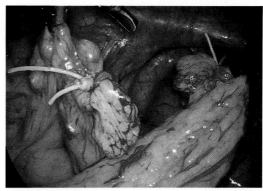

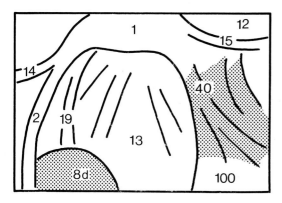

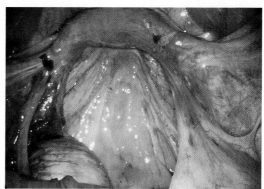

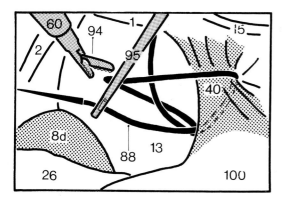

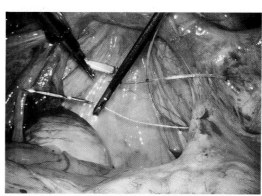

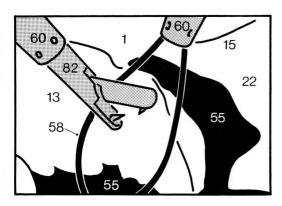

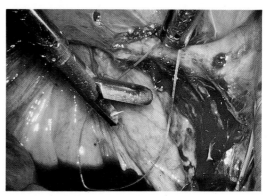

Plate 357. **Lysis of bowel adhesions after hemostasis with peritoneal suture: End result**
Findings: This is an overview of the pelvic structures after a left salpingo-oophorectomy and adhesiolysis on the right side with ligation of the peritoneal pedicle and a peritoneal defect, as demonstrated in Plates 354–357.

Plate 358. **Bowel adhesiolysis without prior hemostatic precautions**
History: A 28-year-old patient with primary sterility had previously had an appendectomy.
Findings: Intra-abdominal bowel adhesions are most commonly diagnosed in the area of the appendix. In this case, a loop of the ascending colon is broadly adherent to the parietal peritoneum.
Operation: The adhesions are kept under tension with atraumatic grasping tongs so that the attachment zone, which is usually poorly vascularized or avascular, can be clearly demonstrated and separated, step by step, with hook scissors.

15.3. ENDOSCOPIC APPENDECTOMY

Plate 359. **Endoscopic appendectomy, indication (see also Plate 46)**
History: A 34-year-old patient with sterility had a history of pelvic peritonitis.
Findings: The appendix is quite distorted due to its adhesion to the right adnexa and the posterior wall of the uterus.
Operation: The atraumatic grasping tongs were used to demonstrate the adhesive bands before a decision was made to correct this condition by performing an endoscopic appendectomy. The endoscopic operative procedure corresponds to the classic appendectomy technique according to McBurney and Sprengel.

Plate 360. **Endoscopic appendectomy, indication**
History: A 38-year-old patient had a laparotomy with a tubal sterilization by Madlener's technique about 4 years before the current presentation.
Findings: There is a retention cyst of 3.5–4 cm diameter in the left ovary. The appendix had apparently been fixed to the right fallopian tube by the permanent suture placed at the time of sterilization.
Operation: Lysis of these adhesions was done without difficulties, followed by an endoscopic appendectomy.

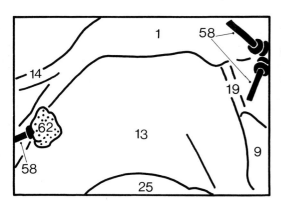

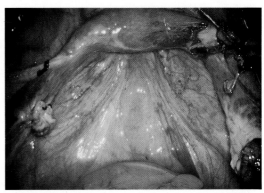

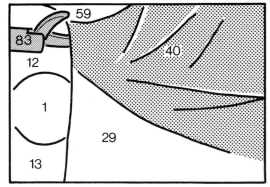

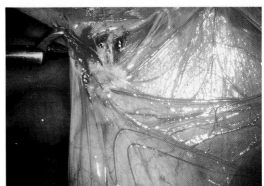

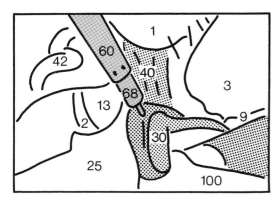

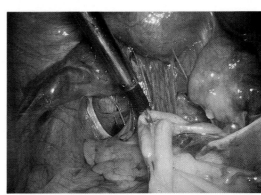

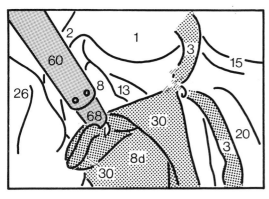

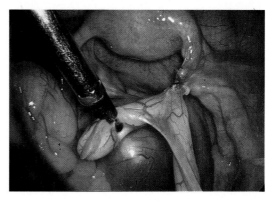

Plate 361. **Endoscopic appendectomy, indication**
History: A 32-year-old patient was being evaluated for sterility
Findings: During chromopertubation, it was noted that the appendix was grossly contorted and attached to the right adnexa by broad adhesions.
Operation: After completion of the sterility operation with bilateral salpingoplasty, the decision was made to perform an endoscopic appendectomy.
See also Plates 362–377, in which the appendectomy is demonstrated.

Plate 362. **Endoscopic appendectomy**
History: A 32-year-old patient was seen with sterility.
Findings: The grossly contorted appendix, shown in Plate 361, has been separated from its adhesions to the right adnexa.
Operation: The tip of the appendix is pulled into an endoloop, which will later be used as a traction suture. Atraumatic grasping tongs assist in the placement of the traction suture.

Plate 363. **Endoscopic appendectomy**
Operation: The retention suture, which had been applied close to the tip of the appendix and shortened to about 5–6 cm in length, is grasped with a biopsy forceps or needleholder to pull the appendix into an appendix extractor.

Plate 364. **Endoscopic appendectomy**
Operation: The appendix is pulled in the direction of the appendix extractor and elevated with atraumatic grasping tongs. At the base of the mesentery of the appendix, further adhesions can be recognized, which will be sharply dissected with hook scissors and without prior hemostasis.

436

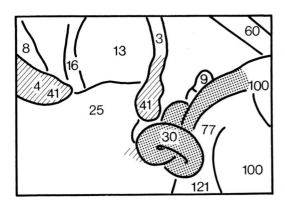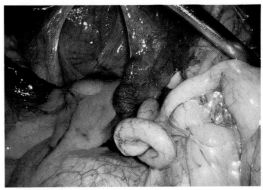

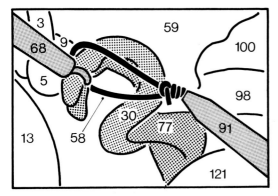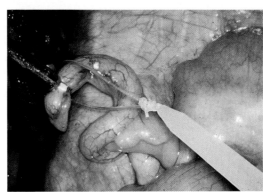

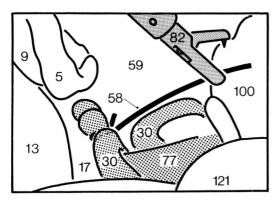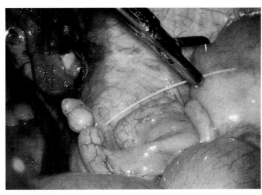

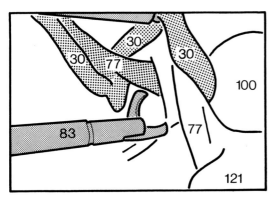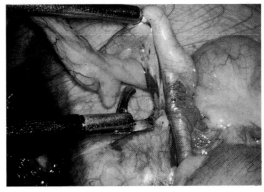

Plate 365. **Endoscopic appendectomy**

Operation: After the base of the mesentery of the appendix has been sufficiently mobilized, the appendiceal artery will be ligated with an endosuture. With the 3-mm needleholder, the needle has been passed behind the appendiceal artery close to the base of the appendix and is just being grasped by the 5-mm needleholder. After another 50 cm of the suture material is introduced, the needle and the suture will be pulled with the 3-mm needleholder through the applicator sleeve so that the slipknot can be tied externally.

Plate 366. **Endoscopic appendectomy**

Operation: After the slipknot has been tied externally, it is pushed into the abdominal cavity with the plastic push rod until the appendiceal artery is ligated with the endosuture. The long end of the suture is cut immediately.

Plate 367. **Endoscopic appendectomy**

Operation: The appendix is elevated by simultaneous traction on the guide suture (which was applied to the tip of the appendix) and the atraumatic grasping tongs. The appendix can then be skeletonized by dissecting it off its mesentery with hook scissors.

Plate 368. **Endoscopic appendectomy**

Operation: After the appendix has been completely skeletonized, it will be pulled through an endoloop, which has been introduced through the right suprapubic trocar sleeve. The ligature is applied directly to the cecal origin of the appendix. Then the free end of the suture will be cut.

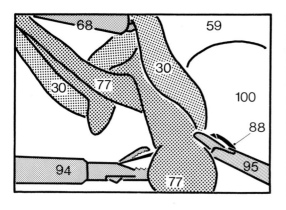
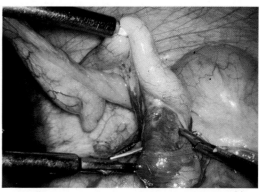

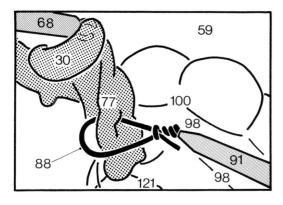
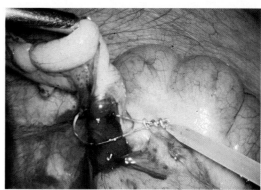

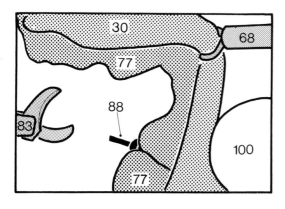
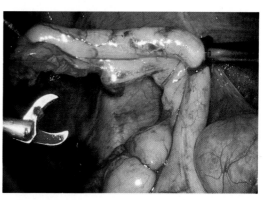

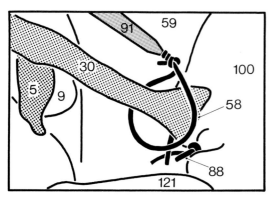
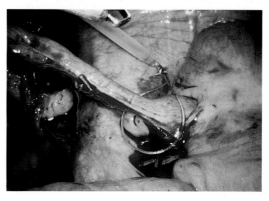

Plate 369.   Endoscopic appendectomy

Operation: After the suture, shown in Plate 368, has been cut, the appendix will be crushed with the crocodile forceps distal to the ligature to displace fecal matter from the area in which the appendix will be severed. The crocodile forceps will then be heated to 90° C for about 20 seconds to "sterilize" the area of the future transection of the appendix.

Plate 370.   Endoscopic appendectomy

Operation: Another endoloop has been introduced and the appendix will be pulled by its guide suture through the endoloop, which will be applied immediately above the crocodile forceps. This accomplishes the second ligature of the appendix so that the crocodile forceps can then be removed.

Plate 371.   Endoscopic appendectomy

Operation: The appendix is kept under tension by retracting it into the appendix extractor while the hook scissors transect the appendix between the two ligatures. The scissors are then immediately withdrawn and removed from the operating table. To avoid any contamination, the appendix is immediately pulled into the appendix extractor and removed with this instrument from the abdominal cavity. The cut surfaces are de facto already devoid of bacteria after the crocodile forceps has been used both for heating and crushing of the appendix. However, for safety's sake, . . .

Plate 372.   Endoscopic appendectomy

Operation: . . . the ligated appendiceal stump is again disinfected with an iodone-soaked gauze applicator, as is routinely done in an appendectomy through a laparotomy incision. The iodone-soaked applicator has been introduced through a *new* appendix extractor.

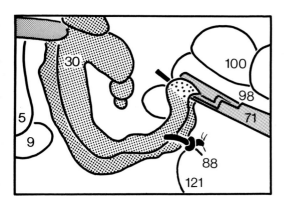

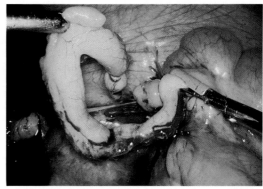

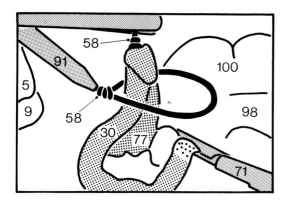

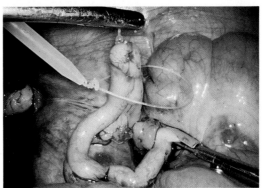

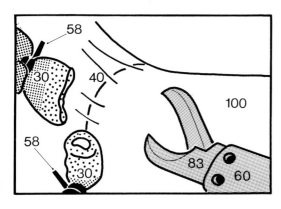

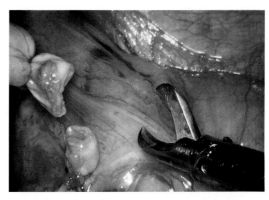

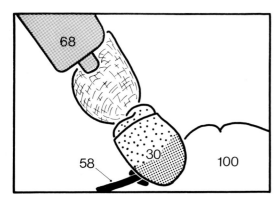

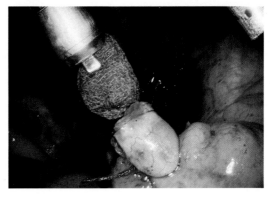

Plate 373.   Endoscopic appendectomy

Operation: A 3-mm needleholder, which has been introduced through a 5-mm trocar sleeve in the right upper abdomen, is used to begin the classic purse string suture. The 5-mm needleholder assists by grasping the serosa of the cecum. As suture material, absorbable Ethicon PDS 4-0 is used because of its long absorption time of approximately 200 days.

Plate 374.   Endoscopic appendectomy

Operation: The purse string suture has been applied with 7 hitches and the surgical knot has been prepared. A plastic push rod, left over after application of the endoloops (shown in Plates 362, 366, or 370), is reintroduced through the appendix extractor and its conical tip will be used to invaginate the appendiceal stump (see Plates 371 and 372) before the purse string suture is closed between the two needleholders. Since this is a monofilament suture material, at least three knots will be tied, as demonstrated in the Z-suture in Plate 376.

Plate 375.   Endoscopic appendectomy

Operation: After invagination of the appendiceal stump by the purse string suture, it will be reinforced by a classic Z-suture. The needle, held by the 3-mm needleholder, is just penetrating the serosa of the ascending colon, again assisted by the 5-mm needleholder. Under these almost microsurgical conditions, both the purse string suture and the Z-suture can be applied with much more precision than can be done through a small McBurney incision.

Plate 376.   Endoscopic appendectomy

Operation: The first double half-hitch of the Z-suture has already been tied and the second double half-hitch of the surgeon's knot is being tied and locked by strong traction between two needleholders. The 4-0 PDS suture will be absorbed in 5–7 months.

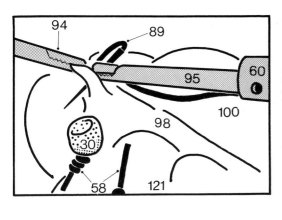

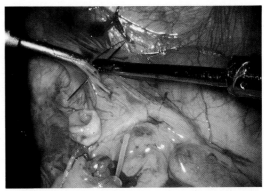

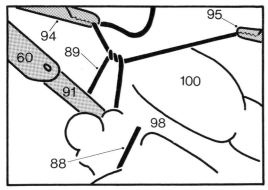

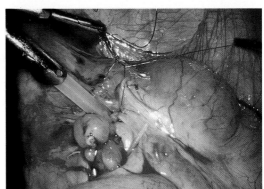

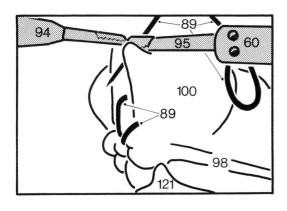

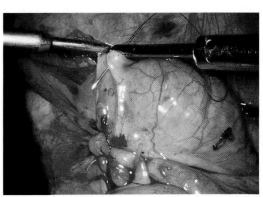

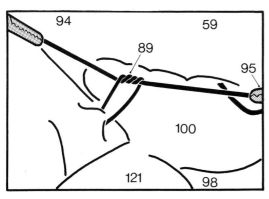

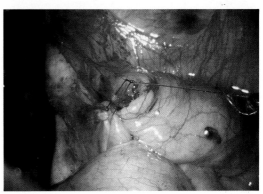

443

Plate 377.   Endoscopic appendectomy: End result

Findings: This is the end result after the endoscopic appendectomy demonstrated in Plates 361–376. The appendiceal stump has been invaginated and doubly oversewn in a classic manner.

Comment: Since there is no corresponding peritoneal wound in the parietal peritoneum, postoperative adhesions after endoscopic appendectomy are practically impossible. If pelviscopy is repeated months or years after the original operation, no adhesions or scars will be present. Microscopic examination of the operative sites has confirmed that the PDS sutures have been completely absorbed.

15.5. BIOPSY OF PERITONEAL METASTASES

Plate 378.   Biopsy of peritoneal metastases

History: A 73-year-old patient had a metastasizing signet ring cell tumor and suspicion of a carcinoma of the appendix.

Findings: There are massive metastases all over the abdominal cavity.

Operation: With the biopsy forceps, which has a spike in each of its jaws, tissue samples are obtained from several metastases.

Caution: If such biopsies are taken from areas adjacent to bowel, one must use great caution to prevent bowel perforation. Such perforations may not be immediately obvious, because the biopsy site within such a metastatic area may not completely penetrate the intestinal wall but only predispose to its perforation at a later time.

Plate 379.   Biopsy of peritoneal metastases

History: A 42-year-old patient had an appendectomy at age 16 years and, 3 years before the current presentation, a total abdominal hysterectomy with salpingo-oophorectomy for ovarian carcinoma. This was followed by chemotherapy, monitored by diagnostic pelviscopy at intervals of 6 months.

Operation: At the time of a diagnostic pelviscopy, suspicious peritoneal nodules are excised with biopsy forceps.

Caution: Such biopsies must be taken with great caution, as already mentioned in Plate 378.

15.6. LIVER BIOPSY

Plate 380.   Needle biopsy of liver

Operation: In addition to suspicious liver scans, grossly abnormal biochemical liver profiles, etc., it is occasionally necessary to biopsy specific areas of the liver. In this photograph, the Menghini needle is introduced into the large right lobe of the liver to punch out a cylinder of tissue for histologic evaluation.

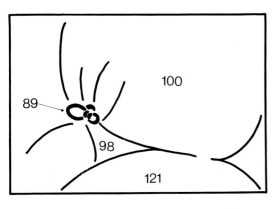

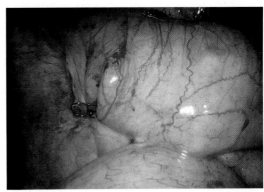

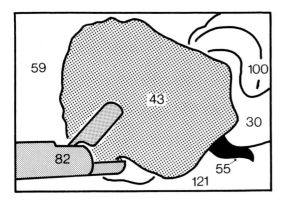

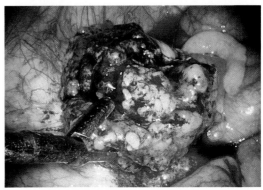

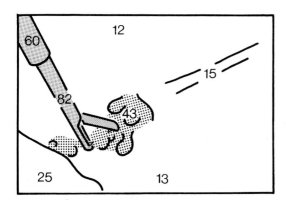

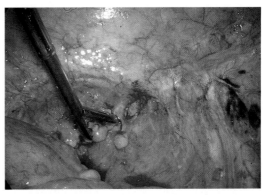

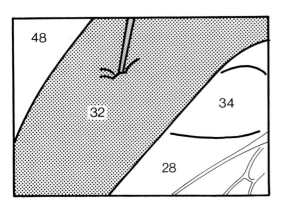

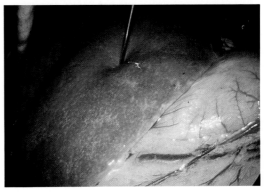

Plate 381. **Needle biopsy of liver**

Operation: Withdrawal of the Menghini needle, shown in Plate 380, has caused some bleeding from the puncture site. It is recommended that this bleeding be stopped by . . .

Plate 382. **Needle biopsy of liver: End result**

Operation: . . . coagulation with the point coagulator. This instrument is heated to 110° C and pressed against the puncture site for about 20 seconds, accomplishing complete hemostasis. The heated point coagulator is presently applied for hemostasis of the second biopsy site.

15.7. LYSIS OF PERIHEPATIC ADHESIONS

Plate 383. **Transection of liver adhesions**

History: The 28-year-old patient with secondary infertility had had a previous laparotomy for correction of sterility.

Findings: There are extensive strings and sail-like adhesions between the liver and the peritoneum of the diaphragm

Operation: Such avascular bridges of adhesions can be cut without difficulty with hook scissors. However, this cannot usually be accomplished through suprapubic incisions. It is recommended that one use the classic puncture site for laparoscopy of the liver: three to five fingerbreadths below the right costal margin.

Comment: Lysis of such adhesions will frequently relieve the patient of "abdominal discomfort of unknown etiology," which may have been present for many years.

[An additional puncture in the right upper quadrant of the abdomen is usually unnecessary if an operating laparoscope is introduced through the umbilical trocar sleeve. Long scissors of 3 mm or 5 mm diameter can be introduced through its operating channel and usually allow transection of the adhesions without difficulties.—*Ed.*]

Plate 384. **Lysis of liver adhesions**

History: A 36-year-old patient had had a laparotomy and salpingo-oophorectomy 5 years earlier for a tubal pregnancy. She had complained of upper abdominal discomfort for many years.

Findings: There is a solid, fibrous adhesive band of 4 mm diameter and 3 cm length between the liver and parietal peritoneum on the diaphragm.

Operation: This vascular bridge has just been carefully coagulated close to the surface of the diaphragm by the crocodile forceps heated to 110° C and applied for 20 seconds, in preparation for . . .

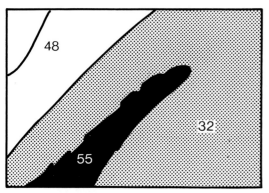
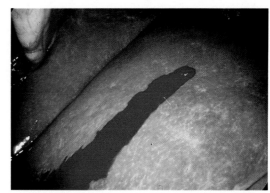

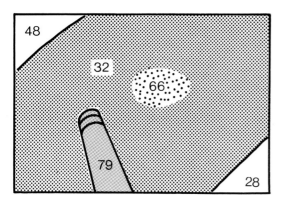
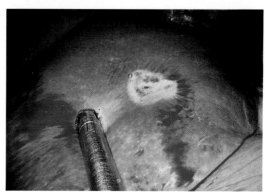

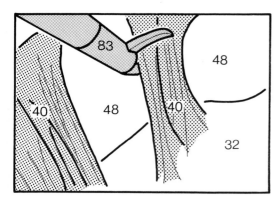
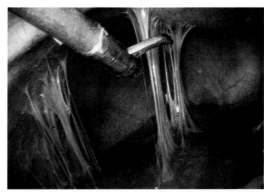

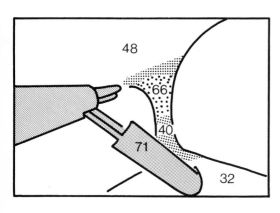
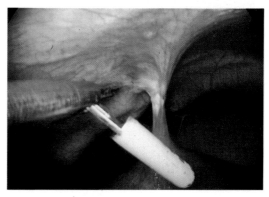

Plate 385. Lysis of liver adhesions

Operation: . . . its transection with hook scissors, which could be accomplished without difficulties and without any loss of blood. For safety's sake, the dissection site in the parietal peritoneum has been recoagulated with the point coagulator.

Comment: This simple procedure relieves the patient of the upper abdominal discomfort from which she has been suffering for many years.

Plate 386. Pelvic endometriosis and thermocolor test: Findings

History: A 28-year-old patient had primary infertility; her original status was shown in Plate 76. Pooled blood in the cul-de-sac had been interpreted as retrograde menstruation and her ampullary phimosis was corrected by bilateral salpingoplasty and blunt dilatation. Since she failed to conceive, a pelviscopic reevaluation was done 11 months later.

Findings: There is another pool of blood in the cul-de-sac. On close inspection of the abdomen and pelvis, several endometriotic implants are noted in the cul-de-sac. Other endometriotic implants in the appendix have been shown in Plate 46. Therefore, an appendectomy was performed during the same laparoscopic procedure.

Plate 387. Pelvic endometriosis and thermocolor test

Operation: The thermocolor test made it obvious that extensive endometriotic implants in the cul-de-sac were responsible for the pool of blood. Their presence also explained why the patient failed to conceive, although her tubes remained patent 11 months after bilateral salpingoplasty.

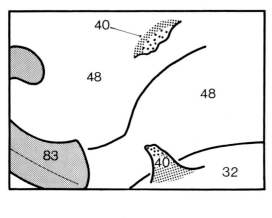
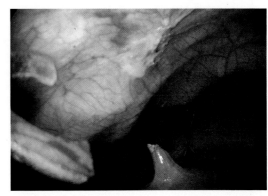

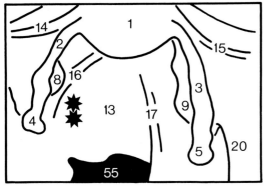
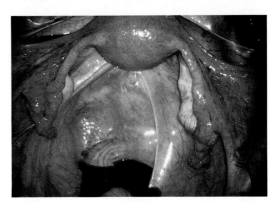

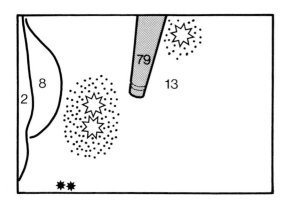
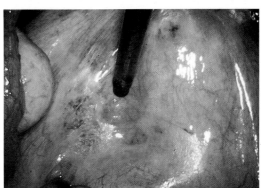

449

24   Literature References

The general literature accumulated in 24.2 is the continuation of the literature cited in the *Atlas of Gynecologic Laparoscopy and Hysteroscopy*, published in 1976 (German edition) and 1977 (English edition). The new references encompass publications since 1975. *For better clarity and utility, the references have been divided by main subjects. It is obvious that certain subjects may be listed under two or more main categories.*

24.1.	Literature Cited in Text	450
24.2.	General Survey of the Literature.	455
24.2.1.	Books and Monographs	455
24.2.2.	Journals	459
I.	History	459
II.	Instruments for Pelviscopy	459
III.	Pelviscopy/Statistics/Methods	460
IV.	Diagnostic Pelviscopy	462
V.	Sterility	465
VI.	Pelviscopy and Carcinoma (Tumor Diagnosis)	467
VII.	Hysterosalpingography and Pelviscopy	468
VIII.	Pelviscopy and Tuberculosis	468
IX.	Anesthesia and CO_2-Gas Metabolism	468
X.	Pneumoperitoneum (Without Complications)	470
XI.	Operative Pelviscopy	470
XII.	Operative Pelviscopy—Complications	473
XIII.	Sterilization by Pelviscopy	476
XIV.	Complications With Sterilization by Pelviscopy	481
XV.	Pelviscopy in Children	482
XVI.	Pelviscopy—Appendectomy	482
XVII.	Hystero-fetoscopy	483
XVIII.	Photo Documentation and Training.	484

24.1. LITERATURE CITED IN TEXT

AAGL (American Association of Gynecologic Laparoscopists) – Entschließung auf dem International Congress on Female Endoscopic Sterilization, Williamsburg, Virginia 1980, 20.–23. Juli.

ACOSTA, A., V. C. BUTTRAM, P. K. BESCH, L. R. MALINAK, R. R. FRANKLIN, J. D. VAN DER HEYDEN: A proposed classification of pelvic endometriosis. Obstet. and Gynec. *42:* 19 (1973).

ALBANO, V., E. CITTADINI: La laparoscopia in ginecologia. Riv. Ostet. Ginec. *17:* 201 (1962).

ANTONOWITSCH, E.: Zölioskopie, insbesondere Douglasskopie. Zbl. Gynäk. *9:* 896–897 (1949).

AHARBANEL, A.: An explained infertility and culdoscopy; observations in fifty consecutive cases. Urol. Rev. *53:* 339 (1951).

AUBINAIS zit. GARNIER, P.: Revue obstétricale-utéroscopie. L'union medicale *24:* 591 (1864).

BAILY, H. A., L. L. GOSSACK: External endometriosis and abnormal uterine bleeding. Am. J. Obstet. Gynec. *72:* 147 (1956).

BENAIM PINTO, V., A. ORTEGA BORJAS, A. DIAZ BRUZAL: Gynecological Coelioscopy. Rev. Obstet. Gynec. *20:* 285–296 (1960).

BEN-NUN, I., R. B. GREENBLATT: Infertility associated with endometriosis. In: SEMM, K., R. B. GREENBLATT, L. METTLER: Genital Endometriosis in Infertility. – X. World Congress of Fertility and Sterility, Madrid 1980. Thieme, Stuttgart – New York 1982.

BHATT, R. V.: 18 Months Follow-up of 7000 cases of Laparoscopic Camp Sterilisation. Persönliche Mitteilung – First Asian Congress on Gynaecological Endoscopy, Bombay 21.–22. Februar 1981.

BHATT, R. V.: Mortality in Camp Sterilisation Using Falope Ring in Rural Camps. Pers. Mitteilung – First Asian Congress on Gynaecological Endoscopy, 21.–22. Februar. Bombay 1981.

BISMUTH, E.: La Coeliscopie Gynécologique, son Application à l'Etude de la Stérilité. Thèse, Paris 45 (1945).

BLEIER, W.: Transvaginaler Tubenverschluß mit Kunststoff-Clip. In: R. KADEN, F. LÜBKE, C. SCHIRREN: Fortschritte der Fertilitätsforschung III – Bericht der Vorträge auf der 8. Tagung der Deutschen Gesellschaft zum Studium der Fertilität und Sterilität, Berlin 1975, Grosse, Berlin 1976.

BOESCH, P. F.: Laparoskopie. Schweiz. Z. Krankenhaus- u. Anstaltsw. *6:* 62 (1936).

BOTELLA-LLUSIA, J., J. M. BEDOYA, Y. F. LA FUENTE: La coelioscopie transvaginale. Acta ginec. (Madr.) *3:* 481 (1952).

BROSENS, I., R. WINSTON: Reversal of Sterilization. 1. Vol. Academic Press, London 1978.

BUMM, E.: In: Diskussion über die Endometritis, S. 524. In: Verhandlungen der Deutschen Gesellschaft für Gynäkologie. 6. Kongreß, Wien. Breitkopf & Hartel, Leipzig 1895.

BUXTON, C. L., W. HERMANN: An analysis of one hundred culdoscopies. Am. J. Obstet. Gynec. *68:* 786 (1954).

CITTADINI, E., P. QUARTARO: L'apporto della laparoscopia alla diagnosi dell' endometriosi externa. Aggiorn. Ostet. e Ginec. (Palermo) *3:* 221 (1961).

CLAUSS, J.: Douglasskopie und Sterilität. Dtsch. med. Wschr. *22:* 886–888 (1954).

CLYMAN, M. J.: A new panculdoscope – Diagnostic, photographic and operative aspects. Obstet. and Gynec. *21:* 343 (1963).

COHEN, M. R.: The role of culdoscopy in infertility. Am. J. Obstet. Gynec. *78:* 266 (1959).

COHEN, M. R.: Laparoscopy, Culdoscopy and Ginecography: Technique, and Atlas. Saunders, Philadelphia 1970.

DALEY, J., H. KOTZ, R. HAUSKNECHT, L. MASTROIANNI, D. C. DAVIS, I. FRIEDMANN: Culdoscopy, colpostomy or culdocentesis as diagnostic procedures. Which one? Trans. New Engl. obstet. gynaec. Soc. *14:* 47–68 (1960).

DAVID, C.: L'Endoscopie de l'utérus après l'avortement et dans le suites de couches à l'état normal et à état pathologique Bull. Soc. Obstét de Paris 1908.

DAVID, C.: L'Endoscopie Utérine (Hystéroscopie). Applications au Diagnostic et au Traitement des Affections Intrautérines. Dissertation, Univers. Paris. G. Jaques, Paris 1908.

DEJABINA, E. J.: Metod peritoneoshkopii i ginekologii. Zsurn. akus. i ginekol. 5 (1957).

DECKER, A.: Pelvic culdoscopy. In: J. V. MEIGS, S. H. STURGIS: Progress in Gynecology, S. 95. Grune & Stratton, New York 1946.

DESORMEAUX, A.-J.: De l'Endoscope et de ses Applications au Diagnostic et au Traitement de Affections de l'Urètre et de la Vessie. Baillière, Paris 1865.

DONALDSON, J. K., J. H. SANDERLIN, W. B. HARREL, jun.: Method of suspending uterus without open abdominal incision; use of peritoneoscope and special needle. Am. J. Surg. *55:* 537–543 (1942).

DOYLE, J. B.: Exploratory culdotomy for observation of tuboovarian physiology at ovulation time. Fertil. and Steril. *2:* 477 (1951).

EDSTRÖM, K., I. FERNSTRÖM: The diagnosis possibilities of a modified hysteroscopic technique. Acta obstet gynec. scand. *49:* 327 (1970).

EISENBURG, J.: Über eine Apparatur zur schonenden und kontrollierbaren Gasfüllung der Bauchhöhle für die Laparoskopie. Klin. Wschr. *44:* 593–594 (1966).

ELERT, R.: Der Mechanismus der Eiabnahme im Laparoskop. Zbl. Gynäk. *1:* 38–43 (1947).

ENDICOTT, E. T.: Peritoneoscopy. J. Am. Women's Ass. *3:* 192–194 (1948).

FIKENTSCHER, R., K. SEMM: Beitrag zur Methodik der utero-tubaren Pertubation. Geburtsh. u. Frauenheilk. *15:* 213–219 (1955).

FIKENTSCHER, R., K. SEMM: Ein Portio-Adapter für Persufflation und Hysterosalpingographie. Geburtsh. u. Frauenheilk. *19:* 868–870 (1959).

FIKENTSCHER, R., K. SEMM: Diagnostik und Therapie der weiblichen Sterilität – technische Neuerungen. Fortschr. Med. *88:* 1052–1056 (1970).

FRANGENHEIM, H.: Die Bedeutung der Laparoskopie für die gynäkologische Diagnostik. Fortschr. Med. *76:* 451 (1958).

FRANGENHEIM, H.: Ein neues Insufflationsgerät zur Anlage des Pneumoperitoneums bei der Zölioskopie. Geburtsh. u. Frauenheilk. *11:* 950 (1964).

FRANGENHEIM, H.: Die Tubensterilisation unter Sicht mit dem Laparoskop. Geburtsh. u. Frauenheilk. *24:* 470 (1964).

FRANGENHEIM, H.: Die Laparoskopie in der Gynäkologie, Chirurgie und Pädiatrie mit einem Beitrag von H.-J. LINDEMANN – Hysteroskopie. Thieme, Stuttgart 1976.

FRANGENHEIM, H.: Diagnostische und operative Laparoskopie in der Gynäkologie. Marseille, München 1980.

FRANKE, G.: Der Aufbau moderner Endoskope. Feinwerktechnik *74:* 382–385 (1970).

FRANKE, G.: Endoskope – Prinzipien und Probleme ihrer Optik. Medizinal-Markt – Acta medicotech. *16:* 372–374 (1968).

FRIEDRICH, E.: Laparoscopy. In: MARTIN, P: Ambulatory Gynecologic Surgery, PSG Publishing Co., Littleton, Ma. 1979, pp. 219–283.

FRIEDRICH, E., S. SAIFEE and F. ARIAS: Volonelgesia (Outpatient tubal sterilization with the laparoscope under VOcal-LOcal-NEuroLept-analGESIA). In: PHILLIPS, J.: Endoscopy in Gynecology, The American Association of Gynecologic Laparoscopists, Downey, Calif. 1978, pp. 469–477.

GAUSS, C. J.: Hysteroskopie. Arch. Gynäk. *133:* 18 (1928).

GOETZE, O.: Die Röntgendiagnostik bei gasgefüllter Bauchhöhle; eine neue Methode. Münch. med. Wschr. *65:* 1275 (1918).

GOLUBEV, V. A.: Use of culdoscopy and laparoscopy in gynecological practice. Akush. Ginec. *37:* 71–74 (1961).

GONZALEZ-LOBO, R.: Culdoscopy, presentation of 80 cases. Gynec. Obstet. mex. *15:* 409–412 (1960).

GORGA, R. S.: La Endoscopia Abdomino Pelviana. Ortiz, São Paulo 1955.

GREWE, H.-E., K. KRÄMER: Appendektomie nach MacBurney und Sprengel in: Chirurgische Operationen, Bd. II, Thieme, Stuttgart 1977.

GUGGISBERG, W.: Bericht über 170 Laparoskopien. Gynaecologica (Basel) *142:* 290–295 (1956).

HASSON, H. M.: Clinical applications of the wing sound device. Obstet. and Gynec. *43:* 498–506 (1974).

HAYDEN, T.: Exploration of the uterus with the endoscope. Dublin quart. J. med. Sci. *XL:* 497 (1965).

HIRSCH, H. A.: Operative Verfahren zur Sterilisation der Frau – Sicherheit – Komplikationen. Geburtsh. u. Frauenheilk *36:* 297–307 (1976).

HIRSCH, H. A.: Schwangerschaft nach fehlgeschlagener Tubensterilisation – Häufigkeit, Ursachen, Vermeidbarkeit. Dtsch. Ärztebl. *78:* 1669–1672 (1983).

HOPE, R. B.: The differential diagnosis of ectopic gestation by peritoneoscopy. Surg. Gynec. Obstet. *64:* 229–234 (1937).

HOPKINS, H. H.: On the diffraction theory of optical images. Proc. roy. Soc. A *217:* 408 (1953).

HULKA, J. F.: Laparoscopic sterilization with spring clips. Chapel Hill, North Carolina, Carolina Population Center, Intern. Fert. Res. Progr. 1973, S. 60.

IRVING: Tubal sterilisation. Am. J. Obstet. Gynec. *60:* 1101 (1950).

IZAWA, I.: Pract. Gynec. Obstet. *4:* 8 (1951).

JAMAIN, B., A. LETESSIER, J. BONHOMME: Tubal pregnancy, celioscopy. Rev. franc. Gynec. Obstet. *55:* 663–668 (1960).

JAMAIN, B., A. LETESSIER, J. BAILLIF: La coelioscopie dans le diagnostic des grossesses extrautérines. Bull. Féd. Soc. Gynéc. franç. *12:* 140–143 (1960).

KALK, H.: Erfahrungen mit der Laparoskopie (zugleich mit Beschreibung eines neuen Instrumentes). Z. Klin. Med. *111:* 303–348 (1929).

KALK, H.: Leitfaden der Laparoskopie und Gastroskopie. Thieme, Stuttgart 1951.

KASTENDIECK, E.: Zur Anlage des Pneumoperitoneums bei der gynäkologischen Laparoskopie. Geburtsh. u. Frauenheilk. *33:* 376–378 (1973).

KASTENDIECK, E., W. MESTWERDT: Tierexperimentelle und klinische Aspekte zur Technik der laparoskopischen Tubensterilisation. Geburtsh. u. Frauenheilk. *33:* 971–978 (1973).

KELLY, J. C., J. ROCK: Culdoscopy for diagnosis in infertility. A report of 492 cases. Am. J. Obstet. Gynec. *72:* 523 (1956).

KLAFTEN, E.: Die Kolpolaparoskopie; eine Methode zur direkten Betrachtung der Organe der Becken-Bauchhöhle vom hinteren Scheidengewölbe. Wien. klin. Wschr. *59:* 829–831 (1947).

KOCKS, J.: Eine neue Methode der Sterilisation der Frau. Zbl. Gynäk. *2:* 617 (1978).

KOENIG, U. D.: Technik der offenen Pelviskopie – eine neue Methode für bessere Sicherheit in der Laparoskopie. Fortschr. Med. *97:* 1850–1853 (1979).

DE KOK, H. J.: A new technique for resecting the non-inflamed not-adhesive appendix through a mini-laparotomy with the laparoscope. Arch. Chir. Nederl. *29:* 195–198 (1977).

KORBSCH, R.: Lehrbuch und Atlas der Laparoskopie und Thorakoskopie. Lehmann, München 1927.

LENZI, G., C. B. CAVASSINI, E. LENZI: La Laparoscopie. Masson, Paris 1960.

LINDEMANN, H.-J.: Second look Pelviskopie nach Tubensterilisierung durch Elektrokoagulation. Zbl. Gynäk. *95:* 578 (1973).

LINDEMANN, H.-J.: Eine neue Untersuchungsmethode für die Hysteroskopie. Endoscopy *4:* 196–199 (1971).

Lindemann, H.-J.: Atlas der Hysteroskopie. Fischer, Stuttgart 1980.

Lübke, F.: Die Laparoskopie als diagnostisches Hilfsmittel in der Gynäkologie. Zbl. Gynäk. *86:* 260 (1964).

Madlener, M.: Über sterilisierende Operationen an den Tuben. Zbl. Gynäk. *43:* 380–384 (1919); Zbl. Gynäk. *56:* 2731 (1932).

Magendie, J., J. P. Secousse, M. Regnier: Sur l'intérèt de la coelioscopie en gynécologie (à propos de 45 laparoscopies effectuées dans service de clinique gynécologique). J. méd. Bordeaux *133:* 265–268 (1956).

Marchesi, F., E. Cittadini: Quadri celioscopici ovarici nella menopausa precoce. Atti Soc. ital. Obstet. Ginec. *51:* 25 (1965).

Menken, F. C.: Photokolposkopie und Photodouglasskopie – Indikation und Technik. Girardet, Wuppertal 1955.

Menken, F. C.: Fortschritte der gynäkologischen Endoskopie. In: Ottenjann, R.: Fortschritte der Endoskopie. Schattauer, Stuttgart–New York 1969.

Mikulicz Radecki, F. von, A. Freund: Das Tuben-Hysteroskop und seine diagnostische Verwendung bei Sterilität und Sterilisierung und Tubenerkrankungen. Arch. Gynäk. *132:* 68 (1927).

Mikulicz-Radecki, F. von: Ein neues Hysteroskop und seine praktische Anwendung in der Gynäkologie. Zbl. Gynäk. *92:* 13 (1927).

Mintz, M.: La biopsie d'ovaire à la pince sous coelioscopie en particulier dans les aménorrhées. C. R. Soc. franç. Gynéc. *32:* 634–658 (1962).

Mintz, H., H. Elmach, J. de Brux: Cancer de l'ovaire décelépar ponction d'un kyste sous coelioscopie. XXe Congrès des Fed. de. Gyn. et Obst. de langue Française, Lille 1963. Masson, Paris 1964.

Mintz, M.: La coelioscopie dans le syndrome de Stein-Leventhal. Gynéc. prat. *18:* 96–101 (1967).

Mintz, M., J. Dupre-Froment, J. de Brux: Ponctions de 94 kysts parautérins sous coelioscopie et étude cystologique des liquides. Gynaecologia *163:* 61 (1967).

Müller-Hermann, E., H. Weerda, P. Pedersen: Computergesteuerte, endoskopische Fotodokumentation im HNO-Bereich – eine neue Methode. Laryng. Rhinol. Otol. *61:* 402–405 (1982).

Naujoks, H.: Das Problem der temporären Sterilisierung der Frau. Enke, Stuttgart 1925.

Naujoks, H.: Reversible (»temporäre«) Sterilisierung der Frau durch Quetschung der Ampulla tubae. Zbl. Gynäk. *55:* 81–88 (1931).

Neumann, H. H., H. C. Frick: Occlusion of the Fallopian tubes with tantalum clips. Am. J. Obstet. Gynec. *81:* 803 (1961).

Nitze, M.: Über die Behandlungsmethode der Höhlen des menschlichen Körpers. Wien. med. Wschr. *24:* 851–858 (1879).

Norment, W. B.: Improved instruments for diagnosis of lesions by hysterogram and waterhysterscope. N. C. med. J. *10:* 646 (1949).

Palmer, R.: La celioscopie gynécologique. Rapport du Prof. Mocquot. Acad. de Chir. *72:* 363–368 (1946).

Palmer, R., A. M. Dourlen-Rollier, A. Audebert, R. Geraud: La Stérilisation Volontaire en France et dans de monde. Masson, Paris 1981.

Philipp, E., K. Semm: Die diagnostische Wertstellung der gynäkologischen Pelviskopie. Geburtsh. u. Frauenheilk. *32:* 46–50 (1972).

Phillips, J. M. et al.: American Association of Gynecologic Laparoscopists. 1976 membership survey. J. Reprod. Med. *21:* 3–6 (1978).

Phillips, J. M. et al.: American Association of Gynecologic laparoscopists. 1977 membership survey. J. Reprod. Med. *23:* 61–64 (1979).

Pomeroy: Zit. nach Lull, C. B., R. M. Mitschell: The Pomeroy method of sterilization. Am. J. Obstet. Gynec. *59:* 1119 (1950).

Power, S. H., A. C. Barnes: Sterilization by means of peritoneoscopic tubal fulguration. A preliminary report. Am. J. Obstet. Gynec. *41:* 1038–1043 (1941).

Pschyrembel, W.: Klinisches Wörterbuch. De Gruyter, Berlin 1982.

Pye, A., M. Fourestier: La culdoscopie (Exploration de la cavité pelvienne chez la femme par voie vaginale). Presse méd. *72:* 679–683 (1964).

Ravina, A.: La coelioscopie par voie vaginale. Presse méd. *58:* 81–82 (1950).

Reidenbach, H.-D.: Hochfrequenz- und Lasertechnik in der Medizin. Springer, Berlin 1983.

Rettenmaier, G.: Bewertung und Einschränkung des Risikos bei der Laparoskopie. Ergebnisse einer Umfrage. Endoscopy *1:* 115–116 (1969).

Riedel, H.-H., K. Semm: Vorzeitiges Auftreten menopausaler Beschwerden in Abhängigkeit von verschiedenen Sterilisationstechniken – ein Vergleich zwischen dem Endokoagulations- und HF-Verfahren. Arch. Gynec. *232:* 229–230 (1981).

Riedel, H. H., P. Conrad, K. Semm: Die deutsche Pelviskopiestatistik der Jahre 1978. bis 1982. Geburtsh. Frauenheilk. *45:* 656–663 (1985).

Rimkus, V., K. Semm: Sterilization by carbon dioxide hysteroscopy. In: Phillips, J. M., L. Keith: Gynecological Laparoscopy-Principles and Techniques, S. 75–84. Symposia Specialists, Miami 1974.

RINGLEB, O.: Das Kystoskop. Leipzig 1910.

ROKITANSKY, C.: Lehrbuch der pathologischen Anatomie, III. Auflage. Wien 1981.

RUBIN, I. C.: Uterine endoscopy, endometroscopy with the aid of uterine insufflation. Am. J. Obstet. Gynec. *10:* 313 (1925).

RUDDOCK, J. C.: Peritoneoscopy. West J. Surg. *42:* 392–405 (1934).

SAMPSON, J. A.: Verschleppung von Menstruationsdesquamaten. Arch. Surg. *3:* 245 (1921).

SCHMIDT-MATTHIESEN, H.: Die Hysteroskopie als klinische Routinemethode. Geburtsh. u. Frauenheilk. *26:* 1498 (1966).

SCHREINER, W. E.: Die operative Sterilisation der Frau. Schweiz. Rdsch. Med. (Praxis) *63:* 260 (1974).

SCHROEDER, C.: Über den Ausbau und die Leistung der Hysteroskope. Arch. Gynäk. *156:* 407 (1934).

SCHWALM, H.: Die Laparoskopie in der gynäkologischen Diagnostik. In: SCHWALM, H., G. DÖDERLEIN: Klinik der Frauenheilkunde und Geburtshilfe, Bd. I, S. 315. Urban & Schwarzenberg, München 1964.

SCHWEPPE, K. W., R. M. WYNN, F. K. BELLER: Ultrastructural comparison of ectopic and extopic endometrium. Am. J. Obstet. Gynec. 1983 (1984) i. Druck.

SEMM, K.: Zur Technik der Eileiterdurchblasung. Z. Geburtsh. Gynäk. Beilageheft *162:* 48–53 (1964).

SEMM, K.: Die Laparoskopie in der Gynäkologie. Geburtsh. u. Frauenheilk. *27:* 1029 (1967).

SEMM, K.: Das Pneumoperitoneum mit CO_2. Visum *6:* 1, 30 (1967).

SEMM, K.: Prüfung der Tubendurchgängigkeit. In: Gynäkologie und Geburtshilfe, Bd. I, S. 857. Thieme, Stuttgart 1969.

SEMM, K.: Tubal sterilization finally with cauterization or temporary with ligation via pelviscopy. In: PHILIPS, J. M., L. KEITH: Gynaecological Laparoscopy: Principles and Techniques. New York, London 1974.

SEMM, K.: Methoden der Sterilisierung der Frau. Therapiewoche *26:* 3931–3941 (1976).

SEMM, K.: Die pelviskopische Chirurgie in der Gynäkologie. Geburtsh. u. Frauenheilk. *37:* 909–920 (1977).

SEMM, K.: Pelviskopie und Hysteroskopie – Farbatlas und Lehrbuch. Schattauer, Stuttgart – New York, 1976. *Englisch:* Saunders, Philadelphia – London – Toronto, 1977. *Französisch:* Masson, Paris – New York – Toronto, 1977. *Spanisch:* Toray-Masson, S. A./Barcelona, 1977. *Portugiesisch:* Schattauer, Stuttgart – New York, 1977.

SEMM, K.: Statistischer Überblick über die Bauchspiegelung in der Frauenheilkunde bis 1977 in der Bundesrepublik Deutschland. Geburtsh. u. Frauenheilk. *39:* 537–544 (1979).

SEMM, K.: Dia-Atlas zur Pelviskopie, Hysteroskopie und Fetoskopie (mit 240 Farb-Dias und Textbuch). Hrsg. K. SEMM, Kiel 1980 (Französisch, Englisch, Kiel, 1981, Spanisch, Kiel, 1984).

SEMM, K.: Physical and Biological Considerations, militating against the use of endoscopically applied high-frequency current in the abdomen. Endoscopy *15:* 238–288 (1983).

SEMM, K., E. PHILIPP: Vermeidung von Spontanrekanalisation des Eileiters post sterilisationem. Gynäk. Prax. *4:* 63–74 (1980).

SEMM, K., V. RIMKUS: Technische Bemerkungen zur CO_2-Hysteroskopie. Z. Geburtsh. u. Frauenheilk. *34:* 451–460 (1974).

SEYMOUR, H. F.: A method of endoscopic examination of the uterus with its indications. Proc. roy. Soc. Med., 19 Sect. Obstet. Gynec. *74* (1926).

SIEDE, W., H. SCHNEIDER: Leitfaden und Atlas der Laparoskopie. Lehmann, München 1962.

SILANDER, R.: Hysteroscopy with carcinoma of the uterine endometrium. Surg. Gynec. Obstet. *114* (1962).

STEIN, S.: The endoscope as an aid in the diagnosis and treatment of granular urethritis and stricture. East River med. Assoc. 1st Oct. The Med. Record, New York 1868. Vol. 2, S. 416.

STEIN, A., W. H. STEWART: Roentgen-ray study of abdominal cavity. Radiology *28:* 391 (1919).

STEIN, O.: Oxygen peritoneal inflation before x-ray. Ann. Surg. *70:* 95 (1919).

STEIN, I. F.: Why pneumoperitoneum? Radiology *28:* 391–398 (1937).

STEIN, I. F., M. R. COHEN, R. ELSON: Results of bilateral ovarian wedge resection in 47 cases of sterility. Am. J. Obstet. Gynec. *29:* 181–191 (1949).

STEIN, S.: Das Photo-Endoskop. Berl. klin. Wschr. H. *3* (1974).

STEPTOE, P. C.: Laparoscopy in Gynaecology, S. 75. Livingstone, Edinburgh 1964.

STEPTOE, P. S.: Laparoscopy for infertility and fertility. In: BERCI, G.: Endoscopy, S. 518–535. Appleton-Century Crofts, New York 1976.

STEPTOE, P. C.: Retrospective and prospective studies in laparoscopy. Proc. roy. Soc. Med. *69:* 143 (1976).

TE LINDE, R. W., F. N. RUTLEDGE: Culdoscopy, a useful gynecological procedure. Am. J. Obstet. Gynec. *55:* 102 (1948).

TETON J. B.: Diagnostic culdoscopy. Am. J. Obstet. Gynec. *60:* 665–670 (1950).

THOMSEN, K.: Erfahrungen und Fortschritte bei der Douglasskopie. Geburtsh. u. Frauenheilk. *11:* 587 (1951).

THOYER-ROZAT, J.: Electronic flash photography in the course of coelioscopy. Gynec. Obstet. *59:* 71–73 (1960).

VALTCHEV, K. L. et al.: A new uterine mobilizer for laparoscopy; its use in 513 patients. Am. J. Obstet. Gynec. *127:* 738–740 (1977).

VERESS, J.: Ein neues Instrument zur Ausführung von Brust- oder Bauchpunktionen und Pneumothoraxbehandlung. Dtsch. med. Wschr. *41:* 1480 (1938).

VERESS, J.: Eine Nadel zur gefahrlosen Anlegung des Pneumoperitoneums. Elöadas a zürichi Gastroenterologiai Kongresszuson, 1960 szeptember 30-àn. Gastroenterologia (Basel).

WALCH, E., H. GRÜNAGL: Praktische Erfahrungen mit der Douglasskopie. Zbl. Gynäk. *76:* 397 (1954).

WALZ, O.: Sterilitätsoperationen an der Tube mit Hilfe eines Operationsmikroskopes. Z. Geburtsh. Gynäk. *153:* 49–55 (1959).

WENNER, R.: Was kann man in der Gynäkologie von der Coelioscopie erwarten? Gynaecologia (Basel) *125:* 264–267 (1948).

WERNER, R.: Sterilisierung der Frau durch Tubenverkochung. Chirurg 6: 843–845 (1934).

WILDHIRT, E.: Mediastinalemphysem bei Laparoskopie und zur Luftembolie bei Laparoskopie. Münch. med. Wschr. *98:* 58 (1956).

WILDHIRT, E., H. KALK: Bedeutung und Wert der Laparoskopie und gezielte Leberpunktion. Thieme, Stuttgart 1965.

WITTMOSER, R.: Fortschritte der selektiven endoskopischen Chirurgie großer Körperhöhlen. In: RÖSCH, W.: Fortschritte in der Endoskopie, S. 25. Straube, Erlangen 1976.

24.2. GENERAL SURVEY OF THE LITERATURE

24.2.1. Books and Monographs

BERCI, G. : Endoscopie. Appleton-Century-Crofts, New York 1976.

BLANDAU, R. J.: Mechanism of tubal transport: comparative aspects. In: BROSENS, I., R. M. L. WINSTON (eds.): Reversibility of Female Sterilization. S. 1–15. Academic Press, London 1978.

BROOKS, P. G.: Economic considerations in tubal microsurgery. In: PHILLIPS, J. M. (ed.): Microsurgery in Gynecology. Proc. of the Fallopian Tube; the 1st International Congress of Gynecologic Microsurgery, Irvine Calif. 1977. S. 206–207. American Association of Gynecologic Laparoscopists, Downey, Calif. 1977.

BROSENS, I., R. M. L. WINSTON (eds.): Reversibility of Female Sterilization. Academic Press, London 1978.

BUNCKE, H. J., N. CHATER, Z. SZABO: The Manual of Microvascular Surgery. San Francisco, Calif. 1980.

CHRIST, F., H. P. KLEISSL, F. EBERLEIN, B. KUSCH: Die Laparoskopie bei Jugendlichen und Kindern in der Gynäkologie. In: RÖSCH, W.: Fortschritte der Endoskopie. S. 199–209. Straube, Erlangen 1976.

CORSON, S. L.: A survey of attitudes toward gynecologic microsurgery. In: SCIARRA, J. J., G. I. ZATUCHNI, J. J. SPEIDEL (eds.): Reversal of Sterilization. Proceedings of a Workshop on Reversal of Sterilization. San Francisco, Calif. S. 177–180. Harper and Row, Hagerstown, Maryland 1980.

CORSON, S. L.: A survey of opinions and attitudes toward gynecologic microsurgery. In: PHILLIPS, J. M. (ed.): Endoscopy in Gynecology. Proceedings of the 3rd International Congress on Gynecologic Endoscopy, San Francisco, Calif. 1977. S. 420–422. American Association of Gynecologic Laparoscopists, Downey, Calif. 1978.

CRAFT, I., A. A. YUZPE: Discussion summary (microsurgery). In: SCIARRA, J. J., G. I. ZATUCHNI, J. J. SPEIDEL (eds.): Reversal of Sterilization. Proceedings of a Workshop on Reversal of Sterilization, San Francisco Calif. S. 181-182 (PARFR Serie on Fertility Regulation). Harper and Row, Hagerstown, Maryland 1977.

CROSIGNANI, P. G., B. L. RUBIN (eds.): Microsurgery in Female Infertility. Proceedings of the Serono Clinical Colloquia on Reproduction, No. 1, S. 134. Academic Press, London 1980.

DIAMOND, E.: Microsurgery in infertility: instrumentation and technique. In: PHILLIPS, J. M. (ed.): Microsurgery in Gynecology. Proceedings of the Fallopian Tube and the 1st International Congress of Gynecologic Microsurgery Irvine, Calif. 1977. S. 20–30. American Association of Gynecologic Laparoscopists, Downey, Calif. 1977.

DIAMOND, E.: A microsurgical study of the blood supply to the uterine tube and ovary. In: PHILLIPS, J. M.: Microsurgery in Gynecology. Proceedings of the Workshop for Laparoscopy and Microsurgical Repair of the Fallopian Tube and the 1st International Congress of Gynecologic Microsurgery, Irvine Calif. 1977. S. 69–76. American Association of Gynecologic Laparoscopists. Downey, Calif. 1977.

DROEGMUELLER, W., M. CHVAPIL, C. D. CHRISTIAN: Modern modified Aldridge procedure. In: SCIARRA, J. J., G. I. ZATUCHNI, J. J. SPEIDEL: Reversal of Sterilization. Proceedings of a Workshop on Reversal of Sterilization, San Francisco, Calif. S. 224–225 (PARFR Series on Fertility Regulation). Harper and Row, Hagerstown, Maryland 1978.

EDDY, C. A., D. A. ARCHER: Tubal electrophysiology after microsurgical anastomosis. In: PHILLIPS, J. M.: Endoscopy in Gynecology. Proceedings of the 3rd International Congress on Gynecologic Endoscopy, San Francisco, Calif. 1977. S. 428–431. American Association of Gynecologic Laparoscopists. Downey, Calif. 1978.

EL KADY, A. A., G. SAMI, K. A. LAURENCE, S. BADAWI: The tubal hood: a potentially reversible sterilization technique. In: SCIARRA, J. J., G. I. ZATUCHNI, J. J. SPEIDEL: Reversal of Sterilization. Proceedings of a Workshop on Reversal of Sterilization, San Francisco Calif. S. 232–240 (PARFR Series on Fertility Regulation). Harper and Row, Hagerstown, Maryland 1978.

FRANGENHEIM, H.: Komplikationen bei der Laparoskopie und Vorschläge zu ihrer Verhütung. In: OBOLENSKY, W., O. KÄSER: Ovulation und Ovulationsauslösung. Perioperative Probleme. S. 202–225 a. Huber, Bern 1975.

FRANGENHEIM, H.: Die Laparoskopie bei der Diagnostik und Therapie maligner und benigner Tumoren im Genital-Bereich. S. 203–208. In: W. RÖSCH: Fortschritte der Endoskopie. Straube, Erlangen 1976.

Frangenheim, H.: Die Laparoskopie in der Gynäkologie, Chirurgie und Pädiatrie und Atlas mit einem Beitrag »Hysteroskopie« von H.-J. Lindemann. 3. überarb. u. erw. Aufl. Thieme, Stuttgart 1977.

Frangenheim, H.: Die Laparoskopie in der Chirurgie. S. 285–294. In: Demling, L., W. Rösch: Operative Endoskopie. Acron, Berlin 1979.

Gomel, V., P. McComb: Microsurgery in gynecology. In: Solber, S. J. (ed.): Microsurgery, S. 143–183. Williams and Wilkins, Baltimore, Maryland 1979.

Gonzales, B.: Physicians' attitudes toward sterilization reversal. In: Phillips, J. M.: Endoscopy in Gynecology. Proceedings of the 3rd International Congress on Gynecologic Endoscopy, San Francisco, Calif. 1977. S. 166–167. American Association of Gynecologic Laparoscopists. Downey, Calif. 1978.

Hasson, H. M.: Open laparoscopy: In: Phillips, J. M., S. L. Corson, L. Keith: Laparoscopy. S. 145–149. Williams and Wilkins, Baltimore 1977.

Hausswald, H.-R., G. Seidenschnur: Gynäkologische Laparoskopie. J. A. Barth, Leipzig 1976.

Hepp, H., G. Reisach, W. Goldhofer: Komplikationen der gynäkologischen Laparoskopie – ein Erfahrungsbericht über 20 Jahre. In: W. Rösch: Fortschritte der Endoskopie. S. 215–221. Straube, Erlangen 1976.

Hoffmann, J. J.: The synthesis between experimental and clinical microsurgery. In: Phillips, J. M.: Microsurgery in Gynecology. Proceedings of the Workshop for Laparoscopy and Microsurgical Repair of the Fallopian Tube and the 1st International Congress of Gynecologic Microsurgery, Irvine, Calif. 1977. S. 63–68. American Association of Gynecologic Laparoscopists. Downey, Calif. 1977.

Hosseinian, A. H., S. Lucero, L. J. D. Zanefeld: Hysteroscopically delivered tubal plugs. In: Sciarra, J. J., G. I. Zatuchni, J. J. Speidel: Reversal of Sterilization. Proceedings of a Workshop on Reversal of Sterilization, San Francisco, Calif. S. 241–248. Harper and Row, Hagerstown, Maryland 1978.

Hulka, J. F.: Tubal damage in elective sterilization. In: Phillips, J. M.: Microsurgery in Gynecology. Proceedings of the Workshop for Laparoscopy and Microsurgical Repair of the Fallopian Tube and the 1st Intern. Congr. of Gynecologic Microsurgery, Irvine 1977. S. 109–112. American Assoc. of Gynecologic Laparoscopists. Downey, Calif. 1977.

International Project of the Association for Voluntary Sterilization, Inc.: A Comprehensive Set of Bibliographies on Voluntary Sterilization. The Assoc. for Vol. Steril., Inc. 208 Third Avenue, New York 1976.

International Planned Parenthood Federation (IPPF). Central Medical Committee. – Statements on policy matters, trends in family planning and new medical developments made by the central Medical Committee, March 1977. S. 1–4. IPPF Med. Bull. *11:* (1977).

International Project/Association for Voluntary Sterilization, Inc. (IP/AVS). A selected bibliography on voluntary sterilization: medical/scientific and general. S. 63. New York IP/AVS 1977.

Jung, H., G. Kubli, K. H. Wolf: Gynäkologie und Geburtshilfe. Kurzgefaßte Darstellung aktueller Neuentwicklungen zur Weiterbildung. Enke, Stuttgart 1980.

Kaback, M. M., C. Valenti: Intrauterine Fetal Visualization: A Multidisciplinary Approach. S. 297. Proceedings. Amer. Elsevier Publ. Excerpta Medica, Amsterdam – Oxford – New York, 1976.

Koch, J., H. J. Kümper, V. Terruhn: Laparoskopische Tubensterilisation mit einer neuen bipolaren Zange. In: Rösch, W.: Fortschritte der Endoskopie. S. 215–221. Straube, Erlangen 1976.

Laufe, L. E.: The fimbrial prosthesis. In: Sciarra, J. J., G. I. Zatuchni, J. J. Speidel: Reversal of Sterilization. Proceedings of a Workshop on Reversal of Sterilization, San Francisco, Calif. S. 220–223. Harper and Row, Hagerstown, Maryland 1978.

Laufe, L. E.: Reversible methods of fimbrial enclosure. In: Zatuchni, G. I., M. Labbok, J. J. Sciarra: Research Frontiers in Fertility regulation. Proceedings of the Workshop, Mexico City 1980. Harper and Row, Hagerstown, Maryland 1980.

Lindemann, H.-J.: Atlas der Hysteroskopie. Fischer, Stuttgart 1980.

Lueken, R. P., H.-J. Lindemann: Der erweiterte Penetrationstest per hysteroskopiam. In: Fortschritte der Fertilitätsforschung, Tagungsbericht der Deutschen Gesellschaft zum Studium der Fertilität und Sterilität FDF 8. S. 223–225. Grosse, Berlin 1979.

Mastroianni, L., jr.: Tubal occlusion. In: Keller, P. J.: Female Infertility, Vol. 4, S. 114–131. Karger, Basel 1978.

Mastroianni, L., jr.: Structure and function of the Fallopian tube as it pertains to microsurgical reconstruction. (Abstract). S. 3. Symposon on Tubal Microsurgery, 10th World Congress on Fertility and Sterility, Madrid 1980.

Menken, F. C.: Neue operative Techniken der gynäkologischen Laparoskopie. In: Rösch, W.: Fortschritte der Endoskopie. S. 211–214. Straube, Erlangen 1976.

Menken, F. C.: Der Mehrzweck-Portioadapter zur Anwendung während der Pelviskopie. In: Fortschritte der Fertilitätsforschung FDF 8, der Deutschen Gesellschaft zum Studium der Fertilität und Sterilität. Grosse, Berlin 1979.

Mettler, L., K. Semm: Laparoscopic surgery in the treatment of peripheral tubal occlusion and endometriosis in female infertility. In: J. M. Phillips: Microsurgery in Gynecology II. S. 166–171. American Association of Gynecologic Laparoscopists. Downey, Calif. 1981.

MEYER, J. H. et. al.: A randomized study of outpatient tubal sterilization by mini-laparotomy and laparoscopy. In: SCIARRA, J. J., G. I. ZATUCHNI, J. J. SPEIDEL: Advances in Female Sterilization Techniques. S. 660. Harper and Row, Hagerstown, Maryland 1976.

NORDENSKJÖLD, F., M. AHLGREN: Laparoskopische Behandlung bei Infertilität. In: Fortschritte der Fertilitätsforschung FDF 8, der Deutschen Gesellschaft zum Studium der Fertilität und Sterilität. S. 220–222. Grosse, Berlin 1979.

PAI, D. N.: The need for sterilization reversal in India. In: SCIARRA, J. J., G. I. ZATUCHNI, J. J. SPEIDEL: Reversal of Sterilization. Proceedings of a Workshop on Reversal of Sterilization, San Francisco, Calif. (PARFR Series on Fertility Regulation). S. 264–273. Harper and Row, Hagerstown, Maryland 1978.

PAI, D. N.: A Study of Recanalization. Parel Bombay, India. WHO Clinical Research Centre, Department of Preventive and Social Medicine Research 1978, S. 8.

PALMER, R., A.-M. DOURLEN ROLLIE, A. AUDEBERT, R. GÉRAUD: La Stérilisation Voluntaire en France et dans le Monde. Masson, Paris 1981.

PAR H., G. ROBERT, R. PALMER, C. BOURY-HEYLER, J. COHEN: Précis de Gynécologie. Masson, Paris 1974.

PATERSON, P.: Microsurgery of the oviduct. In: SCIARRA, J. J., G. I. ZATUCHNI, J. J. SPEIDEL: Reversal of Sterilization. Proceedings of a Workshop on Reversal of Sterilization. San Francisco, Calif. S. 162–169. Harper and Row, Hagerstown, Maryland 1978.

PATERSON, P.: Update on Tubal Anastomosis Experience. Monash University, Department of Obstetrics and Gynaecology, Victorial Medical Centre Australia. Personal Communication 1980.

PHILLIPS, J. M.: Laparoscopy. Williams & Wilkins, Baltimore, Maryland 1977.

PHILLIPS, J. M., W. J. WINCHESTER: Teaching microsurgery in the vivarium workshop. In: PHILLIPS, J. M.: Microsurgery in Gynecology. Proceedings of the Workshop for Laparoscopy and Microsurgical Repair of the Fallopian Tube and the 1st International Congress of Gynecologic Microsurgery, Irvine Calif. 1977. S. 194–205. American Assoc. of Gynecologic Laparoscopists, Downey, Calif. 1977.

PHILLIPS, J. M.: Microsurgery in Gynecology. Proceedings of the Workshop for Laparoscopy and Microsurgical Repair of the Fallopian Tube and the 1st International Congress of Gynecologic Microsurgery. Irvine, Calif. 1977. American Association of Gynecologic Laparoscopists. Downey, Calif. 1977.

PHILLIPS, J. M.: Endoscopy in Gynecology. Proceedings of the 3rd International Congress on Gynecologic Endoscopy, San Francisco, California 1977. American Association of Gynecologic Laparoscopists. Downey, Calif. 1978.

PHILLIPS, J. M.: Female Sterilization. A Comparison of the Methods. American Association of Gynecologic Laparoscopists. Downey, Calif. 1980.

RIOUX, J. E. et al.: Bipolar electrosurgery for laparoscopic sterilization. In: SCIARRA, J. J. et al.: Advances in Female Sterilization Techniques. S. 24–29. Harper and Row, Hagerstown, Maryland 1976.

SCIARRA, J. J., G. I. ZATUCHNI, J. J. SPEIDEL: Reversal of Sterilization. Proceedings of a Workshop on Reversal of Sterilization, San Francisco, Calif. Harper and Row, Hagerstown, Maryland 1978.

SCIARRA, J. J.: Hysteroscopic approaches for tubal closure. In: ZATUCHNI, G. I., M. LABBOK, J. J. SCIARRA: Research Frontiers in Fertility Regulation. Proceedings of the Workshop, Mexico City 1980. Harper and Row, Hagerstown, Maryland 1980.

SCIARRA, J. J.: Survey of tubal sterilization procedures. In: SCIARRA, J. J., G. I. ZATUCHNI, J. J. SPEIDEL: Reversal of Sterilization. Proceedings of a Workshop on Reversal of Sterilization, San Francisco, Calif. S. 117–133. Harper and Row, Hagerstown, Maryland 1978.

SEMM, K.: Tubal sterilization finally with cauterization or temporary with ligation via pelviscopy. In: PHILLIPS, J. M., L. KEITH: Gynecological Laparoscopy – Principles and Techniques. S. 337–359. Symposia Specialists, Miami, Florida 1975.

SEMM, K.: Elektronisch gesteuerter Schwachstrom als Ersatz des Hochfrequenzstromes in der Endoskopie. In: OTTENJANN, R.: Fortschritte der Endoskopie, Bd. 6, S. 17–21. Thieme, Stuttgart 1975.

SEMM, K.: Endokoagulation – eine neue Technik für blutungsfreies, intraabdominelles endoskopisches Operieren. In: RÖSCH, W.: Fortschritte in der Endoskopie. S. 21–24. Straube, Erlangen 1976.

SEMM, K.: Pelviskopie und Hysteroskopie – Farbatlas und Lehrbuch. Schattauer, Stuttgart – New York 1976.
Englisch: (Übersetzer: ALLAN LAKE RICE) W. B. Saunders, Philadelphia, London – Toronto 1977.
Französisch: (Übersetzer: PH. GRIMAIL, J.-C. POULET) Masson, Paris – New York – Barcelona — Mailand 1977.
Spanisch: (Übersetzer: J. J. FUSTER, MERCADE) Toray-Masson, S. A. Barcelona 1977.
Portugiesisch: (Übersetzer: H. MATARE, F. MUELLER) Schattauer, Stuttgart – New York 1977.

SEMM, K.: Gynecologic surgical interventions with the laparoscope. In: PHILLIPS, J. M.: Endoscopy in Gynecology. Proceedings of the 3rd International Congress on Gynecologic Endoscopy, San Francisco 1977. S. 514–521. American Association of Gynecologic Laparoscopists, Downey, Calif. 1977.

SEMM, K.: Bildbeitrag zum »Color-Atlas« In: PHILLIPS, J. M.: Endoscopy in Gynecology. Proceedings of the 3rd International Congress on Gynecologic Endoscopy, San Francisco 1977. S. 34–66. American Association of Gynecologic Laparoscopists, Downey, Calif. 1977.

SEMM, K.: Diagnostik und operative Therapie des Tubenfaktors. In: Fortschritte der Fertilitätsforschung, Bd. V, S. 1–6. Grosse, Berlin 1977.

SEMM, K.: Gynäkologische Mikrochirurgie per pelviskopiam. In: HUSSLEIN, H.: Gynäkologie und Geburtshilfe – Forschung und Erkenntnisse. Tagungsband der VIII. Akademischen Tagung deutschsprechender Hochschullehrer in der Gynäkologie und Geburtshilfe. S. 761–764. Egermann, Wien 1977.

SEMM, K.: Fetoskopie. In: TOLKSDORF, M., J. SPRANGER: Klinische Genetik in der Pädiatrie. S. 114–122. Thieme, Stuttgart 1979.

SEMM, K.: Adhäsiolyse: Endoskopische Intraabdominal-Chirurgie. In: DEMLING, L., W. RÖSCH: Operative Endoskopie. S. 303–310. Acron, Berlin 1979.

SEMM, K.: Die Bedeutung der Endoskopie für die weibliche Sterilität. In: Fortschritte der Fertilitätsforschung FDF 8. S. 217–219. Grosse, Berlin 1979.

SEMM, K.: Instruments for surgical therapeutic pelviscopy. In: Proceedings of the Vth European Congress on Sterility, Venedig 1978. S. 651–655. Edizioni Internazionali Gruppo Edit. Medico, Rom 1980.

SEMM, K.: Dia-Atlas zur Pelviskopie, Hysteroskopie und Fetoskopie (mit 240 Dias und Textbuch). Hrsg. K. SEMM, Kiel 1980 (*Französisch:* Kiel 1981, *Englisch:* Kiel 1981, *Spanisch:* Kiel 1982).

SEMM, K.: Hysteroscopy – A new aid in gynecological intrauterine diseases. Estratto dal Volume degli Atti del 59° Congresso Nazionale della Societa Italiana di Ostetricia e Ginecologia, Parma 1978. S. 459–460. Tipolito Mattioli, Fidenza 1980.

SEMM, K.: Tubal sterilization and ovary. In: K. SEMM, L. METTLER: Human Reproduction – Proceedings of the III. World Congress of Human Reproduction, Berlin 1981. S. 418–420. Excerpta Medica, Int. Congr. Series 551. Amsterdam – Oxford – Princeton 1981.

SEMM, K.: The importance of surgical pelviscopy in sterility for tubal treatment. In: SEMM, K., L. METTLER: Human Reproduction – Proceedings of the III. World Congress of Human Reproduction, Berlin 1981. Excerpta Medica, Intern. Congr. Series 551. S. 76–85. Amsterdam – Oxford – Princeton 1981.

SEMM, K.: Endoskopijà, U. Ginekologiji I Opstetriciji (Übersetzung SRECO SIMIC). Jugoslavenska Medicinska Naklada, Zagreb 1981.

SEMM, K.: Advances in Pelviscopic Surgery. In: Current Problems in Obstetrics and Gynecology, Vol. V., Nr. 10. Year Book Medical Publishers Inc., Chicago – London 1982.

SEMM, K.: Diagnostik der Sterilität und Infertilität. In: DA RUGNA, D.: Festschrift Prof. Dr. Otto Käser – ausgewählte Kapitel der Geburtshilfe und Gynäkologie, Nr. 14. Schwabe, Basel – Stuttgart 1982.

SEMM, K.: Diagnostic Tools: Instruments and Techniques for Endoscopic Ovarian Surgery. In: SERRA, S. B.: The Ovary (Series Comprehensive Endocrinology; Ed. L. MARTINI), S. 159–176. Raven Press, New York 1983.

SEMM, K.: Die operative Pelviskopie. In: SCHWALM, H., G. DÖDERLEIN, H. WULF: Klinik der Frauenheilkunde und Geburtshilfe, S. 375–421/1. Urban u. Schwarzenberg, München – Wien – Baltimore; 1. Folge 1970; 1976; 2. Folge, München; 3. Folge 1983.

SEMM, K., W. DITTMAR: Besonderheiten der postoperativen Therapie nach Sterilitätsoperationen: In: OBOLENSKY, W., O. KÄSER: Ovula und Ovulationsauslösung – perioperative Probleme. S. 237–245. Huber, Bern – Stuttgart – Wien 1975.

SHAHROK, V. M., Z. SZABO: A microsurgical technique for reanastomosis of the human Fallopian tube. In: PHILLIPS, J. M.: Microsurgery in Gynecology. Proceedings of the Workshop for Laparoscopy and Microsurgical Repair of the Fallopain Tube and the 1st International Congress of Gynecologic Microsurgery, Irvine, Calif. 1977. S. 145–152. American Association of Gynecologic Laparoscopists. Downey, Calif. 1977.

SIEGLER, A. M.: Microsurgery for tubal reconstruction. In: PHILLIPS, J. M.: Microsurgery in Gynecology. Proceedings of the Workshop for Laparoscopy and Microsurgical Repair of the Fallopian Tube and the 1st International Congress of Gynecologic Microsurgery, Irvine Calif. 1977. S. 82–95. American Association of Gynecologic Laparoscopists. Downey, Calif. 1977.

SIEGLER, A. M.: Reversibility of tubal sterilization. In: BROSENS, I., R. M. L. WINSTON: Reversibility of Female Sterilization. S. 73–78. Academic Press, London 1978.

SIEGLER, A. M., V. KONTOPOULOS: Reversal of tubal sterilization: implications, techniques, and results. In: SCIARRA, J. J., G. I. ZATUCHNI, J. J. SPEIDEL: Reversal of Sterilization. Proceedings of a Workshop on Reversal of Sterilization. San Francisco, Calif. S. 134–142. Harper and Row, Hagerstown, Maryland 1978.

SILBER, S. J., R. S. COHEN: Microsurgical reversal of female sterilization: techniques and comparison to vasectomy reversal. In: SILBER, S. J.: Microsurgery. S. 185–242. Williams and Wilkins, Baltimore, Maryland 1979.

SILBER, S. J.: Microsurgery. Williams and Wilkins, Baltimore, Maryland 1979.

SIRBU, P.: Celioscopia. In: SIRBU, P., J. CHIRICUTA, A. PANDELE, D. SETLACEC: Chirurgia Ginecologicà. S. 153–176. Medicalà, Bukarest 1981.

STEPTOE, P. C.: Restoration of Fertility Following Sterilization: Preoperative Evaluation of the Female. S. 5. 4th Intern. Conference on Vol. Sterilization, Seoul, Korea 1979.

United States Agency for International Development (USAID) Family planning statistics, India. S. 3 (Mimeo). Washington, D. C. USAID, 1977.

United Nations (UN.) Department of International Economic and Social Affairs. Statistical Office. Statistical Yearbook 1977, 29. Ed. New York UN 1978.

United States. Center for Disease Control (CDC). Family Planning Evaluation Division. Surgical Sterilization Surveillance: Tubal Sterilization 1970–1975. S. 22. Atlanta, Georgia (CDC 1979 – 8378).

VALLE, R. F.: Training for microsurgery. In: SCIARRA, J. J., G. I. ZATUCHNI, J. J. SPEIDEL: Reversal of Sterilization. S. 151–161. San Francisco, Calif. Harper and Row, Hagerstown, Maryland 1978.

WILLIAMS, E. A.: Aspects of Falliopian tube surgery. In: STALLWORTHY, J., G. BOURNE: Recent Advances in Obstetrics and Gynaecology. S. 219–236. London, Churchill Livingstone 1977 (No. 12).

WHEELESS, C. R., jr.: The past, present, and future use of the laparoscope in female sterilization. In: SCIARRA, J. J. et al.: Advances in Female Sterilization Techniques. S. 30–36. Harper and Row, Hagerstown, Maryland 1979.

WELEY, A. T., R. T. RAVENHOLT, W. H. BOYTON, J. J. SPEIDEL: Reversal of tubal ligation in AID-funded population programs. In: PHILLIPS, J. M.: Microsurgery in Gynecology. Proceedings of the Workshop Laparoscopy and Microsurgical Repair of the Fallopian Tube and the 1st International Congress of Gynecologic Microsurgery, Irvine, Calif 1977. S. 250–251. American Association of Gynecologic Laparoscopists. Downey, Calif. 1977.

WILLIAMS, E. A.: Aspects of Fallopian tube surgery. In: STALLWORTHY, J., G. BOURNE (eds.): Recent Advances in Obstetrics and Gynecology. S. 219–236. London, Churchill Livingstone 1977.

WILLIAMS, E. A.: Results of reversal of female sterilization. In: BROSENS, I., R. M. L. WINSTON: Reversibility of Female Sterilization. S. 89–95. Academic Press, London 1978.

WINSTON, R. M. L.: Tubal anastomosis for reversal for sterilization in 45 women. In: BROSENS, I., R. M. L. WINSTON: Reversibility of Female Sterilization. S. 55–67. Academic Press, London 1978.

WINSTON, R. M. L., R. A. MARGARA: Techniques for the improvement of microsurgical tubal anastomosis. In: CROSIGNANI, P. G., B. L. RUBIN: Microsurgery in Female Infertility. S. 25–34. Proceedings of the Serono Clinical Colloquia on Reproduction, No. 1. Academic Press, London 1980.

WINSTON, R. M. L.: Microsurgery in the treatment of female infertility. Proceedings of the Xth World Congress of Fertility and Sterility, Madrid 1980.

WORTMANN, J. S.: A review of complications of laparoscopic sterilisation. In: SCIARRA, J. J. et al.: Advances in Female Sterilization Techniques. S. 37–47. Harper and Row, Hagerstown, Maryland 1976.

23.2.2. Journals

I. History

CUMMING, D. C. et al.: Historical predictability of abnormal laparoscopic findings in the infertile woman. J. Reprod. Med. *23:* 295–298 (1979).

KOCK, W.: Early history of laparoscopy, thoracoscopy and thoracocautery. Neue Münch. Beitr. Gesch. Med. (Medizinhist.) *7–8:* 517–527 (1978).

LEVINSON, J. M.: The introduction of laparoscopy in the People's Republic of China. Delaware med. J. *52:* 147–151 (1980).

SEMM, K.: Change in the classic gynecologic surgery. Int. J. Fertil. *24:* 13–20 (1979).

SEMM, K.: Schlußwort zur Stellungnahme von Herrn Frangenheim. Geburtsh. u. Frauenheilk. *40:* 167–169 (1980).

SOWA, J.: History of laparoscopic examination. Wiad. Lek. *28:* 343–344 (19975).

WHEELESS, C. R. jr.: Laparoscopy. Clin. Obstet. Gynec. *19:* 277–278 (19976).

II. Instruments for Pelviscopy

AORN J.: Guidelines for preparation of laparoscopic instrumentation. AORN J. *32:* 65–66, passim. (1980).

ATANOV, I. P. et al.: Manipulator for laparoscopy. Vestn. Khir. *125:* 141–142 (1980).

BENVENISTE, D. et al.: An uterus introductor for gynecologic laparoscopy. Fertil. and Steril. *28:* 594–595 (1977).

BROOKS, P. G.: Magnification systems alternative to the operating microscope. J. Reprod. Med. *24:* 265–268 (1980).

CORSON, S. L.: The new laparoscopic instruments: bipolar sterilizing forceps and uterine manipulator. Am. J. Obstet. Gynec. *124:* 434–436 (1976).

CORSON, S. L.: Two new laparoscopic instruments: bipolar sterilizing forceps and uterine manipulator. Med. Lastr. *11:* 7–8 (1977).

CORSON, S. L. et al.: Sterilization of laparoscopes. Is soaking sufficient? J. Reprod. Med. *23:* 49–56 (1979).

DINGFELDER, J. R. et al.: The needlescope and other small diameter laparoscope for sterilization and diagnostic procedures. Int. J. Gynaec. Obstet. *14:* 53–58 (1976).

DINGFELDER, J. R.: Direct laparoscope trocar insertion without prior pneumoperitoneum. J. Reprod. Med. *21:* 45–47 (1978).

Editorial – The laparoscope: useful tool or dangerous weapon? Brit. med. J. *6128:* 1650–1651 (1978).

ERB, R. A., T. P. REED: 3rd. hysteroscopic oviductal blocking with formed-in-place silicone rubber plugs. 1. Method and apparatus. J. Reprod. Med. *23:* 65–68 (1979).

GOLDSTEIN, A. L. et al.: Experience with the use of the Carboflator for establishing pneumoperitoneum. J. Reprod. Med. *16:* 126–128 (1975).

DE GRANDI, P.: A new uterine manipulator for gynecologic laparoscopy. Int. J. Gynaec. Obstet. *18:* 248–250 (1980).

HASSON, H. M.: Effective uterine fundal elevation in laparoscopy. J. Reprod. Med. *15:* 76 (1975).

HASSON, H. M.: Malpronged laparoscopic forceps. J. Reprod. Med. *16:* 167–170 (1976).

HASSON, H. M.: Safeguards in operative laparoscopy. J. Reprod. Med. *15:* 82–83 (1975).

HASSON, H. M.: Fail-safe laparoscope cannula: Ob-Gyn. Observer *15* No. 5 (1976).

HAYS, C.V.: Making laparoscopy electrically safer. An engineer's approach. J. Reprod. Med. *23:* 91–93 (1979).

HULKA, F. et al.: A discussion: laparoscopic instrument sterilization. Med. Instrum. *11:* 122–123 (1977).

JAKUBOWSKI, A.: Permanent intraperitoneal defogging of the optics during laparoscopy (letter). Obstet. and Gynec. *49:* 128 (1977).

KLEPPINGER, R. K.: Ancillary uses of bipolar forceps. J. Reprod. Med. *18:* 254–256 (1977).

KOENIG, U. D.: A mobile laparoscopy unit. J. Reprod. Med. *17:* 253–254 (1976).

LAMMES, F. B.: The hysterophore: a new instrument for uterine manipulation during laparoscopy. Eur. J. Obstet. Gynaec. Reprod. Biol. *12:* 243–246 (1981).

LANYI, E. et al.: Manufacture of a single toothed forceps for the elevation of the uterus (like a tenaculum) during laparoscopy. Cesk. Gynek. *43:* 285 (1978).

LOFFER, F. D.: Disinfection vs. sterilization of gynecologic laparoscopy equipment. The experience of the Phoenix surgic-center. J. Reprod. Med. *25:* 263–266 (1980).

MANN, W. J. et al.: Uterine suspension through the laparoscope. Obstet. and Gynec. *51:* 563–566 (1978).

MARKOV, M.: Laparoscopy equipment. Khirurgia (Sofia) *31:* 257–258 (1978).

MARLOW, J.: History of laparoscopy, optics, fiberoptics, and instrumentation. J. clin. Obstet. Gynec. *19:* 261–275 (1976).

MASTROIANNI, L., jr: When is the operating microscope necessary? Int . J. Fertil. *23:* 255–256 (1978).

MENGHINI, G., G. P. MISCUSI: Increased safety and diagnostic availability of laparoscopy with a new trocar. Acta endoscop. *12:* 85–89 (1982).

MILLS, B.: Operating microscopes (Carl Zeiss, Inc., New York, N. Y.). Personal communication, May 15, 1980.

MOORE, D. T.: Laparoscopy: the »eyes« of gynecology. J. nat. med. Assoc. *67:* 45–48 (1975).

PALMER, A. S.: A new uterine mobilizer for laparoscopy. JAMA *78:* 524–525 (1979).

PALMER, J. R.: Laparoscopic instruments have end piece problem (letter) J. med. J. Aust. *21:* 320 (1981).

PHILLIPS, J. M.: Gynecologic endoscopy. Med. Instrum. *11:* 6 (1977).

PILKA, L. et al.: Oocytes obtained by an aspiratory apparatus during laparoscopy. Cesk. Gynek. *44:* 723–726 (1979).

SCHULTZ, J. K.: AORN endorses cleaning, disinfection of laparoscopes. AORN J. *32:* 1028–1030 (1980).

SEMM, K.: Suction pulp – a new aid for pelviscopy. Endoscopy *7:* 85–88 (1975).

SEMM, K.: Endocoagulation: a new and completely safe medical current for sterilization. Int. J. Fertil. *22:* 238–242 (1977).

SEMM, K.: Tissue-puncher and loop-ligation – new aids for surgical therapeutic pelviscopy (laparoscopy) = endoscopic intraabdominal surgery. Endoscopy *10:* 119–124 (1978).

SEMM, K.: New methods of pelviscopy (gynecologic laparoscopy) for myomectomy, ovariectomy, tubectomy and adnexectomy. Endoscopy *11:* 85–93 (1979).

SEMM, K.: Die endoskopische intraabdominelle Naht. Geburtsh. u. Frauenheilk. *42:* 56–57 (1982).

SEMM, K.: Diagnostic tools: instruments and techniques for endoscopic ovarian surgery. In: G. B. SERRA: The Ovary, S. 159–175. Raven Press, New York 1983.

SEMM, K., L. METTLER: Technical progress in pelvic surgery via operative laparoscopy. Am. J. Obstet. Gynec. *138:* 121–127 (1980).

SILBERTRUST, N.: Care and maintenance of rigid endoscopes. Karl Storz Endoscopy-America, Inc. General Manager. 1976.

SMITH, D. B. et al.: The laparoscope in gynecologic diagnosis and evaluation. J. Arkansas med. Soc. *73:* 235–239 (1976).

SOGBANMU, M. O.: Laparoscope. A useful diagnostic instrument in gynaecological oncology and gynaeco-andrology. Niger med. J. *9:* 555–556 (1979).

TAYLOR, H. W.: A comparative evaluation of the 5 mm laparoscope in gynecological endoscopy. J. Reprod. Med. *15:* 65–68 (1975).

TITTELT, J. F.: Le système 110 mm oldelft, standardisation de l'enregistrement diagnostic sur film simple 110 mm. Acta endoscop. *IX:* 49–51 (1979).

VALTCHEV, K. L. et al.: A new uterine mobilizer for laparoscopy; its use in 513 patients. Am. J. Obstet. Gynec. *127:* 738–740 (1977).

WHEELES, C. R.: An inexpensive laparoscopy system for female sterilization. J. Obstet. Gynec. *123:* 727–733 (1975).

WILLIAMS, P. F.: Review of laparoscopic instrumentation. In: J. J. SCIARRA et al.: Advances in Female Sterilization Techniques. S. 12–23. Hagerstown Med., Harper and Row, Hagerstown, Maryland 1976.

WINSTON, R. M. L.: Evaluating instrumentation for gynecologic microsurgery. Contemp. Ob/Gyn *15:* 153–164 (1980).

III. Pelviscopy/Statistics/Methods

ATANOV, I. P.: Laparoscopy in the emergency surgery of abdominal organs. Vestn. Khir. *126:* 9–14 (1981).

BADELL URDANETA, A.: Abdominal laparoscopy, experience in 1400 cases studied. Gen. *30:* 243–250 (1976).

BAILER, P., R. RAUSKOLB: Gynäkologische Laparoskopie. Geburtsh. u. Frauenheilk. *35:* 747–753 (1975).

BLAIR, R. A. et al.: Gynecological laparoscopy in a large private practice. J. Ky. Med. Assoc. *74:* 503–506 (1976).

BRUN, G. et al.: The evolution of the indications for laparoscopy between 1973 and 1977. 1758 cases. J. Gynec. Obstet. Biol. Reprod. (Paris) *8:* 299–306 (1979).

BURMUCIC, R., R. KÖMETTER: Die Laparoskopie bei der adipösen Frau. Geburtsh. u. Frauenheilk. *40:* 1006–1008 (1980).

BUYTAERT, P. et al.: Gynecological laparoscopy: a harmless intervention: Ned. Tijdschr. Geneeskd. *121:* 397–401 (1977).

CASTRO-MARIN, A. et al.: Pelvic laparoscopy at the Mount Sinai Hospital: A report of 384 consecutive cases at the Mount Sinai Medical Center, 1973–1974. Mt. Sinai J. Med. Ny. *43:* 143–146 (1976).

CAROL, W., W. BÖHM: Zur Stellung und Bedeutung der gynäkologischen Laparoskopie. Zbl. Gynäk. *97:* 494–502 (1975).

CHAMBERLAIN, G.: Confidential inquiry into gynaecological laparoscopy (letter). Brit. med. J. *2:* 563 (1978).

CIBILS, L. A.: Laparoscopy in gynecology. Ginec. Obstet. Mex. *37:* 337–350 (1975).

McCORRISTON, C. C.: Positioning the patient to make laparoscopy easier. Trans. Pac. Coast Obstet. Gynaec. *844:* 69 (1975).

Editorial – Safety to laparoscopy. Lancet *I (8068):* 807 (1978).

FAIRBANKS, W. L. et al.: Laparoscopy in family practice. Nebr. Med. J. *60:* 11–12 (1975).

FRANGENHEIM, H.: Zum Stellenwert der Laparoskopie in der heutigen Gynäkologie. Arch. Gynäk. *232:* 51–52 (1981).

FRIMBERGER, E.: Laparoscopy – neue Möglichkeiten und Perspektiven. Münch. med. Wschr. *121:* 29–30 (1979).

GARCEA, N. et al.: Timing of ovulation by laparoscopy and evaluation of some physico-chemical parameters. Acta eur. fertil. *7:* 63–73 (1976).

GHOSH, J. K.: Laparoscopies with the help of culdoscope. J. Ind. Med. Assoc. *65:* 93–94 (1975).

GLINTER, K. P. et al.: Gynecologic endoscopy: Laparoscopy or culdoscopy? J. Am. Osteopath. Assoc. *73:* 986–994 (1974).

GRIMES, E. M.: Open laparoscopy with conventional instrumentation. Obstet. Gynec. *57:* 375–378 (1981).

HARRISON, G. G.: Death attributable to anaesthesia: a 10-year survey: 1967–1976. Brit. J. Anaesth. *50:* 1041–1046 (1978).

HAVLICEK, S., R. POLJANSEK: Die sogenannte »Second-Look« Laparoskopie. Geburtsh. u. Frauenheilk. *39:* 309–310 (1979).

HEPP, F. H., W. GOLDHOFER, G. REISACH: Gynäkologische Laparoskopie von 1952–1975 – eine kritische Analyse. Arch. Gynäk. *224:* 275–276 (1977).

HILFRICH, H.-J.: Gedanken zur Stellung der Laparoskopie in der Gynäkologie. Geburtsh. u. Frauenheilk. *38:* 594–597 (1978).

HILFRICH, H.-J.: Der Wert der Laparoskopie in der Gynäkologie. Fortschr. Med. *97:* 2143–2148 (1979).

HOLT, E. M.: Laparoscopy in gynaecology. Brit. J. Hosp. Med. *18:* 150–152 (1977).

HORWITZ, S. T.: Laparoscopy in gynecology. Obstet. Gynec. Surv. *27:* 1–13 (1978).

HULKA, J. F.: Laparoscopy (letter). Obstet. Gynec. *51:* 514 (1978).

IMPERIAL-HIZON, A. et al.: The impact of laparoscopy in the community hospital. Ill. Med. J. *147:* 47–49 (1975).

JOHNSON, C. E.: Laparoscopy (700 cases). Clin. Obstet. Gynec. *19:* 707–719 (1976).

JORDAN, J. A.: The role of laparoscopy. Clin. Obstet. Gynaec. *1:* 395–407 (1974).

KLEISSL, H. P., F. CHRIST, F. EBERLEIN: Bericht über 700 Laparoskopien in der gynäkologischen Diagnostik. 1975.

KLEPPINGER, R. K.: Laparoscopy at a community hospital: an analysis of 4300 cases. J. Reprod. Med. *19:* 353–363 (1977).

KOENIG, U. D.: Technik der offenen Pelviskopie – eine neue Methode für bessere Sicherheit in der Laparoskopie. Fortschr. Med. *97:* 1850–1853 (1979).

LACEY, C. G.: Laparoscopy. A clinical sign for intraperitoneal needle placement. Obstet. Gynec. *47:* 625–627 (1976).

LETCHWORTH, A. T. et al.: Obstet. Gynec. *56:* 119–121 (1980).

LIMB, D. G. et al.: The use of laparoscopy in gynaecological practice. Practitioner *219:* 719–722 (1977).

LOFFER, F. D. et al.: Hospitalization for laparoscopy. The exception rather than the rule. Obstet. Gynec. *49:* 625–627 (1977).

LÜRMANN, K.: Beitrag zur Stellung der Laparoskopie im Untersuchungsrepertoire kleiner und mittlerer gynäkologischer Abteilungen. Zbl. Gynäk. *99:* 85–90 (1977).

MANDUJANO, L. et al.: Laparoscopy as a coadjuvant method in gynecological clinical diagnosis. Rev. Chil. Obstet. Ginec. *43:* 121–123 (1978).

MANLEY, J. W.: Laparoscopy technique (letter). Obstet. Gynec. *45:* 236 (1975).

MILLAR, D. R.: The use of laparoscopy in gynecology. Clin. Obstet. Gynaec. *5:* 571–590 (1978).

MINTZ, M.: Risks and prophylaxis in laparoscopy: a survey of 100,000 cases. J. Reprod. Med. *18:* 269–272 (1977).

MIRKOV, K.: Our experience with the laparoscopic examination of gynecologic patients. Akush. Ginekol. (Sofia) *14:* 298–306 (1975).

PENT, D. et al.: Laparoscopy as an ambulatory procedure. Clin. Obstet. Gynec. *17:* 231–247 (1974).

PHILLIPS, J. et al.: Survey of gynecologic laparoscopy for 1974. J. Reprod. Med. *15:* 45–50 (1975).

PHILLIPS, J. et al.: Laparoscopic procedures: a national survey for 1975. J. Reprod. Med. *18:* 219–226 (1977).

PHILLIPS, J. M. et al.: Gynecologic laparoscopy in 1975. J. Reprod. Med. *16:* 105–117 (1976).

PHILLIPS, J. M.: The impact of laparoscopy, hysteroscopy, fetoscopy and culdoscopy on gynecologic practice. J. Reprod. Med. *16:* 187–190 (1976).

PIÉRON, R. et al.: Laparoscopy in black African immigrants. Apropos of 60 cases. Sem. Hop. Paris *55:* 130–136 (1979).

The Report of the Working Party of the Confidential Enquiry into Gynaecological Laparoscopy. Brit. J. Obstet. Gynaec. *85:* 401–403 (1978).

RODRIGUEZ, N. et al.: Laparoscopy. Rev. Chil. Obstet. Ginec. *43:* 145–149 (1978).

RUIZ-VELASCO, V. et al.: Laparoscopy in infertility evaluation: findings and clinical management of two groups of patients. Reproduccion *4:* 157–163 (1980).

SANTAMARIA, R. et al.: Laparoscopy in gynecology and obstetrics. Current possibilities. Rev. Clin. Esp. *15:* 333–336 (1980).

SCHWIMMER, W. B.: Laparoscopy in family planning. J. Reprod. Med. *13:* 218–222 (1974).

SCOTT, D. B.: Gynaecological laparoscopy (letter). Brit. med. J. *1:* 1695 (6128) (1978).
SEMCHYSHYN, S. et al.: Laparoscopy: is it replacing clinical acumen? Obstet. Gynec. *48:* 615–618 (1976).
SEMM, K.: Statistical survey of gynecological laparoscopy/pelviscopy in Germany till 1977. Endoscopy *11:* 101–106 (1979).
SEMM, K.: Statistischer Überblick über die Bauchspiegelung in der Frauenheilkunde bis 1977 in der Bundesrepublik Deutschland. Geburtsh. u. Frauenheilk. *39:* 537–544 (1979).
SMITH, D. B. et al.: Laparoscopic uterine suspension. J. Reprod. Med. *18:* 98–102 (1977).
SODERSTROM, R. M.: Unusual uses of laparoscopy. J. Reprod. Med. *15:* 77–78 (1975).
STAMER, S.: Laparoscopy and peritoneoscopy. Ugeskr. Laeger *138:* 914–916 (1976).
STARK, G. et al.: Zehn Jahre Erfahrung mit der Laparoskopie in der Städtischen Frauenklinik Nürnberg. Fortschr. Med *97:* 457–458 (1979).
STEPTOE, P. C.: Research and other horizons in laparoscopy. J. Reprod. Med. *16:* 79–83 (1976).
STEPTOE, P. C.: Retrospective and prospective studies in laparoscopy. Proc. roy. Soc. Med. *69:* 143 (1976).
STRUBEN, F.: Zur Effektivität der gynäkologischen Laparoskopie – ein Erfahrungsbericht. Geburtsh. u. Frauenheilk. *34:* 956–959 (1974).
TAYLOR, P. J. et al.: Laparoscopy. Compr. Ther. *2:* 48–54 (1976).
TAYLOR, P. J.: et al.: Instrumentation for laparoscopic tubal sterilization. Med. Instrum. *11:* 9–12 (1977).
TAYLOR, P. J.: Gynecologic laparoscopy. Obstet. Gynec. Annu. *8:* 333–367 (1979).
TRAMONTANA, S. et al.: The importance of celioscopic examination. Minerva Ginec. *30:* 223–224 (1978).
UHER, J., V. RACLAVSKA: Notes on the technic of laparoscopy in gynecological practice Cesk. Gynekol. *41:* 621–623 (1976).
WEBERG, E.: Culdoscopy – an alternative to gynecological laparoscopy? Ugeskr. Laeger *139:* 1997–2000 (1977).
WILLIAMS, E.: Laparoscopy in Colon, Panama. J. Reprod. Med. *17:* 333–334 (1976).
ZHANG, J. K.: Clinical application of fibroperitoneoscope – a report of 192 cases. Chang Hua Nel Ko Tsa C'nih *20:* 71–74 (1981) (China).

IV. Diagnostic Pelviscopy

AHN, Y. W. et al.: Techniques for laparoscopy on patients with previous abdominal surgery. Int. J. Fertil. *24:* 264–266 (1979).
ANTEBY, S. O. et al.: The value of laparoscopy in acute pelvic pain. Ann. Surg. *181:* 484–486 (1975).
ANDERSON, J. L. et al.: Laparoscopy in the diagnosis of acute lower abdominal pain. Aust. N. Z. J. Surg. *51:* 462–464 (1981).
ANDERSEN, O. J. et al.: Laparoscopy in obesity. Tidsskr. Nor. Laegeforen *101:* 1337 (1981).
ATANOV, I. P.: Laparoscopy in the emergency surgery of abdominal organs. Vestn. Khir. *126:* 9–14 (1981).
ATLAS, M. et al.: Acute adnexitis in pregnancy. Harefuah *90:* 273–276 (1976).
BAILER, P., R. RAUSKOLB: Gynäkologische Laparoskopie. Geburtsh. u. Frauenheilk. *35:* 747–753 (1975).
BAK, V. et al.: Significance of laparoscopy in the diagnosis of extrauterine pregnancy. Cesk. Gynek. *39:* 106–108 (1974).
BAUERMEISTER, D. E.: Diagnostic laparoscopy from the pathologist's viewpoint. J. Reprod. Med. *18:* 273–274 (1977).
BEREK, J. S. et al: Laparoscopy for second-look evaluation in ovarian cancer. Obstet. Gynec. *58:* 192–198 (1981).
BERKOWITZ, R. S. et al.: Laparoscopy in the management of gestational trophoblastic neoplasms. J. Reprod. Med. *24:* 261–264 (1980).
BLUM, F. et al.: Severe acute genital infections (based on 100 cases). A clinical study and the contribution of laparoscopy. J. Gynec. Obstet. Biol. Reprod. (Paris) *8:* 771–721 (1979).
BOGINSKAIA, I. N. et al.: Importance of laparoscopy in the diagnosis of gynecologic diseases. Akush. Ginek. (Moskau) *2:* 23–24 (1979).
BOGINSKAIA, L. N. et al.: Comparative evaluation of the use of endoscopic and X-ray contrast study methods in diagnosing tubular sterility. Akush. Ginek. (Moskau) *5:* 12–14 (1981).
BRAILSKI, K.: Laparoscopy in the diagnosis of diseases of the internal female genitalia. Vutr. Boles *17:* 29–35 (1978).
BRACKEBUSCH, H.-D., K. SEMM: Die biophysikalischen Prinzipien bei der diagnostischen und therapeutischen Anwendung des elektrischen Stromes in der Endoskopie. Acta endosc. radiocinematograph. *VI:* 41–54 (1976).
BRATASH, B. M.: Laparocentesis and laparoscopy in closed abdominal trauma. Khirurgiia (Moskau) *4:* 14–17 (1977).
BUCHHOLZ, F., E. PHILLIPP, K. SEMM: Die pelviskopische Diagnostik und Therapie der Endometriosis genitalis externa. Schleswig-Holst. Ärztebl. *30:* 597–598 (1977).
BURMUCIC, R.: Hauptindikationen und Ergebnisse der diagnostischen Laproskopie an der Geburtshilflich-Gynäkologischen Universitätsklinik Graz. Wien. med. Wschr. *127:* 532–534 (1977).
CHAPARRO, M. V. et al.: Laparoscopy for the confirmation and prognostic evaluation of pelvic inflammatory disease. Int. J. Gynaec. Obstet. *15:* 307–309 (1978).
CHELLI, M. et al.: Celioscopies performed at the maternity unit of the Charles Nicoile Hospital from 1968 to 1978. Tunis Med. *59:* 193–199 (1981).
COOK, W. A.: Needle laparoscopy in patients with suspected bowel adhesions. Obstet. Gynec. *49:* 105–106 (1978).
CRAFT, I. et al.: Laparoscopy, clip occlusion, and uterine cancer. Lancet *2 (8094):* 835 (1978).
CUMMING, D. C. et al.: Combined laparoscopy and hysteroscopy in the investigation of the ovulatory infertile female. Fertil. Steril. *33:* 475–478 (1980).

DESHMUKH, M. A. et al.: Laparoscopy in primary amenorrhea. J. postgrad. Med. *24:* 106–108 (1978).

DIEHL, J. T. et al.: The role of peritoneoscopy in the diagnosis of acute abdominal conditions. Cleveland Clin. Q. *48:* 225–230 (1981).

DUBUISSON, J. B. et al.: Early control laparoscopy after tubal microsurgery. J. Gynec. Obstet. Biol. Reprod. (Paris) *8:* 655–657 (1979).

DVORAK, K. et al.: Laparoscopy in the diagnostic and control of conservative treatment of anovulatory sterility. Cesk. Gynek. *40:* 189–190 (1975).

EL KATEB, Y. et al.: The role of laparoscopy in evaluation of acute pelvic pain in young women. J. Egypt. Med. Assoc. *61:* 593–596 (1978).

ESCHENBACH, D. A.: Epidemiology and diagnosis of acute pelvic inflammatory disease. Obstet. Gynec. *55:* 142–153 (1980).

ESPOSITO, J. M.: Ectopic pregnancy: the laparoscope as a diagnostic aid. J. Reprod. Med. *25:* 17–24 (1980).

FATHALLA, M. F. et al.: Laparoscopy in gynaecological diagnosis. J. Egypt. Med. Assoc. *56:* 760–767 (1973).

FRIEDMAN, I. H. et al.: The value of laparoscopy in general surgical problems. Surg. Gynec. Obstet. *144:* 906–908 (1977).

FUCHS, E. et al.: The place of emergency laparoscopy in trauma surgery. Unfallheilkunde *81:* 601–603 (1978).

GADŹHIEV, I. S. et al.: Effectiveness of laparoscopy in the diagnosis of diseases of the internal female genitalia. Akush. Ginek. (Moskau) *6:* 57 (1978).

GADŹHIEV, I. S. et al.: Combined laparoscopy in emergency surgery of the abdominal cavity. Khirurgiia (Moskau) *2:* 17–19 (1979).

GARCIA, N. et al.: Timing of ovulation by laparoscopy and evaluation of some physico-chemical parameters. Acta eur. fertil. *7:* 63–73 (1976).

GOLDSTEIN, D. P. et al.: Laparoscopy in the diagnosis and management of pelvic pain in adolescents. J. Reprod. Med. *24:* 251–256 (1980).

GOMEL, V.: Laparoscopy prior to reconstructive tubal surgery for infertility. J. Reprod. Med. *18:* 251–253 (1977).

GOODNOUGH, J. E. et al.: Gonococcal peritonitis following uterine manipulation at laparoscopy. Am. J. Obstet. Gynec. *15:* 218–219 (1981).

GORSHKOV, S. Z. et al.: Role of laparoscopy in the diagnosis of closed injuries in the abdominal organs. Khirurgiia (Moskau) *3:* 47–50 (1976).

HEIN, K. et al.: Laparoscopy for presumed nonacute salpingitis: a new look at an old problem. J. Adolesc. Health Care *1:* 96–100 (1981).

HENRY-SUCHET, et al.: Bacteriological cultures by laparoscopy in salpingitis J. Gynec. Obstet. Biol. Reprod. (Paris) *9:* 341–346 (1980).

HERBSINAN, H. et al.: The value of laparoscopy in general surgery. J. Reprod. Med. *18:* 235–240 (1977).

JATZKO, G. et al.: Indications of laparoscopy in abdominal diseases. Wien. med. Wschr. *130:* 790–792 (1980).

KEITH, L.: Presidentials address. The importance of clinical investigation in laparoscopy. J. Reprod. Med. *24:* 236–238 (1980).

KHAN, P. K.: Laparoscopic observation of the female pelvis following abortions by suction curettage. Int. Surg. *62:* 77–78 (1977).

KOCHNEV, O. S. et al.: Laparoscopy in surgical emergencies. Khirurgiia (Moskau) *8:* 79–83 (1983).

KONDSTAAL, J., A. C. JÖBSIS: Enzyme histochemistry of the human ovary. J. Obstet. Gynec. *4, Suppl:* 51–57 (1974).

KING, I. R., et al.: Diagnosis of unruptured ectopic pregnancy by the use of the laparoscope. J. Tenn. Med. Assoc. *71:* 19–21 (1978).

KOENIG, U. D.: Expansion of the indication range for laparoscopy by the method of open pelviscopy. Arch. Gynäk. *228:* 279–281 (1979).

KOLMORGEN, H., R. HAUSWALD, O. HAVEMANN: Chronische Unterbauchbeschwerden der Frau, eine postlaparoskopische Analyse. Zbl. Gynäk. *98:* 1434–1440 (1976).

KOLMORGEN, K., et al.: Significance of gynecological laparoscopy for the differential diagnosis of doubtful acute and chronic lower abdominal disorders in the women. Z. ärztl. Fortbild *71:* 705–710 (1977).

KOLMORGEN, K., O. HAVEMANN: Zur Diagnostik und Klinik der ektopischen Gravidität beim Einsatz der Laparoskopie. Zbl. Gynäk. *100:* 818–824 (1978).

KOLMORGEN, K., G. SEIDENSCHNUR, G. WERGIEN: Diagnostik und Therapie des akuten Adnexprozesses beim Einsatz der Laparoskopie. Zbl. Gynäk. *100:* 1103–1109 (1978).

KRIEK, V. et al.: Laparoscopy in ascites. Cas Lek. Cesk. *120:* 739–742 (1981).

KUSHCH, N. L. et al.: Use of laparoscopy in primary peritonitis. Klin. Khir. *11:* 52–54 (1975).

LANG, J. H.: The use of laparoscope in gynecological diagnosis. Chung Hua Fu Chan Ko Tsa Chih. *15:* 239–241 (1980).

LEDGER, W. J.: Laparoscopy in the diagnosis and management of patients with suspected salpingo-oophoritis. Am. J. Obstet. Gynec. *38:* 1012–1016 (1980).

LEVINSON, J. M.: The role of laparoscopy in intra-abdominal diagnosis. Del. med. J. *50:* 267–270 (1978).

LIPENSKY, S. et al.: Concerning the use of laparoscopy in differential diagnosis of adnexitis. Bratisl. Lek. Listy *72:* 382–385 (1979).

van Lith, D. A. et al.: Diagnostic miniculdoscopy preceding laparoscopy when bowel adhesions are suspected. J. Reprod. Med. *23:* 87–90 (1979).

Loffer, F. D. et al.: Laparoscopy in the obese patient. J. Obstet. Gynec. 104–107 (1976).

Lürmann, K.: Der spastische Tubenverschluß im laparoskopischen Bild. Zbl. Gynäk. *101:* 1195–1199 (1979).

Lürmann, K.: Das laparoskopische Bild der testikulären Feminisierung. Zbl. Gynäk. *102:* 357–361 (1980).

Madelenat, P., C. Boury-Heyler, J. Dupre-Froment, A. Proust: Quel est l'avenir des ponctions per-coelioscopiques des cystes ovariens? J. Gynéc. Obstét. *7:* 1359–1375 (1978).

Magursky, V. et al.: Use of laparoscopy in the diagnosis of inflammations of the internal genitalia under the conditions of a small department. Cesk. Gynek. *43:* 538 (1978).

Makarenko, T. P. et al.: Laparoscopy in the diagnosis of acute inflammatory diseases and injuries of the abdominal organs. Sov. Med. *8:* 108–112 (1974).

McBride, N. et al.: Diagnostic laparoscopy. Int. J. Gynaec. Obstet. *15:* 556–558 (1978).

McJunkim, M. L. et al.: Radiographic appearance of laparoscopic tubal ring. AJR *132:* 297–298 (1979).

Mettler, L.: Extreme Verläufe in der Routine-Pelviskopie. Fortschr. Med. *96:* 1657–1659 (1978).

Mizzoni, M., M. Faggiono, G. P. Jori, G. Lombardi: Laparoscopy in endocrine genetic disorders of the gonads. A cytogenetic endocrine and endoscopic approach to differential diagnosis: report of cases and atlas. Acta endocr. (Kbh.) *78 Suppl. 192:* 124 (1975).

Mirkov, K. et al.: Diagnosis and treatment of inflammatory adnexal diseases using laparoscopy. Akush. Ginekol. (Sofia) *19:* 500–504 (1980).

Mizzoni, M., M. Faggiono, G. P. Jori, G. Lombardi: Laparoscopy in endocrine genetic disorders of the gonads. A cytogenetic endocrine and endoscopic approach to differential diagnosis: report of cases and atlas. Acta endocr. (Kbh,) *78 Suppl. 192:* 124 (1975).

Moghissi, K. S.: Correlation between hysterosalpingography and pelvic endoscopy for the evaluation of tubal factor. Fertil. Steril. *26:* 1778–1784 (1975).

Morris, J. A. et al.: Sampling the fetoplacental circulation II. Combined laparoscopy-fetoscopy in the pregnant bovine. Am. J. Obstet. Gynec. *128:* 279–286 (1977).

Mühlnickel, D., W. Weise, B. Bernoth: Stein-Leventhal-Syndrom: Erste Differentialdiagnose im laparoskopischen Bild. Zbl. Gynäk. *103:* 569–576 (1981).

Murphy, A. et al.: Diagnostic laparoscopy: role in management of acute pelvic pain. Med. J. Aust. *30:* 571–573 (1981).

O'Herlihy, C. et al.: Preovulatory follicular size: a comparison of ultrasound and laparoscopic measurements. Fertil. Steril. *34:* 24–26 (1980).

Palatynski, A.: Laparoscopy in the diagnosis of genital adenomyosis. Ginek. Pol. *Suppl.:* 136–137 (1979).

Palatynski, A., A. Komorowska: Laparoscopy in the diagnosis of hematoma localized in the upper segment of the vagina. Ginek. Pol. *51:* 335–337 (1980).

Palatynski, A. et al.: Role of laparoscopy in the diagnosis of the early stages of tubal pregnancy. Ginek. Pol. *51:* 999–1002 (1980).

Palme, G.: Prämedikation mit Tramal bei Laparoskopie. Med. Welt *32:* 28–30 (1981).

Panariello, S. et al.: Value of celioscopy in the diagnosis of pelvic pain syndromes. Min. Ginec. *30:* 222 (1978).

Philipp, E., K. Semm: Zur Frage der Grenzen der pelviskopischen Diagnostik des Ovarial-Carcinoms. Schleswig Holst. Ärztebl. (1977).

Pieperkov, T. et al.: Inflammatory changes in the lesser pelvis as a laparoscopic finding. Akush. Ginek. (Sofia) *19:* 504–506 (1980).

Pierowski, Z. et al.: Role of laparoscopy in the diagnosis of causative factors of infertility undetectable by other technics. Ginek. Pol *45:* 1407–1410 (1974).

Piver, M. S. et al.: Second-look laparoscopy prior to proposed second-look laparotomy. Obstet. Gynec. *55:* 571–573 (1980).

Pleissner, I., H. Berndt, H.-J. Gütz: Laparoscopy following operations. Endoscopy *10:* 187–191 (1978).

Polak, M. et al.: Lymphatic cysts in the parietal peritoneum: diagnostic significance of laparoscopy. Ref. Hosp. Clin. Fac. Med. (Sao Paulo) *31:* 345–347 (1976).

Portoundo, J. A., A. Agustin, C. Jerran et al.: Das Corpus luteum infertiler Patientinnen bei pelviskopischer Beobachtung in der Lutealphase. Fertil. Steril. *36:* 37–40 (1981).

Prigg, D. H.: Laparoscopy in early diagnosis of ectopic pregnancy. J. Am. Osteopath. Assoc. *75:* 671–678 (1976).

Ragni, G. et al.: Laparoscopic diagnosis of sterility: evaluation of the results of surgical operations on the pelvis minor. Ann. Ostet. Ginec. Med. Perinat. *101:* 168–172 (1980).

Reichert, J. A., Valle, R. F.: Fitz-Hugh-Curtis syndrome. A laparoscopic approach. JAMA *236:* 266–268 (1976).

Riddick, D. H.: A single disappearing incision for diagnostic laparoscopy. Am. J. Obstet. Gynec. *130:* 109–110 (1978).

Rosenfeld, D. L. et al.: Laparoscopy prior to tubal reanastomosis. J. Reprod. Med. *17:* 247–248 (1976).

Rousselet, J. et al.: Spleen study in laparoscopy. Sem. Hop. Paris *50:* 1961–1966 (1974).

Samsula, M. et al.: Is the diagnosis of adnexitis without laparoscopic verification reliable? Cesk. Gynek. *43:* 374–375 (1978).

Sapunar, J. et al.: Laparoscopic aspects in abdominal hydatid disease. Rev. Med. Chil. *103:* 184–188 (1975).

Savel'eva, G. M. et al.: Importance of laparoscopy in the diagnosis and treatment of acute inflammation of the internal female genitalia. Akush. Ginek. (Moskau) *7:* 28–30 (1979).

Scaling, S. T. et al.: The correlation of pelvic ultrasound and laparoscopy in the diagnosis and management of gynecologic disorders. J. Reprod. Med. *21:* 53–56 (1978).

Scarpa, F. et al.: Critical evaluation of the use of laparoscopy in gynecological diagnosis. Min. Ginec. *30:* 859–864 (1978).

Scarpa, F. et al.: Laparoscopy and ovarian biopsy as ovarian function studies in primary and secondary amenorrhea. Min. Ginec. *30:* 871–880 (1978).

Schmidt, K. et al.: Experience with laparoscopy and its contribution to the diagnosis of extrauterine gravidity. Cesk. Gynec. *39:* 685–686 (1974).

Schmidt, K. et al.: Second-look laparoscopy and adhesiolysis in pretreated gynecologic inflammations. Cesk. Gynec. *43:* 603–605 (1978).

Selezneva, N. D. et al.: Use of laparoscopy and echography in the diagnosis of gynecologic disease. Akush. Ginek. (Moskau) *7:* 44–47 (1981).

Steenblock, U. et al.: Diagnosis of intra-abdominal bleeding, comparison of peritoneal lavage and laparoscopy. Helv. chir. Acta. *46:* 707–710 (1980).

Strizhakov, A. N. et al.: Importance of laparoscopy in the diagnosis of gynecologic diseases. Akush. Ginek. (Moskau) *4:* 44–46 (1981).

Sugarbacker, P. H. et al.: Preoperative laparoscopy in diagnosis of acute abdominal pain. Lancet *II (7904):* 442–445 (1975).

Sweet, R. L. et al.: Use of laparoscopy to determine the microbiologic etiology of acute salpingitis. Am. J. Obstet. Gynec. *134:* 68–74 (1979).

Tan, A. K. et al.: Laparoscopy as a diagnostic aid in women with localized ureteral obstruction due to endometriosis. Urology *16:* 47–50 (1980).

Taylor, P. J. et al.: Temperature gradients at various points within the human pelvis as measured during laparoscopy. J. Reprod. Med. *16:* 163–166 (1976).

Templeton, A. A. et al.: An assessment of laparoscopy as the primary investigation in the subfertile female. Brit. J. Obstet. Gynaec. *84:* 760–762 (1977).

Uher, J. et al.: Laparoscopic diagnosis of gynecologic inflammations Cesk. Gynek. *43:* 536–566 (1978).

Wadhwa, R. K. et al.: Preoperative laparoscopy (Letter). Lancet *I (7912):* 924–925 (1975).

Wildhirt, E.: The diagnostic value of laparoscopy – a prospective study. Tokai J. exp. Clin. Med. *6:* 223–227 (1981).

Wildt, D. E. et al.: Laparoscopic exposure and sequential observation of the ovary of the cycling bitch. Anat. Rec. *189:* 443–449 (1977).

Woodworth, E. S.: Further observation on diagnostic and therapeutic use of laparoscopy. Clin. med. *81:* 13–16 (1974).

Zabarskil, L. T. et al.: Laparoscopy in acute surgical pathology of the abdominal cavity organs. Klin. Khir. *7:* 55–57 (1977).

Zielske, F., V. Jaluvka: Die Bedeutung der gynäkologischen Laparoskopie bei Erkrankungen des Colon sigmoideum im Alter. Fortschr. Med. *96:* 1129–1132 (1978).

Zilberman, M. N. et al.: Therapeutic and diagnostic use of retroperitoneoscopy in kidney and upper urinary tract diseases. Sov. Med. *12:* 113–115 (1978).

V. Sterility

Allocca, G. et al.: Celioscopic examination in the study of female sterility. Min. Ginec. *30:* 227 (1978).

Ariga, S. et al.: Recovery of preimplantation blastocysts in the squirrel monkey by a laparoscopic technique. Fertil. Steril *28:* 577–580 (1977).

Asch, R. H.: Laparoscopic recovery of sperm from peritoneal fluid in patients with negative or poor Sims-Huhner-test. *27:* 1111–1114 (1976).

Audebert, A. J.: The place of laparoscopy in unexplained infertility. Acta europ. fertil *11:* 269–791 (1980).

Baron, J. et al.: Endocrinological laparoscopy in gynecologic disease. Endokrynol. Pol. *26:* 547–557 (1975).

Bellina, J. H.: Infertility diagnosed by laparoscopy: review of 324 cases. South Med. J. *68:* 485–488 (1975).

Berger, M. J. et al.: Laparoscopic recovery of mature human oocytes. Fertil. Steril. *26:* 513–522 (1975).

Bernaschek, G.: Rifamycin chromopertubation unter laparoskopischer Kontrolle. Wien. klin. Wschr. *90:* 658–660 (1978).

Boginskain, L. N. et al.: Comparative evaluation of the use of endoscopic and x-ray contrast study methods in diagnosing tubular sterility. Akush. Ginek. (Moskau) *2:* 12–14 (1981).

Broekhuizen, F. F. et al.: Laparoscopic findings in twenty-five failures of artificial insemination. Fertil. Steril. *34:* 351–355 (1980).

Bruhat, M. A. et al.: The indication for laparoscopy in female infertility. J. Gynec. Obstet. Biol. Reprod. (Paris) *9:* 337–340 (1980).

de Brux, J.: Tentative d'evaluation du potential évolutif des lésions cervicales. Acta endoscop. *XI:* 45–51 (1981).

COHEN, M. R.: Laparoscopic diagnosis and pseudomenopause treatment of endometriosis with danazol. Clin. Obstet. Gynec. *23:* 901–915 (1980).

COLAU, I. C. et al.: Celioscopy in the systematic examination of the sterile couple. Min. Ginec. *31:* 761–771 (1979).

COLE, L. P. et al.: Tubal occlusion via laparoscopy in Latin America: an evaluation of 8186 cases. Int. J. Gynaec. Obstet. *17:* 253–259 (1979).

CORSON, S. L.: The role of laparoscopy in the infertility work-up. J. Reprod. Med. *18:* 127–131 (1977).

CORSON, S. L.: Use of the laparoscope in the infertile patient. Fertil. Steril. *32:* 359–369 (1979).

CROXATTO, H. B., M.-E. ORTIZ, S. DIAZ, R. HESS, J. BALMACEDA, H.-D. CROXATTO: Studies on the duration of egg transport by the human oviduct. 2. Ovum location at various intervals following luteinizing hormone peak. Am. J. Obstet. Gynec. *132:* 629–634 (1978).

CUMMING, D. C. et al.: Combined laparoscopy and hysteroscopy in the investigation of the ovulatory infertile female. Fertil. Steril. *33:* 475–478 (1980).

DMOWSKI, W. P., M. R. COHEN: Treatment of endometriosis with an antigonadotrophin Danazol. A laparoscopic and histologic evaluation. Obstet. Gynec. *46:* 147–154 (1975).

DRAKE, T. S. et al.: The unsuspected pelvic factor in the infertility investigation. Fertil. Steril. *34:* 27–31 (1980).

DRASNAR, J. et al.: Results of microbiological diagnosis in complicated female gonorrhea with tubal sterility using laparoscopy. Cesk. Gynek. *43:* 538–539 (1978).

DUPONT, P. et al.: Laparoscopy in the study of infertility. Union Med. Can. *109:* 599–600 (1980).

DVORÁK, K. et al.: Laparoscopy in the diagnostic and control of conservative treatment of anovulatory sterility. Cesk. Gynek. *40:* 189–190 (1975).

FEICHTINGER, W., S. SZALAY, A. BECK, P. KEMETER, H. JANISCH: Die Gewinnung reifer menschlicher Eizellen mittels Laparoskopie zum Zwecke der In vitro-Fertilisierung. Geburtsh. Frauenheilk. *41:* 400–403 (1981).

FEICHTINGER, W., S. SZALAY, P. KEMETER, A. BECK, H. JANISCH: Zwillingsschwangerschaft nach laparoskopischer Eizellgewinnung, In vitro-Fertilisierung und Embryotransfer. Geburtsh. Frauenheilk. *42:* 197–199 (1982).

FLORSHEIM, Y.: Mikrochirurgische Behandlung der weiblichen Sterilität. Schweiz. med. Rdsch. *69:* 1780–1785 (1980).

GARCEA, N., A. CARUSO, E. MONETA: Timing laparoscopico dell ovulazione in rapporto alla temperatura basale. Min. Ginec. *28:* 133–138 (1976).

GIELWANOWSKI, W.: Laparoscopic examination in female sterility. W. Wiad. Lek. *31:* 1509–1514 (1978).

GILL, B. P. jr.: Investigation of the utero-tubal factor: laparoscopy. Ir. J. med. Sci. *148 Suppl. 1:* 55–57 (1979).

GOLDENBERG, R. L., H. G. MAGENDANTZ: Laparoscopy and the infertility evaluation. Obstet. Gynec. *47:* 410–414 (1976).

HAAKE, K. W.: Die Gewinnung und Klassifizierung menschlicher Eizellen bei gynäkologischen Operationen. Zbl. Gynäk. *103:* 10–18 (1981).

ISRAEL, R., CH. M. MARCH: Diagnostic laparoscopy: a prognostic aid in the surgical management of infertility. Am. J. Obstet. Gynec. *125:* 969–975 (1976).

LAURITSEN, J. G.: Aspiration of human oocytes by laparoscopy and laparotomy. Ugeskr. Laeger *142:* 158–161 (1980).

LERIDON, H. : Permanent sterility. In: LERIDON, H.: Human Fertility: the Basic Components. S. 96–103. Chicago, Illinois University of Chicago 1977.

LÜRMANN, K.: Schwangerschaft bei endoskopisch diagnostizierter, nichtbehandelter tubarer Sterilität. Zbl. Gynäk. *104:* 357–363 (1982).

MADELENAT, P. et al.: Laparoscopic treatment of stenoses and phimosis of the ampulla of the tube. A critical study of the results. J. Gynec. Obstet. Biol. Reprod. (Paris) *8:* 445–450 (1979).

McDOUGALL: Laparoscopy in the investigation of infertility. Ann. Scott. med. J. *20:* 209–216 (1976).

METTLER, L., M. SEKI, V. BAUKLOH, K. SEMM: Human ovum recovery via operative laparoscopy and in vitro fertilization. Fertil. Steril. *38:* 30–37 (1982).

METTLER, L., K, SEMM: Laparoscopic surgery in the treatment of peripheral tubal occlusion and endometriosis in female infertility. Microsurgery in Gynecology *II,* z.Zt. i. Druck.

MINOZZI, M., M. FAGGIANO, G. P. JORI, G. LOMBARDI: Laparoscopy in endocrine and genetic disorders of the gonads: A cytogenetic endocrine and endoscopic approach to differential diagnosis – Report of cases and atlas. Acta endocr. (Kbh.) *(Suppl.) 78:* 1–124 (1975).

MINTZ, H.: La liberation per-coelioscopique d'adherences dans 55 cas de sterilité feminine. Technique, resultats, indications. Gynécol. *26:* 277–284 (1975).

MUDGE, T. J. et al.: Alice through the laparoscope: the place of laparoscopy in an infertility service. Med. J. Aust. *30:* 589–590 (1981).

PEXIEDER, T.: Microscopie électronique á balayage dé l'épithelium de la trompe utérine aprés la chirurgie tubaire restauratrice à chaud. Rev. méd. Suisse rom. *101:* 535–541 (1981).

PSHENICHNIKOVA, T. et al.: Comparative study of uterine tube patency using laparoscopy and hysterosalpingography. Akush. Ginek. (Moskau) *3:* 44–46 (1980).

ROLAND, M. D.: A new classification for surgical procedures for tuboperitoneal abnormalities in infertility. Int. J. Fertil. *27:* 27–28 (1982).

RUIZ-VELASCO, V. et al.: Preparations indications and findings of laparoscopy in sterility in 2 groups of patients. Ginec. Obstet. Mex. *44:* 451–458 (1978).

SCARPA, F. et al.: Diagnostic and therapeutic importance of celioscopic ovarian biopsy in female sterility. Min. Ginec. *30:* 739–748 (1978).

SCHMID, R. et al.: The place of laparoscopy in the investigation of infertility. Wien. klin. Wschr. *90:* 130–133 (1978).

SEMM, K.: Therapie der tubaren Sterilität 1. Indikation und Diagnostik. Gynäkol. Prax. *1:* 437–443 (1977).

SULEWSKI, J. M., F. D. CURCIO, C. BRONITSKY, V. G. STENGER: The treatment of endometriosis at laparoscopy for infertility. Am. J. Obstet. Gynec. *138:* 128–132 (1980).

TAYLOR, P. J.: Correlations in infertility: symptomatology, hysterosalpingography, laparoscopy and hysteroscopy. J. Reprod. Med. *18:* 339–342 (1977).

TRAMONTANA, S. et al.: Laparoscopic and radiological correlations in sterility of tubal origin. Arch. Obstet. Ginec. *83:* 31–36 (1978).

UHER, J. et al.: Pseudoinclusion of the ovary (bursa penovarica) in the laparoscopic picture of sterility. Cesk. Gynek. *45:* 24–26 (1980).

UHER, J. et al.: Adhesions in laparoscopic picture of sterility. Cesk. Gynek. *46:* 443–451 (1981).

URDAPILLETA, J. D. et al.: Laparoscopy in the study of female sterility (500 cases). Ginec. Obstet. Mex. *37:* 185–196.

WINSTON, R. M. L.: Microsurgical restoration of fertility following tubal ligation. (presented at the 4th Intern. Conf. on Voluntary Sterilization, Seoul, Korea, May 1979, S. 12.

VI. Pelviscopy and Carcinoma (Tumor Diagnosis)

BADER, J. P.: Pourquoi individualiser la cancerologie digestive. Acta endoscop. *XI:* 459–461 (1981).

BERNER, J. et al.: Value of simultaneous laparoscopy and needle biopsy for detection of neoplastic metastases in the abdominal cavity. Nowotwory *30:* 255–260 (1980).

BEREK, J. S. et al.: Laparoscopy for second-look evaluation in ovarian cancer. Obstet. Gynec. *58:* 192–198 (1981).

CHERENKOV, B. G.: Laparoscopy in the diagnosis of ovarian tumours. Vopr. Onkol. *26:* 63–67 (1980).

COSSARD, F. et al.: The indications for laparoscopy in malignant tumours of the ovary. J. Gynec. Obstet. Biol. Reprod. (Paris) *8:* 497–504 (1979).

COUPLAND, G. A. et al.: Peritoneoscopy-use in assessment of intra abdominal malignancy. Surgery *89:* 645–649 (1981).

CRAFT, I., et al.: Laparoscopy, clip occlusion and uterine cancer. Lancet *II (8094):* 835 (1978).

DAGNINI, G.: Considérations à propos de la surveillance laparoscopique des localisations abdominales des tumeurs malignes sans traitement. Acta endoscop. *12:* 91–96 (1982).

FRANGENHEIM, H.: Der Einfluß der Laparoskopie auf die Diagnose und Therapie maligner und benigner Tumore im Unterbauch. Arch. Gynäk. *224:* 280–281 (1977).

GIARDINA, G. et al.: Usefulness of a 2nd laparotomy and laparoscopy in the follow-up of patients receiving ovarian tumor therapy. Min. Gynec. *52:* 708–712 (1978).

GITSCH, E., E. KUBISTA: Ergebnisse der operativen Therapie des Ovarialkarzinoms der Jahre 1948–1968. Gynäk. Rundsch. *16:* 35–46 (1976).

LACEY, C. G., C. P. MORRIS, P. J. DISAIA, P. C. LUCAS: Laparoscopy in the evaluation of gynecologic cancer. J. Obstet. Gynec. *52:* 712 (1978).

LEITSMANN, H., K. EBELING: Zur Bedeutung der Laparoskopie für die postoperative Behandlung des Ovarialkarzinoms. Zbl. Gynäk. *101:* 716–721 (1979).

LINHART, P., F. ROCA-MARTINEZ, H. WÄHLENBERG: Die Bedeutung der endoskopischen Untersuchung für die Differentialdiagnose abdomineller Tumoren. Gyn. Prax. *5:* 465 (1981).

MANGIONI, C. et al.: Indications, advantages, and limits of laparoscopy in ovarian cancer. Gynec. Oncol. *7:* 47–55 (1979).

MARTI VICENTE, A. et al.: Laparoscopy and its possibilities in the diagnosis of abdominal cancer. Rev. Esp. Enferm Apar. Dig. *48:* 271–280 (1976).

MEYER-BURG, J., U. ZIEGLER: The intra-abdominal inspection and biopsy of lymph nodes during peritoneoscopy. Endoscopy *10:* 41–43 (1978).

OZOLS R. F., R. R. FISCHER, T. ANDERSON: Peritoneoscopy in the management of ovarian cancer. Am. J. Obstet. Gynec. *140:* 611–619 (1981).

PENT, D.: Small bowel incarceration (Letter). Obstet. Gynec. *45:* 356–357 (1975).

QUINN, M. A. et al.: Laparoscopic follow-up of patients with ovarian carcinoma. Brit. J. Obstet. Gynaec. *87:* 1132–1139 (1980).

REHMANN, J.: Die Laparoskopie in der Krebsdiagnostik. Krebsgeschehen *11:* 169–171 (1979).

SMITH, W. G. et al.: The use of laparoscopy to determine the results of chemotherapy of ovarian cancer. J. Reprod. Med. *18:* 257–260 (1977).

SOTNIKOV, V. N. et al.: Laparoscopic diagnosis of intra-abdominal metastases of extra-abdominal tumors. Vopr. Onkol. *13:* 38–44 (1977).

Spinelli, P. et al.: Laparoscopy in staging and restaging of 95 patients with ovarian carcinoma. Tumor *62:* 493–501 (1976).

Spinelli, P., S. Pilotti, A. Luini, G. B. Spatti, P. Pizzetti, G. de Paol de Palo: Laparoscopy combined with peritoneal cytology in staging and restaging ovarian carcinoma. J. Tumori *65:* 601–610 (1979).

Zoltán, D. et al.: Incidence of metastatic tumor of the abdominal wall after laparoscopy. Orv. Hetil. *118:* 1291–1292 (1977).

Zóltowski, M.: Evaluation of laparoscopy in early detection of ovarian tumors and gonadal dysgenesis. Patol. Pol. *30:* 275–280 (1979).

Zóltowski, M.: Role of laparoscopy in the complex diagnosis of ovarian tumors. Ginek. Pol. *51:* 153–156 (1980).

VII. Hysterosalpingography and Pelviscopy

Boginskaia, L. N. et al.: Comparative evaluation of the use of endoscopic and x-ray contrast study methods in diagnosing tubular sterility. Akush. Ginek. (Moskau) *2:* 12–14 (1981).

Brolin, I et al.: Comparison between hysterosalpingorapic findings and lesions observed by laparoscopy and laparotomy. ROFO *133:* 510–513 (1980).

Davidson, S. et al.: Hysterosalpingographic control of patients sterilized by laparoscopy. Ugeskr. Laeger *11:* 434–435 (1980).

Delgado Urdapilleta, J. et al.: Correlation of hysterosalpingographic and laparoscopic findings with respect to tubal patency. Ginec. Obstet. Mex. 48: 77–85 (1980).

El-Minawi, M. F. et al.: Comparative evaluation of laparoscopy and hysterosalpingraphy in infertile patients. Obstet. Gynec. *51:* 29–32 (1978).

Gabos, P.: A comparison of hysterosalpingography and endoscopy in evaluation of tubal function in infertile women. Fertil. Steril. *27:* 238–242 (1976).

Hutchins, C. J.: Laparoscopy and hysterosalpingography in the assessment of tubal patency. Obstet. Gynec. *49:* 325–327 (1977).

Idris, W. et al.: A comparative study of hysterosalpingography and laparoscopy in the investigation of infertility. Int. J. Gynaec. Obstet. *14:* 428–430 (1976).

Korzon, T. et al.: Diagnostic conclusions arrived at on the basis of hysterosalpingography and laparoscopy in sterile women. Ginek. Pol *45:* 1181–1184 (1974).

Lapido, O. A.: Tests of tubal patency: comparison of laparoscopy and hysterosalpingography. Brit. med. J. *2* (6047): 1287–1298 (1976).

Leeton, J. et al.: The tortuous tube: pregnancy rate following laparoscopy and hydrotubation. Aust. NZ J. Obstet. Gynaec. *18:* 259–262 (1978).

Omsjö, I. et al.: Hysterosalpingography and laparoscopy in the study of female sterility. Tidsskr. Nor. Laegeforen *98:* 735–737 (1978).

Oroján, J., Gy. Godó J. Ökrös: Laparoskopie und Hysterosalpingographie in der Untersuchung der Sterilität. Zbl. Gynäk. *102:* 53–58 (1980).

Philipsen, T. et al.: Comparative study of hysterosalpingography and laparoscopy in infertile patients. Acta obstet. gynec. scand. *60:* 149–151 (1981).

Sheikh, H. H.: Hysterosalpingographic follow-up of laparoscopic sterilization. Am. J. Obstet. Gynec. *126:* 181–185 (1976).

Servy, E. J. et al.: Tubal patency: hysterosalpingography compared laparoscopy. South. med. J. *71:* 1511–1512 (1978).

Tramontana, S. et al.: Correlations between laparoscopic and radiological findings in sterility of tubal origin. Min. Ginec. *30:* 225–226 (1978).

VIII. Pelviscopy and Tuberculosis

Geake, T. M. et al.: Peritoneoscopy in the diagnosis of tuberculous peritonitis. Gastrointest. Endosc. *27:* 66–68 (1981).

Harris, W. H.: Diagnosis of pelvic tuberculosis at laparoscopy. Can. med. Assoc. J. *111:* 393 (1974).

Lewis, A.: Tuberculous peritonitis and laparoscopy. Lancet *I (8125):* 1084 (1979).

Mendis, K. L. et al.: Laparoscopy in diagnosis of pelvic tuberculosis. Lancet *I (8128):* 1240 (1979).

Sutherland, A. M.: Laparoscopy in diagnosis of pelvic tuberculosis. Lancet *II (8133):* 95 (1979).

Wolfe, J. H. et al.: Tuberculous peritonitis and role of diagnostic laparoscopy. Lancet *I (8121):* 852–853 (1979).

Yamada, S. et al.: Four cases of tuberculous peritonitis diagnosed by laparoscopy. Kekkaku *52:* 223–228 (1977).

IX. Anesthesia and CO₂-Gas Metabolism

Aldrete, J. A. et al.: Analgesia for laparoscopic sterilization. Anesth. Analg. (Clevel.) *55:* 177–181 (1976).

Bridenbaugh, I. D. et al.: Lumbar epidural block anesthesia for outpatient laparoscopy. J. Reprod. Med. *23:* 85–86 (1979).

BROWN, D. R. et al.: Ventilatory and blood gas changes during laparoscopy with local anesthesia. Am. J. Obstet. Gynec. *124:* 741–745 (1976).

CHLUMSKÝ J. et al.: Cardiovascular system reaction in laparoscopy. Cas. Lek. Cesk. *116:* 785–788 (1977).

DAVIDSON, E. C. jr. et al.: Sampling the fetoplacental circulation III. Combined laparoscopy-fetoscopy in the pregnant macaque for hemoglobin identification. Am. J. Obstet. Gynec. *132:* 833–844 (1978).

DOCTOR, N. H., Z. HUSSAIN: Bilateral pneumothorax associated with laparoscopy. Anaesthesia *28:* 75–81 (1973).

DODSON, M. E.: Laparoscopy and suxamethonium muscle pain (letter). Brit. J. Anesth. *50:* 84 (1978).

DRUMMOND, G. B. et al.: Pressure-volume relationships in the lung during laparoscopy. Brit. J. Anaesth. *50:* 261–270 (1978).

DUFFY, B. L.: Regurgitation during pelvic laparoscopy. Brit. J. Anaesth. *51:* 1089–1090 (1979).

DUFFY, B. L.: Regurgitation during laparoscopy (letter). Brit. J. Anaesth. *52:* 960–961 (1980).

ELLUL, J. M. et al.: Paralysis of the circumflex nerve following general anesthesia for laparoscopy. Anesthesiology *41:* 520–521 (1974).

EL MINAWI, M. F. et al.: Physiologic changes during CO_2, and N_2O pneumoperitoneum in diagnostic laparoscopy. A comparative study. J. Reprod. Med. *26:* 338–346 (1981).

FERNÁNDEZ-LÓPEZ DE HIERRO, M. D. et al.: Changes in the concentration of CO_2, O_2, pH, bicarbonaic and excess base in patients subjected to gynecologic laparoscopic examination under general anesthesia. Rev. Esp. Anestesiol. Reanim. *28:* 15–20 (1981).

FIGALLO, E. M. et al.: Ketamine as the sole anaesthetic agent for laparoscopic sterilization. The effects of premedication on the frequency of adverse clinical reactions. Brit. J. Anaesth. *49:* 1159–1165 (1977).

FISHBURNE, J. L. jr.: Office laparoscopic sterilization with local anesthesia. J. Reprod. Med. *18:* 233–234 (1977).

FISHBURNE, J. L.: Anesthesia for laparoscopy: considerations, complications and techniques. J. Reprod. Med. *21:* 37–40 (1978).

GAGNON, D. et al.: Laparoscopy: anesthesia and central venous pressure. Union Med. Can. *103:* 1608–1610 (1974).

GARCEA, N. et al.: Laparoscopy. Evaluation of its diagnostic possibilities and anesthesiological problems. Min. Ginec. *28:* 124–132 (1976).

GEBBIE, D.: Anaesthesia and death. Can. Anaesth Soc. J. *13:* 390–396 (1966).

GOMEL, V.: Laparoscopy in general surgery. Am. J. Surg. *131:* 319–323 (1976).

GORDH, T., J. W. MOSTERT: Anesthetic accidents: cases studies. Intern. Anesth. Clin. *16:* 1–193 (1978).

KEATS, A. S.: What do we know about anesthetic mortality? J. Anesth. *50:* 387–392 (1979).

KLEINDIENST, W. et al.: Ketamine – HCI-diazepam anesthesia for laparoscopy. J. Reprod. Med. *23:* 299–303 (1979).

LEE, C. M.: Acute hypotension during laparoscopy: a case report. Anesth. Analg. (Clevel.) *54:* 142–143 (1975).

LENZ, R. J., T. A. THOMAS, G. W. WILKINS: Cardiovascular changes during laparoscopy; studies of stroke volume and cardiac output using impedance cardiography. Anesth. *31:* 4–12 (1976).

LEWIS, G. B. et al.: Sodium bicarbonate treatment of ventricular arrhythmias during laparoscopy (letter). Anesthesia *41:* 416 (1974).

MAGNO, R. et al.: Acid-base balance during laparoscopy. The effects of intraperitoneal insufflation of carbon dioxide and nitrous oxide on acid base balance during controlled ventilation. Acta obstet. gynec. scand. *58:* 81–85 (1979).

McKENZIE, R. et al.: Noninvasive measurement of cardiac output during laparoscopy. J. Reprod. Med. *24:* 247–250 (1980).

MEYER-BURG, V. J. et al.: Prämedikation mit Valoron (Tilidin) während der Laparoskopie. Fortschr. Med. *94:* 91–94 (1976).

PAPATHEODOSSIU, N.: Gynecological laparoscopy under general anesthesia. Rev. Med. Suisse rom. *99:* 389–391 (1979).

PIECHOWIAK, Z. et al.: Evaluation of extrameningeal anesthesia in laparoscopy. Ginek. Pol. *46:* 1191–1193 (1976).

ROBINSON, H. B. et al.: Applications for laparoscopy in general surgery. Surg. Gynec. Obstet. *143:* 829–834 (1976).

SCOTT, D. B.: Regurgitation during laparoscopy. Brit. J. Anaesth. *52:* 599 (1980).

SIMPSON, J. M.: Suxamethonium pains following laparoscopy (letter). Anaesthesia *31:* 956–957 (1976).

SMITH, I. et al.: Proceedings: Central venous pressure charges during laparoscopy. Anaesthesia *30:* 117 (1975).

SUPPAN, P.: Besonderheiten der Anaesthesie in Gynäkologie und Geburtshilfe. Therap. Umschau *38:* 531–541 (1981).

TAY, H. S. et al.: Acid aspiration during laparoscopy. Anaesth. Intens. Care *6:* 134–137 (1978).

TOURUNEN, E.: et al.: Haemodynamic effects produced by insufflation of carbon dioxide into the abdominal cavity during laparoscopy. Ann. Chir. Gynaec. *65:* 385–387 (1976).

VOIGT, E.: Necessity to control endexpiratory CO_2-concentration during laparoscopic sterilisation under general anaesthesia with controlled ventilation. Anästhesist *27:* 219–222 (1978).

WHEELER, A. S. et al.: Local anesthesia for laparoscopy in a case of myotonia dystrophica (letter). Anesthesiology *50:* 169 (1979).

ZEVALLOS, H. et al.: Outpatient laparoscopy with local anesthesia. Int. J. Gynaec. Obstet. *17:* 379–381 (1980).

ZIVNY, J. et al.: Laparoscopy: anesthesia and its complications. Cesk. Gynek. *44:* 368–373 (1979).

X. Pneumoperitoneum (Without Complications)

ANSARI, A. H.: Vaginal induction of pneumoperitoneum for laparoscopy. Obstet. Gynec. *48:* 251–252 (1976).

BUECHNER, H. A.: Pneumopericardium following laparoscopy. Chest *77:* 811–812 (1980).

CORSON, S. E.: Routine pneumoperitoneum. Obstet. Gynec. *47:* 638 (1976).

HASSON, H. M.: Safe Pneumoperitoneum in Laparoscopy: Principles and Techniques, S. 265–267. Hrsg.: PHILLIPS, J. M., L. KEITH: Ed. Stratton Intercont. Med. Book Corp., New York 1974.

LEMAY, M. et al.: Post-laparoscopy pneumoperitoneum. Clin. Invest. Med. *1:* 211–212 (1978).

MORGAN, H. R.: Laparoscopy: induction of pneumoperitoneum via transfundal puncture. Obstet. Gynec. *54:* 260–261 (1979).

NEELY, M. R. et al.: Laparoscopy: routine pneumoperitoneum via the posterior fornix. Obstet. Gynec. *45:* 459–460 (1975).

NICHOLSON, R. D. et al.: Pneumopericardium following laparoscopy. Chest *76:* 605–607 (1979).

SANDERS, R. R. et al.: Transfundal induction of pneumoperitoneum prior to laparoscopy. J. Obstet. Gynaec. Brit. Cwlth. *81:* 829–830 (1974).

SEMM, K.: Die Automatisierung des Pneumoperitoneums für die endoskopische Abdominalchirurgie. Arch. Gynäk. *232:* 738–739 (1980).

XI. Operative Pelviscopy

ALFONSIN, A., A. ARRIGHI, E. RETAMOSA: A propos de la biopsie d'ovaire per ceolioscopqique. Gynécologie *XXVI:* 121–127 (1975).

AMMAN, J. et al.: The precision of laparoscopy in blunt abdominal injuries. Helv. chir. Acta *44:* 89–91 (1977).

ANSELMO, J.: Curigia reconstructora tubaria postesterilizacion quirurgica. Rev. Chil. Obstet. Ginec. *42:* 256–260 (1977).

ANSARI, A. H.: Tubal reanastomosis using absorbable stent. Int. J. Fertil *23:* 242–243 (1978).

ANSARI, A. H.: End-to-end tubal anastomosis using absorbable stent. Fertil. Steril *32:* 197–201 (1979).

ARNDT, H. J. et al.: Abdominal pain caused by adhesions and their removal at laparoscopy. Dtsch. med. Wschr. *101:* 395–398 (1976).

BALFOUR, T. W. et al.: The use of laparoscopy in surgical diagnosis. Practitioner *217:* 539–541 (1976).

BARNETT, R. M. et al.: Laparoscopic removal of a foreign body from the bladder. Amer. J. Obstet. Gynec. *130:* 364–365 (1978).

BATTIG, C. G.: Electrosurgical burn injuries and their prevention. J. Am. med. Assoc. *204:* 1045–1046 (1976).

BATTY, L. H. et al.: Laparoscopic repair of the prolapsed fallopian tube. J. Reprod. Med. *24:* 244–246 (1980).

BENVENISTE, D. et al.: A uterus mobilizing device for gynecologic laparoscopy. Ugeskr. Laeger *14:* 471 (1978).

BEREZOV, I. et al.: Laparoscopy in the diagnosis and treatment of acute surgical diseases of the abdominal organs. Klin. Khir. *9:* 18–23 (1976).

BLANDAU, R. J.: Comparative aspects of tubal anatomy and physiology as they relate to reconstructive procedures. J. Reprod. Med. *21:* 7–15 (1978).

BOECKX, D., G. VASQUEZ, J. A. BROSENS: Reversibility of tubal ring sterilization. Contraception. *15:* 505–512 (1977).

BRUHAT, M. A. et al.: Trial treatment of extra-uterine pregnancy during celioscopy (letter). Nouv. Presse méd. *6:* 2606 (1977).

BRUHAT, M. A. et al.: Treatment of ectopic pregnancy by means of laparoscopy. Fertil. Steril. *33* (1980), 411–414.

BRUCKMAN, R. F., jr., P. D. BRUCKMAN, H. V. HUFNAGEL, A. S. GERVIN: A physiologic basis for the adhesions-free healing of deperitonealized surface. J. Surg. Res. *21:* 67–76 (1976).

CANDY, J. W.: Modified Gilliam uterine suspension using laparoscopic visualization. Obstet. Gynec. *47:* 242–243 (1976).

CARREL, A.: The surgery of blood vessels etc. Johns Hopk. Hosp. Bull. *18:* 18–28 (1907).

CARTWRIGHT, A.: Reversal of sterilisation (letter). Brit. med. J. *2:* 641–642 (1977).

COHEN, M. R.: Laparoscopy and the management of endometriosis. J. Reprod. Med. *23:* 81–84 (1979).

DANIELL, J. F.: Microsurgical techniques in reconstructive surgery of the fallopian tube. Southern med. J. *72:* 585–587 (1979).

DIAMOND, E.: Microsurgical reconstruction of the uterine tube in sterilized patients. Fertil. Steril. *28:* 1203–1210 (1977).

DIAMOND, E.: Lysis of postoperative pelvic adhesions in infertility. Fertil. Steril. *31:* 287–295 (1979).

DIAMOND, E.: A comparison of gross and microsurgical techniques for repair of cornual occlusion in infertility: a retrospective study 1968–1978. Fertil. Steril. *32:* 370–376 (1979).

DIZERGA, G. S., G. D. HODGEN: Prevention of postoperative tubal adhesions: comparative study of commonly used agents. Amer. J. Obstet. Gynec. *136:* 173–178 (1980).

DUBUISSON, J. B. et al.: Early control laparoscopy after tubal microsurgery. J. Gynec. Obstet. Biol. Reprod. (Paris) *8:* 655–657 (1979).

EGGER, H., K. KINDERMANN, F. EBERLEIN: Laparoskopische Ovarialbiopsie bei 71 amenorrhoischen Patientinnen. Arch. Gynäk. *220:* 43–54 (1975).

Esposito, J. M.: Removal of polyethylene catheters under laparoscopic supervision. J. Reprod. Med. *14:* 174–175 (1975).

Esposito, J. M.: The laparoscopist and electrosurgery. Am. J. Obstet. Gynec. *126:* 633–637 (1976).

Esposito, J. M.: Laparoscopy and electrosurgery (letter). Am. J. Obstet. Gynec. *129:* 930–931 (1977).

Fayez, J. A, R. Gutknecht: Microscopic tubouterine anastomosis with and without splints. Fertil. Steril. *30. (6 Suppl):* 735–736 (1978).

Fogart, J. A. jr.: Removal of an unusual foreign body from the peritoneal cavity via laparoscopy: report of a case. J. Am. Osteopath. Assoc. *74:* 62–64 (1974).

Frangenheim, H.: Effect of laparoscopy on current indications for conservative and surgical therapy in gynecology. ZFA *53:* 130–135 (1977).

Gaisford, W. D.: Peritoneoscopy: a valuable technique for surgeons. Am. J. Surg. *130:* 671–678 (1975).

Gawecki, F. M. et al.: Removal of an extrauterine IUD by combined laparoscopy and colpotomy. Nebr. med. J. *62:* 99–101 (1977).

Gayän, P. et al.: Extraction of an ectopic intrauterine device by laparoscopy. Rev. Chil. Obstet. Ginec. *43:* 305–311 (1978).

Gentile, G. P. et al.: Inadvertent intestinal biopsy during laparoscopy and hysteroscopy: a report of two cases. Fertil. Steril. *36:* 402–404 (1981).

Gomel, V.: Laparoscopic tubal surgery in infertility. Obstet. Gynec. *46:* 47–48 (1975).

Gomel, V.: Tubal reanastomosis by microsurgery. Fertil. Steril. *28:* 59–65 (1977).

Gomel, V.: Salpingostomy by laparoscopy. J. Reprod. Med. *18:* 265–268 (1977).

Gomel, V.: Profile of women requesting reversal of sterilization. Fertil. Steril. *30:* 39–41 (1978).

Gomel, V.: Microsurgical reversal of female sterilization: a reappraisal. Fertil. Steril. *33:* 587–597 (1980).

Gomel, V., P. McComb: Microsurgery in Gynecology. In: Solber, S. J. (ed.): Microsurgery, S. 143–183. Williams and Wilkins, Baltimore, Maryland 1979.

Gomel, V.: Causes of failed reconstructive tubal microsurgery. J. Reprod. Med. *24:* 239–243 (1980).

Hak, V. et al.: How operative laparoscopy contributes to decreasing work disability. Cesk. Gynek. *46:* 112–114 (1981).

Harris, F. W.: Electrosurgery in laparotomy. J. Reprod. Med. *21:* 48–52 (1978).

Hasson, H. M.: Electrocoagulation of pelvic endometriotic lesions with laparoscopic control. Am. J. Obstet. Gynec. *135:* 115–121 (1979).

Hasson, H. M.: Window for open laparoscopy. Am. J. Obstet. Gynec. *137:* 869–870 (1980).

Henderson, S. R.: Refertilisierung und Tubensterilisation. Vergleiche zwischen mikro- und makrochirurgischer Technik für Tubenanastomosen. Am. J. Obstet. Gynec. *139:* 73–79 (1981).

Henry-Suchet, J. et al.: Prevention of recurring adhesions after tuboblasties. Interest of early laparoscopy, 8 days after surgery. J. Gynec. Obstet. Biol. Reprod. (Paris). *8:* 451–454 (1979).

Hernandez Ayup, S. et al.: Value of ovarian biopsy by laparoscopy in endocrine-gonadal pathology. Ginec. Obstet. Mex. *47:* 321–328 (1980).

Hochuli, E., H. Gehring: Tubare Sterilität und operative Behandlung. Geburtsh. u. Frauenheilk. *38:* 921–931 (1978).

Hodari, A. A., S. Vibhasiri, A. Y. Isaac: Reconstructive surgery for midtubal obstruction. Fertil. Steril. *28:* 620–623 (1977).

Hoffmann, J.-J.: A practical classification of the risk factor in restorative surgery of the fallopian tube. Fertil. Steril. *28:* 1006–1007 (1977).

Hoffmann, J.-J.: A simple solution to five of the major problems of the microsurgical reversal of sterilization. Fertil. Steril. *30:* 480–481 (1978).

Hoffmann, J. J.: Routine for microsurgical tubal reanastomosis. Int. J. Fertil. *23:* 257–259 (1978).

Holtz, G.: Anastomosis of fallopian tubes. Personal communication; University of Oklahoma Health Sciences Center, Oklahoma City, Juli 1980.

Holtz, G.: Prevention of postoperative adhesions. J. Reprod. Med. *24:* 141–146 (1980).

Holtz, G., E. Baker, C. Tsai: Effect of thirty-two per cent dextran 70 on peritoneal adhesion formation and re-formation after lysis. Fertil. Steril. *33:* 660–662 (1980).

Hoynck van Papendrechten, H. P. et al.: Antefixation of the uterus using laparoscopy. Ned. Tijdschr. Geneesk. *119:* 301–304 (1975).

Jones, H. W. jr., J. A. Rock: On the reanastomosis of fallopian tubes after surgical sterilization. Fertil. Steril. *29:* 702–704 (1978).

Joshi, C. K., S. Maheshwari, A. Soangara, M. R.: A follow-up study of tubectomy acceptors in Bikaner. J. Ind. med. Ass. *73:* 1–4 (1979).

Junker, H.: Lagekorrektur des hypermobilen retroflektierten Uterus durch Ligamenta rotunda-Doppelung per laparoskopiam. Arch. Gynäk. *224:* 281–288 (1977).

Kleppinger, R. K.: Ovarian cyst fenestration via laparoscopy. J. Reprod. Med. *21:* 16–19 (1978).

Koenig, U. D.: Die offene Pelviskopie – ein Beitrag zur Erhöhung der Sicherheit bei der Pelviskopie. Gynäkologie *15:* 30–34 (1982).

KOLMORGEN, K., H. R. HAUSSWALD, O. HAVEMANN, G. WERGIEN: Ergebnisse nach Ovarialzystenpunktion unter laparoskopischer Sicht. Zbl. Gynäk. *100:* 289–293 (1978).

LADIPO, O. A.: Laparoscopic removal of extra-uterine Lippes-loop. J. nat. med. Assoc. *72:* 701–702 (1980).

LEYTON, R., L. ARANEDA: Laparoscopia un metoto diagnostico y quirurgico. Rev. Chil. Obstet. Ginec. 80–88 (1975).

MADELENA, P. et al.: A critical study on freeing peri-adnexial adhesions using the laparoscope. J. Gynec. Obstet. Biol. Reprod. (Paris) *8:* 347–352 (1979).

MENKEN, F. C.: Die Mikro-Endoskopie der Cervix uteri. Geburtsh. u. Frauenheilk. *41:* 192–193 (1981).

MCCORMICK, W. G., J. TORRES, L. R. MCCANNE: Tubal reanastomosis: an update. Fertil. Steril. *31:* 689–690 (1979).

METTLER, L., H. GIESEL, K. SEMM: Treatment of female infertility due to tubal obstruction by operative laparoscopy. Fertil. Steril. *32:* 384–388 (1979).

MOSHER, W.: Reproductive impairements among currently married couples. United States 1976. Advancedata *55:* 1–11 (1980).

MOTASHAW, N. D. et al.: Laparoscopy for resolving Müllerian abnormalities. J. Reprod. Med. *21:* 20–23 (1978).

NEUFELD, G. R.: Principles and hazards of electrosurgery including laparoscopy. Surg. Gynec. Obstet. *147:* 705–710 (1978).

NORIEGA, C. et al.: Surgical and diagnostic endoscopy in gynecology. Rev. Chil..Obstet. Ginec. *40:* 212–215 (1975).

OWEN, E. R., A. A. PICKETT-HEAPS: The microsurgical basis of fallopian tube reconstruction. Austr. N. Z. J. Surg. *47:* 300–305 (1977).

PALMER, R.: Safety in laparoscopy. J. Reprod. Med. *13:* 1–5 (1974).

PATERSON, P.: Tubal microsurgery: a review. Austr. N. Z. J. Obstet. Gynec. *18:* 182–184 (1978).

PATERSON, P., C. WOOD: The use of microsurgery in the reanastomosis of the rabbit fallopian tube. Fertil. Steril. *25:* 757–761 (1974).

PATERSON, P. C. WOOD, B. DOWNING: Microsurgical tubal anastomosis for sterilization reversal. Med. J. Austr. *2:* 560–561 (1977).

PATTON, D. L., S. A. HALBERT: Electron microscopic examination of the rabbit oviductal ampulla following microsurgical end-to-end anastomosis. Fertil. Steril. *32:* 691–696 (1979).

PETERSON, E. P. J. R. MUSICH, S. J. BEHRMAN: Uterotubal implantation and obstetric outcome after previous sterilization. Amer. J. Obstet. Gynec. *128:* 662–667 (1977).

PHILLIPS, J. M.: Gynecologic microsurgery: a déjà vu of laparoscopy. J. Reprod. Med. *22:* 135–143 (1979).

POWERS, J. S. et al. Removal of intraperitoneal Dalkon Shields (letter). Am. J. Obstet. Gynec. *120:* 569 (1974).

RADWANSKA, E., G. S. BERGER, J. HAMMOND: Luteal deficiency among women with normal menstrual cycles, requesting reversal of tubal sterilization. Obstet. Gynec. *54:* 189–192 (1979).

RIEDEL, H.-H., L. MÜLLER, H. MOSLER, K. SEMM: Devitalisierung und Hämostase durch destruktive Wärme. Ergebnisse enzymhistochemischer und histologischer Untersuchungen an Eileiterpräparaten nach Gewebekoagulation mit Endokoagulation oder Hochfrequenzstrom. Zbl. Gynäkol. *104:* 489–501 (1982).

RIEDEL, H.-H., K. SEMM: There is no place in gynecological endoscopy for unipolar or bipolar high-frequency current. Endoscopy *14:* 51–54 (1982).

ROBERT, B., J. JUNT, C. STEPHEN: Laparoscopy in the diagnosis of occult inguinal Hernia. Am. J. Obstet. Gynec. *142:* 924–925 (1982).

ROCK, J. A., Z. ROSENWAKS, E. Y. ADASHI, H. W. JONES, jr., T. M. KING: Microsurgery for tubal reconstruction following Fallope-ring sterilization in swine. J. Microsurg. *1:* 61–64 (1979).

ROSENFELD, D. L., C.-R. GARCIA: Laparoscopy prior to tubal reanastomosis J. Reprod. Med. *17:* 247–248 (1976).

SCARPA, F. et al.: Diagnostic and therapeutic importance of celioscopic ovarian biopsy in female sterility. Min. Ginec. *30:* 739–748 (1978).

SCHMIDT, K. et al.: Possibility of timely treatment of twisted cysts by means of laparoscopy. Cesk. Gynek. *39:* 669–670 (1974).

SEKI, K., C. A. EDDY, N. K. SMITH, C. J. PAUERSTEIN: Comparison of two techniques of suturing in microsurgical anastomosis of the rabbit oviduct. Fertil. Steril. *28:* 1215–1219 (1977).

SEMM, K.: Endo-coagulation: Une nouvelle ressource pour la chirurgie endoscopique par pelviscopie. Gynécologie *27:* 9–15 (1976).

SEMM, K.: Endocoagulation: a new field of endoscopic surgery. J. Reprod. Med. *16:* 195–203 (1976).

SEMM, K.: Die Mikrochirurgie in der Gynäkologie – Endokoagulation, ein neues Hilfsmittel für operative Eingriffe per pelviskopiam. Geburtsh. u. Frauenheilk. *37:* 93–102 (1977).

SEMM, K.: Therapie der tubaren Sterilität 2. Operative pelviskopische Therapie. Gynäk. Prax. *1:* 625–636 (1977).

SEMM, K.: Pelviskopische Chirurgie in der Gynäkologie. Geburtsh. u. Frauenheilk. *37:* 909–920 (1977).

SEMM, K.: Operative Pelviskopie/Laparoskopie (Serie »Im Dienste der Chirurgie«). Ethicon, Hamburg 1978.

SEMM, K.: New methods of pelviscopy (gynecologic laparoscopy) for myomectomy, ovariectomy, tubectomy and adnectomy. Endoscopy *11:* 85–93 (1979).

SEMM, K.: Technical progress in pelvic surgery via operative laparoscopy. Am. J. Obstet. Gynec. *138:* 121–127 (1980).

Semm, K.: Die endoskopische intraabdominelle Naht. Geburtsh. u. Frauenheilk. *42:* 56–57 (1982).

Semm, K., L. Mettler: Technical progress in pelvic surgery via operative laparoscopy. Am. J. Obstet. Gynec. *138:* 121–127 (1980).

Semm, K.: Neue Möglichkeiten der endoskopischen Chirurgie am inneren weiblichen Genitale. Notabene medici *10:* 801–808 (1982).

Semm, K.: Endoskopische Intraabdominal-Chirurgie in der Gynäkologie. Wien. klin. Wschr. *95:* 353–366 (1983).

Semm, K., F. W. Dittmar, L. Mettler: Das voroperierte Abdomen: Möglichkeiten und Grenzen der Pelviskopie (Kasuistik von 1970–1975). Arch. Gynäk. *224:* 276–280 (1977).

Shain, R. N.: Acceptability of reversible versus permanent tubal sterilization: an analysis of preliminary data. Fertil. Steril. *31:* 13–17 (1979).

Siegler, A. M., R. J. Perez: Reconstruction of Fallopian tubes in previously sterilized patients. Fertil. Steril. *26:* 383–392 (1975).

Siegler, A. M.: Surgical treatment for tuboperitoneal causes of infertility since 1967. Fertil. Steril. *28:* 1019–1032 (1977).

Siegler, A. M.: Selection of patients for tuboplasty. J. Reprod. Med. *18:* 333–335 (1977).

Silber, S. J., R. S. Cohen: Microsurgical reversal of female sterilization: the role of tubal length. Fertil. Steril. *33:* 598–601 (1980).

Smith, D. C.: Irrigation solutions for gynecologic microsurgery. Presented at the 3rd International Workshop on Laparoscopy and Microsurgery in Gynecology, Anaheim and Irvine, California, Oct. 12–15, 1978.

Sulewski, J. M. et al.: The treatment of endometriosis at laparoscopy for infertility. Am. J. Obstet. Gynec. *138:* 128–132 (1980).

Swolin, K.: Laparoscopy as an operative tool in female sterility. J. Reprod. Med. *19:* 167–170 (1977).

Tesarik, J., M. Dvorak, L. Pilkar, M. Uher, J. Soska: Die Wirkung der laparoskopischen Aspiration des Graaf'schen Follikels auf die Ultrastruktur von Oozyten. Zbl. Gynäkol. *102:* 641–644 (1980).

Utian, W. H., J. M. Goldfarb, G. C. Starks: Role of dextran 70 in microtubal surgery. Fertil. Steril. *31:* 79–82 (1979).

Valle, R. F.: Laparoscopic removal of translocated retroperitoneal IUD's Gastrointest. Endoscopy *27:* 28–30 (1981).

Vammen, A. N., W. P. Giedon, J. P. Elkins: Reanastomosis of the previously ligated fallopian tube. Fertil. Steril. *32:* 652–656 (1979).

Wheeless, C. R. jr.: Problems with tubal reconstruction following laparoscopic sterilization using the electrocoagulation and resection technique. Fertil. Steril. *28:* 723–727 (1977).

Williams, G. F. J.: Tubo-uterine implantation with special reference to reversal of sterilisation. Lancet *I:* (1969).

Wilson, P. C. M.: Microsurgical repair of fallopian tubes. Med. J. Austr. *1:* 1013 (1976).

Winston, R. M. L.: Microsurgical reanastomosis of the rabbit oviduct and its functional and pathological sequelae. Brit. J. Obstet. Gynaec. *28:* 513–522 (1975).

Winston, R. M. L.: Reconstructive tubal surgery (letter). Fertil. Steril. *28:* 1264–1265 (1977).

Winston, R. M. L.: Microsurgical tubocornual anastomosis for reversal of sterilisation. Lancet *I (8006):* 284–285 (1977).

Winston, R. M. L.: The future of microsurgery in infertility. Clin. Obstet. Gynaec. *5:* 607–622 (1978).

Yuzpe, A. A. et al: The value of laparoscopic ovarian biopsy. J. Reprod. Med. *15:* 57–59 (1975).

XII. Operative Pelviscopy—Complications

van Assen, F. J. et al.: Patients with intestinal perforation following coagulation of the tubes by means of laparoscopy. Ned. Tijdschr. Geneeskd. *119:* 304–306 (1975).

Bak, V.: Complications in gynecologic laparoscopy. Cesk. Gynek. *45:* 493–498 (1980).

Bal, H.: Complications in laparoscopic interventions and how to prevent them. Ned. Tijdschr. Geneesk. *119:* 307–309 (1975).

Bartsich, E. G. et al.: Injury of superior mesenteric vein; laparoscopic procedure with unusual complication. N. Y. State J. Med. *81:* 933 (1981).

Bell, J. G. et al.: Complication of laparoscopic tubal banding procedure: case report. Am. J. Obstet. Gynec. *131:* 908–910 (1978).

Bisler, H., J. Sinde, J. Alemany, J. Kunde: Verletzungen der großen Gefäße bei gynäkologischen Laparoskopien. Geburtsh. u. Frauenheilk. *40:* 553–556 (1980).

Boer, C. H., C. J. Hutchin: Complications of laparoscopy. Brit. med. J. *2:* 137 (1975).

Burmucic, R.: Late manifestation of a burn of intestine caused by laparoscopic tubal sterilization. Wien. med. Wschr. *129:* 157–158 (1979).

Chapin, J. W. et al: Hemorrhage and cardiac arrest during laparoscopic tubal ligation. Anesthesiology *53:* 342–343 (1980).

Cheng, Y. S.: Ureteral injury resulting from laparoscopic fulguration of endometriotic implant. Am. J. Obstet. Gynec *126:* 1045–1046 (1976).

Chiu, H. H. et al.: Complication of laparoscopy under general anaesthesia. Anaesth. Intensive Care *5:* 169–171 (1977).

Clark, C. C. et al.: Venous carbon dioxide embolism during laparoscopy. Anesth. Analg. (Clevel.) *56:* 650–652 (1977).

COGNAT, M., D. GERALD, A. VIGNAUD: Le risque d'arrêt Cardiaque au cours de la coelioscopie. Etude à partie de 50000 coelioscopies et d'une expérimentation animale. J. Gynéc. obstet. *5:* 925–940 (1976).

COON, W. W.: Risk factors in pulmonary embolism. Surg. Gynec. Obstet. *14:* 385–390 (1976).

CORALL, I. M. et al.: Laparoscopy explosion hazards with nitrous oxide (letter). Brit. med. J. *4:* 288 (1975).

CORALL, I. J. et al.: Laparoscopy explosion hazards with nitrous oxide. Brit. med. J. *1 (6006):* 397 (1976).

CORSON, S. L.: Major vessel injury during laparoscopy (letter). Am. J. Obstet. Gynec. *38:* 589–590 (1980).

CRAWFORD, J. W.: Complications of laparoscopy (letter). Brit. med. J. *2 (5964):* 191 (1975).

CREMERS, N. P. et al.: Complications of laparoscopic operations (letter). Ned. Tijdschr. Geneeskd. *119:* 807–808 (1975).

DAMIANO, A. et al.: Cardiac arrhythmias during laparoscopy. Rev. Clin. Esp. *135:* 123–126 (1974).

DEBRAY, C. et al.: Complications of laparoscopy. Ann. med. Interne (Paris) *127:* 689–692 (1974).

DÖBRÖNTE, Z., T. WITTMANN, G. KARÁCSONY: Rapid development of malignant metastases in the abdominal wall after laparoscopy. Endoscopy *10:* 127–130 (1978).

DRUMMOND, G. B. et al.: Laparoscopy explosion hazards with nitrous oxide. Brit. med. J. *1 (6009):* 586 (1976).

DRUMMOND, G. B. et al.: Laparoscopy explosion hazards with nitrous oxide (letter). Brit. med. J. *1 (6024):* 1513 (1976).

DULBERY M. et al.: Advantage of laparoscopy in uterine perforation. Harefuah *89:* 309–313 (1975).

ENDLER, G. C. et al.: Perforation during pelvic laparoscopy. Obstet. Gynec. *47:* 40–42 (1976).

EREMENKO, V.P.: Complication of a peritoneoscopy performed in portal hypertension. Vestn. Khir *121:* 126–127 (1978).

ERKRATH, K. D., G. WEILER, G. ADEBAHR: Zur Aortenverletzung bei Laparoskopie in der Gynäkologie. Geburtsh. u. Frauenheilk. *39:* 687–689 (1979).

FATHALLA, M. F. et al.: Laparoscopic ventrosuspension in the treatment of backward displacement of the uterus. J. Egypt. med. Assoc. *57:* 202–205 (1974).

GAUJOUX, J., R. PORTO, C. VALLETTE: Incidents and accidents in laparoscopy. (Apropos of 2335 cases.) J. Gynéc. Obstet. *4:* 5–28 (1975).

GEORGITIS, J. W.: Two late complications of laparoscopic tubal ligation. J. Maine med. Assoc. *68:* 352–353 (1977).

GEORGY, F. M. et al.: Complication of laparoscopy: two cases of perforated urinary bladder. Am. J. Obstet. Gynec. *120:* 1121–1122 (1974).

GIROTTI, M., A. E. SCHAER: Zwischenfälle bei der gynäkologischen Laparoskopie. Riv. ital. Ginec. *56:* 49–54 (1975).

GORSHKOV, S. Z. et al.: Laparoscopy in closed injuries of the abdomen. Vestn. Khir *112:* 84–86 (1974).

GUNATILAKE, D. E.: Case report: fatal intraperitoneal explosion during electrocoagulation via laparoscopy. Int. J. Gynaec. Obstet. *15:* 353–357 (1978).

HAVEMANN, O., K. KOLMORGEN, H.-R. HAUSWALD, G. WERGIEN: Komplikationen bei der gynäkologischen Laparoskopie. Zbl. Gynäk. *99:* 1186–1189 (1977).

HERRERIAS, J. M. et al.: Unusual complications of laparoscopy. Rev. Esp. Enferm. Apar. Dig. *49:* 83–92 (1977).

HO, Y. H.: Changes of the heart axis with in flow occlusion through intraabdominal pressure (an unusual complication during laparoscopy). Prakt. Anaesth. *12:* 423 (1977).

HOMBURG, R. et al.: Perforation of the urinary bladder by the laparoscope. Amer. J. Obstet. Gynaec. *130:* 597 (1978).

HOUSE, M. J.: Abdominal actinomycosis. Complication of laparoscopy? Case report. Brit. J. Obstet. Gynaec. *66:* 459–460 (1981).

IMRAN, M. et al.: Laparoscopy and some of its hazards. Del. med. J. *48:* 71–74 (1976).

IVASENKO, I. D., V. B. SBABELIANSKIJ: Complications in laparoscopy. Khirurgiia (Moskau) *7:* 78–81 (1979).

JANSEN, R. P. S.: Abortion incidence following Fallopian tube repair. Obstet. Gynec. (in press).

KAKKAR, V. V., T. P. CORRIGAN, D. P. FOSSARD, I. SUTHERLAND, J. THIRWELL: Prevention of fatal postoperative pulmonary embolism by low doses of heparin. Lancet *II (8011):* 567–569 (1977).

KAPIŃSKI, J. et al.: Rare complications of laparoscopy. Wiad. Lek. *32:* 1151–1155 (1979).

KAPLAN, L. R.: Operator anesthesia as a complication of laparoscopy (letter). Gastrointest. Endosc. *24:* 185 (1978).

KARAM, K. S. et al.: Mesenteric hematoma – Meckel's diverticulum: a rare laparoscopic complication. Fertil. Steril. *28:* 1003–1005 (1977).

KATZ, M. et al.: Major vessel injury during laparoscopy: anatomy of two cases. Am. J. Obstet. Gynec. *135:* 544–545 (1979).

KENT, S. W.: Retention of detective Veress needle sheath in abdominal cavity after laparoscopy. Fertil. Steril *28:* 499 (1977).

KHUNDA, S. et al.: Laparoscopy explosion hazards with nitrous oxide (letter). Brit. med. J. *1 (6018):* 1147 (1976).

KOLMORGEN, H., R. HAUSWALD, O. HAVENMANN: Chronische Unterbauchbeschwerden der Frau, eine postlaparoskopische Analyse. Zbl. Gynäk. *98:* 1434–1440 (1976).

LENZ, R. J., T. A. THOMAS, D. G. WILKINS: Cardiovascular changes during laparoscopy studies of stroke volume and cardiac output using impedance cardiography. Anaesthesia (Lond.) *31:* 4–12 (1976).

LEVINSON, C. J.: Laparoscopy is easy – except for the complications: a review with suggestions. J. Reprod. Med. *13:* 187–194 (1974).

LOFFER, F. D. et al.: Indications, contraindications and complications of laparoscopy. Obstet. Gynec. Surv. *30:* 407–427 (1975).

Loffer, F. D. et al.: Sciatic nerve injury in a patient undergoing laparoscopy. J. Reprod. Med. *21:* 371–372 (1978).

Lübke, F.: Complicationen in der Laparoskopie. Arch. Gynäk. *224:* 282–283 (1977).

Lysholm, J. et al.: Hemorrhage from the hilus of the spleen after Laparoskopy. Lakartidningen *75:* 3918–3919 (1978).

MacLaughlin, W. S. jr. et al.: Four years experience with laparoscopy and its complications at the Maine Medical Center. J. Maine. med. Assoc. *66:* 307–310 (1975).

Makauji, H. H., H. R. Elliot: Rupture of spleen at laparoscopy: Case report. Brit. J. Obstet. Gynaec. *87:* 73–74 (1980).

Mazchenko, N. S. et al.: Complications of laparoscopy. Sov. Med. *11:* 106–107 (1979).

McCausland, A.: High rate of ectopic pregnancy following laparoscopic tubal coagulation failures. Incidence and etiology. Am. J. Obstet. Gynec. *136:* 97–101 (1980).

Menken, F. C.: Failures and hazards of surgical laparoscopy. Fortschr. Med. *93:* 1773–1774 (1975).

Menken, F. C.: Vermeidung von Fehlern und Gefahren in der operativen Pelviskopie. Arch. Gynäk. *228:* 284–295 (1979).

Mintz, M.: Le risque et la prophylaxie des accidents en coelioscopie gynécologique. Enquête portant sur 100.000 cas. J. Gynéc. Obstét. *5:* 681–695 (1976).

Montalva, M. et al.: Carbon dioxide hemostasis during laparoscopy. South Med. J. *69:* 602–603 (1976).

Moreira, V. F. et al.: Intestinal mechanical obstruction after laparoscopy. Rev. Clin. Esp. *30:* 291–292 (1979).

Morison, D. H. et al.: Cardiovascular collapse in laparoscopy. Can. med. Assoc. J. *111:* 433–437 (1974).

Nichols, S. L. et al.: Probable carbon dioxide embolism during laparoscopy; case report. Wiss. Med. *80:* 27–29 (1981).

Nuyens, A., J. W. Andrews: Hazards of laparoscopic tubal sterilization. J. Obstet. Gynec. *4:* 221–225 (1975).

Parewijck, W. et al.: Serious complications of laparoscopy. Med. Sci. Law. *19:* 199–201 (1979).

Pent, D., F. D. Loffer: Avoiding Medical and surgical complications of laparoscopy. Contemp. OB/GYN *14:* 75–86 (1979).

Phillips, J. M.: Complications in laparoscopy. Int. J. Gynaec. Obstet. *15:* 157–162 (1977).

Pongthai, S. et al.: Laparoscopic complication: bowel injury from direct trocar puncture. J. med. Assoc. Thal. *60:* 231–233 (1977).

del Pozo Camaron, A. et al.: Laparoscopy: complications and evaluation of the risk in a series of 700 explorations. Rev. Esp. Enferm. Apar. Dig. *47:* 85–92 (1976).

Pressl, J. et al.: Heart arrest during laparoscopy. Cesk. Gynek. *30:* 229 (1974).

Pressl, J.: Laparoscopy and heart arrest. Cesk. Gynek. *39:* 553 (1974).

Prian, D. V.: Ruptured spleen as a complication of laparoscopy and pelvic laparotomy. Report of an unusual complication. Am. J. Obstet. Gynec. *120:* 983–984 (1974).

Rawlings, E. E., B. Balgobin: Complications of laparoscopy. Brit. med. J. *1 (5960):* 727–728 (1975).

Riedel, H.-H., K. Semm: Das postpelviskopische (laparoskopische) subphrenische Schmerzsyndrom. Arch. Gynäk. *228:* 283–284 (1979).

Robinson, J. S., J. M. Thompson, J. W. Wood: Laparoscopy explosion hazards with nitrous oxide (letter). Brit. med. J. *4 (5986):* 760–761 (1975).

Robinson, J. S., J. M. Thompson, J. W. Wood: Laparoscopy explosion hazards with nitrous oxide (letter). Brit. med. J. *1 (6020):* 1277 (1976).

Roopnarinesingh, S. et al.: Laparoscopic trocar point perforation of the small bowel. Int. Surg. *62:* 76 (1977).

Root, B. et al.: Gas embolism death after laparoscopy delayed by »trapping« in portal circulation. Anesth. Analg. (Clevel.) *57:* 232–237 (1978).

Rust, M. et al.: Injury to retroperitoneal vessels, a serious complication of gynaecological laparoscopy. Anaesth. Intens. Nofallmed. *15:* 356–359 (1980).

Ryan, G. B., J. Grobety, G. Mahno: Postoperative peritoneal adhesions: a study of the mechanisms. Am. J. Pathol. *65:* 117–138 (1971).

Schapira, M. et al.: Urinary ascites after gynaecological laparoscopy (letter). Lancet *I (8069):* 871–872 (1978).

Sherwood, R., G. Berci, E. Austin, L. Morgenstern: Minilaparoscopy for blunt abdominal trauma. Arch. Surg. *115:* 672–673 (1980).

Semm, K.: Physical and biological considerations militating against the use of endoscopically applied high-frequency current in the abdomen. Endoscopy *15:* 282–288 (1983).

Sivanesaratnam, V.: Obeyed small bowel perforation following laparoscopic tubal cauterization. Int. Surg. *64:* 560–561 (1975).

Steptoe, P.: Laparoscopic explosion hazards with nitrous oxide (letter). Brit. med. J. 833 (1976).

Tasseron, E. W. et al.: Simultaneous curettage and laparoscopy following perforation of the uterus. Ned. Tijdschr. Geneeskd. *119:* 1306–1308 (1975).

Trofimov, V. M. et al.: Risk and complications in peritoneoscopy. Vestn. Khir. *120:* 117–119 (1978).

Wadhwa, R. K. et al.: Gas embolism during laparoscopy. Anesthesiology *48:* 74–76 (1978).

White, M. K. et al.: A case-control study of uterine perforations documented at laparoscopy. Am. J. Obstet. Gynec. *129:* 623–625 (1977).

XIII. Sterilization by Pelviscopy

ALDERMAN, B.: Women who regret sterilisation (letter). Brit. med. J. *2 (6089):* 766 (1977).

ALEXANDER, C.: Laparoscopic sterilization without electrocautery. J. Reprod. Med. *14:* 176–177 (1975).

ALI, M. N., D. H. HUBER, A. R. KHAN, S. WILLIAMS: Sterilization campaign of 1977: a national long term follow-up survey. Dacca Bangladesh, Bangladesh Fertility Research Programme July 1979, Technical Report *25:* 49 (1979).

Anonymous: Reversal of female sterilization. IPPF Med. Bull. *12:* 1–2 (1978).

Anonymous: Expert looks at tubal sterilization. AVS Newsletter *22:* 1, 2, 4 (1979).

Anonymous: International Fertility Research Program sponsors effort in 43 lands to develop new, safer methods. Int. Family Planning Perspectives *5:* 128–129 (1979).

Anonymous: Non-surgical sterilization techniques tested. Lankenau Hospital Reporter 1–2 (1979).

Anonymous: The problem of reversal. International Project. Assoc. Vol. Steril. Inc. Newsletter *21:* 1–2 (1979).

Anonymous: Female sterilisation: no more tubal coagulation. Brit. med. J. *280 (6220):* 1037 (1980).

ANSARI, A. H. et al.: Silicone rubber band for laparoscopic tubal sterilization. Fertil. Steril. *28:* 306–309 (1977).

ANSARI, A. H.: Georgia Baptist Medical Center: Estimated proportion of women requesting sterilization reversal. Personal communication 1980.

ARANDA, C. et al.: Laparoscopic sterilization immediately after term delivery: a preliminary report. J. Reprod. Med. *14:* 171–173 (1975).

ARANDA, C., A. BROUTIN, D. A. EDELMAN, A. GOLDSMITH, T. MANGEL, C. PRADA, A. SOLANO: A comparative study of electrocoagulation and tubal occlusion at laparoscopy. Int. J. Gynaec. Obstet. *14:* 411–415 (1976).

ARGUETA, G., E. HENRIQUEZ, M. AMADOR et al.: Comparison of laparoscopic sterilization via spring-loaded clip and tubal ring. Int. J. Gynec. Obstet. *18:* 115–118 (1980/81).

ARIBARG, A., S. ARIBARG: Emotional reaction to interval and postpartum sterilization. Int. J. Gynaec. Obstet. *16 (1):* 40–41 (1978).

ARIBARG, A.: Chulalongkorn Hospital Medical School Bangkok, Thailand; Sterilization regret and reversal. Personal communication 1980, 1.

BALMER, J. A. et al.: Falope-ring: a laparoscopic sterilization. Technical handling, action and experiences. Praxis *66:* 1314–1320 (1977).

BARNES, A. C., F. P. ZUSPAN: Patient reaction to puerperal surgical sterilization. 1. General considerations. Am. J. Obstet. Gynec. *75:* 65–71 (1958).

BARTSCH, E. G. et al.: Coagulation of the infundibulopelvic ligament during laparoscopic tubal sterilization: a report of an unusual complication. Am. J. Obstet. Gynec. *127:* 888 (1977).

BHATT, R. V. et al.: A comparative study of the tubal ring applied via minilaparotomy and laparoscopy in post-abortion cases. Int. J. Gynaec. Obstet. *16:* 162–166 (1978).

BHIWANDIWALA, P. P. et al.: Laparoscopic sterilization using a needle-puncture technique. J. Reprod. Med. *18:* 69–73 (1977).

BIRNBAUM, M. D.: Complications of laparoscopic sterilisation. Lancet *I (8210):* 43 (1981).

BLACK, W. P., A. B. SCLARE: Sterilization by tubal ligation: a follow-up study. J. Obstet. Gynaec. Brit. Cwlth. *75 (2):* 219–224 (1968).

BRANDL, E., K. SEMM, L. METTLER: Pelviskopische Sterilisation mittels Plastik-Clip im Tierversuch (Kaninchen). Arch. Gynäk. *224:* 43–44 (1977).

BRENNER, G.: Rechtliche Zulässigkeit der Sterilisation. Geburtsh. u. Frauenheilk. *42:* 226–230 (1982).

BUYTAERT, P. et al.: Laparoscopic sterilization with electrocautery, silastic bands and spring-loaded clips: report of our experience with 790 patients. Eur. J. Obstet. Gynaec. Repr. Biol. *10:* 109–118 (1980).

CAHILL, A. M.: Sterilization: it has a role in quality care. Aorn J. *12:* 73–80 (1970).

CAMPANELLA, R., J. R. WOLFF: Emotional reaction to sterilization. Obstet. Gynec. *45:* 331–334 (1975).

CANTOR, B., F. C. RIGGALL: The choice of sterilizing procedure according to its potential reversibility with microsurgery. Fertil. Steril. *31:* 9–12 (1979).

CHAMBERLAIN, G. et al.: Long-term-effects of laparoscopic sterilization on menstruation. South. Med. J. *69:* 1474–1475 (1976).

CHAN, W. F. et al.: The place of laparoscopic tubal sterilisation in Malaysia. Med. J. Mal. *29:* 57–59 (1974).

CHATMAN, D. L.: Laparoscopic Falope ring sterilization. Two years of experience. Am. J. Obstet. Gynec. *131:* 291–294 (1978).

CHENG, M. C. E., J. CHEONG, K. S. KHEW, S. S. RATNAM: Psychological sequelae of sterilization in women in Singapore. Intern. J. Gynaec. Obstet. *15:* 44–47 (1977).

CHENG, M. C. E., S. C. CHW, J. CHEONG, H. T. CHOO, S. S. RATNAM, M. A. BELSEY, K. E. EDSTROM: Safety of post-abortion sterilisation compared with interval sterilisation: a controlled study. Lancet *II (8144):* 682–685 (1979).

CHI, I.-C., L. E. LAUFE, S. D. GARDNER, M. A. TOLBERT: An epidemiologic study of risk factors associated with pregnancy following female sterilization. Am. J. Obstet. Gynec. *136:* 768–773 (1980).

CHI, I. C. et al.: Pregnancy risk following laparoscopic sterilization in nongravid and gravid women. J. Reprod. Med. *26:* 289–294 (1981).

VAN COEVERDEN, DE GROOT, et al.: Laparoscopic sterilization on a day-case basis. S. Afr. med. J. *58:* 61–64 (1980).

CORSON, S. L.: Studies in sterilization of the laparoscope: II. J. Reprod. Med. *23:* 57–59 (1979).

COX, M. L., I. M. CROZIER: Female sterilization: long-term follow-up with particular reference to regret. J. Reprod. Fertil. *35:* 624–626 (1973).

CUNANAN, R. G., jr. et al.: Combined laparoscopic sterilization and pregnancy termination: II. Further experiences with a larger series of patients. J. Reprod. Med. *13:* 204–205 (1974).

DIAMOND, E.: Sterilization reversal (St. Barnabas Medical Center). Personal communication 1980.

DIAZ, M. O. et al.: Laparoscopic sterilization with room air insufflation. Preliminary report. Int. J. Gynaec. Obstet. *18:* 119–122 (1980).

DONNEZ, J., F. CASANAS-ROUX, J. FERIN: Macroscopic and microscopic studies of Fallopian tube after laparoscopic sterilization. Contraception *20:* 497–509 (1979).

DONNEZ, J., M. WANTERS, C. LECART: Complications et échees de 600 stérilisations laparoscopiques por agrafes de HULKA-Clemens. Acta endoscop. *12:* 69–77 (1982).

EAKES, M.: Laparoscopic sterilization. Ned. Tijdschr. Geneesk. *124:* 729–734 (1980).

EDELMAN, D. A., A. GOLDSMITH, W. E. BRENNER: Esterilización femenina por laparoscopia en el periodo puerperal y de intervalo. Rev. Obstet. Ginec. Venez. *27:* 17–25 (1976).

EDWARDS, T. K.: Permanent sterilization by the laparoscopic method at the Bluefield Sanitarium 1973. W. Va. med. J. *70:* 253–255 (1974).

ENGEL, T. et al.: The electrical dynamics of laparoscopic sterilization. J. Reprod. Med. *15:* 33–42 (1975).

EMENS, J. M., J. E. OLIVE: Timing of female sterilisation. Brit. med. J. *2 (6145):* 1126 (1978).

ENOCH, M. D., K. JONES: Sterilization: a review of 98 sterilized women. Brit. J. Psych. *127:* 583–587 (1975).

FAN, G. Y.: Tubal ligation via laparoscope: report of 84 cases. Chung Hua Fu Chan Ko Tsa Chih. *15:* 110–111 (1980).

FATHALLA, M. F. et al.: Outpatient female sterilization via laparoscopy (a preliminary report of 63 cases). J. Egypt. med. Assoc. *57:* 23–29 (1974).

FISHBURNE, J. I. et al.: Outpatient laparoscopic sterilization with therapeutic abortion versus abortions alone. Obstet. Gynec. *45:* 665–668 (1975).

FISHBURNE, J. I. jr. et al.: Tubal healing following laparoscopic electrocoagulation. J. Reprod. Med. *16:* 129–134 (1976).

FLORES, R. Sterilization by laparoscopic route. Gynec. Obstet. Mex. *38:* 99–104 (1975).

FOSTER, H. W. jr.: J. nat. med. Assoc. *72:* 567–570 (1980).

FRANGENHEIM, H.: Laparoscopic results and risk. ZFA (Stuttgart) *52:* 1613–1617 (1976).

FRANGENHEIM, H.: Laparoskopische Tubensterilisation. Methoden und ihre Sicherheit. Gynäk. Rdsch. *20:* 142–143 (1980).

FRANGENHEIM, H.: Probeexcision bei der Tubensterilisation. Gynäk. Prax. *5:* 459–460 (1981).

GARCEÁ FLORES, R.: Sterilization by laparoscopic route. Ginec. Obstet. Mex. *38:* 99–104 (1975).

GLEW, R. H. et al.: Tuboovarian abscess following laparoscopic sterilization with silicone rubber bands. Obstet. Gynec. *55:* 760–762 (1980).

GOH, T. H. et al.: A study of menstrual patterns following laparoscopic sterilization with silastic rings. Int. J. Fertil. *26:* 116–119 (1981).

GREEN, C. P.: Voluntary sterilization worlds' leading contraceptive method. Populat. Rep. *2:* 35 (1978).

GREENWOOD, J., jr.: Two-point or interpolar coagulation: review after a twelve-year period with notes on addition of a sucker tip. J. Neurosurg. *12:* 196–197 (1955).

GRUNDERT, G. M.: Late tubal patency following tubal ligation. Fertil. Steril *35:* 406–408 (1981).

GUNNING, J. E. et al.: Laparoscopic tubal sterilization using thermal coagulation. Obstet. Gynec. *54:* 505–509 (1979).

HALL, J., et al.: Laparoscopic tubal sterilization: a report on 300 cases. St. Elmo. West Ind. med. J. *26:* 187–196 (1977).

HANSEN, P. et al.: Laparoscopic sterilization with a silicone rubber ring. (Falope-ring). Ugeskr. Laeger *142:* 438–440 (1980).

HASSLER, R. E.: Laparoscopic sterilization as an outpatient procedure. Wis. med. J. *73:* 113–114 (1974).

HENDERSON, S. R.: Refertilization following fallopian tube sterilization. Comparison between micro- and macrosurgical technique for tubeanastomosis. Am. J. Obstet. Gynec. *139:* 73–79 (1981).

HENRY-SUCHET, J. et al.: The surgical treatment of tubal sterility. Value of free peritoneal graft and of early coelioscopy in the prevention of adhesions. Nouv. Presse méd. *26:* 311–314 (1980).

HERNANDEZ, I. M. et al.: Postabortal laparoscopic tubal sterilization. Results in comparison to interval procedures. Obstet. Gynec. *50:* 356–358 (1977).

HERRERIAS, J. M. et al.: An unusual complication of laparoscopy. Endoscopy *12:* 254–255 (1980).

HIRSCH, H. A. et al.: Changing methods of sterilization as influenced by laparoscopy. J. Reprod. Med. *16:* 325–328 (1976).

HULKA, J. F.: Preclinical and clinical testing of laparoscopic sterilization techniques. Med. Instrum. *11:* 17–19 (1977).

HULKA, J. F.: Current status of elective sterilization in the United States. Fertil. Steril. *28:* 515–520 (1977).

HULKA, J. F.: Current status of the reversibility of sterilization. Res. Reprod. *10:* 1–2 (1978).

HULKA, J. F. et al.: Laparoscopic sterilization with the spring clip instrumentation: development and current clinical experience. Am. J. Obstet. Gynec. *135:* 1016–1020 (1979).

HULKA, J. F., J. P. MERCER, J. I. FISHBURNE, TH. KUMARASAMY, K. F. OMRAN, J. M. PHILLIPS, H. T. LEFLER, jr.: Spring clip sterilization: one-year follow-up of 1079 cases. Am. J. Obstet. Gynec. *125:* 1039–1043 (1976).

IRVIN, T. T. et al.: Injury to the ureter during laparoscopic tubal sterilization. Arch. Surg. *110:* 1501–1503 (1975).

JOSHI, C. K.: Sardar Patel Medical College, Bikaner, India: Sterilization regret study by P. Misra. Personal communication 1980.

KEITH, L.: Laparoscopic sterilization in the puerperium: a review of international experience. Int. J. Gynaec. Obstet. *14:* 407–410 (1976).

KLEPPINGER, R. K.: The operating laparoscope and the optimal positions for tubal coagulation. J. Reprod. Med. *15:* 60–64 (1975).

KLEPPINGER, R. K.: Regeln und Risiken der Laparoskopie. Zur instrumentellen operativen Technik der Tubensterilisation. Sexualmedizin *6:* 489–492 (1977).

KOETSAWANG, S. et al.: Comparison of culdoscopic and laparoscopic tubal sterilization. Am. J. Obstet. Gynec. *124:* 601–606 (1976).

KOETSAWANG, S. et al.: A comparison of laparoscopy and culdoscopy for internal sterilization. Int. J. Gynaec. Obstet. *14:* 217–223 (1976).

KOYA, Y.: Sterilization in Japan. Eugenics Quart. *8:* 135–141 (1961).

KUMARASAMY, T. et al.: Laparoscopic sterilization with a spring-loaded clip. J. Obstet. Gynaec. Brit. Cwlth. *81:* 913–920 (1974).

KUMARASAMY, T. et al.: Laparoscopic sterilization with silicone rubber bands. Obstet. Gynec. *50:* 351–355 (1977).

KWAK, H. M. et al.: Timing of laparoscopic sterilization in abortion patients. Obstet. Gynec. *56:* 85–89 (1980).

LACKRITZ, R. : Cost of sterilization reversals (University of Texas Health Center, San Antonia). Personal communication 1980.

LAUFE, L. E.: Suprapubic endoscopy for interval female sterilization. Am. J. Obstet. Gynec. *136:* 257–259 (1980).

LEE, W. K., M. S. BAGGISH: Laparoscopic sterilization with an elasticated silicone ring. Brit. J. Obstet. Gynaec. *83:* 809–813 (1976).

LETCHWORTH, A. T., B. A. LIEBERMAN: Successful reversal of clip sterilisation (letter). Lancet. *II (7991):* 904 (1976).

LEYTON, H. et al.: Sterilization by laparoscopy. Use of Yoon's ring. Rev. Chil. Obstet. Ginec. *42:* 187–191 (1977).

LIEBERMAN, B. A. et al.: Evaluation of laparoscopic sterilization using a spring-loaded clip. J. Obstet. Gynaec. Brit. Cwlth. *81:* 921–932 (1974).

LIEBERMAN, B. A.: A clip applicator for laparoscopic sterilization. Fertil. Steril. *27:* 1036–1039 (1976).

LIEBERMAN, B. A. et al.: Laparoscopic sterilization with a spring-loaded clip. Proc. roy. Soc. Med. *69:* 143–144 (1976).

LIEBERMAN, B. A. et al.: Laparoscopic sterilization with spring-loaded clip, – double-puncture technique. J. Reprod. Med. *18:* 241–245 (1977).

LIEBERMAN, B. A., M. C. ANDERSON: Reversal of female sterilization following tubal occlusion by a spring clip. In: I. BROSENS, R. M. I. WINSTON (eds.): Reversibility of Female Sterilization. S. 123–134. Academic Press, London 1978.

LETCHWORTH, A. T., L. RUSHTON, A. D. NOBLE: Late complications of female sterilization (letter). Lancet *I (7965):* 906 (1976).

LIMPAPHAYOM, A. T., L. RUSHTON, A. D. NOBLE: Late complications of female sterilization (letter). Lancet *I (7965):* 906 (1976).

LIMPAPHAYOM, K. et al.: Laparoscopic tubal electrocoagulation for sterilization: 5000 cases. Int. J. Gynaec. Obstet *18:* 411–413 (1980).

LOFFER, F. D. et al.: Risks of laparoscopic fulguration and transection of the fallopian tube. Obstet. Gynec. *49:* 218–222 (1977).

LOFFER, F. D. et al.: Pregnancy after laparoscopic sterilization. Obstet. Gynec. *55:* 643–648 (1980).

MADRIGAL, V. et al.: Laparoscopic sterilization as an outpatient procedure. J. Reprod. Med. *18:* 261–264 (1977).

MALHOTRA, R. P. et al.: Evaluation of the fallopian tube section obtained at laparoscopic fulguration. J. Reprod. Med. *18:* 38–40 (1977).

MARIK, J. J. et al.: A simple technique of laparoscopic tubal sterilization. J. Reprod. Med. *15:* 109–113 (1975).

McCANN, M. F., L. P. COLE: Laparoscopy and minilaparotomy: two major advances in female sterilization. Studies in Family Planning *11:* 119–127 (1980).

McDONNELL, C. F. jr.: Puerperal laparoscopic sterilization. Am. J. Obstet. Gynec. *137:* 910–913 (1980).

METHA, P. V.: Laparoscopic sterilization with the Falope ring: Experience with 10,000 women in rural camps. Obstet. Gynec. *57:* 345–350 (1981).

MORAD, M. et al.: Indication of abortion by intrauterine administration of prostaglandin via laparoscopy with concurrent sterilization. Int. J. Gynaec. Obstet. *15:* 256–257 (1977).

MUELLER, R. L. et al.: Puerperal laparoscopic sterilization. J. Reprod. Med. *16:* 307–309 (1976).

MUSICH, J. R., J. S. PAGANO, S. J. BEHRMAN, E. P. PETERSON: Uterotubal implantation and successful pregnancy following laparoscopic tubal cauterization. Obstet. Gynec. *50:* 507–509 (1977).

DiMUSTO, J. C., E. B. OWENS, K. A. KLOMPARENS: A follow-up study of 100 sterilized women. J. Reprod. Med. *12:* 112–116 (1974).

MUZSNAI, D., E. CARILLO, T. HUGHES: New laparoscopic sterilization with exteriorization of tubes (cauterization, ligation): a preliminary report. Europ. J. Obstet. Gynec. *11:* 281–289 (1981).

NAKAMURA, M.: Reversal of tubal sterilization (Sao Paulo Family Planning Center, Brazil). Personal communication 1980, 9 p.

NAHMANOVICI, C. et al.: Tubal sterilization by a combined laparoscopic and external technique: preliminary report on 75 cases. Fertil. Steril. *30:* 534–537 (1978).

NEUWIRTH, R. S.: Tubal sterilizations via laparoscopy and hysteroscopy. Acta europ. fertil. *6:* 265–269 (1975).

NEUWIRTH, R. S.: Restoration of Fertility Following Sterilization (presented at the 4th Internat. Conf. on Voluntary Sterilization, Seoul, Korea), Mai 1979, S. 2.

NILSEN, P. A. et al.: Tubal sterilization with special reference to electrocoagulation through the laparoscope. Acta obstet. gynec. scand. *55:* 349–353 (1976).

NOYER, A. et al.: 1st report of pelviscopic sterilization in the Lausanne University Hospital Department of Gynecology and Obstetrics. Rev. med. Suisse rom. *94:* 813–818 (1974).

NOVY, M. J.: Reversal of Kroener fimbrioectomy sterilization. Amer. J. Obstet. Gynec. *137 (2):* 198–206 (1980).

OBER, K. G.: Zur Methodik der laparoskopischen Sterilisierung und zu möglichen Mißerfolgen. Geburtsh. u. Frauenheilk. *38:* 593 (1978).

ORTIZ, MARISCAL, J. D. et al.: Tubal occlusion by laparoscopy with unipolar current. Ginec. Obstet. Mex. *48:* 191–197 (1980).

PALMER, R.: Reversibility as a consideration in laparoscopic sterilization. J. Reprod. Med. *21:* 57–58 (1978).

PELLAND, P. C.: The application of lidocaine to the fallopian tubes during tubal fulguration by laparoscopy. Obstet. Gynec. *47:* 501–502 (1976).

PELLAND, P. C.: Patient acceptance of laparoscopic tubal fulguration via falope-ring banding. Obstet. Gynec. *50:* 106–108 (1977).

PENFIELD, A. J.: Laparoscopic sterilization under local anesthesia. 1200 cases. Am. J. Obstet. Gynec. *49:* 725–727 (1977).

PETERSON, H. B., J. R. GREENSPAN, F. DE STEFANO: The impact of laparoscopy on tubal sterilization in United States Hospitals, 1970 and 1975 to 1978. Am. J. Obstet. Gynec. *140:* 811–814 (1981).

PHILLIPS, J., L. KEITH: The evolution of laparoscopic sterilization. Int. J. Gynaec. Obstet. *14:* 59–64 (1976).

POUS-IVERN, L.: Estado actual de la esterilizactión tubárica por via laparoscópica. Rev. Esp. Obstet. Gynec. *39:* 1–37 (1980).

POWE, C. E., J. A. McGEE: Combined outpatient laparoscopic sterilization with therapeutic abortion. N. C. J. Am. J. Obstet. Gynec. *126:* 565–567 (1976).

QUAN, A. et al.: Laparoscopic sterilization after spontaneous abortion. Int. J. Gynaec. Obstet. *15:* 258–261 (1977).

RADWANSKA, E., G. S. BERGER, J. HAMMOND: Luteal deficiency among women with normal menstrual cycles, requesting reversal of tubal sterilization. Obstet. Gynec. *54:* 189–192 (1979).

RAHMAN, M., D. HUBER, J. CHAKRABORTY: A follow-up survey of sterilization acceptors in Matlab. Bangladesh. Dacca, Bangladesh, Cholera Research Laboratory, Working Paper *No. 9:* 29 (1978).

REED, T. P., R. A. ERB: Tubal occlusion with silicone rubber. J. Reprod. Med. *25:* 25–28 (1980).

RIEDEL, H.-H., H. AHRENS, K. SEMM: Spätkomplikationen nach Anwendung unterschiedlicher Sterilisationstechniken – ein Vergleich zwischen unipolarer Hochfrequenzsterilisation und dem Endokoagulationsverfahren nach Semm. Geburtsh. u. Frauenheilk. *42:* 273–279 (1982).

ROCK, J. A.: Female sterilization reversals. (Johns Hopkins University). Personal communication 1980.

ROCK, J. A., T. H. PARMLEY, T. M. KING, L. E. LAUFE, B. HSU: Endometriosis and the development of tubo-peritoneal fistulae after tubal ligation. Res. Triangel Park, North Carolina, Intern. Fertil. Res. Progr. 1980 (AID-DSPE-C-0054) 9.

ROITMAN, M. J.: Laparoscopic sterilization: falope ring technique. JAMA *76:* 735–738 (1977).

RUBINSTEIN, L. M., L. BENJAMIN, V. KLEINKOPF: Menstrual patterns and women's attitudes following sterilization by Falope Rings. Fertil. Steril. *31:* 641–646 (1979).

RUBINSTEIN, L. M., T. B. LEBHERZ, V. KLEINKOPF: Laparoscopic tubal sterilization: long-term postoperative follow-up. Contraception *13:* 631–638 (1976).

SAIDI, M. H. et al.: Laparoscopic tubal sterilization in unselected outpatients. Tex. Med. *74:* 55–57 (1978).

SCHARLAU, L.: Die laparoskopische Tubensterilisation – Methoden, Indikationen, Resultate von 500 Eingriffen. Med. Welt *27:* 1469–1472 (1976).

SCHLUND, G. H.: Nochmals: Zu Rechtsfragen bei der freiwiligen Sterilisation. Geburtsh. u. Frauenheilk. *38:* 587–590 (1978).

SEILER, J. S. et al.: Tubal sterilization by bipolar laparoscopy: report of 232 cases. Obstet. Gynec. *58:* 92–95 (1981).

SEMM, K.: Eileitersterilisation mittels Schwachstrom. Arch. Gynäk. *219:* 41 (1975).

SEMM, K.: Thermo-Coagulation avec l'Endo-Coagulator. Une nouvelle méthode pour la stérilisation pelviscopique. Gynécologie *27:* 279–282 (1976).

SEMM, K.: Methoden der Sterilisierung der Frau. Therapiewoche *26:* 195–203 (1976).

SEMM, K.: Sterilisierung im Wochenbett. Z. Geburtsh. Perinat. *160:* 167–182 (1976).

SEMM, K.: Conclusions d'une experimentale sur la stérilisation thermique transutérine. Gynécologie *27:* 283–385 (1976).

SEMM, K.: Endocoagulatio: a new and completely safe medical current for sterilization. Int. J. Fertil. *22:* 238–242 (1977).

SEMM, K.: Gefälligkeitssterilisation. Gynäc. Prax. *1:* 403 (1977).

SEMM, K., F. W. DITTMAR: Pelviskopische Sterilisation. Dtsch. Ärztebl. Mitt. *73:* 1–4 (1976).

SEMM, K., E. PHILIPP: Eileiterregeneration post sterilisationem. Geburtsh. u. Frauenheilk. *39:* 14–19 (1979).

SEMM, K., E. PHILIPP: Vermeidung von Spontanrekanalisation des Eileiters post sterilisationem. Gynäk. Prax. *4:* 63–74 (1980).

SEMM, K., V. RIMKUS, F. W. DITTMAR, L. METTLER: Komplikationen der pelviskopischen und hysteroskopischen Sterilisation. Arch. Gynäk. *224:* 38–39 (1977).

SHAIN, R. N.: Acceptability of reversible versus permanent tubal sterilization: an analysis of preliminary data. Fertil. Steril. *31:*13–17 (1979).

SIEGLER, A. M., R. J. PEREZ: Reconstruction of fallopian tubes in previously sterilized patients. Fertil. Steril *26:* 383–392 (1975).

SIEGLER, A. M.: Sterilization reversal (State University of New York, Downstate Medical Center), Personal communication 1980.

SINGH, K. B.: Tubal sterilization by laparoscopy. Five-year experience in university hospitals. N. Y. State J. Med. *76:* 1488–1492 (1976).

SINGH, K. B.: Tubal sterilization by laparoscopy. Simplified technique. N. Y. State J. Med. *77:* 194–196 (1977).

SMITH, A. M.: Laparoscopic sterilisation with silastic bands (letter). Brit. med. J. *1 (6071):* 1281 (1977).

SMITH, D. B. et al.: Sterilization by laparoscopic tubal electrocoagulation. A report of 1000 private patients. J. Arkansas Med. Soc. *73:* 384–387 (1977).

SODERSTROM, R. M. et al.: The snare method of laparoscopic sterilization: an analysis of 1000 cases with 4 failures. J. Reprod. Med. *18:* 246–250 (1977).

SOONAWALLA, F. P.: Reversal of male sterilization. IPPF Medical Bull. *12:* 3–4 (1978).

SPANN, W., W. BRAUN: Sterilisation: Die Pflicht des Arztes? Geburtsh. u. Frauenheilk. *38:* 591–592 (1978).

STOCK, R. J.: Evaluation of tubal ligation. Fertil. Steril. *29:* 169–174 (1978).

TATUM, H. J., F. H. SCHMIDT: Contraceptive and sterilization practices and extrauterine pregnancy: a realistic perspective. Fertil. Steril *28:* 407–421 (1977).

THATCHER, R. A.: Reversal of sterilization of the female (letter). Med. J. Austr. *1 (2):* 102 (1978).

THOMPSON, P., A. TEMPLETON: Characteristics of patients requesting reversal of sterilization. Brit. J. Obstet. Gynaec. *85:* 161–164 (1978).

UCHIDA, J.: Uchida Tubal Sterilization (on the basis of 24.000 operations). Presented at the 4th International Conference on Voluntary Sterilization, Seoul Korea, Mai 1979, S. 76.

URIBE-RAMIREZ, L. C. et al.: Female sterilization by laparoscopy. Ginecol. Obstet. Mex. *38:* 105–111 (1975).

URIBE-RAMIREZ, L. C. et al.: Outpatient laparoscopic sterilization: a review of complications on 2000 cases. J. Reprod. Med. *18:* 103–108 (1977).

URIBE-RAMIREZ, L. C. et al.: Bipolar coagulation. Technique of female sterilization by laparoscopy. Preliminary report of 100 cases. Ginec. Obstet. Mex. *43:* 243–249 (1978).

VÁGNER, Z.: Contribution to electrocoagulative sterilization of ovarian cysts by laparoscopy. Gynek. *41:* 681–682 (1976).

VASQUEZ, G., R. M. L. WINSTON, W. BOECKX: Tubal lesions subsequent to sterilization and their relation to fertility after attempts at reversal. Am. J. Obstet. Gynec. *138:* 86–92 (1980).

VERMA, L. B., H. N. AWASTHI, R. N. SRIVASTAVA: A follow-up study of sterilised cases in an urban community. Med. Surg. 19–22 (1977).

WATKINS , R. A., J. F. CORREY, D. A. WISE, G. J. PERKIN: Social and psychological changes after tubal sterilization: a reevaluation study on 425 women. Med. J. Austr. *2 (7):* 251–254 (1976).

WEIL, A.: Laparoscopic sterilization with therapeutic abortion versus sterilization or abortion alone. Obstet. Gynec. *52:* 79–82 (1978).

WHEELESS, C. R., jr.: Laparoscopically applied hemoclips for tubal sterilization. Obstet. Gynec. *44:* 752–756 (1974).

WHITELAW, R. G.: 10 year survey of 485 sterilisations. 2 Patients views on their sterilisation. Brit. med. J. *1 (6155):* 34–35 (1979).

WILLIAMS, G. F.: Tubocornual anastomosis for reversal of sterilisation (letter). Lancet *I (18008):* 422 (1977).

WILSON, P. C. M.: (North Parramatta, New South Wales Australia) Results of Australia sterilization reversal series. Personal communication 1980.

WINSTON, R. M. L.: Why 103 women asked for reversal of sterilisation. Brit. med. J. *2 (6082):* 305–307 (1977).

WINSTON, R. M. L.: Reversal of female sterilization. IPPF Medical Bull. *12:* 1–2 (1978).

WOOD, C., J. LEETON: Stérilisation par ovariotexie: une technique réversible. Gynec. Invest. *21:* 299–305 (1970).

YOON, I. B., C. R. WHEELESS, jr., T. M. KING: Preliminary report on a new laparoscopic sterilization approach: the silicone rubber band technique. Am. J. Obstet. Gynec. *120:* 132–136 (1976).

YOON, I. B. et al.: A two-year experience with the Falope ring sterilization procedure. Am. J. Obstet. Gynec. *127:* 109–112 (1977).

YOON, I. et al.: Laparoscopic tubal ligation. A follow-up report on the Yoon falope ring methodology. J. Reprod. Med. *23:* 76–80 (1979).

YUZPE, A. A. et al.: A review of 1.035 tubal sterilizations by posterior colpotomy under local anesthesia or by laparoscopy. J. Reprod. Med. *13:* 106–109 (1974).

YUZPE, A. A.: Choosing a sterilization procedure: laparoscopic tubal sterilization. J. Reprod. Med. *15:* 119–122 (1975).

ZABRANSKÝ, F.: Laparoscopic sterilization with the aid of the Yoon ring Cesk. Gynek. *45:* 231–233 (1980).

ZAKUT, H. et al.: Tubal sterilization with a clip applicator under laparoscopic control. Harefuah *94:* 262–264 (1978).

ZIEGLER, J. S. et al.: A comparison of the Falope ring and laparoscopic tubal cauterization. J. Reprod. Med. *20:* 237–238 (1978).

XIV. Complications With Sterilization by Pelviscopy

TE BREUIL, W., F. BOEMINGHAUS: Harnleiterläsion bei laparoskopischer Tubensterilisation. Geburtsh. u. Frauenheilk. *37:* 572–576 (1977).

CHAMBERLAIN, G. et al.: Late complications of sterilisation by laparoscopy. Lancet *II (7940):* 878 (1975).

CHAPIN, J. W. et al.: Hemorrhage and cardiac arrest during laparoscopic tubal ligation. Anesthesiology *53:* 342–343 (1980).

CHI, J., L. P. COLE: Incidence of pain among women undergoing laparoscopic sterilization by electrocoagulation, the spring-loaded clip, and the tubal ring. Am. J. Obstet. Gynec. *135:* 397–401 (1979).

CHI, I.-C., L. E. LAUFE, S. D. GARDNER, M. A. TOLBERT: An epidemiologic study of risk factors associated with pregnancy following female sterilization. Am. J. Obstet. Gynec. *136:* 768–773 (1980).

CHI, I. et al.: Uterine perforation during sterilization by laparoscopy and minilaparotomy. Am. J. Obstet. Gynec. *139:* 735–736 (1981).

CUNANAN, R. G., N. G. COUREY, J. LIPPES: Complications of laparoscopic tubal sterilization. Obstet. Gynec. *55:* 501–506 (1980).

DONNEZ, J., F. CASANAS-ROUX, J. FERIN: Lésions microscopiques tubaires après stérilisation laparoscopique: Gynéc. Obstet. *9:* 193–199 (1980).

EDGERTON, W. D.: Late complications of laparoscopic sterilization. J. Reprod. Med. *18:* 275–277 (1977).

EDGERTON, W. D.: Late complications of laparoscopic sterilization 2. J. Reprod. Med. *21:* 41–44 (1978).

FREILICH, T. H.: Possibility of burns during laparoscopic tubal sterilization. Am. J. Obstet. Gynec. *129:* 708–709 (1977).

GEORGITIS, J. W.: Two late complications of laparoscopic tubal ligation. J. Maine med. Assoc. *68:* 352–353 (1977).

HEJL, B. L. et al.: Immediate and late complications of laparoscopic sterilization. Ugeskr. Laeger *142:* 436–438 (1980).

HENKEL, B.: Typische Komplikationen bei der Tubensterilisierung per laparoscopiam mit dem Tupla Clip, Maßnahmen zu ihrer Vermeidung. Geburtsh. u. Frauenheilk. *39:* 892–896 (1979).

HIRSCH, H. A.: Verbrennungen bei der laparoskopischen Tubensterilisation und Möglichkeiten ihrer Vermeidung. Geburtsh. u. Frauenheilk. *34:* 345–349 (1974).

HULKA, J. F.: Studies in simpler tubocclusion methods. J. Obstet. Gynec. *122:* 337–348 (1975).

IRVIN, T. T., J. C. GLIGHER, J. S. SCOTT: Injury to the ureter during laparoscopic tubal sterilization. Arch. Surg. *110:* 1501–1503 (1975).

KOLMORGEN, K., H. R. HAUSWALD, O. HAVEMANN: Chronische Unterbauchbeschwerden der Frau, eine postlaparoskopische Analyse. Zbl. Gynäk. *98:* 1434–1440 (1976).

LAWSON, S., R. A. COLE, A. A. TEMPLETON: The effect of laparoscopic sterilization by diathermy or silastic bands on post-operative pain, menstrual symptoms and sexuality. J. Obstet. Gynec. *86:* 659–663 (1979).

LEIDAL, O.: Electric injuries during diathermy sterilization using the laparoscope. Tidsskr. Nor. Laegeforen *97:* 450–452 (1977).

LOW, L. C. et al.: Shoulder-hand syndrome after laparoscopic sterilization. Brit. med. J. *2 (6144):* 1059–1060 (1978).

LÜRMANN, K.: Der spastische Tubenverschluß im laparoskopischen Bild. Zbl. Gynäk. *101:* 1195–1199 (1979).

Maudsley, R. F. et al.: Thermal injury to the bowel as a complication of laparoscopic sterilization. Canad. J. Surg. *22:* 232–234 (1979).

McCausland, A.: High rate of ectopic pregnancy following laparoscopic tubal coagulation failures: incidence and etiology. Am. J. Obstet. Gynec. *136:* 97–101 (1980).

Mertz, A., R. Wiedemann, R. Eschbach: Effets éloignés de la stérilisation tubaire endoscopique. J. méd. Strasbourg *10:* 29–34 (1979).

Nilsen, P. A., F. Jerve: Tubensterilisation mit spezieller Berücksichtigung der Elektrokoagulation durch das Laparoskop. Acta obstet. gynec. scand. *55:* 349–353 (1976).

Peterson, H., H. B. Ory, J. R. Grenspan et al.: Todesfälle bei laparoskopischer Tubensterilisation durch monopolare Hochfrequenzkoagulation im Jahre 1978/79. Am. J. Obstet. Gynec. *139:* 141–143 (1981).

Phillips, J., L. Keith: The evolution of laparoscopic sterilization. Int. J. Gynaec. Obstet. *14:* 59–64 (1976).

Pigeau, F. et al.: Complications of per-celioscopic tubal sterilizations (letter). Nouv. Presse méd. *34:* 2251 (1976).

Pulido, M., J. M. Briceno: Hallazgos, accidentes y complicationes tardias en 3000 mujeres esterilizadas por el método de laparoscopia en forma ambulatoria. Rev. Colomb. Obstet. Ginec. *27:* 341–346 (1976).

Riedel, H.-H., K. Semm: Vorzeitiges Auftreten menopausaler Beschwerden in Abhängigkeit von verschiedenen Sterilisationstechniken – ein Vergleich zwischen dem Endokoagulations- und HF-Verfahren. Arch. Gynec. *232:* 229–230 (1981).

Riedel, H.-H., H. Ahrens, K. Semm: Spätkomplikationen nach Anwendung unterschiedlicher Sterilisationstechniken – ein Vergleich zwischen der unipolaren Hochfrequenzsterilisation und dem Endokoagulationsverfahren nach Semm. Geburtsh. u. Frauenheilk. *42:* 273–279 (1982).

Schneller, E., K. Felshart, S. Fischermann, U. Schwartz, K. H. Bruntsch: Operative Komplikationen der laparoskopischen Tubensterilisation mit dem Bleier-Clip (prospektive Studie). Geburtsh. u. Frauenheilk. *42:* 379–384 (1982).

Schwimmer, W. B.: Electrosurgical burn injuries during laparoscopic sterilization. Treatment and prevention. Obstet. Gynec. *44:* 526–530 (1974).

Shah, A. et al.: Pregnancy following laparoscopic tubal electrocoagulation and division. Am. J. Obstet. Gynec. *129:* 459–460 (1977).

Singh, K. B.: Laparoscopic tubal sterilization. Radiofrequency burns. N. Y. State J. Med. *77:* 190–192 (1977).

Sivanesaratnam, V.: Obeyed small bowel perforation following laparoscopic tubal cauterization. Int. Surg. *51:* 560–561 (1975).

Stengel, J. N. et al.: Ureteral injury. Complication of laparoscopic sterilisation. Urology *4:* 341–342 (1974).

Thompson, B. H. et al.: Failures of laparoscopy sterilization. Obstet. Gynec. *45:* 659–664 (1975).

Uribe-Ramirez, L. C. et al.: Outpatient laparoscopic sterilization: a review of complications in 2000 cases. J. Reprod. Med. *18:* 103–108 (1977).

Weil, A., U. Baumann, W. Schenk: Langzeiteffekt der bipolaren laparoskopischen Tubensterilisation auf die Menstruation. Arch. Gynäk. *227:* 141–146 (1979).

XV. Pelviscopy in Children

Christ, F. H., P. Kleissl, F. Eberlein, B. Kusch: Die Laparoskopie bei Jugendlichen und Kindern. In: W. Rösch: Fortschritt der Endoskopie. Straube, Erlangen 1976.

Gans, S. L.: A new look at pediatric endoscopy. Postgrad. Med. *61:* 91–98 (1977).

Karamehmedovic, O. et al.: Laproscopy in childhood. J. pediat. Surg. *12:* 75–81 (1977).

Kleinhaus, S. et al.: Laparoscopy for diagnosis and treatment of abdominal pain in adolescent girls. Arch. Surg. *112:* 1178–1179 (1977).

Leape, L. L. et al.: Laparoscopy in children. Pediatrics *66:* 215–220 (1980).

XVI. Pelviscopy—Appendectomy

de Kok, H. J.: A new technique for resecting the non-inflamed not-adhesive appendix through a mini-laparotomy with the laparoscope. Arch. Chir. Nederl. *29:* 195–198 (1977).

Kolmorgen, K. et al.: Akute und chronische Appendizitis; gynäkologische Laparoskopie. Zbl. Chir. *102:* 531–539 (1977).

Leape, L. L., M. L. Ramenofsky: Laparoscopy for questionable appendicitis: Can it reduce the negative appendectomy rate? Ann. Surg. *191:* 410 (1980).

Puder, H.: Die Erkrankung der Appendix und ihre Folgen aus gynäkologischer Sicht. (Erfahrungsbericht unter Berücksichtigung laparoskopischer Ergebnisse) Zbl. Gynäk. *103:* 902–908 (1981).

Schmidt, K. et al.: The contribution of laparoscopy in the differential diagnosis of adnexitis and appendicitis and in the conditions post-appendectomy. Cesk. Gynek. *39:* 664–665 (1974).

SEMM, K.: Die endoskopische Appendektomie. Gynäkol. Prax. *7:* 26–30 (1982).

SEMM, K.: Endoscopic appendectomy. Endoscopy *15:* 59–64 (1983).

XVII. Hystero-fetoscopy

BARBOT, J.: Hysteroscopie de Contact. Thése pour le Doctorat den Médecine, Paris 1975.

BENZIE, R. J., T. A. DORAN: The »fetoscope« – a new clinical tool for prenatal genetic diagnosis. Am. J. Obstet. Gynec. *121:* 460–464 (1975).

BRUESCHKE, E. E., H. E. FADEL, K. MAYERHOFER, F. C. SCRIBANO, J. T. ARCHIE, G. D. WILBANKS, L. J. D. ZANEVELD: Transcervical tubal occlusion with a steerable hysteroscope: implantation of devices into extirpated human uteri. Amer. J. Obstet. Gynec. *127:* 118–125 (1977).

CIBILS, L. A.: Permanent sterilization by hysteroscopic cauterization. Am. J. Obstet. Gynec. *121:* 513–520 (1975).

COHEN, M. R., W. P. DMOWSKI: Modern Hysteroscopy: diagnostic and therapeutic potential. Fertil. Steril. *24:* 905–909 (1973).

DARABI, K. F., R. M. RICHART: Collaborative study on hysteroscopic sterilization procedures. Obstet. Gynec. *49:* 48–54 (1977).

DAVIDSON, E. C. jr., J. A. MORRIS, J. P. O'GRADY, J. P. HENDRICKX, A. G. ANDERSON, J. KABACK, R. FRAZER: Sampling the fetoplacental. circulation-III combined laparoscopy-fetoscopy in the pregnant macaque for hemoglobin. identification. Am. J. Obstet. Gynec. *132:* 833–843 (1978).

GUSTAVI, B., E. CORDESIUS: Transvaginal Fetoscopy in anterior placentas. Acta obstet. gynec. scand. *59:* 231–235 (1980).

HAMOU, J. E.: Microhysteroscopy – a new technique in endoscopy and its applications. Acta endoscop. *X–N:* 415–422 (1980).

HAMOU, J.: Microhysteroscopy. J. Reprod. Med. *26:* 375–382 (1981).

HAMOU, J.: Hysteroscopy and microhysteroscopy with a new instrument: the microhysteroscope. Acta. europ. fertil. *12:* 29–58 (1981).

HEPP, H., H. ROLL: Die Hysteroskopie. Gynäkologe *7:* 166–170 (1974).

HEPP, H., G. HOFFMANN, R. KREIENBERG, P. BROCKERHOFF: Möglichkeiten und Grenzen der Hysteroskopie in der Diagnostik des Korpuskarzinoms. Fortschr. Med. *95:* 2113–2116 (1977).

HOBBINS, J. C., M. J. MAHONEY, L. A. GOLDSTEIN: New method of intrauterine evaluation by the combined use of fetoscopy and ultrasound. Am. J. Obstet. Gynec. *118:* 1069–1072 (1974).

HOBBINS, J. C., M. J. MAHONEY: Fetoscopy in continuing pregnancies. Am. J. Obstet. Gynec. *129:* 440–442 (1977).

JENSEN, M., V. ZAHN: Fetoskopie, eine neue Methode in der pränatalen Diagnostik. Münch. med. Wschr. *118:* 625–628 (1976).

LANCET, M., N. MASS: Concomitant hysteroscopy and hysterography in Asherman's Syndrome. Int. J. Fertil. *26:* 267–272 (1981).

LEVINE, M. D., D. E. MCNEIL, M.M. KABACK, R. E. FRAZER, D. M. OKADA, C. J. HOBEL: Second-trimester fetoscopy and fetal blood sampling: current limitations and problems. Am. J. Obstet. Gynec. *120:* 937–943 (1974).

LINDEMANN, H.-J., J. MOHR: Ergebnisse von 274 transuterinen Tubensterilisationen per Hysteroskop. Geburtsh. u. Frauenheilk. *34:* 775–779 (1974).

LINDEMANN, H.-J., J. MOHR: CO_2-Hysteroscopy: diagnosis and treatment. Am. J. Obstet. Gynec. *124:* 129–133 (1976).

LINDEMANN, H.-J.: Die Sterilisationsmethoden bei der Frau; Möglichkeiten der hysteroskopischen Sterilisation. Münch. med. Wschr. *118:* 903–906 (1976).

LINDEMANN, H.-J., A. GALLINAT: Physikalische und physiologische Grundlagen der CO_2-Hysteroskopie. Geburtsh. u. Frauenheilk. *36:* 729–737 (1979).

LINDEMANN, H.-J., J. MOHR, A. GALLINAT, M. BUROS: Der Einfluß von CO_2-Gas während der Hysteroskopie. Geburtsh. u. Frauenheilk. *36:* 153–162 (1976).

LINDEMANN, H.-J.: Hysteroskopie. Arch. Gynäk. *232:* 52–53 (1981).

MARCH, C. M., R. ISRAEL, A. D. MARCH: Hysteroscopy management of intrauterine adhesions. Am. J. Obstet. Gynec. *130:* 653–657 (1978).

MORRIS, A., E. C. DAVIDSON, jr., E. MAIDMAN, J. J. ARCE, J. E. BROWN, R. FRAZER: Sampling the fetalplacental circulation. II. combined laparoscopy-fetoscopy in pregnant ovine. Am. J. Obstet. Gynec. *128:* 279–286 (1977).

NEUBÜSER, D., P. BALLER, K. BOSSELMANN: Erfahrungen über die hysteroskopische Tubensterilisation. Geburtsh. u. Frauenheilk. *37:* 809–812 (1977).

PATRICK, J. E., T. B. PERRY, R. A. H. KINCH: Fetoskopie und fetale Blutuntersuchung: eine percutane Methode. Am. J. Obstet. Gynec. *119:* 539–542 (1974).

PHILLIPS, J. M.: The impact of laparoscopy, hysteroscopy, fetoscopy and culdoscopy on gynecologic practice. J. Reprod. Med. *16:* 187–190 (1976).

PHILLIPS, J. M.: Fetoscopy: its genesis and promise. J. Reprod. Med. *21:* 115–122 (1978).

QUINONES, R. G., A. D. ALVARADO, E. LEY: Tubal electrocoagulation under hysteroscopic control (threehundredfifty cases). Am. J. Obstet. Gynec. *121:* 111–113 (1975).

RAUSKOLB, R.: Fetoskopie: Klinische Erfahrungen. Geburtsh. u. Frauenheilk. *37:* 304–311 (1977).

RAUSKOLB, R.: Fetoskopie unter Sichtkontrolle im Ultraschall. Dtsch. med. Wschr. *102:* 1341–1344 (1977).

RAUSKOLB, R., W. FUHRMANN: Die Fetoskopie. Z. Geburtsh. Perinat. *182:* 243–262 (1978).

RAUSKOLB, R.: Die Fetoskopie. Arch. Gynäk. *232:* 53–54 (1981).

REED, T. P., R. A. ERB: Hysteroscopic oviductal blocking with formed-in-place silicone rubber plugs. 2. Clinical studies. J. Reprod. Med. *23:* 6972 (1979).

RIMKUS, V., K. SEMM: Hysteroscopic sterilization – a routine method. Int. J. Fertil. *22:* 121–124 (1977).

RUDECK, C., C. HOLEMAN, J. KARNACKI: Direct intravascular fetal blood transfusion by fetoscopy in severe rhesus isoimmunisation. Lancet *I:* 625–627 (1981).

SCIARRA, J. J., R. F. VALLE: Hysteroscopy: a clinical experience with 320 patients. Am. J. Obstet. Gynec. *127:* 340–348 (1977).

SEKI, M., H.-H. RIEDEL, J. VIEHWEG, L. METTLER, K. SEMM: Ein Vergleich der Flüssigkeits- und CO_2-Hysteroskopie bei Blutungsanomalien im reproduktiven Alter. Arch. Gynäk. *232:* 741–742 (1980).

SEMM, K.: Kontakt-hysteroskopische Fetoskopie. Tägl. Prax. *20:* 93–95 (1979).

SIEGLER, A., E. KEMMANN: Hysteroscopy. Obstet. Gynec. Surg. *30:* 567–588 (1975).

SUGIMOTO, O.: Hysteroscopic diagnosis of endometrial carcinoma. A report of fifty-three cases examined at the women's clinic of Kyoto University Hospite. Am. J. Obstet. Gynec. *121:* 105–113 (1975).

WALLENBURG, H., C. S. JAHODA, M. G. J. JAHODA, E. S. SACHS, M. F. NIERMEIJER: Die Grenzen der Sichtbarmachung des gesamten Feten bei der Fetoskopie im mittleren Schwangerschaftsdrittel. Arch. Gynäk. *222:* 1–4 (1977).

YUKI, T.: Dysfunctional uterine bleeding on diagnostic hysteroscopy. Acta obstet. gynaec. jap. *32:* 225–233 (1980).

ZWINGER, A., J. E. JIRASEK, J. ZIDOVSKY, C. JUNGMANOVA: Fetoscopy in prenatal diagnostics of inborn evolutive anomalies. Cesl. Gynek. *42:* 644–648 (1977).

XVIII. Photo Documentation and Training

CLAPPER, D.: Education in Gynecology and Obstetrics. Change in female sterilization equipment supplies. (Johns Hopkins Program for International Education in Gynecology and Obstetrics). Personal communication, June 24, 1980.

ESPOSITO, J. M.: An inexpensive method for documenting laparoscopic findings. J. Reprod. Med. *16:* 269–270 (1976).

EPSTEIN, L. C.: Orientation in endoscopy. Endoscopy *13:* 77–80 (1981).

HULKA, J. F., J. P. MERCER, J. K. FISHBURNE, TH. KUMARASAMY, J. R. DINGFELDER: Regional training program of laparoscopy: Impact on regional care. Fertil. Steril. *28:* 29–31 (1977).

KATZ, D. L. et al.: The use of a flexible teaching head for video laparoscopy. J. Med. Educ. *52:* 859–860 (1977).

KEMP, J.: Photography as a method of recording and improving skill in laparoscopy. J. Med. Aust. *2:* 491–493 (1977).

LANGLOIS, P.: Coeliophotographies. Bull. Src. Sci. med. Luxemburg: 104–105 (1967).

LEVENTHAL, J. M.: Documentation of laparoscopy with polaroid cinematography. J. Reprod. Med. *26:* 5–9 (1981).

OH, C.: Johns Hopkins Program for International Education in Gynecology and Obstetrics—Supply of Minilaparotomy Kits. Personal communication 1980.

OTT, W. J. et al.: Diagnostic laparoscopy in a university training program. Case report. Mo. Med. *72:* 545–549 (1979).

PENT, D. et al.: Documents and documentation in laparoscopy. J. Reprod. Med. *18:* 90–94 (1977).

POLAK, M.: Laparoscopic photography on infra-red sensitive film. Z. Gastroenterol. *13:* 679–680 (1975).

ROCK, J. A.: Training Program in Microsurgery for Tubal Reconstruction. Baltimore, Maryland, Johns Hopkins Hospital 1979, S. 29 (unveröffentlicht).

ROLAND, M., ST. M. KURZER, D. V. M. JOHN, J. M. LEVENTHAL: Automated still photography for endoscopy. Int. J. Fertil. *26:* 245–249 (1981).

SEMM, K.: Die Geschichte des endoskopischen Fotos. Dtsch. Ärztebl. – Ärztl. Mittlg. *79:* 132–134 (1982).

SEMM, K.: Das endoskopische Foto als Schrittmacher der endoskopischen Abdominal-Chirurgie. Dtsch. Ärztebl. *80:* 70–71 (1983).

TITTELT, J. F.: Le système 110 mm oldelft, standardisation de l'enregistrement diagnostic sur film simple 110 mm Acta endoscop. *IX:* 49–51 (1979).

ULBRICH, R. et al.: Necessity of training and safety in gynecological laparoscopy – a contradiction? Fortschr. Med. *97:* 2129–2131 (1979).

WARNER, E. et al.: Increasing image size in laparoscopic photography. J. Biol. Photogr. *48:* 27–29 (1980).

Key to Endoscopic Color Photographs

SYMBOLIC CODES IN LINE DRAWINGS

▨ = Instruments

▦ = Anatomical site before or after surgery

■ = Blood

✷ = Endometriotic implants

✺ = Endometriotic implants after coagulation

▨ = Blue dye solution from chromopertubation

NUMERALS IN LINE DRAWINGS

1 = Uterine corpus
2 = Left fallopian tube
3 = Right fallopian tube
4 = Left tubal ampulla
5 = Right tubal ampulla
6 = Sactosalpinx (clubbed tube)
7 = Hydrosalpinx
8 = Left ovary
9 = Right ovary
    a = Maturing follicle
    b = Corpus luteum
    c = Ovarian endometriosis (chocolate cyst)
    d = Retention cyst
    e = Convoluted ovarian surface
10 = Epoophoron, Parovarium

11 = Parovarian cyst
12 = Uterovesical pouch
13 = Cul-de-sac of Douglas
14 = Left round ligament
15 = Right round ligament
16 = Left uterosacral ligament
17 = Right uterosacral ligament
18 = Infundibulo-ovarian ligament
19 = Utero-ovarian ligament
20 = Infundibulopelvic ligament
21 = Lateral umbilical ligament
22 = Broad ligament of uterus
23 = Mesosalpinx
24 = Dome of bladder
25 = Rectal ampulla
26 = Sigmoid colon
27 = Loop of small intestines
28 = Greater omentum
29 = Ascending colon
30 = Appendix
31 = Fatty tissue
32 = Liver (right lobe)
33 = Liver (left lobe)
34 = Gallbladder
35 = Myoma (subserous)
36 = Myoma (intramural)
37 = Hydatid cyst of Morgagni
38 = Genital ridge
39 = Emphysema caused by CO_2 insufflation
40 = Adhesions
41 = Blue dye solution (chromopertubation)
42 = Varicosities
43 = Metastatic carcinoma
44 = Scars in broad ligament (Allen-Masters syndrome)

45 = Ascitic fluid
46 = Myometrial infiltration of dye solution
47 = Varicocele
48 = Diaphragm
49 = Ureter
50 = Extrauterine pregnancy
51 = Contents of ''chocolate cyst''
52 = Bladder catheter
53 = Arcuate line of pelvis
54 = Exudate in cul-de-sac of Douglas
55 = Blood
56 = Tubal stump (also 110)
57 = Physiologic saline solution
58 = Endoloop
59 = Parietal peritoneum
60 = Trocar sleeve
61 = Fascia of muscle
62 = Ovarian pedicle
63 = Dermoid cyst
64 = Arcuate uterus
65 = Bicornuate uterus
66 = Coagulated tissue
67 = Falope-Ring (Yoon ring)
68 = Atraumatic grasping forceps
69 = Falciform ligament of the liver
70 = Transverse colon
71 = Crocodile forceps
72 = Adenomyosis of the tube
73 = Obturator nerve
74 = External iliac artery
75 = Transection of tube after coagulation
76 = Corpus luteum of pregnancy
77 = Mesenteriolum of appendix
78 = Rudimentary uterine horn
79 = Point coagulator
80 = Uterine aplasia
81 = Atraumatic suction probe
82 = Biopsy forceps
83 = Hook scissors
84 = Threaded dilator
85 = Pelviscope/Laparoscope

86 = Curette
87 = Tissue punch
88 = Endosuture with knot tied externally
89 = Endosuture with knot tied internally
90 = Endoligature
91 = Push rod for slipknot
92 = Right external iliac artery
93 = Fetus
94 = Needle holder: 5 mm diameter
95 = Needle holder: 3 mm diameter
96 = Aspiration needle
97 = Claw forceps
98 = Taenia of colon
99 = Purse string suture
100 = Cecum
101 = Veress needle
102 = Epiploic appendix
103 = Tip of trocar
104 = Large needle in abdominal wall
105 = Spoon forceps
106 = Guide rod for threaded dilator
107 = Blood vessel
108 = Irrigation fluid
109 = Hematosalpinx
110 = Tubal stump (also 56)
111 = Ovarian biopsy
112 = IUD
113 = Chorionic tissue
114 = Irrigation-suction cannula
115 = Ovum at time of spontaneous ovulation
116 = Bipolar coagulation forceps for high-fre-
      quency current
117 = Mesovarium with ovarian plexus
118 = Clip
119 = Clip applicator
120 = Ring applicator
121 = Ileum
122 = Uterine cavity
123 = Tubal ostium
124 = IUD tail
125 = Vaginal stent of dilator

Index

A

Abdomen, irrigation of, 76–77
Abdominal cavity, reasons for
    not using, 82–88
Abdominal-pelvic endoscopy, 2
Abdominal surgery, endoscopic
    (*See* Endoscopic abdom-
    inal surgery)
Abdominal wall, preparation of,
    for diagnostic procedure,
    131
Abdominoscopy, 2
Abortion
  tubal, 190, 191
Acidosis, 41
  during insufflation, 65
Adenoma
  cervical, 187
    enucleation of, with suture
     of uterus, 374
  cornual, 278
Adenomyomas, 161
Adenomyosis, 79, 306
  tubal, 280
  of tubal cornu, 161
  uterine, 278
Adhesiolysis, 13
  bleeding with, 264
  bloodless, 215
  of bowel, after hemostasis,
    424
  endoscopic, in preparation for
    laparotomy, 270, 272,
    274
  intestinal, 215–216
    and enucleation of myoma,
     376
    intestinal suture and,
     420–434
    without prior hemostasis,
     420, 421
  intra-abdominal, 10

omental, 152, 214–215
omental and intestinal, and
    enucleation of myoma,
    376
pelviscopic in preparation for
    laparotomy, 156
postoperative, 260
  intestinal, 14
with and without prior he-
    mostasis, 274
with prophylactic hemostasis,
    154–156, 266
without prophylactic hemosta-
    sis, 152–154, 262
salpingostomy and, 302,
    304
of small intestine, 320
uterine, 378, 380
Adhesion prophylaxis, 216
Adhesions
  abdominal
    in patients awaiting in vitro
     fertilization, 198
    after surgery to correct ste-
     rility, 304
  after appendectomy, 216
  of bowel
    lysis of, after hemostasis,
     428, 430, 432
    lysis of, after hemostasis
     with peritoneal suture,
     432, 434
  after chocolate cyst excision,
    320
  after endometriosis operation,
    235
  fundal, 156
  after gallbladder surgery,
    216
  intestinal
    lysis of, 420 (*see also* Ad-
     hesiolysis, intestinal)
  intestinal-ovarian, 215

lysis of
  with hemostasis, 266, 268,
    270
  without prior hemostasis,
    264, 266, 272
omental, 152, 154, 270, 274,
    296
  lysis of, with and without
    hemostasis, 424, 426,
    428
perihepatic, 216
  lysis of, 224, 446, 448
peritoneal, 94, 274, 302
postoperative intestinal/omen-
    tal, 155
tubo-ovarian, 290
in umbilical region, 150
vascular bridges of, 96
velamentous, 139, 163, 288
Adnexa
  biologic changes in area of,
    after high-frequency co-
    agulation, 88–90
  resection of, 328
Adolescent, indications for en-
    doscopic abdominal sur-
    gery in, 29–32
Ambulation, patient, 40
American Fertility Society clas-
    sification of Endometrio-
    sis, 157–160
Ampullary phimosis, 292
Ampullary stenosis, 292
Anastomosis
  end-to-end, 156
Anesthesia
  administered by anesthesiolo-
    gist, 40–41
  administered by surgeon,
    37–40
  caudal block, 40
  endotracheal, psychological
    preparation of patient

Anesthesia *(cont.)*
  for, 21
  endotracheal inhalation, 241
  epidural block, 40
  general inhalation, 40–41
  intubation, 228
  local
    effectiveness of, 39
    in presence of abdominal
      pain, 22
    reasons for selecting, 38
    safety of, 39
  patient agreement about, 17
  patient intolerance of, 35
  patient's fear of, 21
  pneumoperitoneum factors af-
    fecting choice of, 66
  regional block, 40
  spinal block, 40
  topical, 39
Anesthesia incident
  incorrect diagnosis of, 146
  procedure following, 146
Anesthesiologist
  anesthesia administration and,
    17
Animal electricity, 83
Antibiotic therapy
  preoperative, 36
Antigonadotropin therapy, 306
Aorta
  abdominal, palpation of, 68
  bifurcation of, 66
Aorta palpation test, 133
Appendectomy, 14
  adhesions following, 216
  endoscopic, 216–222, 434,
    444
    indications for, 217, 434,
      436
    instruments for, 222–224
    postoperative care, 238
  endoscopic operative proce-
    dures applicable to, 32
  orthograde, 217–221
  prophylactic, 217
  retrograde, 221–222
  therapeutic, 217
Appendicitis
  diagnosis of, 32
Appendix
  endometriosis in, 161
  indications for endoscopic re-
    moval of, 32
  instruments for extracting,
    118, 120
  perforation of, 264
    discovered by laparoscopy,
      32

vermiform, 216
Appendix extractor, 118–120,
  218, 219, 220
Aquapurator aspiration apparatus, 76, 77, 117, 124,
  312, 314, 330
Aquapurator aspiration flash,
  172
Aspiration
  instruments for, 108, 110,
    111
  of ovarian cyst, 310, 312
  of ovum
    for in vitro fertilization,
      79–80
Aspiration needle, 108, 110
Aspiration test, 134–135
Atraumatic suction manipulator,
  108
Autoclaving
  of endoscope, 59, 60

B

Baths
  warm water, 124
Biopsy
  after cytostatic chemotherapy,
    224
  forceps, 107, 108
  gonadal, 212
  of liver, 224, 444, 446
  ovarian, 11
    pelviscopic, 169–171, 308,
      310
  of peritoneal metastases, 224,
    444
  tubal, 202
Bipolar forceps, 82
Bladder dome
  coagulation of, 162
  endometriotic implants in,
    286
  enucleation of myoma from,
    378
  injury to, 114
  perforation in peritoneum of,
    260
Bleeding (*See also* Hemorrhage)
  with adhesiolysis, 264
  from endometriotic implants,
    292
  after myoma removal, 186
  in omentum, 154
  postoperative, pelviscopy in
    diagnosis of, 33
  from right ovarian artery,
    338

withdrawal, after endometriosis, 236
Bleeding disorders
  severe, as contraindication to
    endoscopic surgery, 35
Bleier clip, 208, 209
  for tubal sterilization, 414
Blind puncture method, 147
  safety tests with, 132–133
Blood pressure, drop in, 146
Blood vessels
  ovarian, damage of, in sal-
    pingectomy, 274
  uterine, blue dye in, 79
Bowel
  adhesiolysis of, after hemo-
    stasis, 424
  adhesions of
    lysis of, after hemostasis,
      428, 430, 432
    lysis of, after hemostasis
      with peritoneal suture,
      432, 434
    lysis of, with and without
      hemostasis, 424, 426,
      428
  endometriotic implants on,
    161
  preoperative evacuation of
    18, 22–23
  preoperative preparation of,
    237
Breast carcinoma, 344, 350

C

Cameras
  movie, 247
  reflex, 58, 244
  single-tube video, 247
  triple-tube color television,
    248
Candida salpingitis, 18
Cannula(s)
  for abdominal or pelvic irri-
    gation, 76
  single-channel/dual-purpose
    irrigation/aspiration, 76,
    108, 174
  vacuum intra-uterine, 77, 78,
    103, 104, 131
Carbon dioxide
  for insufflation, 65
    effects of, 65
    volume used, 74
  subphrenic collection of,
    230
    discomfort from, 230
Carbonization effect, 87, 94

Carcinoma
   breast, 344, 350
   ovarian
      as contraindication to en-
         doscopic surgery, 35–36
Cardiac arrest
   during insufflation, 66
   during laparoscopy, 146
   procedure following, 146,
      147
   during surgery, 120
Cardiac insufficiency, 36
Castration, 200
   by bilateral oophorectomy,
      334
Catgut suture, 96, 114
   in pelviscopic salpingostomy,
      168
Catheter
   cervical balloon, 124
   transfer, 118
Caudal block anesthesia, 40
Cautery
   Paquelin's, 80
Celioscopy, 2
Celiotonometer, development
   of, 63
Cervical adenoma, 187
   enucleation of, with suture of
      uterus, 374
Cervical balloon catheter,
   124
Cervical coagulator, 94
Chocolate cysts, 171, 172
   excision of, 318, 320, 322
      and treatment of sterility,
         320, 322
Chorionic tissue, removal of,
   191–193
Chromopertubation, 124, 278
Chromosalpingoscopy, 18, 79,
   131, 278
α-Chymotrypsin powder, 231
Cinematographic documenta-
   tion, 57–58, 242–248
Cinematographic recording
   light source for, 51–53
Clamps, vascular, 120, 121
Claw forceps, 107, 108
Clips
   Blier, 208, 209
   hemostasis by, 102–103
   Hulka (*see* Hulka clip)
   tantalum, 206–207
Coagulation, 85, 86
   bipolar high-frequency, tubal
      sterilization by,
      202–203, 408
   of bladder dome, 162

blood
   use of destructive heat for,
      81–82
   of endometriotic implants,
      13, 161–163, 280, 282,
      284, 286, 330
   of fallopian tubes, 199
   high-frequency, 2, 258
      biologic changes in adnexa
         area following, 88–90
      in general surgery, 82
   instruments for, 117
   interval tubal sterilization by,
      203–205
   of retro-ovarian endometriotic
      implants, 162–163
   thermal, endometriotic im-
      plants and, 286
   of tubal pedicle, 362
   unipolar, high-frequency
      tubal sterilization by,
      201–202, 406, 408
Coagulation circuit, high-frequency, 6, 7
Coagulation forceps, 86
Coagulation necrosis, 87
Coagulation temperature, selection of, 93
Coagulation time, selection of,
   93
Coagulator
   cervical, 94
   point, 93, 94, 117, 158
Communication
   vocal, with use of volonelge-
      sia, 38
Conception
   products for removal of, 388,
      392
Conductors for electromagnetic
   waves, 82–83
CO_2 gas insufflation, 164
CO_2 PNEU Automatic Insuffla-
   tor, 62, 72
Consent, patient, preoperative,
   21
Cornual adenoma, 278
Cortisone
   for adhesion prophylaxis,
      216
   after gynecologic surgery,
      230
Critical temperature, 87
Crocodile forceps, 93, 94, 117
   in interval tubal sterilization,
      203
Cul-de-Sac of Douglas
   insufflation of, 69–70, 256
Culdoscopy, development of, 5

Currents
   eddy, effects of, 83, 85
   high-frequency
      biophysical reasons for not
         using, 82–88
      bipolar, 87
      burns from, 93
      coagulation by, 258
      effect of heat produced by,
         86
      medical reasons for not us-
         ing, 90–92
      in ovarian biopsy, 170
      problems with, 80
      in removal of coagulation
         necrosis, 87
      risks of, 3, 211
      tubal sterilization by,
         88–89, 199
   unipolar high-frequency, 7
      tubal sterilization by, 256
Cutting, instrument for, 111
Cystic endometrioma, 310
Cystic teratoma, 314, 326
Cysts
   avascular (serosal), 197
   chocolate (*see* Chocolate
      cyst)
   dermoid (*see* Dermoid cyst)
   endometrial, 318
   granulosa-theca cell, 312
   hydatid, of morgagni
      excision of, 195–197, 398
   ovarian (*see* Ovarian cyst)
   parovarian
      excision of, 197, 400, 402
      pelviscopic excision of,
         402
   serosal, excision of, 400
   serous cyst-adenoma, 171
   theca-lutein, 171, 172
Cytostatic chemotherapy
   biopsy following, 224

D

D & C procedure
   following tubal sterilization,
      89
Dermoid cysts, 171–173
   enucleation of, 316, 322,
      324, 326
Diagnosis
   differential
      pelviscopy in, 33
   endoscopes for, 53–54
   in endoscopic abdominal sur-
      gery, 130–151
   endoscopic procedures in, 20

Diagnosis *(cont.)*
  endoscopic, questions leading
    to, 28–29
  intra-abdominal, endoscopes
    for, 53
  second and third punctures to
    establish, 150–151
Diagnostic pelviscopy
  indications for endoscopic
    abdominal surgery based
    on, 28–29
Diagnostic phase
  preparing patient for, 21
Diagnostic scan
  second, 147–149
Diagnostic set for endoscopy,
  125–126
Diaphragm
  elevation of, 41
  uncontrolled elevation of,
    65
Diet
  before surgical procedure,
    22
Differential diagnosis, pelvis-
    copy in, 33
Dilatation
  of abdominal incision, 116
  blunt
    salpingoplasty/salpingos-
      tomy by, 296, 300
    of tubal ampulla, 294
  instruments for, 114–117,
    260
  trocar sleeve, risk of, 260
  of tubal ampulla, 290
Dilatation sets, 151
Dilatation trocar
  in salpingectomy for hydro-
    salpinx, 364
Dilator
  threaded, 114, 116
Dissemination of endometrial
  particles, 18
Documentation
  cinematographic, 57–58
  of endoscopic abdominal sur-
    gery, 242–248
  intra-abdominal
    endoscope for, 57–58
Douglas, Cul-de-Sac of
  insufflation of, 69–70

E

Ectopic pregnancy *(See also*
    Tubal pregnancy)

  conservative treatment of,
    190
  in distal tubal ampulla, 191
  middle segment of tube,
    191–193
  conservative operation for,
    386, 388, 390, 392,
    394
Eddy currents, effects of, 83,
  85
Electric knife, 85
Electricity
  animal, 83
Electrolysis, 83
Electromagnetic imaging,
  247
Electronic insufflator, 15
Electrotomy, 85, 86
Embolism
  risk of during insufflation,
    65
Embryo, transfer of, 118
Embryo transfer set, 118
Emergency laparoscopy,
  226–227
Emphysema
  mediastinal, 134
  peritoneal, 67
  preperitoneal, 133
Endocoagulation, 46
  advantage of, 163
  controlled, equipment for,
    92–93
  in endometriosis, 286
  hemostasis by, 258
  interval tubal sterilization by,
    408, 410
  and pelviscopic operations on
    uterus, 184
  postoperative follow-up of,
    89–91
  and poststerilization syn-
    drome, 199–200
  tubal sterilization by, 88–89
    postoperative condition af-
      ter, 410, 412
Endocoagulator, 93, 124
Endoligature, 46, 156
  hemostasis by, 96–98
Endoloop, 95, 97
  in adhesiolysis, 153
  hemostasis by ligation with,
    258, 260
  tubal ligation by, 206
Endoloop ligation, 46, 113
Endometrial particles
  dissemination of, 18
Endometrioma, cystic, 310

Endometriosis
  American Fertility Society
    classification of,
    157–160
  endoscopic tubal surgery in
    presence of, 169
  genital, 169
  genital tract, 292, 294
  hormonal therapy of, 236
  intestinal, 278
  intramural nodule of, 292
  ovarian, 284
    salpingo-oophorectomy for,
      350
  paracervical, 161
  pelvic
    procedures to treat, 19
    and thermocolor test, 448
    postoperative care for,
      235–237
  retrocervical, 276
  retrovaginal, 161
  sterility caused by, 235
  superficial, 288
  superficial pelvic
    endoscopic operative man-
      agement of, 157–163
  theories on development of,
    157
  thermocolor test for identify-
    ing, 286
  tubal patency in presence of,
    308
  tubal surgery in presence of,
    308, 310
Endometriotic implants, 235
  in bladderdome, 286
  bleeding from, 292
  coagulation of, 13, 161–163,
    280, 282, 284, 286, 330
  excision of, 158, 161, 276,
    278, 280
  hormonal suppression of, 157
  ovum nidation on, 195
  peritoneal, 163
  removal of, 280, 282, 284
  retrocervical
    excision of, 308
  retro-ovarian, 284
    coagulation of, 162–163
  superficial abrasion and bi-
    opsy of, 276
Endoscope
  blind introduction of trocar
    for, 141–144
  cleansing of, 124
  exchange of diagnostic for
    operative, 151

headband accessory for, 55, 56
for intra-abdominal diagnosis, 53–54
introduction of, 144–147
limitations of, 24
manually supported by assistant, 56–57
operating, 54–55
  advantages of, 54
  Palmer-Jacobs type, 54, 55
preparation of, 58–59
sleeves for, 106–107
sterilization and maintenance of, 59–61
support of, for bimanual operation, 55–57
for surgery, 54–55
warming of, 124
warming device for, 124–125
Endoscopic abdominal surgery
absolute contraindications to, 35
anesthesia for, 37–41
catalog of possible procedures, 151–152
complications of, preparing patient for, 21
course of, 130–213
decision for, 151
diagnostic phase of, 130–151
  preparing patient for, 21
documentation of, 242–248
endoscopes for, 54–55
general, 214–224
  postoperative care after, 237–238
general surgical procedures in, 19
gynecologic elective procedures, 18
indications for, 28–34
  on adnexa, 29–31
  in adolescents and infants, 31–32
  catalog of, 33
  correction of sterility, 31
  on uterine corpus, 29
informing patient about, 16–17, 20
informing patient of risks of, 17
instrument preparation for, 126–129
instruments for, 106–123
legal decisions affecting, 16
medical requirements for, 24–26

operating team for, 27
operative phase of, 151–212
postoperative care, 228–238
preparing patient for, 20–23
recovery and restoration to working capacity after, 239–240
relative contraindications to, 35–36
repeated, 241
requirements for, 25
restrictions affecting, 24
risk assessment in, 249–250
timing of, 18–19
training levels in, 249
Endoscopic adapter device, 129
Endoscopic endometriosis classification, 157–161
classification I, 158
classification II, 158
classification III, 158
classification IV, 158
  postoperative treatment of, 235
Endoscopic fimbrioplasty, 163–164
Endoscopic image
low-power loupe magnification of, 57
Endoscopic microsurgery, 57
Endoscopic procedure(s)
as diagnostic measure, 20
Endoscopic salpingostomy, 164–168
Endoscopy
diagnostic set for, 125–126
establishing operating room for, 124–129
flexible, in abdominal surgery, 54
historical review, 5–15
transition from, to laparotomy in same operation, 225–227
Endoscopy cart, 124
Endosutures, 96, 97, 114, 156
hemostasis by, 98–102
in pelviscopic salpingostomy, 168
in salpingoplasty/salpingostomy, 298
Endotracheal anesthesia
psychological preparation of patient for, 21
Epidural block anesthesia, 40
Equipment
for controlled endocoagulation, 92–93

for endoscopic abdominal surgery, 46–53
for intra-abdominal irrigation, 76–80
for thermal hemostasis, 80–95
Evaluation imonocular (*see* Monocular evaluation)
Exsiccation effect, 87, 94, 201

F

Fallopian tube
anatomy of, 200, 203
coagulation of, 199
distention of, 296
Falope-Ring, 209–210
Faraday's law, 83, 84
Fertilization, in vitro (*see* In vitro fertilization)
Fiberglass cables, coherent, 47
Fiber optic light cable, integrated, 50, 57
Fibrinogenemia, 33
Fimbrial suture, 102
Fimbriolysis, blunt, 292
Fimbrioplasty, 10, 198
endoscopic, 163–164, 292, 294, 296
Fistula, tubal, 192, 201, 308
Flashtube, spherical, 50
Flexible optical attachment, 24, 25
Follicle
mature, puncture and aspiration of, 198
puncture of for oocyte aspiration, 402, 404
spontaneous rupture of, 404
Follicle puncture
instruments for, 117–118
Forceps
atraumatic grasping, 107
biopsy, 107, 108
bipolar, 82
claw, 107, 108
coagulation, 86
crocodile (*see* Crocodile forceps)
heated tubal, 9
spoon, 107, 109
Formalin tablets, 59
Fulguration, 85

G

Galvanic current, 81
Gas
inadequate absorption of, 229

Gas *(cont.)*
  insufflation, volume of, 65
  selection of, for pneumoperi-
    toneum, 64–66
Gastric ptosis, 41
Generator
  high-frequency, 81, 85
Genital endometriosis, 169
Genitalia
  external
    preparation of, for diag-
      nostic procedure,
      130–131
  internal
    endometriosis of, 19
    monocular evaluation of,
      25
Genital tract
  endometriosis of, 292, 294
Germany, Federal Republic of
  laparoscopic/pelviscopic op-
    erations in, 2
Granulosa-theca cell cyst, 312
Grasping forceps
  atraumatic, 107
Gynecologic endoscopic proce-
    dures
  typical, 152–154
Gynecologic endoscopic surgery
  postoperative care after,
    229–231
Gynecologic laparoscopy, 2
Gynecologic pelviscopy, 2
Gynecologic surgical proce-
    dures, 10–15
Gynecology
  diagnostic questions in,
    28–29
  endoscopic diagnosis in, 3
  specialty training in, 25

H

Healing, wound *(see* Wound
  healing)
Heat
  destructive
    in endometriotic implant
      excision, 158
    highest degree of, 86
    in high-frequency steriliza-
      tion, 90
    in intra-abdominal surgery,
      94
    tubal sterilization by,
      200–206
  produced by high-frequency
    current, 86

Heat shield, 47
Hematoma, retroperitoneal, 144
Hematosalpinx, 184
  with torsion of stalk, 358
Hemorrhage *(See also* Bleeding)
  during adhesiolysis, 216
  adnexal, ligature control of,
    96
  control of with straight liga-
    ture carrier, 113–114,
    115
  delayed, risk of, 95
  diagnosis of, in pelviscopy,
    33
  omental, ligature control of,
    96
  in ovarian biopsy, 170
  in postpartums period, 205
  retroperitoneal, 146
  during salpingectomy for
    tubal pregnancy, 194
Hemosiderin effect, 163, 280,
    284, 286, 330
Hemostasis
  adhesiolysis with and with-
    out, 274
  prophylaxis, 216
  thermal, equipment for,
    80–95
  transabdominal, 262
Hemostatic methods
  development of new, 46
Hepatic decompensation, 36
Hernia
  hiatal, as contraindication to
    endoscopic surgery, 36
Hiatal hernia, as contraindica-
    tion to endoscopic sur-
    gery, 36
Hissing phenomenon, 134
Hook scissors, 111
Hormonal stimulation
  salpingo-oophorectomy to
    eliminate, 350, 352, 354
Hormone withdrawal therapy,
    344
Hose clamps, 76
Hospitalization, psychological
    preparation of patient
    for, 22
Hulka clip
  tubal sterilization by,
    207–209
Hydatid cysts of Morgagni, 398
Hydatid cysts of Morgagni
  excision of, 195–197
Hydropertubation, 79
  postoperative, 236

prolonged, 19
  solution, 231–234
Hydrosalpinx, salpingectomy
    for, 183–184, 354, 356,
    358
Hyperventilation during insuf-
    flation, 66
Hypotension caused by regional
    blocks, 40
Hysterectomy
  after endocoagulation method
    of sterilization, 89
  after high-frequency current
    sterilization, 89
  salpingo-oophorectomy fol-
    lowing, 182
  total
    oophorectomy after, 340,
      342
    salpingo-oophorectomy af-
      ter, 346, 348
Hysterosalpingogram, 164, 296
Hysteroscope
  for removing lost IUD, 380
Hysteroscopy
  development of, 8–9
  for lost IUD, 188

I

Imaging, electromagnetic, 247
Imaging techniques
  liver scintigraphy, 2
  nuclear molecular response/
    nuclear magnetic reso-
    nance, 2
Incision
  abdominal, dilation of, 116
  longitudinal, 146
  ovarian, closure of, 316
  psychological preparation of
    patient for, 22
Inductance
  magnetic, 83
Infant
  indications for endoscopic
    abdominal surgery in,
    31–32
Infection
  preoperative treatment of, 23,
    131
Inflammatory process
  presurgical management of,
    18
Infundibulopelvic ligament
  ligation of, 328
  transection of, 180–181, 342
Infusion rate, IV, 46

Inhalation anesthesia, general, 40
Instrument set for appendectomy, 222, 223
Instruments
  for asperation, 108, 110, 111
  for clamping large vessels, 120
  for coagulation, 117
  for cutting, 111
  for dilatation, 114–117, 260
  for endoscopic abdominal surgery, 46–53
    preparation of, 126–129
  for endoscopic appendectomy, 222–224
  for extracting appendix, 118, 120
  for follicle puncture, 117–118
  for grasping and holding, 107
  for ligation, 113
  for morcellation, 111–113
  for skin closure, 120–123
  for suturing, 113–114
  for vaginal mobilization of uterus, 103–106
Instrument table, 124
Insufflation, CO_2, 61, 164
  CO_2 PNEU Automatic, 62, 72
  of cul-de-sac of Douglas, 256
  electronic, 15
  equipment for establishing pneumoperitoneum, 61–64
  needle, 61
  by open laparoscopy, 70–71
  OP-PNEU Electronic, 72–73
  of pneumoperitoneum, 138–139
  problems of, 62
  system, single-channel/dual purpose, 73–74
  transabdominal, of pneumoperitoneum, 66–69
  transvaginal, of pneumoperitoneum, 69–70
  transvaginal gas, to establish pneumoperitoneum, 256
  tubing, 144
Insulation effect, 87
Intestinal obstruction, symptoms of, 155–156
Intestine
  adhesiolysis of, 215–216
  endometriosis of, 278

lysis of, and enucleation of myoma, 376
  small, adhesiolysis of, 320
Intra-abdominal hemostasis, 9
Intrauterine device (IUD)
  Copper-T, 189
  CU-7, 188, 380, 382
  lost
    pelviscopic removal of, 188–189
    removal of, with hysteroscope, 380
    transabdominal removal of, 380, 382
In vitro fertilization, 169
  ovum aspiration for, 79–80, 198–199, 400
Irrigation
  abdominal or pelvic equipment for, 76–77
  intra-abdominal equipment for, 76–80
  reasons for, 76
  tubal or transuterine equipment for, 77–79
Irving's technique, 206
Isthmic salpingostomy, 168–169, 306, 308
IV infusion rate, 40

K

Knife, electric, 85
Knots, internal tying of, 102
  (*See also* Slip knot)
Koiloscopy, 2

L

Laparoscope
  operating, 106
  second operation, 55
Laparoscopy
  diagnostic, postoperative care after, 228–229
  fatal accidents during, 146
  gynecologic, 2
    chronological development of, 6
    complications of, 6
  inaccuracy of term, 2
  of liver, 2
  open, 135, 141
    insufflation by, 70–71
  pelvic, 2
  replacement of, by ultrasound, in diagnostic phase, 21

Laparotomy
  adhesiolysis in preparation for, 270, 272, 274
  avoiding, 21
  classic indications for, 15
  emergency, 226–227
  informing patient about, 16–17
  physical stress of, 22
  preparing patient for, 20
  reduced frequency of, 15
  replacement of, by pelviscopy, 4
  transition from endoscopy to, in same operation, 225–227
Leiomyoma, 372, 378
  with focal hyalination, 374
  removal of, 184
Lens, telephoto zoom, 58
Ligament
  infundibulopelvic, transection of, 180–181
Ligation
  endoloop, 113
  of infundibulopelvic ligament, 328, 342
  instruments for, 113
  tubal sterilization by, 206–207
  of utero-ovarian ligament, 328
Ligature
  loop, hemostasis by, 95–96, 258
  after sharp lysis of adhesions to ovary, 153
Light
  external
    for photographic documentation, 50–51
    total internal reflection of, 47, 49
  transmission of, 47, 49
Light cable, integrated fiber optic, 57
Light-conduction fibers, nonoriented, 47
Light intensity, loss of, 49
Light source, 124
  for cinematographic and videotape recording, 51–53
  combination, 51
  endoscopic, 46–53
  external, for diagnostic and operative procedures, 46–47

Light source *(cont.)*
  photographic, 247
    checking illumination ca-
      pacity of, 245
    high-intensity, 248
Light-transmitting cable, flexible, 49
Liver
  adhesions of, lysis of, 446,
    448
  biopsy of, 224
  laparoscopy of, 2
  needle biopsy of, 444, 446
  as orientation point, 148, 150
  scintigraphy, 2
  techniques for visualizing, 2
Loop, Roeder, 96, 113
Loop ligature, hemostasis by,
  95–96
Loupe
  low-power, in diagnosis of
    pelvic endometriosis, 19
  for magnification of endo-
    scopic image, 57
Lysis
  of perihepatic adhesions, 224

M

Madlener's technique, 206, 217
Magnetic inductance, 83
Magnification, loupe attachment
  for, 244
Malpractice suits
  adequate patient information
    and, 16
Manometer
  insufflation pressure, 63, 64
  on OP-PNEU Electronic In-
    sufflator, 74
  static intra-abdominal pres-
    sure, 64
Manometer test, 135, 136
Mediastinal emphysema, 134
Menghini needle, 444
Menopause
  premature onset of following
    tubal sterilization, 89
Menstrual blood, removal of,
  308
Menstrual disturbances
  from partial castration, 202
  after tubal sterilization, 89
Mesosalpinx, 177
  following endocoagulation
    technique, 204
Mesovarium/mesosalpinx
  indications for endoscopic
    operations on, 30

Metal push rod, 114
Metastases, peritoneal
  biopsy of, 224, 444
Microknives, 111
Microsurgery, endoscopic, 57
Minilaparotomy, 71
Mitoses in Fallopian tubes following sterilization, 210
Monocular evaluation, 24, 25
  operating team's compensa-
    tion for, 27
Morcellation
  instruments for, 111–113
  and oophorectomy, 338
  of ovarian tissue, 179, 356
  of ovaries, 336
  of pedunculated myoma,
    186–187
Motion pictures for teaching endoscopic procedures,
  247
Myoma
  enucleation of, 366
    from bladder dome, 378
    and intestinal adhesiolysis,
      376
    and omental and intestinal
      adhesiolysis, 376
    and ovarian biopsy and bi-
      lateral salpingoplasty,
      376, 378
    with suture of uterus, 368,
      370, 374
  intramural
    enucleation of, with suture
      of uterus, 368, 370
  pedunculated, 186
    enucleation of, 372, 374
  pelviscopic enucleation of,
    184–188
  subserous intramural, 186
Myoma enucleator, 93, 94, 117
Myomata
  pedunculated or subserous,
    excision of, 11
Myometrium
  adenomatous infiltration of, 161

N

Nasogastric tube
  to prevent stomach disten-
    tion, 40–41
Necrobiosis, 201
  thermal, 199
Necrosis
  coagulation, 87
  thermal, 87, 202, 408
  thermobiologic, 158

Needle
  aspiration, 108, 110
  for follicle puncture, 117
  insufflation, 61
    consequences of placement
      of, 68
    insertion of, 67
  Menghini, 444
  spring mechanism of, 133
  Veress, modified, 63
Needleholders, 114, 115
Needle test, 133
Neosalpingostomy, isthmic,
  306, 308
Neovagina, construction of,
  418, 420
  pelviscopic monitoring of,
    212–213
Neuroleptanalgesia, 39
Nitrous oxide
  risks of using for insufflation,
    65
Nuclear molecular response/nu-
  clear magnetic resonance
  (NMR) imaging, 2

O

Obstruction
  intestinal, symptoms of,
    155–156
  tubal, 190
Omenectomy, partial, 384
Omental adhesiolysis, 152
Omentum
  adhesiolysis of, 214–215
  adhesions of, 270, 274, 296
    lepis of, with and without
      hemostasis, 424, 426,
      428
  resection of, 152, 156,
    214–215
Oocytes
  aspiration of, for in vitro fer-
    tilization, 198–199, 400
  resulting from hMG/hCG or
    clomiphene stimulation,
    198
Oophorectomy, 12
  with complications, 338
  endoloop ligation in, 113
  and morcellation, 338
  ovarian cyst removal by, 174
  pelviscopic, 175–180, 334,
    336, 338, 340, 342
  risk of complications in,
    179–180
  after total abdominal hyster-
    ectomy, 340, 342

Operating room for endoscopy, 124–129
Operating team for endoscopic abdominal surgery, 27
Operating technique, bimanual, 128–129
Operative report, 242
OP-PNEU Electronic device, 124
OP-PNEU Electronic Insufflator, 72–73, 135
Optical systems, endoscopic, 53
Organoscopy, 2
Orthograde appendectomy, 217–221
Ovarian biopsy, 11
    pelviscopic, 169–171, 308, 310
Ovarian carcinoma as contraindication to endoscopic surgery, 35–36
Ovarian cyst
    aspiration of, 172, 310, 312
    benign, 171
    enucleation of, 171
    excision of, 12, 312, 314, 316
    pelviscopic puncture and excision of, 171–175
    puncture of, 310, 312
    removal of
        by oophorectomy or salpingo-oophorectomy, 175
        by salpingo-oophorectomy, 326, 328, 330, 332
    sebaceous material in, 316
Ovarian endometriosis, 284
Ovarian follicle (*see* Follicle)
Ovarian suture, 314, 316
Ovarian tissue
    without germinal elements, 340
    morcellation of, 356
Ovarian tumors, 346
    as contraindication to endoscopic surgery, 35
Ovariolysis, 10, 198
Ovary
    accessory, 330
    arterial network supplying, 88
    blood supply to, 199
    indications for endoscopic operations on, 30
    morcellation of, 179, 336
    streak, 171
    supported by uterus and pelvic wall

biopsy of, 308, 310
    suspended by ligaments biopsy of, 310
Oviduct
    indications for endoscopic operation on, 29–30
Ovum
    aspiration of for in vitro fertilization, 79–80
    collection vessel for, 117
    nidation of, on endometriotic implants, 195
Oxygen
    risk of using for insufflation, 65

P

Pain, abdominal,
    effect on diagnostic phase, 21
Palmer-Jacobs endoscope, 54, 55
Paquelin's cautery, 80
Paralysis
    intestinal, caused by laparotomy, 102
    postoperative intestinal, 168
    vascular, caused by laparotomy, 102
Parovarian cysts, excision of, 197, 400, 402
Patient
    ambulation of, 40
    consent, preoperative, 21
    as consumers, 240
    fears of, 37
    informing about endoscopic abdominal surgery, 16–17, 20
    physical needs of, during surgery, 39
    physical preparation of, for endoscopic abdominal surgery, 22
    position for endoscopic gynecologic surgery, 42
    position for general surgery, 42–45
    preoperative counseling of, 211
    preparing for endoscopic abdominal surgery, 20–23
    psychological guidance and education of, 20–22
    psychological needs of, during surgery, 39
Pedicle, torsion of, salpingectomy after, 358, 360, 362

Pelvic cavity, irrigation of, 330
Pelvic laparoscopy, 2
Pelvis
    structures in, indications for endoscopic operations on, 30–31
Pelviscope, optical deflection of, 53
Pelviscopy
    diagnostic
        indications for endoscopic abdominal surgery based on, 28–29
    emergency, in gynecology and general surgery, 33–34
    gynecologic, 2
    indifferential diagnosis, 33
    informing patient about, 17
    number and types of, at Women's Hospital, Kiel University, 3
    second-look, 28, 36, 181, 236
    statistics on, 231
Pelviscopy/laparoscopy
    diagnostic, instrument preparation for, 124–126
Pelviscopy/laparotomy, 23
Pelvi-Trainer, 102, 251–254
    description of, 251
    practice on, 251–253
    recommended training program with, 253–254
Perforation, limiting risk of, 132–147
Peristalsis
    intestinal, resumption of, 102
Peritoneal adhesions, 94
Peritoneal defects, 157
Peritoneal emphysema, 67
Peritoneal metastases
    biopsy of, 444
Peritoneoscopy, 2
Peritoneum, adhesions of, 274, 302
Peritonitis
    acute, preoperative treatment of, 36
    of upper abdomen, as contraindication to endoscopic surgery, 35
Pertubation apparatus, 77, 78
    universal, 124
Phemosis
    ampullary, 292
    preampullary, 308
    tubal, 376
    of tubal ampulla, 292, 294

Photographic documentation, 242–248
  external light for, 50–51
Photographs
  instant, 58, 246
  panoramic, 245
Pneumoperitoneum
  CO$_2$ gas, 41
  electronic and mechanical control, for intra-abdominal diagnosis, 72
  expansion media to establish, 64–66
  insufflation of, 138–139
  insufflation equipment to establish, 61–64
  monitor for, 15
  N$_2$O gas, 41
  transabdominal insufflation of by blind puncture and Veress needle, 66–69
  transvaginal gas insufflation to establish, 256
  transvaginal insufflation of, through posterior vaginal fornix, 69–70
Pneumoroentgenography of female pelvic organs, 68
Point coagulator, 93, 94, 117, 158
Poiseville's law, 138
Polydioxanon, 102
Pomeroy's technique, 206, 412
Portal venous collapse, 36
Position, patient (*see* Patient position)
Postoperative care, after endoscopic abdominal surgery, 228–238
Postpartum period, tubal sterilization during, 205–206
Poststerilization syndrome, 199, 202
  following sterilization with clips, 209
Pregnancy
  abdominal, operation for, 195
  ectopic (*see* Ectopic pregnancy)
  fear of, 205
  poststerilization, legal consequences of, 88
  tubal (*see* Tubal pregnancy)
  after tubal sterilization, 210
  after tubal sterilization with tantalum clips, 207
  after tubal sterilization by unipolar high-frequency coagulation, 410

Pressure
  insufflation, 135, 138
  intra-abdominal
    relationship to intra-abdominal gas accumulation, 61
    static, 135, 137, 138, 141
  kinetic insufflation, 63
  negative, 234
  static intra-abdominal, 63
Probe
  unipolar high-frequency, 8
Probing/Sounding test, 139–141
Protein
  coagulation of, 117
  denaturation of, 201
  heat transformation of, 88
Psychological preparation of patient, 21–22
Pubic area, introduction of trocar sleeves in, 150
Pulse rate
  acceleration of, 41
Puncture
  second and third to establish diagnosis, 262
Purse string suture
  in appendectomy, 216

R

Recanalization, 203
Recording, videotape, 58
Rectal tube to aspirate intestinal gas, 22
Reflex camera, 58, 244
Regional anesthesia, 40
Regional block anesthesia, 40
Relaxing seat, 127, 128
Resection, omental, 152, 156
Respiratory insufficiency, 36
Respiratory volume, reduced, 41
Retrocervical endometriosis, 276
Retrocervical endometriotic implants, removal of, 280, 282, 284
Retrograde appendectomy, 221–222
Retro-ovarian endometriotic implants, 284
Rod lens system, 53
Roeder loop, 96, 113
Roeder slipknot, 96
Rokitansky-Küster-Mayer-Hauser syndrome, 212

S

Sactosalpinx, 165, 288, 298, 300, 302
  manual inflation of, 77
Salpingectomy, 11, 157
  endoloop ligation for, 113
  for hydrosalpinx, 183–184, 354, 356, 358
  after torsion of pedicle, 358, 360, 362
  for tubal pregnancy, 193–195, 394, 396
  for tubal pregnancy, 394, 396
Salpingitis, *Candida,* 18
Salpingitis isthmica nodosa, 161, 280, 292
Salpingolysis, 10, 198
Salpingoplasty
  bilateral, 322
  bilateral blunt, 308
  by blunt dilatation, 296
Salpingoplasty/salpingostomy, 296
  by blunt dilatation, 300
  with suture, 298
Salpingo-oophorectomy, 12, 181–183, 344, 346
  to eliminate hormonal stimulation, 350, 352, 354
  endoloop ligation in, 113
  ovarian cyst removal by, 175, 326, 328, 330, 332
  for ovarian endometriosis, 350
  pelviscopic, 180–183
  after total hysterectomy, 346, 348
Salpingo-ovariolysis, endoscopic, 288, 290
Salpingostomy, 198, 306
  distal, 164–168, 296, 298, 300, 302, 304, 306
  endoscopic, 164–168, 296, 298, 300, 302, 304, 306
  and extensive adhesiolysis, 302, 304
  follow-up findings of, 156
  isthmic, 168–169, 306, 308
  pelviscopic, 168
  with suture, 298, 300, 302
Scar tissue
  repeated operative procedures and, 241
Scintigraphy, liver, 2
Scissors
  hook, 111

serrated, 111
Semicastration effect, 406
Sensitivity tests, 36
Serosal cysts, excision of, 400
Serous cyst-adenoma, 171, 172
Sexual intercourse following tubal sterilization, 205
Siderophages, with chocolate cyst, 318
Silicone ring for tubal sterilization, 209–210, 416, 418
Single-entry technique, of clip application, 208, 209
Skin, closure of, instruments for, 120–123
Skin effect, 83, 84, 86, 202
  in high-frequency sterilization, 90
Slipknot
  external, 98
    in adhesiolysis, 154, 155
    in excision of ovarian cyst, 174
    tying technique, 99–101
  Roeder, 96
Snap test, 133–134
Soap-boiler effect, 117
Spinal block anesthesia, 40
Splanchnoscopy, 2
Spoon forceps, 107, 109
"Spy" (*see* Teaching attachment)
Spring mechanism of needle, 133
Staple guns, 122
  disposable, 120
Stein-Levanthal Syndrome, 310, 320
Stenosis
  ampullary, 292
  preampullary, 308
Sterility
  correction of
    indications for endoscopic surgery for, 31
    with pelviscopic tubal surgery, 18
  lysis of adhesions in patient with, 272
  pelviscopic diagnosis of, 163
  retro-ovarian endometriotic implants and, 284
  surgery to correct, abdominal adhesions after, 304
  three-phase therapy of, 235–237
  treatment of, and chocolate cyst excision, 320, 322

Sterility operations
  pelviscopic, 163–169
Sterilization
  of endoscope, 59–61
  gas, 59
  high-frequency
    postoperative follow-up of, 89–91
    risks of, 90
Sterilization (*see* Tubal sterilization)
Stomatoplasty, bilateral, 306
Streak ovaries, 171
Suction manipulator, atraumatic, 108
Surgeon
  gynecologic, anesthesia administration and, 17
  requirements of, 24
  seating and support possibilities for, 128–129
Surgery, general
  endoscopic abdominal operative applications to, 32–33
Surgical procedures, gynecologic, 10–15
Suture
  catgut, 96
  fimbrial, 102
  intestinal, 215–216
  ovarian, 172, 314, 316
  purse string, 102, 216
  subcutaneous-subcuticular absorbable, advantages of, 122
Suture applicator, 96, 97, 114
Suture technique, endoscopic, 181
Suturing, instruments for, 113–114

T

Tantalum clips, 206–207
Teaching attachment, 242, 244
  articulated, 56
  flexible, 39
Teaching films, 247
Telephoto zoom lens, 58, 246
Temperature, critical, 87
Teratoma, cystic, 314, 326
Theca-lutein cysts, 171, 172
Thermal hemostasis, equipment for, 80–95
Thermal necrobiosis, 199
Thermal necrosis, 87, 202, 408
Thermobiologic necrosis, 158

Thermobionecrosis, 256
Thermocolor test, 163, 235, 280, 284
  in diagnosis of pelvic endometriosis, 19
  for identifying endometriosis, 286
  pelvic endometriosis and, 448
  in salpingo-oophorectomy, 330
Thermoprobe technique, modified, 8
Three-puncture technique in postpartum or postabortal sterilization, 205
Tissue punch, 111, 112
  in oophorectomy, 179
Transfer catheter, 118
Transuterine tubal occlusion, 9
Trendelenburg position, 42
  to prevent vasodilation and hypotension, 40
  reversed, 45
Triple-loop technique, 96, 175
  for oophorectomy, 176
  for removing hydrosalpinx, 183
  in salpingectomy, for hydrosalpinx, 354
  in salpingo-oophorectomy, 180, 328, 332
Trocar
  blind introduction of, for endoscope, 141
  conical, 142
  dilatation, in salpingectomy for hydrosalpinx, 364
  introduction of, 256
  pyramidal, 144
  secondary, 302
Trocar sleeve, 106
  dilatation, 260
    risk of, 260
  with trumpet valves, 106
  wounds, 120
Tubal abortion, 190, 191
Tubal adenomyosis, 280
Tubal ampulla
  bloodless eversion of, 304
  blunt dilatation of, 294
  dilatation of, 290, 300
  everted, 300
  phimosis of, 292, 294
Tubal biopsy, 202
Tubal fistula, 192, 308
Tubal forceps, heated, 9
Tubal fragments, 190

Tubal ligation, ring method of, 110

Tubal obstruction, 190

Tubal occlusion
intramural, 156
transuterine, 9

Tubal patency
grade I, 164
grade III, 306
in presence of endometriosis, 308

Tubal phimosis, 376

Tubal pregnancy, 157 (*See also* Ectopic pregnancy)
conservative management of, 190–193
conservative operation for, 11
pelviscopic operations for, 189–195
radical operation for, 394, 396
rupture of, 193
salpingectomy for, 193–195, 394, 396
after sterilization, 200

Tubal reimplantation, 157

Tubal sterilization, 5, 199–210
by bipolar high-frequency co-agulation, 202–203, 408
by Bleier clip application, 414, 416
by clips, local anesthesia or volonelgesia for, 209
by coagulation, during post-partum or postabortal phase, 205–206
complications of, 6
by destructive heat, 200–206
effectiveness of, 200
effects of differing techniques of, 88–89
endocoagulation method of, 88–89
postoperative condition af-ter, 410, 412
high-frequency current in, 199
by Hulka clip, 207–209
hysteroscopic, 201
conclusions about, 211
interval
by coagulation, 203
by endocoagulation, 408, 410
legal considerations in, 88, 211
by ligation, 206–207

by ligation (Pomeroy's tech-nique), 412
pelviscopic, conclusions about, 211
by plastic clips, foreign body reaction to, 416
postoperative care, 231–237
preoperative patient counsel-ing, 211
reversal of, 211
tubal surgery in preparation for, 169
with sharp transection, 13
by silicone ring application, 209–210, 416, 418
tubal pregnancy following, 200
unipolar high-frequency method of, 88–89, 201–202, 256, 406, 408
by unipolar high-frequency coagulation
pregnancy following, 410

Tubal surgery
endoscopic, with endometrio-sis, 169
in presence of endometriosis, 308, 310
prior to microsurgical rees-tablishment of fertility, 169

Tube, arterial network supply-ing, 88

Tubo-ovarian adhesions, 290

Tumor
large
as contraindication to en-doscopic surgery, 35
ovarian, 346
as contraindication to en-doscopic surgery, 35
tubo-ovarian conglomerate, 190

Tunica albuginea, 318, 320

U

Ultrasound
for confirming ectopic preg-nancy, 190
for locating lost IUD, 188
as replacement for pelvis-copy, 3
as replacement for laparos-copy
in diagnostic phase, 2

Umbilicus
identification of, 67

preparation of, for diagnostic procedure, 131

Unipolar high-frequency cur-rent, 7

Unipolar high-frequency probe, 8

Universal pertubation apparatus, 124

Uterine adenomyosis, 278

Uterine corpus
indications for endoscopic operative procedures on, 29

Uterine sound, 106

Uterine wall
suture of after perforation with curette, 384, 386

Utero-ovarian ligament
ligation of, 328

Uterus
elevation of, 131
lysis of adhesions of, 378, 380
pelviscopic operation on, 184–189, 366, 368, 370, 372, 374, 376, 378, 380, 382, 384
retroflexed, and insertion of vacuum intrauterine can-nula, 105
risk of perforation of, 103, 105
suture of, after perforation with curette, 189
vaginal mobilization of, in-struments for, 103–106

Uterus mobilizer, 79

V

Vacuum intrauterine cannula, 103, 104, 131

Vagina, artificial
construction of, 212–213, 418, 420

Vascular clamps, 120, 121

Vasodilation caused by regional blocks, 40

Velamentous adhesions, 139, 163, 288

Veress needle, 256
introduction of, 256
modified, 63
test, 133
in transabdominal insufflation of peritoneum, 66–69

Vermiform appendix, 216

Vessels, large
  instruments for clamping,
    120
Venous collapse, portal, 36
Ventroscopy, 2
Videotape documentation,
    242–248
Videotape recording, 58
  light source for, 51–53
Volonelgesia
  patient agreement about, 17
  reasons for selecting, 38
Volume test, 135, 138

W

Warming apparatus for endo-
    scope, 59
Wellness, emphasis on, 240
Wound healing
  duration of hospitalization,
    22
  pathophysiology of, postoper-
    ative hospitalization and,
    239
Wounds, endoscopic trocar, 122

Z

Z-insertion technique, 142, 143
Zona pellucida
  protection of, during oocyte
    aspiration, 198
Zoom lens
  telephoto, 58
Z-suture
  in appendectomy, 216